A SHORT COURSE IN
PATHOLOGY

A SHORT COURSE IN
PATHOLOGY

NANCY STANDLER, M.D., Ph.D.

Department of Pathology
University of Pittsburgh School of Medicine
Pittsburgh, Pennsylvania

CHURCHILL LIVINGSTONE
New York, Edinburgh, London, Madrid, Melbourne, Tokyo

Library of Congress Cataloging-in-Publication Data

Standler, Nancy
    A Short course in pathology / Nancy Standler.
       p.   cm.
    Includes bibliographical references and index.
    ISBN 0-443-08955-8
    1. Pathology   I. Title
    [DNLM: 1. Pathology. QZ 140 S785s 1994]
  RB25.S78   1994
  616.07 — dc20
  DNLM/DLC
  for Library of Congress   94 – 3037
                                                   CIP

© Churchill Livingstone Inc. 1994

Distributed in the United Kingdom by Churchill Livingstone, Robert Stevenson House, 1–3 Baxter's Place, Leith Walk, Edinburgh EH1 3AF, and by associated companies, branches, and representatives throughout the world.

Acquisitions Editor: *Kerry Willis*
Copy Editor: *Elizabeth Bowman-Schulman*
Production Supervisor: *Christina Hippeli*
Desktop Coordinator: *Robert Quattro*
Cover Design: *Jeanette Jacobs*

Printed in the United States of America

First published in 1994   7 6 5 4 3 2 1

This book is dedicated to all the medical students who are working too hard to have fun. My desires for this book will be satisfied if having A Short Course in Pathology *helps you to spend a little more time with your family, sleep a little later, or sit for an hour in the sun.*

Preface

A Short Course in Pathology was written for second-year medical students in the general pathology course. It is designed to be both concise enough to be easily read and comprehensive enough to include the details tested in course work and national boards examinations. The textbook includes processes that are not organ specific, such as infections and nutritional disturbances, as well as diseases of different organ systems. Included are short but detailed sections on virtually all the diseases tested by the national boards examination. Common pathophysiologic pathways by which a variety of diseases may produce similar effects on the body are emphasized. Boldface terms highlight important diseases and facilitate skimming of the points for quick review. Enough marginal space has been left to include a reader's own notes as well. To help keep the length of the book short and its price as low as possible, *A Short Course in Pathology* does not include photographs. General and organ-specific pathology atlases with large numbers of photographs are listed in the Suggested Readings section at the end of the text.

Using *A Short Course in Pathology*

A Short Course in Pathology is designed to be used both in a medical school pathology course and in preparation for part I of the national boards. Medical students face the formidable challenge of absorbing a large volume of information about pathology (and all of their other subjects, as well) in what seems to be far too short a time. Ideally, you should read the material pertaining to a lecture the night before, because having some knowledge of a subject often makes a lecturer easier to follow. If this is not possible, the headings, bold terms, and marginal notes in *A Short Course in Pathology* can be skimmed during the few minutes before the lecture starts.

One of the problems many people encounter in medical school is that they find they are spending nearly all their time either in lecture or doing the first reading of the assigned material. I have tried to write *A Short Course in Pathology* in as concise a format as possible to allow you to read or skim the material several times. It is also helpful to explore ways of actively working with the material, such as working old test questions or trying to write down the key features of a disease. The headings and key words can be used as a source of topics for essay questions.

At some point, you should look at photographs, color slides, or actual specimens of gross and microscopic pathologic material. Your pathology department probably has considerable material available. A list of useful general and organ-specific atlases is also given in the back of this text. My experience was that it was most helpful to look at the pathology visual material about halfway between examinations, when I knew enough for the time to be meaningfully spent, and a couple of days before an examination, when the material served as a good review.

As you approach either a course examination or the national boards examination, you can continue to use *A Short Course in Pathology*. Each heading can be used to trigger a minute or so of mental review of the subject covered under the heading. Skimming the paragraphs following the heading after such an exercise in recall will point out the features you have forgotten. For a quick review, I would suggest that you simply skim the headings, marginal notes, key words, and any comments or underlining you may have added.

It is my hope that this text will make more manageable the overdose of information experienced by many students during the preclinical years and permit them to absorb and appreciate the beauty of pathology.

Nancy Standler, M.D., Ph.D.

Acknowledgments

Many people besides the author contribute to the success of a book. The Department of Pathology at the University of Pittsburgh graciously allowed me to spend my research year writing this text. My parents, Guy and Gloria Elliott, have been both financially and emotionally supportive during the writing of this book. Sherry Williams did the bulk of the typing of the manuscript after it became clear that my new daughter, Christiana, would let Mommy write but not type. Kerry Willis and Elizabeth Bowman, together with the rest of the staff at Churchill Livingstone, helped make editing the manuscript pleasant. I also wish to thank Alexandra Nickerson for her excellent index.

Contents

Part I   General Pathology

1. **Congenital and Genetic Diseases   1**
   Congenital Disease / 1
   Immature and Small for Gestational Age
      Infants / 1
   Sudden Infant Death Syndrome / 2
   Chromosomal Diseases / 2

2. **Nontherapeutic Agents, Drug
   Toxicity, and Injury   9**
   Toxicity of Nontherapeutic Agents / 9
   Adverse Drug Reactions / 10
   Adverse Effects of Illicit Drug Use / 11
   Healing Following Injury / 12

3. **Nutritional Disease   13**
   Protein-Energy Malnutrition / 13
   Fat-Soluble Vitamin Deficiencies / 13
   Water-Soluble Vitamins / 15
   Minerals / 17

4. **Immune Diseases   19**
   Autoimmune Disease / 19
   Mechanisms of Immunologic Tissue
      Injury / 19
   Primary Immunodeficiency
      Disorders / 22
   AIDS / 23
   Systemic Lupus Erythematosus / 24
   Other Systemic Autoimmune
      Diseases / 25

5. **Infectious Disease   27**
   Viruses
   Viral Respiratory Disorders / 27
   Viral Disorders of the Digestive
      Tract / 28
   Viral Epithelial Growths / 28
   Viral Disorders with Skin Rashes / 29
   Herpesvirus Diseases / 29
   Arbovirus Diseases / 31

Viral Diseases of Other Organ
   Systems / 31

Bacteria
Chlamydial Diseases / 32
Rickettsial Diseases / 34
Mycoplasmal Diseases / 36
Staphylococcal Infections / 37
Streptococcal Infections / 38
Pneumococcal Infections / 39
Meningococcal Infections / 39
Gonococcal Infections / 40
Gram-Negative Bacilli / 40
Infections of Childhood / 42
Enteropathogenic Bacteria / 43
Clostridia / 46
Zoonotic Bacteria / 47
Treponemes / 52
Mycobacteria / 54
Actinomycetes / 56
Uncommon Bacteria / 56
Sarcoidosis / 58

Fungi
Candidiasis / 59
Mucormycosis / 60
Aspergillosis / 60
Cryptococcosis / 60
Blastomycosis / 61
Paracoccidioidomycosis / 61
Coccidioidomycosis / 61
Histoplasmosis / 62
Unusual Deep Fungal Infections / 62
Superficial Fungi / 62

Parasites
Protozoal Diseases / 63
Luminal Protozoa / 63
Blood and Tissue Protozoa / 65
Intracellular Protozoa / 67
Helminthic Diseases / 68
Intestinal Roundworms / 68
Tissue Roundworms / 70
Cestodes / 72
Trematodes / 73

Part II Systemic Pathology

6. Hematopoietic System 77

Erythrocytes and Hemorrhagic Diatheses

Anemias of Blood Loss / 77
Hemolytic Anemias / 77
Hereditary Hemolytic Anemias / 78
Traumatic Hemolytic Anemia / 78
Anemias of Diminished Erythropoiesis / 78
Iron Deficiency Anemia / 79
Aplastic Anemia / 80
Pure Red Cell Aplasia / 80
Other Forms of Marrow Failure / 81
Polycythemia / 81
Paroxysmal Nocturnal Hemoglobinuria / 81
Autoimmune Hemolytic Anemias / 81
Red Cell Enzyme Deficiency / 83
Disorders of Structurally Abnormal Hemoglobin Synthesis / 83
Thalassemias / 84
Disseminated Intravascular Coagulation / 85
Hemorrhagic Diatheses / 85
Defective Platelet Function / 87
Clotting Factor Abnormalities / 87

Granulocytes and Lymphocytes

Leukopenia / 89
Reactive Proliferations of White Cells and Nodes / 89
Malignant Lymphomas / 91
Lymphocytic Lymphomas / 91
Hodgkin's Disease / 93
Leukemias and Myeloproliferative Diseases / 94
Acute Leukemias / 94
Chronic Leukemias / 96
Chronic Lymphocytic Leukemia / 97
Hairy Cell Leukemia / 97
Morphology of Leukemias / 97
Myeloproliferative Disorders / 98
Plasma Cell Dyscrasias and Related Disorders / 99
Histiocytoses / 101

Spleen

Splenomegaly / 103
Congenital Anomalies / 103
Nonspecific Acute Splenitis / 103
Reactive Hyperplasia of Spleen / 104
Congestive Splenomegaly / 104
Splenic Infarcts / 104
Splenic Neoplasms / 105
Rupture / 105

7. Connective Tissue 107

Skin

Acute Inflammatory Dermatoses / 107
Chronic Inflammatory Dermatoses / 109
Skin Infections and Infestations / 111
Blistering Diseases / 112
Benign Epithelial Tumors / 114
Premalignant and Malignant Epidermal Tumors / 115
Disorders of Skin Pigmentation / 117
Nevi / 117
Tumors of the Dermis / 119
Benign Fibrous Histiocytoma / 119
Other Tumors / 120

Soft Tissue Tumors and Tumorlike Conditions

Soft Tissue Tumors / 122
Tumorlike Conditions / 127

Joint, Tendon, and Muscle

Degenerative Joint Disease / 129
Rheumatoid Arthritis / 129
Variants of Rheumatoid Arthritis / 131
Suppurative Arthritis / 131
Lyme Disease / 132
Gout / 132
Calcium Crystal Deposition Arthritis / 134
Other Forms of Arthritis / 134
Miscellaneous Lesions / 135
Other Forms of Tenosynovitis / 135
Bursitis / 135
Ganglion and Baker's Cyst / 136
Basic Pathologic Reactions of Muscle / 136
Neurogenic Muscle Disease / 136
Myopathic Disease / 137
Other Muscle Diseases / 139

Bone

Bone Infections / 140
Fractures / 141
Osteoporosis / 142
Paget's Disease of Bone / 142
Secondary Bone Diseases / 143
Defects in Bone Maturation / 144
Hereditary Disorders of Bone 145
Tumors of the Skeletal System / 147

8. Head and Neck 151

Ear / 151
Nasal Cavities and Accessory Air Sinuses / 152
Tumors of the Nose, Sinuses, and Nasopharynx / 153
Larynx / 153

Oral Cavity / 154
Eye / 155

9. **Respiratory System   159**
Congenital Anomalies / 159
Atelectasis / 159
Pulmonary Diseases of Vascular
    Origin / 160
Chronic Obstructive Pulmonary
    Disease / 163
Restrictive Lung Diseases / 166
Pulmonary Infections / 167
Lung Tumors / 170
Mediastinal and Pleural Disease / 172

10. **Nervous System   175**
Common Pathophysiologic
    Complications / 175
Malformations and Developmental
    Diseases / 176
Nutritional, Environmental, and
    Metabolic Disorders / 177
Meningitis / 179
Encephalitis / 180
Central Nervous System Trauma / 183
Intracranial Hemorrhage / 184
Vascular Diseases of the Brain / 186
Ischemic Encephalopathy / 187
Demyelinating Diseases / 189
Degenerative Diseases / 190
Central Nervous System Tumors / 193
Peripheral Nervous System / 196
Peripheral Nerve Tumors / 198

11. **Cardiovascular System   199**
Blood Vessels
Congenital Diseases of Arteries / 199
Arteriosclerosis / 199
Aneurysms / 201
Vasculitides / 203
Blood Vessel Tumors / 207
Diseases of Veins and Lymphatics / 209

Heart
Congenital Heart Disease / 212
Ischemic and Hypertensive Heart
    Disease / 215
Cor Pulmonale / 217
Congestive Heart Failure / 218
Myocarditis / 219
Cardiomyopathy / 220
Cardiac Tumors / 222
Rheumatoid Heart Disease / 223
Endocardial and Valvular Disease / 223
Pericardial Disease / 227

12. **Digestive System / 231**
Esophagus
Nontumorous Conditions / 231
Tumors / 233

Stomach
Congenital Anomalies and Miscellaneous
    Lesions / 235
Gastritis / 235
Acute Gastric Erosions and
    Ulcerations / 237
Gastric and Duodenal Peptic Ulcers / 238
Benign Gastric Tumors / 239
Malignant Gastric Tumors / 239

Small Intestine
Congenital Anomalies / 242
Ischemic Bowel Disease / 242
Infective Gastroenterocolitis / 243
Malabsorption Syndromes / 244
Obstructive Lesions of the Small
    Bowel / 246
Crohn's Disease / 247
Tumors of the Small
    Intestine / 248

Colon
Diseases of the Appendix / 249
Congenital Anomalies of the Colon / 249
Miscellaneous Lesions / 250
Diverticular Disease / 250
Inflammations of the Colon / 251
Colonic Polyps / 252
Colon Cancer / 254

Liver
Basic Clinical Patterns of Liver
    Disease / 256
Hepatitis / 258
Alcoholic Liver Disease 262
Postnecrotic Cirrhosis / 263
Other Forms of Cirrhosis / 264
Hepatic Vascular Disease / 266
Hepatic Cysts and Tumors / 268
Hereditary Hyperbilirubinemias / 271
Reye Syndrome / 272
Neonatal Cholestasis / 272
Additional Diseases That Can Affect the
    Liver / 272
Drug-Related Injury / 273

Extrahepatic Biliary System and Exocrine
    Pancreas
Cholecystitis / 274
Cholelithiasis / 275
Tumors of the Gallbladder and
    Extrahepatic Biliary System / 276
Miscellaneous Disorders of the
    Gallbladder / 277

Congenital Disorders of the
    Pancreas / 278
Pancreatitis / 279
Tumors of the Exocrine Pancreas / 281

13. **Urinary Tract   283**

Kidneys

Congenital Anomalies / 283
Cystic Diseases of the Kidneys / 283
Hypertension and Renal Failure / 285
Microangiopathic Hemolytic Anemia and
    Renal Disease / 287
Other Renal Vascular Diseases / 288
Glomerular Diseases / 289
Glomerular Lesions Associated with
    Systemic Disease / 292
Other Forms of Glomerulonephritis / 295
Tubulointerstitial Nephritis / 297
Acute Renal Failure / 298
Tumors of the Kidney / 300
Urinary Tract Obstruction / 302
Urolithiasis / 302
Pyelonephritis and Urinary Tract
    Infections / 303

Lower Urinary Tract

Diseases of the Ureters / 306
Urethral Pathology / 307
Congenital Anomalies of the Bladder / 307
Cystitis / 308
Bladder Tumors / 308

14. **Male Genital System   311**

Penis / 311
Testes and Epididymis / 312
Prostate / 319

15. **Breast and Female Genital System   323**

Breast

Congenital Anomalies / 323
Inflammations / 323
Breast Tumors / 324
Fibrocystic Disease of the Breast / 325
Breast Cancer / 326
Diseases of the Male Breast / 329

Vulva, Vagina, and Cervix

Diseases of the Vulva / 330
Lesions of the Vagina / 332
Diseases of the Cervix / 332

Uterus

Non-Neoplastic Diseases of the Uterus
    and Endometrium / 335

Endometrial Hyperplasia / 337
Uterine Tumors / 337

Ovaries and Fallopian Tubes

Ovarian Tumors / 339
Non-Neoplastic Ovarian Cysts / 342
Diseases of the Fallopian Tubes / 343

16. **Endocrine System   345**

Pituitary Gland

Pituitary Adenomas / 345
Anterior Pituitary Insufficiency / 346
Posterior Pituitary Syndromes / 347

Thyroid Gland

Tumors of the Thyroid Gland / 348
Goiter / 349
Thyroiditis / 350
Hyperthyroidism / 351
Hypothyroidism / 352
Graves Disease / 352
Thyroid Carcinoma / 353
Miscellaneous Thyroid Lesions / 355

Parathyroid Glands

Primary Hyperparathyroidism / 356
Secondary Hyperparathyroidism / 357
Hypoparathyroidism / 357
Pseudo- and
    Pseudopseudohypoparathyroidism / 357

Endocrine Pancreas

Islet Cell Tumors / 358
Diabetes Mellitus / 358

Adrenal Glands

Developmental Anomalies of the Adrenal
    Cortex / 361
Hyperfunction of the Adrenal Cortex / 361
Hypofunction of the Adrenal Cortex / 363
Nonfunctional Mass Lesions of the Adrenal
    Gland / 365
Diseases of the Adrenal Medulla / 365

Pineal Gland and Thymus

Pineal Gland / 367
Thymus / 367

Suggested Readings / 369

Index / 371

1

Congenital and Genetic Diseases

Congenital disorders are present from birth and may or may not have a genetic basis. Genetic disorders may be due to abnormalities in chromosomal number or morphology, single gene mutations, and polygenetic or multifactorial abnormalities.

CONGENITAL DISEASE

Congenital diseases may be genetic or acquired in utero. In utero infections that may have devastating consequences include syphilis, toxoplasmosis, herpes, hepatitis, rubella, cytomegalovirus, coxsackievirus, and tuberculosis. Neoplasms that may develop in utero include neuroblastoma, Wilms tumor, and teratomas. Additionally, the genetically mediated neoplasms of multiple polyposis and retinoblastoma may have developed by birth. In utero organ development may be abnormal. Anomalies in the cardiovascular system, nervous system, respiratory tract, gastrointestinal tract, urinary tract, reproductive organs, and endocrine system may also occur. Each of these disorders is discussed elsewhere in this book.

Congenital diseases may be genetic or acquired.

IMMATURE AND SMALL FOR GESTATIONAL AGE INFANTS

Small or immature infants are vulnerable to diseases that are related to the immaturity of their organ systems. The immature lungs may have insufficient surfactant production and may develop infant respiratory distress syndrome (see p. 160). The kidneys, while not yet fully formed, usually have sufficient numbers of functioning deep glomeruli to permit survival. Vital brain centers may function well enough to sustain life, but have difficulty maintaining homeostasis, so that the infant is vulner-

Immature infants are vulnerable to organ immaturity and birth injuries.

1

able to poor temperature control, vasomotor instability, and irregular respirations. Liver immaturity can cause jaundice and an impaired ability to metabolize some drugs. Small or immature infants are also vulnerable to increased risk of birth injuries, with an intracranial hemorrhage and neonatal asphyxia being particularly apt to have long-term neurologic sequelae.

SUDDEN INFANT DEATH SYNDROME

Sudden infant death syndrome is a major cause of death in infants.

The sudden infant death syndrome is a major cause of death in 2- to 4-month-old infants. The etiology remains undefined despite many years of research, possibly because the sudden death is a common end of several different processes. The infants characteristically suddenly stop breathing and cannot be resuscitated. They have often had a recent upper respiratory infection and die while sleeping or shortly after awakening from sleep, often at night. Autopsy findings, which are subtle and may be absent, include smooth muscle hypertrophy in small pulmonary arteries, brain stem gliosis (which suggests chronic hypoxia), right ventricular hypertrophy, possibly cardiac conduction system abnormalities, extramedullary hematopoiesis, and retained periadrenal brown fat.

CHROMOSOMAL DISEASES

Sex Chromosome Abnormalities

Common sex chromosome abnormalities include Turner syndrome and Klinefelter syndrome.

Turner syndrome (45,X0) is characterized by a phenotypic female with short stature, webbed neck, and immature genitalia. The ovaries are small and fibrotic ("streak" ovaries); coarctation of the aorta may be present. Since only one X chromosome is present, no Barr bodies are observed in nuclei from buccal smears. Patients with mosaic genetics are common and have less pronounced pathologic changes. **Klinefelter syndrome** (47,XXY) is characterized by a phenotypic male with tall stature, gynecomastia, and small testes that do not produce sperm. Klinefelter syndrome is the most common sex chromosome abnormality. Variants include mosaics, XXXY, and XXXXY. Increasing numbers of X chromosomes are associated with increasing mental retardation. The number of X chromosomes can be determined by counting nuclear Barr bodies from buccal smears and adding one. **"Triple X"** females (47,XXX) are phenotypically normal but have mild mental retardation. **47,XYY** patients are tall, mildly retarded males who have been shown in some studies to have an increased incidence in prison populations. The **fragile X syndrome** [Fra(X)] is usually observed in male patients and is associated with mental retardation, enlarged testes, and fragility at the end of the q arm of the X chromosome. **True hermaphrodites** are characterized by the presence of both ovarian and testicular tissue, may have either XX or XY genetics, and are rare. **Male pseudohermaphrodites** have normal XY genetics, are phenotypically female, and often have a testicular feminization syndrome. **Female pseudohermaphrodites** have normal XX genetics, are phenotypically male, and often have either ovarian or adrenal tumors (see pp. 342, 362) that produce virilizing hormones.

Other sex chromosomal disorders include triple X; 47,XYY; and fragile X syndrome.

Hermaphrodites usually have normal chromosomes.

Autosomal Abnormalities

In general, **autosomal** chromosomal abnormalities produce more severe (often lethal) disease than do sex chromosomal abnormalities. **Down syndrome** (trisomy 21, mongolism) is the most common autosomal trisomy, occurs in both sexes, and has a significantly increased risk in children of mothers older than age 40. The usual cause is disjunction of maternal chromosomes. Variants (not associated with increasing maternal age) due to translocation (46,XY-D,+tDqGq) also exist. Affected infants tend to have poor motor tone ("floppy" infants); a distinctive face with mongoloid facies, epicanthic folds, and a flat nose; palmar creases; and cryptorchidism. Patients with Down syndrome are often mildly to moderately retarded; the effects of the retardation can sometimes be limited by mental stimulation and training in very early childhood. Patients with Down syndrome may also have congenital cardiovascular anomalies and an increased incidence of leukemia. **Edwards syndrome** (16–18 trisomy, E trisomy) usually causes death in infancy, is more common among female babies, and has a high prevalence of coexisting cardiac and renal abnormalities. Other features include a distinctive face with low-set ears, epicanthic folds, and micrognathia; rocker-bottom feet; and overlapping second and fifth finger. **Patau syndrome** (13–15 trisomy, D trisomy) affects both sexes, commonly has cardiovascular anomalies, and may have brain anomalies. Other features include low-set ears, cleft palate and lip, and small eyes. **Cri du chat syndrome** (5p-) is a rare syndrome observed more commonly among females that is due to deletion of the p arm of chromosome 5. Infants are retarded, have a distinctive "cat cry," and are prone to cardiovascular anomalies. Other features include a moonface, micrognathia, and an antimongoloid slant to the eyes. **Other chromosomal abnormalities** that are associated with severe anomalies and are often fatal include D13p-, D13q-, E18q-, and triploidy.

> Down syndrome is associated with mental retardation, distinctive fascies, congenital cardiovascular anomalies, and leukemia.

> Other autosomal anomalies tend to include mental retardation and congenital anomalies, and may cause death in childhood.

Autosomal Dominant Genetic Defects

Genetic disorders transmitted by autosomal dominant genetics will express in all individuals who carry the gene, and most affected individuals are heterozygotes for the characteristic. Genes coding for structural proteins tend to cause autosomal dominant defects; in contrast, autosomal recessive defects often involve enzymes. **Achondroplasia** is a form of dwarfism associated with defective endochondral ossification. **Huntington's chorea** manifests with dementia, choreic movements, seizures, and death. **Marfan syndrome** is due to a defect in collagen and elastin synthesis that has variable expression (pleiotropy). Individuals who express the full disorder tend to be tall, with long extremities and fingers (arachnodactyly); are vulnerable to dissecting aortic aneurysm secondary to cystic medial necrosis; and may have subluxation of the lens of the eye. **Gardner syndrome** is an example of a genetic syndrome with neoplastic potential that predisposes for skin cysts, osteomas, colonic polyps, and colon cancer. Some cases of the joint disease **gout** and of the iron deposition disorder **hemochromatosis** also appear to be transmitted by autosomal dominant genetics. Other autosomal dominant diseases include neurofibromatosis (nerve tumors, pigmented skin lesions), spherocytosis (altered erythrocyte membrane leading to spherical shape), some forms of congenital hyperbilirubinemia (Dubin-Johnson syndrome, some cases of Rotor and possibly Gilbert syndromes), and hypophosphatemia (abnormal alkaline phosphatase).

> Autosomal dominant genetic disorders are often related to defective production of structural proteins.

Autosomal Intermediate Abnormalities

Not all autosomal abnormalities have classic dominant or recessive genetics.

The classic description of single gene autosomal defects involves autosomal dominant and autosomal recessive categories, but some diseases are characterized by mild disease in heterozygotes and severe disease in homozygotes. These conditions can be considered as due to autosomal intermediate abnormalities. **Sickle cell anemia** (see also p. 83) is due to an amino acid substitution in the β chain of hemoglobin A that decreases the solubility of the hemoglobin in a deoxygenated environment. Homozygotes have severe anemia and frequently die before age 30. Heterozygotes (sickle cell trait) are common in black populations and have normal longevity, few symptoms, and mild anemia. The **thalassemias** (see also p. 84) are a group of disorders in which decreased amounts of otherwise normal hemoglobin is synthesized. The thalassemias have complex genetics, and affected individuals may have mild to severe anemia depending upon the number of affected genes they carry.

Autosomal Recessive Abnormalities

Autosomal recessive disorders are often due to defective enzyme production.

Autosomal recessive disorders are characterized by phenotypically normal or near normal heterozygotes and severely affected homozygotes. **Cystic fibrosis** (see also p. 278) is the most common autosomal recessive disease in the Caucasian population; is associated with abnormal mucus and sweat production; and causes pancreatic insufficiency and bronchiectasis with predisposition for severe pneumonia. **Galactosemia** is due to a deficiency of galactosyl-1-phosphate uridyltransferase, which is necessary for the metabolism of galactose from milk lactose. It is characterized by galactosemia, galactosuria, gastrointestinal symptoms, cirrhosis that may progress to liver failure, cataracts, and mental retardation. **Wilson's disease** (see also p. 265) (hepatolenticular degeneration) is due to a deficiency of the copper-binding protein ceruloplasmin. Wilson's disease typically presents in adolescence and leads to accumulation of copper in the deep gray matter of the brain, causing convulsions and ataxia. Copper also accumulates in the liver (cirrhosis), eyes (Kayser-Fleischer rings), and renal tubules.

Glycogen storage diseases tend to affect liver, kidneys, striated muscle (including heart), lymph nodes, and leukocytes. Defects in different enzymes produce slightly different patterns.

GLYCOGEN STORAGE DISEASES. The **glycogen storage diseases,** in which glycogen accumulates in tissue cells, are due to autosomal recessive genetic defects. **Type I** glycogen storage disease (von Gierke's disease, hepatorenal form) is caused by deficiency in glucose-6-phosphatase, which leads to glycogen accumulation in liver cytoplasm and nuclei. Both liver and kidneys enlarge. Affected infants have difficulty maintaining serum glucose levels and develop hypoglycemia, hyperlipidemia, lactic acidosis, ketosis, and later gout. **Type Ib** is a clinical variant due to a defect in the transport membrane protein associated with glucose-6-phosphate. **Type II** (Pompe's disease, generalized or cardiac form) is due to a deficiency of lysosomal acid α_1,4-glucosidase and causes an accumulation of glycogen within striated muscle lysozymes, leading to skeletal muscle hypotonia and massive cardiomegaly that causes heart failure. **Type III** (Cori's disease, Forbes disease, limited dextrinosis) is due to deficiency of debrancher enzyme (amylo-1,4-to-1,6-glucosidase), leading to glycogen accumulation in liver cells. The clinical course resembles mild type I disease. **Type IV** (Andersen's disease, amylopectinosis) is a uniformly fatal disease due to a deficiency of brancher enzyme (amylo-1,4-to-1,6-transglucosidase), which leads to accumulation in many tissues (liver, heart, skeletal muscle, lymph nodes) of material that resembles amylopectin, rather than glycogen. Hepatosplenomegaly with cirrhosis causes early death. **Type V** (McArdle's disease, muscle glycogenosis) is due to a deficiency of myophosphorylase. Glycogen accumulation in muscle is associated with muscle weakness, and sometimes myocytolysis, which may cause renal failure secondary to myoglobinuria. **Type VI** (Hers disease, liver glycogenosis) is due to deficiency of liver phosphorylase. Glycogen accumulation in liver cells is associated with hypoglycemia and hepatomegaly. Other uncommon variants of glycogen storage disease affect muscle **(type VII)** and both liver and leukocytes **(type VIII).**

LIPID STORAGE DISEASES. **Lipid storage diseases** are predominantly autosomal recessive genetic defects in lysosomal enzymes. Lipids accumulate in reticuloendothelial cells and neurons. Enzymatic analysis of amniotic fluid cells, cultured fibroblasts, or blood leukocytes can facilitate the diagnosis of these diseases. **Gaucher's disease** is due to deficiency of glucocerebrosidase (β glucosidase), which leads to the accumulation of glucocerebroside in glia, reticuloendothelial cells, and marrow cells. Serum acid phosphatase is usually increased. The chronic form of Gaucher's disease is usually observed in Ashkenazi Jews who slowly develop hepatosplenomegaly, pancytopenia, and sometimes a hemopoietic neoplasm. A rare acute infantile form also exists with prominent brain stem involvement and hepatosplenomegaly. **Niemann-Pick disease** (sphingomyelin lipidosis) is a fatal disease most common among Ashkenazi Jews that is due to a deficiency of sphingomyelinase. This deficiency leads to accumulation of sphingomyelin in neurons and reticuloendothelial cells. Patients have hepatosplenomegaly and neurologic symptoms (infantile psychomotor retardation, blindness, deafness). About one-third of patients have a cherry red spot in the macula. **Krabbe's disease** (globoid cell leukodystrophy) is due to deficiency of β-galactosidase, which leads to accumulation of ceramide galactoside. This material accumulates in multinucleated "globoid" cells in demyelinating white matter in the cerebral cortex and cerebellum. Patients show infantile psychomotor retardation and die at an early age. **Metachromatic leukodystrophy** (sulfatide lipidosis) is due to a deficiency in arylsulfatase A. Sulfatides accumulate in neurons, nerves, kidney, and gallbladder. Patients experience psychomotor retardation, weakness, blindness, and death. **Fabry's disease** (glycosphingolipidosis) differs from other lipid storage diseases by having X-linked rather than autosomal recessive genetics. Fabry's disease is due to a deficiency of α-galactosidase (ceramide trihexosidase), which leads to accumulation of glycosphingolipids in reticuloendothelial cells, ganglion cells, cornea, and vascular endothelium. Patients experience cardiac and renal failure, autonomic instability, skin lesions (angiokeratomas), and impaired vision secondary to corneal opacity.

    Tay-Sachs disease (GM_2 gangliosidosis) is actually a group of diseases characterized by a deficiency of hexosamidase A, which leads to the accumulation of gangliosides in ballooned neurons and foamy macrophages in the reticuloendothelial system. By electron microscopy, the accumulated ganglioside has a distinctive laminated appearance

> Defects in lysomal enzymes lead to cytoplasmic accumulations of partially degraded molecules. Commonly affected are the nervous system, the reticuloendothelial system, the renal system, eyes, skin, and vasculature.

(laminated bodies). The classic infantile form (type I) is seen most often in Ashkenazi Jews, and causes severe psychomotor retardation with convulsions and blindness that progresses to death in early childhood. Similar diseases that present at somewhat later ages are observed in the late infantile (Jansky-Bielschowsky) and juvenile (juvenile amaurotic idiocy of Spielmeyer-Vogt) forms of the disease. Sandhoff's (type II) form of Tay-Sachs disease is due to a deficiency of both hexosamidase A and B, which causes ganglioside and globoside accumulation in kidney, spleen, and liver. The **generalized (GM$_1$) gangliosidoses** are due to deficiency in β-galactosidase. Gangliosides accumulate in neurons, glomeruli (ballooned epithelial cells), and reticuloendothelial cells in liver and bone marrow. Patients experience psychomotor retardation. **Wolman's disease** is due to a deficiency of acid lipase, which leads to an accumulation of neutral lipids and xanthoma formation, adrenal involvement, and hepatosplenomegaly.

Mucopolysaccharidoses are due to defective lysosomal enzymes. Connective tissues, reticuloendothelial cells, and neurons tend to be most severely affected.

MUCOPOLYSACCHARIDOSES. The **mucopolysaccharidoses** are due to genetic deficiencies of lysosomal enzymes involved in the degradation of acid mucopolysaccharides. The prototype of these diseases is **Hurler syndrome** (type I mucopolysaccharidosis), which is characterized by "gargoyle" fascies due to accumulation of mucopolysaccharide (dermatin sulfate and heparin sulfate) in chondrocytes, osteocytes, and fibrocytes. Other skeletal abnormalities include deformed "gibbus" back, claw hand, and stiff joints. Patients also have hearing loss; visual impairment secondary to corneal clouding; cardiac involvement that often leads to cardiac ischemia and death before age 10; and accumulation of mucopolysaccharide in reticuloendothelial cells (hepatosplenomegaly, lymphadenopathy) and glycolipid in neurons (mental retardation). **Scheie syndrome** is a variant of Hurler syndrome in which dermatan sulfate, but not heparin sulfate, accumulates. **Hunter syndrome** differs from other mucopolysaccharidoses by having X-linked rather than autosomal recessive genetics. Hunter syndrome (type II mucopolysaccharidosis) is due to a deficiency of sulfoiduronate sulfatase, which leads to the accumulation of both dermatan sulfate and heparin sulfate. Hunter syndrome clinically resembles Hurler syndrome but does not show the abnormal back or corneal opacity. Most patients die by midadolescence. **Sanfilippo syndrome** (type III mucopolysaccharidosis) is due to deficiency of heparin sulfate sulfatase (or N-acetyl-α-d-glucose amidase). Heparin sulfate accumulates, producing severe mental retardation.

Abnormalities in tyrosine metabolism produce a wide variety of clinical syndromes.

ABNORMALITIES OF TYROSINE METABOLISM. Abnormalities in the metabolism of **tyrosine** and its derivatives produce a variety of autosomal recessive diseases. Tyrosine is synthesized from phenylalanine by action of phenylalanine hydroxylase. Deficiency of this enzyme produces **phenylketonuria,** which is characterized by phenylketone excretion into (musty-smelling) urine; decreased myelinization with mental retardation and convulsions; and fair skin, fair hair, and blue eyes. Decreasing dietary phenylalanine can help to minimize the mental retardation. The skin pigment melanin is synthesized from tyrosine (via dopa) by the action of tyrosinase. Deficiency of tyrosinase produces **albinism** (see also p. 117), characterized by pale skin, blue irises, red pupils, photophobia, and vulnerability to ultraviolet-induced skin cancers. The thyroid hormones triiodothyronine (T_3) and thyroxine (T_4) are also synthesized from tyrosine, and genetic blocks in this synthesis produce **cretinism,** with hypothyroidism, mental retardation, umbilical hernia, and cretin fascies. Tyrosine is degraded to homogentisic acid (which is secreted in urine) by the action of *p*-hydroxyphenylpyruvate oxidase. Lack of this oxidase produces **tyrosinosis,** which manifests with acute or chronic liver disease (cirrhosis) and renal tubular disease. Tyrosinosis has an increased prevalence among French Canadians, and its manifestations can be partially controlled by a diet low in phenylalanine and tyrosine. Homogentisic acid is further degraded to maleilacetoacetic acid by homogentisic acid oxidase. Lack of this oxidase produces **alkaptonuria** (ochronosis), characterized by urine that turns black on standing; blue-black staining of cartilage in ears, nose, and joints; and chronic arthritis.

MUCOLIPIDOSES. The **mucolipidoses** are generalized lysosomal disorders. **I cell disease** (type II mucolipidosis) is due to abnormal N-acetyl-glucosamino-transferase, which prevents the Golgi apparatus from adding the recognition marker mannose phosphate to enzymes destined to enter lysosomes. I cell disease is a severe general disorder that causes death early in life. The milder type III form **(pseudo-Hurler syndrome)** has an enzyme with partial activity that permits survival to adult life.

Mucolipidoses are generalized lysosomal disorders.

X-Linked Genetics

Fewer **X-linked genetic diseases** have been described than autosomal recessive diseases. In these diseases, affected individuals are usually hemizygote males who received the gene from their mothers; heterozygous females are carriers for the gene, and rare homozygous females may have the diseases. **Color blindness** is the most common X-linked disease. **Glucose-6-phosphate dehydrogenase deficiency** is associated with impaired synthesis of the antioxidant glutathione. This deficiency renders erythrocytes vulnerable to oxidant-induced hemolysis by priaquine, infections, fava beans, and other drugs. Both the clotting disorders **classic hemophilia** (see also p. 88) (hemophilia A, factor VIII deficiency) and **Christmas disease** (see also p. 88) (hemophilia B, factor IX deficiency) are transmitted by X-linked genetics and are associated with bleeding into deep tissues and joints. **Duchenne muscular dystrophy** (see also p. 138) produces weakness of heart and proximal skeletal muscle, and usually causes death before age 20.

X-linked disorders are uncommon.

2

Nontherapeutic Agents, Drug Toxicity, and Injury

TOXICITY OF NONTHERAPEUTIC AGENTS

Cigarette smoking is the most dangerous form of tobacco use and is associated with increased risk of emphysema, chronic bronchitis, atherosclerosis, myocardial infarction, cancer (lung, larynx, esophagus, pancreas, kidney, and bladder), acute gastritis, and pregnancy complications (spontaneous abortion, reduced birth rate, perinatal mortality). Passive smoking can cause nasal and small airway irritation. Smokeless forms of tobacco can cause oral cancer.

Acute **ethyl alcohol** ingestion can cause reversible gastritis, hepatic fatty change, and depression of subcortical brain centers. Chronic alcohol ingestion (alcoholism) can cause hepatitis, cirrhosis, gastritis, gastric ulcers, peripheral neuropathies, Wernicke-Korsakoff syndrome (possibly as a result of vitamin B_{12} deficiency in addition to alcohol use), cerebellar degeneration, optic neuropathy, congestive cardiomyopathy, hypertension, pancreatitis, and myopathy. The incidence of cancers of the oropharynx, larynx, and esophagus is increased. Infants of alcoholic mothers may have growth and mental retardation.

Deliberately or accidentally ingested **methyl alcohol** (found in solvents, antifreeze, and the portable fuel Sterno) can cause gastric hemorrhage; inhaled methyl alcohol causes pulmonary edema and hemorrhage. The metabolite formaldehyde can cause coma and blindness secondary to retinal damage. The metabolite formic acid can cause a metabolic acidosis with deranged glucose metabolism.

Lead poisoning sources include leaded gasoline, lead in water pipes, metal fabrication, paint, ingested or burned newspapers, home-distilled liquors, and food from lead-containing cans or leaded pots. Children are particularly vulnerable to lead poisoning, both because they are more apt to ingest toxic material, and because they absorb a greater fraction of the

Smoking affects many organ systems.

Ethyl alcohol damages liver, brain, gastrointestinal tract, and heart.

Methyl alcohol can cause coma, blindness, gastric hemorrhage, and pulmonary hemorrhage.

Lead poisoning can damage brain, nerves, bone marrow, and kidney.

ingested lead. Lead poisoning in children is an important cause of mild to severe brain damage. Severely affected children may have significant sensory, motor, intellectual, and psychological impairment. Seizures, psychosis, blindness, coma, and death occur occasionally. In adults, the nervous system damage tends to be only a peripheral demyelinating neuropathy. Other manifestations of lead poisoning, not present in all patients, include a microcytic anemia with basophilic stippled erythrocytes; severe abdominal pain; Fanconi syndrome (glycosuria, aminoaciduria, and phosphaturia); chronic tubulointerstitial nephritis; hyperuricemia with gout; and arthralgias.

Carbon monoxide causes systemic asphyxiation and damage to the brain.

Carbon monoxide binds tightly to hemoglobin, displacing oxygen and causing systemic asphyxiation. The carboxyhemoglobin characteristically causes a cherry-red discoloration of skin and mucous membranes in acutely poisoned individuals. Chronic low-dose carbon monoxide can cause demyelination of cerebral white matter and damage to basal ganglia and lentricular nuclei. Damage to kidneys, liver, and heart may also occur.

Carcinogens are common.

Environmental and occupational **carcinogens** are common, and include cigarette smoke, metals (arsenic, nickel, cadmium, uranium, chromium), organic compounds (vinyl chloride, benzene, β-naphthylamine), asbestos, and nitrites.

ADVERSE DRUG REACTIONS

Adverse drug reactions can affect bone marrow, skin, kidneys, lung, or liver.

While adverse drug reactions are common, most cause relatively mild, self-limited illnesses. More serious reactions are uncommon. **Blood dyscrasias** (granulocytopenia, thrombocytopenia, hemolytic anemia, aplastic anemia, leukemia) can cause death and have been associated with ibuprofen, quinidine, methyldopa, phenacetin, and antineoplastic therapy. **Skin reactions** may range from relatively benign macules, papules, or urticaria to life-threatening exfoliative dermatitis. The skin reactions have been associated with many drugs including antibiotics, antiepileptic medications, bromides, and antimitotic agents. Serious **renal diseases** can be caused by phenacetin and aspirin (papillary necrosis); penicillamine (glomerulonephritis); sulfonamides (tubulointerstitial nephritis); and cyclosporine (acute tubular damage and glomerular thrombosis). **Lung disease** can include edema (amiodarone and busulfan), diffuse alveolar damage (bleomycin), and interstitial fibrosis (nitrofurantoin). **Liver** manifestations can include fatty change (tetracycline), hepatitis (isoniazide), cholestasis (chlorpromazine), and focal to massive necrosis (halothane).

Systemic and hormonal reactions also occur.

Systemic reactions can include anaphylaxis (penicillin), lupus erythematosus-like syndromes (hydralazine), and vasculitis (allopurinol). **Hormonal reactions** include benign and malignant proliferations (estrogens), thrombotic complications (oral contraceptives), and adrenocortical insufficiency (glucocorticoids).

Some important causes of drug-induced injury include halothane, isoniazid, acetaminophen, and aspirin.

Of the agents mentioned above, only the most important will be discussed in greater detail. The anesthetic **halothane** can produce hepatic necrosis that is occasionally massive enough to be fatal and appears to be in part the result of a hypersensitivity reaction, since the necrosis tends to be greater in subsequent exposures. The antitubercular drug **isoniazid** can cause liver injury that resembles viral hepatitis and appears to be more common in patients who are genetically rapid acetylators of isoniazid. Massive overdose of **acetaminophen** can cause liver failure secondary to centrilobular necrosis, due to the action of a toxic metabolite that is normally detoxified by binding to glutathione. Massive **aspirin** overdose can acutely cause an initial alkalosis that is followed by potentially fatal metabolic acidosis; chronic aspirin toxicity can cause dizziness, gastrointestinal symptoms, gastritis, bleeding symptoms, and central nervous symptoms (drowsiness, hallucinations, convulsions, coma).

Exogenous **estrogens** given postmenopausally are associated with increased risks of endometrial cancer, ovarian cancer, venous thrombosis, and pulmonary embolism. The estrogen **diethylstilbesterol** (formerly given during pregnancy) is associated with vaginal adenosis and subsequent vaginal clear cell carcinoma in the adolescent offspring of treated mothers. High-dose oral contraceptives were associated with increased risks (particularly when compounded with smoking in women over 35) of myocardial infarction and subarachnoid hemorrhage. Liver pathology (adenoma, focal nodular hyperplasia, and hepatocellular carcinoma) and a slightly increased incidence of cervical cancer also are associated with high-dose oral contraceptive use. It is still unclear whether the modern low-dose oral contraceptives are associated with any of these problems.

Estrogens are associated with female pelvic cancers, pulmonary emobli, myocardial infarction, and liver tumors.

Antineoplastic agents commonly cause toxicity, which may affect the heart (doxorubicin), bone marrow (many agents that affect mitosis), or gastrointestinal tract mucosa (many agents). Months to years after chemotherapy, a new tumor, often acute leukemia, can arise. **Antibiotics** can cause mild (skin rash) to life-threatening (anaphylaxis, exfoliative dermatitis) hypersensitivity reactions and can induce superinfection by antibiotic-resistant or opportunistic organisms. **Immunosuppressants** can predispose for life-threatening opportunistic infections and can be toxic to organs including the lungs (azathioprine) and kidneys (cyclosporine, which is also toxic to liver and heart).

Other important causes of toxic injury include antineoplastic agents, antibiotics, and immunosuppressants.

ADVERSE EFFECTS OF ILLICIT DRUG USE

The problems associated with the specific use of different illicit drugs may be difficult to define. Many drug abusers use multiple illicit drugs and may dilute their drugs with toxic material or contaminated water. **Needle users** are vulnerable to bacterial (*Staphylococcus aureus,* others), viral (AIDS, hepatitis, others) and fungal (*Candida, Aspergillus,* others) infections. Common sites of infection include the skin and subcutaneous tissues, an often right-sided endocarditis, liver, and lungs. Needle users are also vulnerable to foreign body granuloma formation (often due to talc or other materials used to "cut" the illicit drugs) that may involve lymph nodes draining the upper extremity, liver, spleen, or lungs. **Heroin** users are additionally at risk for sudden death due to overdose, pulmonary edema, renal disease (amyloidosis, focal glomerulosclerosis), tetanus, peripheral neuropathy, myopathy, osteomyelitis, and vasculitis. **Cocaine** and its purified form **crack** activate the sympathetic nervous system and may predispose for sudden death due to ventricular arrhythmias. Cocaine and crack users are additionally vulnerable to congestive cardiomyopathy, myocardial infarction, and pulmonary edema. **Phencyclidine hydrochloride** ("angel dust") is an hallucinogen that can cause agitation, delirium, convulsions, and accidental death (drowning, motor vehicle accidents). Chronic **marijuana** use, particularly when contaminated by herbicides, appears to cause irritation of the upper and lower respiratory tract, angina in some individuals, impaired

Problems associated with specific illicit drugs may be hard to define.

cell-mediated immunity, and chromosomal damage; it possibly exposes latent schizophrenia. Use of **inhalant** illicit drugs (glue, paint thinners, etc.) has caused occasional deaths from heart failure, apparently by intensifying the effects of epinephrine on the heart.

HEALING FOLLOWING INJURY

Rapid, primary healing is observed in clean cuts that are closely approximated.

Many tissues heal following trauma by formation of a fibrous scar. Clean cuts (e.g., surgical incisions) whose edges can be closely approximated undergo **primary healing** (healing by "first intention"). The incision is initially sealed by a narrow layer of clotted blood. Within 24 hours, the adjacent, minimally damaged tissues become acutely inflamed. During the next several days, the inflammation stimulates fibroblastic activity; fibroblasts migrate into the clot, and the blood clot and inflammatory exudate begin to be resorbed. At the same time, new vascular channels form by ingrowth of endothelial cells. By 2 to 3 days after the injury, the clot has been transformed into richly proliferating fibroblasts. Over the next week, a true scar forms as fibroblasts lay down collagen. The vascularity diminishes as the thin-walled vessels are compressed by contracting collagen. The result is a densely collagenous scar that is relatively avascular and contains relatively large numbers of fibrocytes. Full scar strength (which is usually less than the strength of the original tissue) is only obtained weeks to months after the injury. Remodeling of the scar continues for years. If the rate of collagen production exceeds its breakdown, a hypertrophic scar or keloid may be produced.

Secondary union is slower and produces a larger scar.

In contrast to the primary healing that follows apposition of a clean wound, **secondary union** (healing by "second intention") is a slower process that is observed in the healing of large or ragged wounds. The basic processes are the same, but more debris must be removed, and the size of the scar may be much larger. Large skin defects may require grafting.

Brain does not form fibrous scars.

Epithelia, but not the underlying connective tissues, can regenerate.

The description given above is modified in some organs and tissues. In **brain,** glial cells, which do not produce collagen, are involved in healing instead of fibroblasts. The damaged tissue is removed by dissolution and phagocytosis (sometimes leaving a permanent hole), and astrocyte proliferation may replace damaged cells. In other organs, **epithelial cells** (vascular endothelium, gastrointestinal mucosa, renal tubular cells, etc.) can often regenerate, but the damaged connective tissues (including muscle) heal by fibrous scar formation.

3

Nutritional Disease

PROTEIN-ENERGY MALNUTRITION

Deficient protein in a diet that supplies adequate caloric intake produces **kwashiorkor.** Kwashiorkor is characterized by an enlarged fatty liver; hypoalbuminia secondary to decreased hepatic synthesis; electrolyte disturbances (potassium deficiency and sodium retention); peripheral edema secondary to the hypoalbuminemia and electrolyte disturbances; subcutaneous fat ("moonface"); a variety of hair and skin changes; and anemia. In contrast to kwashiorkor, **marasmus** is classical starvation, characterized by a marked deficiency of both protein and calories. Affected infants and children become "skeletons," with complete loss of subcutaneous fat, severe muscle atrophy, and stunted growth. Edema and liver enlargement are not observed. In practice, kwashiorkor and marasmas can be considered to represent extremes of protein-energy malnutrition, and patients with intermediate findings occur.

Obesity is most commonly the result of eating too much and having too little physical exercise. In some individuals, genetic factors also appear to play a role. Health risks associated with marked obesity include hypertension, type II diabetes, hyperlipoproteinemia, atherosclerosis, stroke, heart disease, osteoarthritis, and cholelithiasis. Additionally, hypersomnolence (pickwickian syndrome) is observed in the morbidly obese, who may have periods of apnea during sleep secondary to the mechanical burden imposed by massively thickened subcutaneous fat. While markedly obese individuals are clearly at greater risk of developing the above-mentioned disorders, the risks of mild to moderate obesity appear to be much less and may not even be statistically significant.

FAT-SOLUBLE VITAMIN DEFICIENCIES

Deficiencies of fat-soluble vitamins occur most commonly worldwide as a result of primary malnutrition. In affluent societies, oil-soluble vitamin deficiencies are observed in patients with biliary tract disease, pancreatic disease, or intestinal malabsorption.

Kwashiorkor is due to protein deficiency; marasmus is due to classical starvation.

Obesity is most commonly the result of too much food and too little exercise.

13

Vitamin A

Vitamin A (retinol and related compounds) has roles in maintaining **vision** in reduced light as a component (11-cis-retinol) of rhodopsin in retinal rods; in the differentiation of mucus-secreting **epithelial cells;** and possibly as an **anticancer agent.** Severe vitamin A deficiency can produce eye disease including blindness, squamous metaplasia of mucosal epithelium, and impaired immunologic responses. Active vitamin A is found in animal-derived foods; its precursor beta-carotene can be found in yellow vegetables. Acute vitamin A toxicity can produce headache and papilledema suggestive of brain tumor, particularly in children. Chronic toxicity produces anorexia, dry skin and mucus membranes, hepatic fibrosis, bony exostoses, and mental disturbances.

Vitamin D

Vitamin D acting alone stimulates intestinal absorption of **calcium** and **phosphorus.** Vitamin D acting with parathormone mobilizes calcium from bone and stimulates renal calcium resorption in distal tubules. Vitamin D is absorbed in the form of vitamin D_2 or D_3 from the intestinal lumen; transported in plasma bound to D-binding protein; stored principally in fat cells; converted in the liver to 25-hydroxy vitamin D; and subsequently converted to the active form 1,25 dihydroxy vitamin D in the kidneys. Dietary sources of vitamin D or its precursors include plants, animal-derived products, and hormonal supplements, often in milk. Vitamin D_3 can also be synthesized in the skin from 7-dehydrocholesterol by the action of ultraviolet light. Deficiency of vitamin D produces rickets in growing children and osteomalacia in adults (see p. 143). Vitamin D deficiency can be produced by multiple mechanisms in addition to inadequate endogenous synthesis coupled with dietary lack, including malabsorption, diffuse liver disease, chronic renal failure, drugs (phenytoin, phenobarbitol, rifampin), genetic lack of 1,α-hydroxylase, and end-organ resistance to vitamin D. Large excesses of vitamin D are well tolerated, but may induce metastatic calcifications and renal stones.

Vitamin E

Vitamin E functions as a lipid-soluble **antioxidant** that limits the damage caused by free radical formation. Vitamin E activity is found in tocopherols and tocotrienols found widely in plants and animal products. Deficiency is usually caused by processes other than dietary lack, including fat malabsorption, immaturity of the liver and gastrointestinal tract in low-birthweight neonates, and abetalipoproteinemia. Vitamin E deficiency can damage the nervous system, producing manifestations that may include ataxia, dysarthria, sensory disturbances, and impaired vision. Vitamin E, together with glutathione, protects erythrocytes from hemolysis by oxidants. Anemia is a feature of vitamin E deficiency in neonates but not in adults. Mild vitamin E excesses are well tolerated; massive overdosage can cause gastrointestinal symptoms (including necrotizing enterocolitis in infants), prolonged prothrombin time, decreased platelet aggregation, and impaired absorption of other oil-soluble vitamins.

Vitamin K

Vitamin K acts as a cofactor for hepatic microsomal carboxylase in the synthesis of **clotting factors** II (prothrombin), VII, IX, and X. The specific role of vitamin K involves formation of a 2,3 epoxide that facilitates conversion of glutamyl residues to γ-carboxyglutamates on the clotting factors. Since vitamin K can be synthesized by intestinal flora, deficiency states are associated with other conditions, including malabsorption, drugs (coumarin, cholestyramine), and diffuse liver disease. Vitamin K deficiency is sometimes observed in neonates. Vitamin K deficiency impairs blood clotting, manifesting as a prolonged prothrombin time with deficient factor VII serum levels. Clinically, vitamin K deficiency can cause ecchymoses and bleeding in the gastrointestinal and genitourinary systems. In hypercoagulable states, the anticoagulant coumarin is used to antagonize the effects of vitamin K.

Vitamin K is needed for the synthesis of some blood clotting factors.

WATER-SOLUBLE VITAMINS

Water-soluble vitamins tend to be widely available and easily absorbed in the small intestine.

Vitamin B Complex

The **vitamin B complex** includes thiamine, riboflavin, niacin, B_6, folic acid, and B_{12}; some authors also include biotin and pantothenic acid, even though well-defined deficiency states do not appear to occur. Rich sources of B vitamins include leafy green vegetables, yeast, liver, and milk.

Most members of the vitamin B complex act as cofactors for enzymes.

Thiamine

Thiamine is a cofactor in the pentose phosphate pathway and the decarboxylation of α-ketoacids. Thiamine deficiency can cause dilated cardiomyopathy (**"wet beriberi"**); a symmetric polyneuropathy (**"dry beriberi"**); and focal degeneration in the mamillary bodies, cerebellum, and other sites in the central nervous system (**Wernicke-Korsakoff syndrome**). Thiamine deficiency is encountered in underdeveloped countries and in chronic alcoholics. Thiamine overdose produces transient dizziness and flushing.

Thiamine deficiency affects the heart, nerves, and brain.

Riboflavin

Riboflavin is a component of the oxidation-reduction coenzymes flavin mononucleotide and flavin adenine dinucleotide. Riboflavin deficiency is encountered in alcoholics; patients with serious chronic disease (cancer, infection); during pregnancy and lactation; and in the economically deprived in developing countries. The deficiency state **ariboflavinosis** is characterized by fissures at the corners of the mouth (cheilosis); red-blue discoloration of the tongue (glossitis); corneal opacities and conjunctivitis; a scaling dermatitis that often involves the nose and cheeks; and erythroid hyperplasia of the bone marrow.

Riboflavin deficiency affects skin, mucus membranes, eyes, and bone marrow.

Niacin

Niacin occurs in the coenzymes nicotinamide adenine dinucleotide and nicotinamide adenine dinucleotide phosphate. Niacin deficiency **(pellagra)** is encountered in developing countries, in alcoholics, and in patients with chronic illnesses (cancer, hepatic cirrhosis, tuberculosis). Additionally, since niacin can be synthesized from endogenous tryptophan, pellagra can be observed in patients with the carcinoid syndrome, as a consequence of consumption of tryptophan during serotonin synthesis; and in Hartnup's disease, in which tryptophan absorption is impaired. Pellagra is characterized by a depigmenting dermatitis, chronic diarrhea, and dementia. Prolonged niacin excess can produce hepatic injury, peptic ulcer, and, possibly, diabetes.

Vitamin B_6

Vitamin B_6 (pyridoxine) is used in the coenzyme pyridoxal 5-phosphate. Overt vitamin B_6 deficiency is uncommon, but **subclinical deficiencies** occur during pregnancy, lactation, hyperthyroidism, with high protein diets, and drug treatment with penicillamine, estrogens, or isoniazide. Several rare genetic disorders are responsive to large doses of vitamin B_6, including a familial form of infantile convulsions, hypochromic pyridoxine-responsive anemia, homocystinuria, and xanthurenic aciduria.

Folic Acid

Folic acid (folate) and compounds derived from it are important as acceptors of 1-carbon fragments. Folic acid deficiency produces **megaloblastic anemia,** which is discussed with anemias (see p. 79).

Vitamin B_{12}

Vitamin B_{12} (cobalamin) deficiency produces megaloblastic anemia (see p. 79), neurologic damage (see p. 177), and infertility in both men and women.

Vitamin C

Vitamin C (ascorbic acid) deficiency produces scurvy. **Scurvy** in children is more severe than in adults, and produces hemorrhages (purpura, hemarthroses, intracranial hemorrhages), skeletal changes (bowed legs, depressed sternum), anemia, gingival inflammation, and poor wound healing. In adults, skeletal changes are not observed, but the other effects are present. Scurvy responds well to replacement therapy. Large doses of vitamin C have been recommended for prevention of the common cold and for cancer, but these potentially beneficial results have not been substantiated by clinical trials. Large-dose vitamin C is relatively nontoxic, but can interfere with clinical chemistry tests (fecal occult blood, urinary glucose); potentiate for iron overload by increasing intestinal absorption of nonheme iron; cause hemolysis in patients with glucose-6-phosphate dehydrogenase deficiency; and induce uricosuria.

MINERALS

Minerals required in large amounts for health include iron, calcium, and phosphorus. The results of calcium and phosphorus deficiency are similar to those of vitamin D deficiency (see p. 14). The elements zinc, copper, selenium, and iodine are required in trace amounts. Deficiency of the trace elements is usually only observed in patients who are on total parenteral nutrition; who have inborn errors of metabolism; or whose diet interferes with absorption of the nutrient.

Iron

Iron deficiency can cause a hypochromic, **microcytic anemia** secondary to inadequate heme synthesis. Severe iron deficiency can also cause a variety of systemic impairments including irreversible cognitive dysfunction, impaired immunity, impaired thermoregulation, and reduced levels of physical activity. Body iron stores are normally tightly regulated. Absorption of iron is principally in the duodenum. Dietary lack is an important cause of iron deficiency in developing countries; in developed countries, dietary lack is observed most frequently in the elderly, infants, children, and the very poor. Impaired absorption of iron is observed in patients with chronic small intestinal disease. Increased requirement for iron is observed in infants, children, adolescents, menstruating women, and pregnant women. Chronic blood loss, often from the gastrointestinal tract, is also an important cause of iron deficiency. The possibility of occult gastrointestinal bleeding, possibly due to malignancy, should be evaluated in patients without an obvious explanation for iron deficiency, particularly in adult men and postmenopausal women.

Iron is needed for heme synthesis.

Zinc

Zinc can be found in meats, fish, cereals, and legumes. Zinc deficiency is usually observed in patients on total parenteral nutrition without zinc supplementation; a rare genetic syndrome that interferes with absorption has also been described. The biochemical role for zinc has not been identified. Zinc deficiency is characterized by **rash** and **growth retardation.** Impairments of immunity, wound healing, mentation, sexual function, and night vision have also been observed. Congenital malformations have been observed in infants of zinc-deficient mothers.

Zinc deficiency causes rash and growth retardation.

Copper

Copper is found in many oxidase enzymes. Excessive absorption of copper is observed in **Wilson's disease** (see p. 265). **Copper deficiency** is associated with anemia, neutropenia, hypotonia, psychomotor retardation, osteoporosis, depigmentation of hair, glucose intolerance, and hypercholesterolemia. Copper deficiency is most often observed in premature or malnourished infants; unsupplemented parenteral nutrition; intestinal malabsorption; and therapy with chelating agents. **Menkes**

Copper deficiency affects bone, bone marrow, brain, hair, and glucose metabolism.

kinky hair disease is a rare X-linked disease that causes early death secondary to progressive neurologic deterioration and appears to be due to a defect in copper absorption by the intestine.

Selenium

Selenium deficiency may produce cardiac and skeletal muscle diseases.

The role of **selenium** in the body remains poorly understood. Dietary selenium deficiency has been described in China, where it produced a congestive **cardiomyopathy** (Keshan disease); patients on parenteral supplementation have developed skeletal muscle degeneration and cardiomyopathy thought to be related to selenium deficiency.

4

Immune Disease

AUTOIMMUNE DISEASE

Disease can be produced by many autoimmune mechanisms, and similar mechanisms may be triggered by exogenous antigens. These mechanisms include complex of an antigen to another molecule (drug-induced hemolytic anemia); exposure of new antigenic determinants (partial enzymatic degradation of thyroglobulin, albumin, and collagen); cross-reaction of antibodies to exogenous and host antigens (rheumatic heart disease); exposure of previously sequestered antigen (spermatozoa, myelin basic protein); and polyclonal B-cell activation (endotoxin). Antibodies may also form to other antibodies, sometimes producing biologically active anti-idiotypic determinants (thyroid-stimulating hormone [TSH]-receptor stimulation in Graves disease). Some patients with systemic lupus erythematosus appear to have (controversial) defects in T-suppressor cell function or numbers; other patients have enhanced T-helper cell function, which manifests with chronic hypersecretion of T-helper factors. Thymic defects and defects of macrophages may also be involved with loss of self-tolerance. Many diseases that are thought to have an autoimmune basis have familial clustering associated with specific HLA (especially class II) antigens. The mechanisms by which such associations produce autoimmune disease are still not fully understood, but apparently involve facilitation of immune responses against autoantigens. Autoimmunity can also be induced by large numbers of microbial agents including bacteria, mycoplasma, and viruses. This section considers diseases with targets in many organs and systems; those autoimmune diseases in which the target is a single tissue are discussed with the appropriate organ.

Autoimmune disease is produced by many mechanisms.

MECHANISMS OF IMMUNOLOGIC TISSUE INJURY

Type I Hypersensitivity

Preformed IgE antibody bound to mast cells or basophils can react with antigen to release vasoactive and spasmogenic substances, causing ana-

19

Type I hypersensitivity involves preformed IgE antibody bound to mast cells and basophils.

phylaxis **(type I hypersensitivity). Systemic anaphylaxis** can occur after administration of even tiny quantities of antigens (typically by injection) in previously sensitized individuals. These antigens may have a variety of sources including antisera, hormones, polysaccharides, and drugs (including penicillin). Minutes after exposure, the patient develops itching, hives, skin erythema, and respiratory distress. Patients dying during systemic anaphylaxis show prominent lung findings, which may include pulmonary edema and hemorrhage. Alternatively, the lungs may be hyperdistended and the right heart dilated, presumably reflecting constricted pulmonary vasculature. **Local anaphylaxis reactions** (atopic allergies) tend to develop at the site of inhalation or ingestion of allergens. The range of diseases included in this category includes urticaria, angioedema, allergic rhinitis (hay fever), and sometimes asthma. These diseases are discussed in the appropriate chapters elsewhere in this book. Positive family histories are common in atopic individuals, and appear to be transmitted by a multifactorial pattern that is not associated with HLA antigens and atopic diseases as a group. While there is no generalized response, particular antigens, such as ragweed allergin 5, have been associated with particular HLA loci (HLA-D2). IgE antibodies protect against some parasitic infections, apparently by degranulation of IgE-sensitized mast cells, which attracts other leukocytes that damage the parasite surface.

Type II Hypersensitivity

Type II hypersensitivity involves surface antigens on cells or other tissue components.

In **type II hypersensitivity,** intrinsic or adsorbed surface antigens on cells or other tissue components react with antibodies. **Complement-mediated reactions** are induced by binding of complement to the antigen–antibody complexes, facilitating phagocytosis and cell lysis. Blood cells are particular targets, and complement-dependent reactions are observed in transfusion reactions, erythroblastosis fetalis, autoimmune hemolytic anemia, agranulocytosis, thrombocytopenia, and some drug reactions.

Antibody-dependent cell-mediated cytotoxicity reactions do not involve the fixation of complement. Instead, the target cells are coated with a very low concentration of IgG antibody, which renders them vulnerable to being killed by cells (monocytes, neutrophils, eosinophils, and natural killer [NK] cells) that react to Fc receptors. IgG antibodies are usually involved in antibody-dependent cell-mediated cell toxicity, but in a few cases, IgE antibodies can be used (e.g., in eosinophil-mediated cytotoxicity against parasites). **Antireceptor antibodies** can be formed that are directed against receptors on the cell surface, and may alter cellular function by either blocking or stimulating the receptor. The muscle weakness observed in myasthenia gravis is a consequence of binding of anti-acetylcholine receptor antibodies to the acetylcholine receptor.

Type III Hypersensitivity

Type III hypersensitivity is due to deposition of circulating antigen-antibody complexes.

Type III hypersensitivity is associated with tissue damage produced by **deposition of circulating antigen-antibody complexes** with resulting activation of serum mediators, including the complement system. The complexes may be either deposited in many organs (generalized immune complex-mediated disease), or localized to organs such as the kidney (glomerulonephritis), joints (arthritis), or small blood vessels of the skin (local Arthus reaction).

Acute serum sickness remains the prototypic disease of this type, even though it is now seen uncommonly because animal sera are no longer used for passive immunization. Circulating antigen–antibody complexes are formed about 5 days after the serum is injected, when newly produced antibodies react with small amounts of antigen remaining in the circulation. Deposition of complexes within microvessel walls induces an acute inflammatory reaction accompanied by microthrombi (platelets and fibrin) formation. The resulting pathologic lesions are similar, independent of type, and can take the form of vasculitis, glomerulonephritis, arthritis, or similar inflammations in other sites. Complement-fixing IgM and IgG are usually involved; IgA-containing complexes can also induce tissue injury, since IgA can activate complement by an alternate pathway. The active phase can be monitored by observing a consumption-related decrease in serum complement factors. Clinically apparent disease typically occurs 10 days after antigen administration, and has features including urticaria, fever, arthralgias, lymph node enlargement, and proteinuria. A **chronic form of serum sickness** is usually associated with continuous antigenemia, as can be present in systemic lupus erythematosus, and probably also occurs in rheumatoid arthritis, polyarthritis nodosum, membranous glomerulonephritis, and some vasculitides. The **Arthus reaction** is a local immune complex disease in which tissue necrosis occurs as a result of acute immune complex vasculitis, which is typically elicited in the skin and is due to antigen precipitation with formation of large immune complexes in the vascular wall. The inflammation induced by the complexes can cause fibrinoid necrosis of vessel walls, which may be accompanied by hemorrhage or thrombosis. The Arthus lesions develop over several hours, and, consequently, differ from the IgE-mediated type I reactions.

Type IV Hypersensitivity

The prototype for **delayed-type hypersensitivity** is the tuberculin reaction, which is seen when mycobacterial protein antigens are injected into the skin. In previously sensitized individuals, the injection site shows induration with reddening 12 hours later. Histologically, a predominantly mononuclear perivascular infiltrate is associated with increased vascular permeability, leading to edema and fibrin deposition in the interstitium. At the injection site, a few previously sensitied CD4+ T lymphocytes (memory T cells) recognize antigens on the surface of antigen-presenting cells and are stimulated to divide and release lymphokines. Most of the pathologic features observed are based on the response by circulatory inflammatory cells to the lymphokines. In contrast to delayed hypersensitivity, in which the bulk of the damage is done by macrophages, **T cell-mediated cytotoxicity** is due to the generation by the immune system of cytotoxic T cells, predominantly belonging to the CD8+ subset of T lymphocytes. These cells recognize cell surface antigens, bind to a target cell, and deliver a lytic signal whose biochemical basis is still being explored. A characteristic feature of cytotoxic T cell-mediated cytolysis is that adjacent "innocent" cells are not damaged. It is thought that class I HLA antigens, which can be modified in some virus-infected or tumorous cells, are important in recognition of target cells.

Type IV hypersensitivity is a delayed, cell-mediated reaction.

Transplant Rejection

Transplant rejection appears to involve a combination of cell-mediated immunity and circulating antibodies directed against antigens from the major histocompatibility (HLA) system. The pathology of rejection is best described for the **kidney. Hyperacute rejection,** due to preformed circulating antibodies, can usually be recognized at the time of transplantation, because the grafted kidney becomes cyanotic and does not produce urine. The kidney appears to experience a classic Arthus reaction, with an initial neutrophil binding to arteriole and capillary endothelium that is followed by fibrinoid necrosis of vessel walls and formation of fibrin–platelet thrombi.

Acute rejection may occur days to months to years after transplantation, often when immunosuppression has been employed and then terminated. **Acute humoral rejection** causes vasculitis. A subacute form of vasculitis with arterial intimal thickening is also seen, which is actually more common than true acute rejection vasculitis, and is characterized clinically by intermittent episodes of clinical rejection with altered renal function. **Acute cellular rejection,** due to activated T cells and sometimes plasma cells, is seen most commonly in the initial months after transplantation, and may cause an abrupt onset of renal failure. In contrast to the humoral-based rejection, which is resistant to therapy, acute cellular rejection responds promptly to immunosuppressive therapy.

Patients who experience **chronic rejection** develop increasing serum creatinine over a period of 4 to 6 months. A prominent feature of chronic rejection is the presence of dense intimal fibrosis of vessels, particularly in the cortical arteries, which is thought to be due to the end stage of proliferative arteritis in acute and subacute stages. The vascular lesions are associated with a pronounced renal ischemia, which produces glomerular damage, interstitial fibrosis, and tubular atrophy. Chronic rejection additionally shows an interstitial mononuclear cell infiltrate with large numbers of plasma cells and eosinophils.

Liver transplantation has two patterns of rejection. Acute rejection usually develops within the first 2 months and is characterized by an infiltrate of lymphocytes, neutrophils, and eosinophils that may occur in the triads or bile ducts. The arterioles in chronic rejection show marked thickening and hyalinization. Continued portal tract inflammation produces fibrosis and destruction of bile ductules. In **bone marrow transplantation,** graft-versus-host disease may arise when immunocompetent T cells received from donor marrow recognize the recipient's tissue as foreign. Common clinical manifestations involve skin, liver, and intestinal mucosa. A graft can also fail from rejection; the source of the cells causing rejection appears to be NK cells and radiation-resistant T cells, which may persist despite the bone marrow having received "lethal doses" of irradiation.

PRIMARY IMMUNODEFICIENCY DISORDERS

Immunodeficiency syndromes can be associated with antibody-mediated or cell-mediated immunity, or both. Antibody-mediated reactions are important in control of common bacterial infections. Cell-mediated reactions are important in a few bacterial (e.g., mycobacterial) and many fungal infections. Both antibody-mediated and cell-mediated reactions are important in control of viral and parasitic diseases.

Some immunodeficiency diseases are characterized by a deficiency that predominantly involves antibody production by B lymphocytes. **Bruton's hypogammaglobulinemia** is an X-linked recessive disease characterized by a lack of B cells and no IgM, IgA, IgD, or IgE production. Small quantities of IgG are produced. **Transient hypogammaglobulinemia of infancy** is a delay observed in some infants in the development of antibody production. **Acquired hypogammaglobulinemia** is observed in adults who have normal numbers of B cells but low serum antibody levels. **Selective IgA deficiency** is a relatively common condition characterized by low levels of IgA with normal levels of other antibodies; selective IgM and IgG deficiencies occur less commonly.

DiGeorge syndrome is a deficiency in cell-mediated (T-cell) immunity that is associated with congenital aplasia or hypoplasia of the thymus. The parathyroids may also be absent. The amount of antibody produced is variable. **Acquired immunodeficiency syndrome (AIDS),** discussed in the next section, is associated with a deficiency of helper T cells secondary to viral infection.

Diseases also exist that have combined B- and T-cell deficiency. **Severe combined immunodeficiency** can have either X-linked recessive or autosomal recessive genetics. This condition is characterized by either a defect in the stem cell or in processing to produce both T and B cells. **Nezelof syndrome** is associated with a dysplastic thymus, deficient cell-mediated immunity with a defect in T-helper function, and variable antibody production. **Ataxia telangiectasia** is an autosomal recessive condition associated with a dysplastic thymus, deficient cell-mediated immunity with a defect in T-helper function, and usually decreased IgA production. **Wiskott-Aldrich syndrome** is an X-linked recessive condition that appears to be related to a surface receptor defect in responsiveness. IgA and IgE serum levels are often high, while IgM (and sometimes IgG) levels are low.

AIDS

AIDS is an autoimmune disease that is initiated by infection with the retrovirus human immunodeficiency virus (HIV, known in older literature as HTLV-III). AIDS is a disease with increasing worldwide frequency. The patient groups originally described as at greatest risk of developing AIDS include homosexuals, drug abusers, and recipients of multiple blood products (e.g., hemophiliacs). However, the incidence in heterosexual populations is already very high in some parts of Africa and is increasing throughout the world. Transmission is almost always either through sexual contact, blood transfusion, or transplacentally.

The AIDS virus damages T-helper cells and other lymphocytes, which damages cell-mediated immunity and predisposes for both serious infections (bacterial, fungal, viral) and some **tumors** (malignant lymphoma, Kaposi's sarcoma). Pathologic features associated with AIDS include lymphoid hyperplasia and thymus involution. Some patients develop malignant lymphoma or the vascular tumor Kaposi's sarcoma (see p. 120). Patients with AIDS are vulnerable to severe, often disseminated, **viral infections,** with cytomegalovirus, herpesviruses, Epstein-Barr virus, and hepatitis B virus being common infecting agents. **Parasitic infections** to which these patients are vulnerable include *Pneumocystis* pneumonia, cryptosporidosis, toxoplasmosis, and giardiasis. The patients experience multiple **bacterial infections,** which may be due to common

The AIDS virus damages T-helper cells, leading to impaired cell-mediated immunity.

pathogens (*Staphylococcus, Mycobacterium tuberculosis,* gram-negative bacilli). These patients are also vulnerable to unusual bacterial infections, notably atypical mycobacterial (*Mycobacterium avium-intracellulare*) intestinal and disseminated infection. Disseminated or deep fungal infections (candidiasis, cryptococcosis, aspergillosis) are common.

The delay between the acquisition of the AIDS virus and development of clinical AIDS may be years. Diagnosis of clinical AIDS is based on the presence of antibodies to the virus, a reduced helper T-cell to suppressor T-cell ratio, and clinical features such as Kaposi's sarcoma and the presence of unusual infections. The AIDS-related complex (ARC) is a cluster of findings, notably lymphoid hyperplasia, observed in individuals who have been infected by the virus but have not (yet) developed marked immunosuppression. Clinical AIDS remains, despite aggressive research, nearly universally fatal as a consequence of uncontrollable infections or tumor.

SYSTEMIC LUPUS ERYTHEMATOSUS

Systemic lupus erythematosus is a multisystem disease characterized by the presence of large numbers of autoantibodies.

Systemic lupus erythematosus is a febrile illness accompanied by injury to many sites, particularly skin, joints, kidney, and serosal membranes. Systemic lupus erythematosus is usually observed in young to middle-aged women but can also manifest in both sexes and at any other age, including early childhood. Large numbers of **autoantibodies,** particularly those directed against nuclei, are produced, possibly as a failure of immunologic regulatory mechanisms. Patients with systemic lupus erythematosus can have antibodies directed against DNA, histones, non-histone proteins, and nucleolar antigens; these antinuclear antibodies can be observed by indirect immunofluorescence. A polyclonal activation of B cells appears to be central to the pathogenesis of systemic lupus erythematosus, and characteristically produces hypergammaglobulinemia with in vivo autoantibody production.

Type II hypersensitivity with deposition of immune complexes leading to tissue (glomeruli, blood vessels) injury appears to be the most common mechanism by which lupus erythematosus produces pathology. Autoantibodies may be directed against red cells, white cells, and platelets. The antinuclear antibodies that form such a prominent role in the diagnosis and monitoring of lupus erythematosus do not appear to penetrate intact cells, but can bind to the nuclei of damaged cells, causing the nuclei to become homogeneous, degenerating masses known as LE bodies. The in vitro production of LE bodies by agitation of blood forms the basis of the LE cell test, which is positive in approximately two-thirds of patients with systemic lupus erythematosus.

Diagnosis is based on the presence of several of many criteria.

The presentation of systemic lupus erythematosus is highly variable. Diagnosis is based on the presence of several of many criteria that include malar or discoid **rash,** photosensitivity, oral ulcers, **arthritis, serositis** (either pleuritis or pericarditis), **renal disorder** (persistent proteinuria or cellular casts), **neurologic disorder** (seizures, psychosis), **hematologic disorder** (hemolytic anemia, leukopenia, lymphopenia, thrombocytopenia), and **immunologic disorder** (positive lupus erythematosus cell preparation, anti-DNA or antinuclear antibody, anti-smooth muscle antibody, false-positive test for syphilis). The most characteristic lesions are found in blood vessels, kidneys, connective tissue, and skin.

An acute vasculitis with fibrinoid necrosis and perivascular lymphocytic infiltrate can affect small arteries and arterioles. The renal pathology can be highly complex and is described elsewhere (see p. 292). The skin is commonly affected by an erythematosus "butterfly" or "wolf-like" malar rash (see also p. 110). The skin lesions may alternatively be bullous, urticarial, or maculopapular and may involve extremities or trunk. Often, the rash is exacerbated by sun exposure. The affected skin shows degeneration of the epidermal basal layer, and immunofluorescence studies will usually demonstrate immunoglobulin and complement in the dermal–epidermal junction. A characteristic feature of systemic, as opposed to localized, lupus erythematosus is the presence of immunoglobulin deposition even in clinically uninvolved skin.

The clinical course of lupus erythema\tosus is very difficult to predict, since some patients die within weeks or months, while others survive for years to decades with only occasional flaring of disease. Roughly three-quarters of treated paitents now survive for 10 years. Common causes of death include renal failure, infections, cardiac failure, pulmonary disease, and central nervous system disease.

Chronic discoid lupus erythematosus produces skin lesions, often on the face or scalp, but does not usually cause systemic manifestations. The skin plaques characteristically show edema, erythema, scaliness, follicular plugging, and skin atrophy surrounded by an erythematous border. Serologic studies rarely show a positive LE test, but may have a positive antinuclear antibody test, although antibodies to double-stranded DNA are rarely present. Skin biopsies show deposition of immunoglobulin and C3 at the dermal–epidermal junction, similar to that of systemic lupus erythematosus, but, unlike systemic lupus erythematosus, uninvolved skin does not show any immunoglobulin and C3 deposition. **Subacute cutaneous lupus erythematosus** has widespread superficial lesions accompanied by mild systemic disease, and it is associated with antibodies to the SS-A nuclear antigen and the HLA-DR3 genotype. This group appears to be intermediate between systemic lupus erythematosus and lupus erythematosus localized to the skin. **Drug-induced lupus erythematosus syndromes** can be observed in patients who have been exposed to hydralazine, procainamide, isoniazid, D-penicillamine, or other drugs. Patients often have antinuclear (particularly antihistone) antibodies, but many patients do not develop symptoms of lupus erythematosus. Remission can often be induced by withdrawal of the offending drug.

Variant forms of lupus are observed.

OTHER SYSTEMIC AUTOIMMUNE DISEASES

Progressive systemic sclerosis is thought to be due to immune complex-mediated small vessel vasculitis that leads to increased collagen deposition throughout the body. A variety of antinuclear antibodies are typically present. The dermal fibrosis (**scleroderma**) in long-standing progressive systemic sclerosis is usually severe and may be associated with mask-like facies, severe contractures ("claw-hand" or sclerodactyly), trophic ulcerations, and dystrophic calcification. Gastrointestinal involvement manifests as dysphagia (esophagus) and stasis of luminal contents (small intestine). Renal involvement (vascular and glomerular

Progressive systemic sclerosis is a small vessel vasculitis that leads to collagen deposition throughout the body.

Polymyositis-dermatomyosis and mixed connective tissue disease are other systemic autoimmune diseases that appear to be related to lupus and scleroderma.

Amyloidosis may be due to deposition of immunoglobulin or proteins produced by chronic inflammatory diseases.

changes, nephrotic syndrome) is a common cause of death in these patients. The lungs may develop severe interstitial fibrosis. The subset of patients with the **CREST syndrome** (calcinosis, Raynaud's phenomen, esophageal hypomotility, sclerodactyly, and telangiectasias) have disease that progresses more slowly but does eventually involve the visceral organs. Forms of scleroderma localized to the skin (**morphea, linear scleroderma**) histologically resemble the dermal involvement of pgoresssive systemic sclerosis but do not appear to be systemic autoimmune diseases.

Polymyositis-dermatomyosis is an uncommon, apparently autoimmune, disorder characterized by a violaceous rash involving the eyelids, accompanied by a myositis that most severely affects limb-girdle muscles. About 10 percent of patients have an associated malignant neoplasm, typically lung or breast carcinoma. **Mixed connective tissue disease** is a rare overlap syndrome with features of systemic lupus erythematosus, progressive systemic sclerosis, and polymyositis. High titers of antibodies directed against ribonucleoprotein are typically present.

Amyloidosis refers to the extracellular deposition of protein with a characteristic β-pleated structure (but variable chemical composition) that stains red with apple-green birefringence with Congo red. In **primary systemic amyloidosis**, immunoglobulin produced by plasma cell or B-lymphocyte neoplasms is deposited preferentially in heart, gastrointestinal tract, tongue, skin, and nerves. In **secondary systemic amyloidosis**, chronic inflammatory disease (tuberculosis, lepromatous leprosy, rheumatoid arthritis) leads to deposition of a protein of unknown origin in kidney, liver, spleen, and adrenals. **Localized amyloidosis** (heart, cerebral vessels, tongue, bladder, eye, lung), **tumor amyloid** (medullary carcinoma of the thyroid, pheochromocytoma, islet cell tumor of the pancreas), and a rare **familial amyloidosis** also occur. Organs involved by amyloid tend to be larger, firmer, and grayer than their normal counterparts. Renal involvement caused by amyloid deposition in glomeruli (nephrotic syndrome, chronic renal failure) is a common cause of death. Amyloid deposition in the subendocardium and between myocardial fibers can cause restrictive cardiomyopathy and heart block. Amyloid deposition in the liver, spleen, and gastrointestinal tract is usually asymptomatic.

5

Infectious Disease

VIRUSES

VIRAL RESPIRATORY DISORDERS

Many viruses cause respiratory disorders ranging from the common cold to pneumonia. Viral respiratory disorders are typically acquired by spread of the virus via respiratory route from a sick, incubating, or convalescing individual. The viruses typically have short incubation times. The pathologic changes produced depend upon the level of the infection and can include nasal mucosal inflammation with mucus production, hyperplasia of Waldeyer's ring, vocal cord swelling, inflammation with mucus production in the trachea and large bronchi, and plugging of small airways. **Upper respiratory viral infections** are usually transient, may impair ventilation, and may be superinfected by bacteria, particularly in infants, the elderly, and persons with pre-existing chronic respiratory disease or diabetes. **Lower respiratory infections** can produce marked hypoxia or dramatic radiographic changes (atypical pneumonia). The milder viral pneumonias are characterized by a patchy, interstitial, inflammatory reaction. More severe pneumonias may cause hyaline membrane formation resembling that of adult respiratory distress syndrome; alveolar consolidation with fibrin and hemorrhage; and parenchymal necrosis. Severe viral pneumonias may heal by organization of alveolar plugs, producing interstitial fibrosis. Patients who are seriously ill from other causes, elderly, or infected with particularly severe strains (such as occurred during the 1918 swine flu epidemic) may acquire a subsequent bacterial pneumonia that may lead to sepsis and death.

Different viral species produce different disease patterns. Rhinoviruses usually cause upper respiratory tract infections; influenza viruses usually involve both the upper and lower respiratory tract. Several viral skin diseases (measles, rubella, chickenpox) produce respiratory symptoms after viremic spread had occurred. Viruses that characteristically produce respiratory infections may also cause other disorders. Coxsackie A viruses cause blistering of the pharynx (herpangina). Coxsackie B viruses cause pleuritis, myocarditis, and Guillain-Barré syndrome. Types A and B influenza virus produce "flu" syndromes characterized by lower respiratory tract infection accompanied by fever, myal-

Viral respiratory disorders tend to cause inflammation and mucus production.

Severe viral pneumonias may scar the lung or become secondarily infected by bacteria.

Different viruses produce different disease patterns.

27

gia, and headaches. Potentially lethal Reye syndrome (see p. 272) occasionally follows aspirin therapy during viral illness, particularly in children. Echoviruses produce pharyngitis, skin rash, and, uncommonly, myocarditis. Infants and children infected by respiratory syncytial virus and parainfluenza viruses may develop lethal bronchiolitis (croup) and pneumonia. Various strains of adenoviruses produce upper respiratory infection, sporadic pneumonia, pharyngoconjunctival fever, keratoconjunctivitis, or a whooping cough-like syndrome.

VIRAL DISORDERS OF THE DIGESTIVE TRACT

Mumps can affect salivary glands, testes, pancreas, central nervous system, or heart.

Mumps is caused by a paramyxovirus, which produces a usually mild infection that is typically an acute contagious disease of childhood. Children and teenagers may be asymptomatic, have mild infection, or may have clinical mumps, which tends to have a 1- to 2-week duration. Mumps parotitis typically involves both parotid glands. The affected glands contain a diffuse infiltration of histiocytes, lymphocytes, and plasma cells, which can compress acini and ducts. Adult patients tend to have more severe disease with more complications than do children. Complications are uncommon and include sterility secondary to orchitis, pancreatitis, nonspecific meningitis or encephalitis, and potentially fatal myocarditis. Childhood vaccination is reducing the incidence of mumps in developed countries.

Acute viral diarrhea is most often caused by rotaviruses, Norwalk agents, or adenoviruses.

Acute diarrheal diseases can be caused by viruses, particularly rotaviruses, Norwalk agents, and adenoviruses. **Rotaviral diarrhea** can be diagnosed either by the use of enzyme-linked immunosorbent assays (ELISAs) or by electron microscopy of stool filtrates. The rotaviruses are usually transmitted by an oral–fecal route, with peak prevalence in winter months in temperate zones, and in the dry season in the tropics. Following a 48-hour incubation period, rotaviruses commonly cause diarrhea that lasts only a few days, but is occasionally fatal secondary to dehydration and electrolyte imbalance as a consequence of fever, vomiting, and loss of appetite. Histologically, the small bowel may show lamina proprial infiltration, shortened villi, and cellular hyperplasia in mucosal crypts. **Norwalk agents** have a short (18-hour) incubation period and are a cause of diarrheal epidemics. The Norwalk agents can be detected by stool electron microscopy and can cause small bowel biopsy changes similar to those observed with rotavirus infection. Most patients experience diarrhea for only 1 or 2 days, although more prolonged diarrhea is experienced by a few patients. **Adenoviruses** are also identified in some childhood diarrheas.

VIRAL EPITHELIAL GROWTHS

Viral epithelial growths may be either benign or malinant.

Viral epithelial growths can involve the epidermal tissues and are discussed in connection with sexually transmitted diseases, since these viruses can cause condyloma (papillomavirus), cervical carcinoma (papillomavirus), and molluscum contagiosum (molluscum virus). These epithelial growths tend to be characterized by exuberant epithelial proliferation with inclusion bodies or koilocytosis involving the maturing epithelial cells. A predominantly mononuclear stromal and basal inflammatory infiltrate may be present.

VIRAL DISORDERS WITH SKIN RASHES

Measles (rubeola) is a formerly common childhood systemic viral infection whose incidence has been reduced in the United States and Europe by extensive vaccination. Cough and conjunctivitis are followed by blistering of cheek mucosa **(Koplik's spots)**, swollen lymph nodes and/or splenic enlargement, and a characteristic morbilliform rash. This rash shows nonspecific pathologic changes, usually begins behind the ears, and subsequently involves the neck, trunk, and extremities with blotchy, reddish-brown patches. The most diagnostic changes occur in lymphoid tissues, which may contain randomly distributed multinucleate **(Warthin-Finkeldey)** giant cells with eosinophilic nuclear and cytoplasmic inclusions. Measles can be complicated by encephalitis or pneumonia, particularly in infants, the elderly, and immunosuppressed patients. Bacterial superinfection of the pneumonia may cause prominent pathologic changes. Measles pneumonia also uncommonly causes severe pulmonary fibrosis, often with prominent giant cells. Measles has been implicated in a variety of chronic problems including subacute sclerosing panencephalitis, minimal change nephrotic syndrome, and thrombocytopenic purpura. Prenatal rubeola infection is not associated with fetal congenital anomalies.

> **Measles can affect skin, lungs, lymphoid tissues, brain, or kidneys.**

German measles (rubella), caused by togavirus infection, is milder than rubeola, but produces a similar rash, which is usually accompanied by swelling of the posterior cervical lymph nodes. Prenatal infection can cause severe congenital malformations, often involving the heart.

> **German measles is usually milder than rubeola, but can cause severe congenital malformations.**

Smallpox (variola) is a formerly commonly fatal infectious vesicular disease caused by a double-stranded DNA virus, which appears to have been completely eradicated by aggressive vaccination. Two additional mild childhood skin rashes are **erythema infectiosum,** caused by a parvovirus, and **roseola infantum,** which is of unknown etiology.

> **Other viral skin rashes include smallpox, erythema infectiosum, and roseola infantum.**

HERPESVIRUS DISEASES

Clinically important **herpesviruses** include herpes simplex I and II; the herpes zoster viruses, which cause both chickenpox and shingles; cytomegalovirus, which causes cytomegalic inclusion disease; and the Epstein-Barr virus, which causes infectious mononucleosis and has been associated with Burkitt's lymphoma and nasopharyngeal carcinoma. The herpesviruses cause latent infection that may later become reactivated, producing clinical disease. The herpesviruses can also produce systemic disease, usually in immunosuppressed hosts. Herpesvirus infections characteristically produce intranuclear (Cowdry type A) inclusions.

> **Herpes virus infection may be acute, latent, reactivated, or systemic.**

Herpes simplex (HSV I) and **herpes genitalis** (HSV II) infections are very similar vesicular diseases. Herpes simplex is usually transmitted by physical contact including kissing; herpes genitalis virus is usually transmitted by sexual contact or during birth. Both strains have long latency periods, during which they reproduce in neural ganglia. Following the initial infection or reactivation of the virus, vesicles form in skin or mucosa. The bases of the vesicles contain infected epithelial cells whose nuclei contain large, eosinophilic viral (Cowdry type A) inclusions. Giant cells (polykaryons) caused by fusion of epithelial cells can also be found in the blister fluid.

> **Herpes simplex and herpes genitalis can affect both the skin and internal organs.**

Chickenpox and shingles are caused by the same virus.

Cytomegalovirus is an important cause of congenital disease and disease in immunocompromised adults.

Immunofluorescence and DNA probes can identify the viruses. Unlike herpes zoster, described below, the distribution of skin, mucosal, and gingival lesions does not characteristically follow a dermatome. Depending upon the site involved and the extent of infection, these viruses can produce cold sores, gingivostomatitis, genital herpes, keratoconjunctivitis (which may cause blindness), severe skin involvement (Kaposi's varicelliform eruption, eczema herpeticum), encephalitis, esophagitis, pneumonitis, or widely disseminated disease. Severe infection is most commonly observed in neonates and immunocompromised adults in whom it may contribute to death.

The varicella-zoster virus can cause both chickenpox (varicella) and herpes zoster. **Chickenpox,** the acute infection, is now the most common childhood rash, since effective vaccines have not yet been developed. The rash produces "crops" of spontaneously rupturing intraepithelial vesicles that begin on the trunk. Infected adults tend to be sicker and have more complications (pneumonitis, encephalitis, transveres myelitis) than infected children. Reactivation of varicella-zoster virus infection produces **herpes zoster** or shingles. Adults with shingles have transmitted chickenpox to children. The virus travels the peripheral nerve to the skin, where it causes a localized vesicular eruption that histologically and clinically resembles that of chickenpox. The eruption causes intense itching or pain, apparently as a consequence of a simultaneous nerve involvement. When the rash involves distribution of the branches of the trigeminal nerve, temporary facial paralysis is sometimes observed **(Ramsay Hunt syndrome).** Typically, only one dermatome, often on one side of the thorax, is involved, but the eruptions may be bilateral or involve multiple dermatomes. Immunosuppressed patients are particularly vulnerable and may also develop disseminated disease, which may contribute to the patient's death. The lesions of herpes zoster resemble those of herpes simplex.

Cytomegalovirus causes latent infection in adults and rarely produces clinical disease, usually in fetuses or immunocompromised patients. Cells infected with cytomegalovirus are often markedly enlarged and have large pleomorphic nuclei that may contain intranuclear inclusions resembling those of herpes simplex virus. Smaller basophilic inclusions may also be seen. Congenital infections usually follow a new maternal infection. Most congenital infections are asymptomatic at birth. Some apparently asymptomatic infants later develop brain damage, failure to thrive, transient hepatitis, purpura, or mild respiratory disease. More severely infected (often premature or low-birth-weight) infants develop classic **cytomegalic inclusion disease** with hemolytic anemia, thrombocytopenia, hepatosplenomegaly, and sometimes lung infection, deafness, visual impairments, or brain damage. These infants often die, but may survive with mental retardation, or in a few fortunate cases, appear to recover completely. In immunocompromised adults (acquired immunodeficiency syndrome [AIDS], transplant recipients), reactivation of latent cytomegalovirus may produce interstitial pneumonitis, intestinal ulcerations, chorioretinitis, encephalitis, or widely disseminated disease. Cytomegalovirus infection can also cause a self-limited infectious mononucleosis-like syndrome, which is typically observed in previously healthy children or adults who received transfusions of blood from donors with latent cytomegalovirus infections.

Epstein-Barr virus causes **infectious mononucleosis,** characterized by a generalized lymphadenopathy that is usually accompanied by fever and sore throat. The spleen, liver, and, less commonly, other organ systems can also be affected. The blood and affected tissues contain atypical activated T lymphocytes (mononucleosis cells) with abundant basophilic cytoplasm, a variably shaped nucleus, and small fenestrations or vacuolations of the cytoplasm. Infectious mononucleosis is most commonly seen in late adolescents and young adults who did not experience a usually asymptomatic childhood infection. Patients are usually sick from 2 to 4 weeks and slowly recover, unless either cardiac or hepatic disease occurs, which may prolong the course. Carriers of Epstein-Barr virus are common. Heterophil (Paul-Bunnell) antibodies transiently rise following infection. The peripheral blood usually shows lymphocytosis, with many atypical lymphocytes. Lymph nodes throughout the body become moderately enlarged, with proliferation of both follicles and paracortical T cells. Occasional binucleate cells may resemble the Reed-Sternberg cells of Hodgkin's lymphoma. The virus may be incorporated into the lymphocyte genome, producing a latent infection that may be later reinitiated, usually in seriously immunocompromised patients. Epstein-Barr virus infection is also associated with African Burkitt's lymphoma and nasopharyngeal carcinoma. An X-linked recessive immunodeficiency state is associated with a familial form of adverse responses to infection by Epstein-Barr virus, including lethal mononucleosis, autoimmune disease, and development of many lymphomas and leukemias.

Infectious mononucleosis affects lymph nodes, spleen, and liver.

Epstein-Barr virus is associated with some malignancies.

ARBOVIRUS DISEASES

The **arthropod-borne** (arbo-) **viruses** are usually carried by insect vectors feeding on animal reservoirs. Human transmission by mosquitoes can occasionally occur. Colorado tick fever, which clinically resembles the rickettsial infection Rocky Mountain spotted fever, appears to be due to an arbovirus transmitted by a tick vector. Dengue fever produces tropical disease resembling influenza that is accompanied by severe bone pain (breakbone fever) and can cause potentially fatal disseminated intravascular coagulation. An efficient dengue vector mosquito has been isolated in Cuba, Puerto Rico, and the southern United States. Other forms of fulminant hemorrhagic fevers transmitted as arboviruses include the Lassa, Marburg, and Ebola viruses. Yellow fever was formerly a problem, but now appears confined to a jungle monkey reservoir. A variety of encephalitis viruses are carried by domestic mosquitos and have caused outbreaks in the United States. The arbovirus diseases tend to cause devastating local outbreaks rather than global epidemics.

Arboviruses are usually transmitted by insects from animal reservoirs.

VIRAL DISEASES OF OTHER ORGAN SYSTEMS

Viral diseases that principally affect the brain, liver, and heart are discussed with these organs. A number of serious human diseases are caused by retroviruses, in which the viral genome becomes incorporated into the human genome. Diseases included in this class are human T-cell leukemia (see p. 92), caused by HTLV-I; the acquired immune deficiency syndrome (see p. 23), caused by the AIDS virus; and Kawasaki syndrome (see p. 206), possibly caused by a reverse transcriptase-producing virus.

Retroviruses can incorporate into the host genome and cause leukemia and AIDS.

BACTERIA

CHLAMYDIAL DISEASES

Chlamydiae live in host cells.

Chlamydiae are obligate intracellular organisms that resemble bacteria, but differ from free-living bacteria in that they cannot synthesize their own adenosine triphosphate (ATP). Chlamydiae live in phagocytic vacuoles of the host cells. Individual chlamydia are called elementary bodies; aggregates of chlamydia form cytoplasmic inclusions. The elementary bodies and inclusions are best visualized by immunofluorescence or on Giemsa-stained smears. Their intracellular habitat protects chlamydia from host antibodies and cellular immunity, and chlamydial infections consequently tend to be protracted.

Ornithosis can cause flu-like illness or pneumonia.

Ornithosis (psittacosis) is a respiratory infection by *Chlamydia psittaci,* which is usually acquired by inhalation of dust contaminated by excreta of infected birds (parrots, seagulls), who do not always appear ill. *Chlamydia psittaci* can cause asymptomatic infection, transient flu-like illness, or potentially fatal pneumonia. Very severe cases typically show interstitial pneumonitis, pulmonary edema, and superinfection by other bacteria. The alveolar septal cells occasionally contain intracytoplasmic bodies that can be identified with Giemsa or immunofluorescent techniques. Hilar lymph nodes may show reticular endothelial hyperplasia and acute lymphadenitis. In severe cases with generalized disease, usually observed in epidemics, other organs (liver, spleen, kidneys, heart, brain) may show focal necrosis or diffuse mononuclear infiltration. Most cases resolve either spontaneously or with chemotherapy after 2 to 3 weeks of illness; carrier states can occur. A rise in the specific antibody to *Chlamydia psittaci* is helpful in diagnosis, and the organism can also be cultured in yolk sac and tissue culture inoculation.

Chlamydial Urethritis and Cervicitis

Chlamydiae are important causes of nongonococcal venereal disease.

Chlamydial urethritis and cervicitis are frequent forms of chlamydial disease that are usually transmitted venereally. These conditions are typically recognized after treatment for gonorrhea fails to alleviate infectious symptoms. Postgonococcal urethritis is most commonly identified, and subsequent follow-up of partners may identify chlamydiae in asymptomatic partners and in women with chronic cervicitis. In this form of chlamydial infection, the histologic hallmark is the presence of inclusions in epithelial cells. Fluorescent antibodies can be used to identify both inclusions and elementary bodies. Definitive identification can be obtained by culture on McCoy cells followed by serotyping by microcomplement fixation. These latter tests are usually available only in specialized venereal diseases centers, and may be used with secretions as well as serum.

Inclusion Conjunctivitis

Newborns can be infected with *Chlamydia trachomatis* from the birth canal of infected mothers. Such **inclusion conjunctivitis** is usually a benign, suppurative conjunctivitis that clears spontaneously. A histologically similar disease, but caused by a different *Chlamydia trachomatis* group, can be acquired by adults swimming or bathing in water that is contaminated by secretions (swimming pool conjunctivitis). In newborns, the incubation time appears to be roughly 1 to 2 weeks, and untreated disease can last several months. Inclusion conjunctivitis in infants is characterized by a monocyte-rich purulent exudate accompanied by conjunctival hyperemia and edema. In adults, lymphocytic, rather than monocytic, infiltration occurs, but the changes observed in trachoma are not observed. Type-specific antiserum can be used for serotyping *Chlamydia trachomatis* strains.

Newborns infected by chlamydia can develop inclusion conjunctivitis.

Trachoma

Several subtypes (A, B, Ba, C) of *Chlamydia trachomatis* can cause the chronic suppurative disease known as **trachoma.** Worldwide, trachoma is a leading cause of blindness; progressive trachoma is seen most commonly among poor people and nomads in dry, endemic areas. Affected individuals have often been repeatedly exposed to the organisms by direct human contact, fomites, and, possibly, flies. Conjunctival infection resembling inclusion conjunctivitis progresses to deep tissue involvement. The conjunctiva may ulcerate, and a pannus can form over the affected cornea, leading to scarring with eventual blindness. Trachoma responds to antibiotics, but these agents are not always available in developing countries.

Children and adults who experience multiple chlamydial eye infections may develop trachoma.

Lymphogranuloma Venereum

Chlamydia trachomatis (serotypes L1, L2, and L3) causes **lymphogranuloma venereum,** which is endemic in tropical countries, and is typically transmitted between sexual partners along with other venereal infections. In early infection, a small skin vesicle bursts to form an ulcer. The ulcer base shows nonspecific chronic inflammation that may eventually progress to granuloma formation. Diagnosis of lymphogranuloma venereum can sometimes be made in these early lesions when specific immunofluorescence or Giemsa-stained smear shows chlamydial inclusions within the epidermal cells. Subsequently, regional lymph nodes show diffuse reticulosis and/or scattered granulomas that eventually, by a combination of necrosis and confluence, form stellate abscesses that may discharge through fistulae to the skin or other surfaces. Stellate abscesses, while distinctive, can also be observed in cat-scratch fever and a few fungal or mycobacterial diseases. Definitive diagnosis at this stage can also be established by demonstrating elementary bodies by immunofluorescence or in a Giemsa-stain smear. The lesions eventually resolve, leaving chronic inflammatory infiltrates and dense fibrosis. Diagnosis in long-standing disease can be difficult, as the chlamydiae may not be microscopically detectable. In neglected disease, severe scarring may produce rectal stenosis in women, and chronic genital lymphedema in both men **(elephantiasis)** and women **(esthiomene).** A serotype-specif-

Lymphogranuloma venereum is a severe chlamydial venereal infection characterized by skin ulcers, regional lymph node necrosis, and severe scarring.

ic microimmunofluorescent test for lymphogranuloma-type chlamydiae has also been developed, but is not yet widely available. Patients with lymphogranuloma venereum should also be evaluated for the presence of other venereal diseases, including latent syphilis.

RICKETTSIAL DISEASES

Rickettsiae are obligate intracellular bacteria that are typically transmitted by arthropod hosts and have a predilection for infecting vasculature.

Rickettsiae are gram-negative, obligate intracellular bacteria. Most rickettsiae that infect humans inhabit natural arthropod hosts including ticks, mites, fleas, or lice, in whom they are passed transovarially to subsequent generations without damage to the host. These arthropods typically infest the hair of animals, who can occasionally be infected by the rickettsiae. Rickettsiae are usually transmitted to animals, including humans, by the bite of a feeding host arthropod. Most rickettsiae that can affect humans tend to have a predilection for infecting small vessel endothelia, and consequently cause disease that is clinically similar, independent of the type of rickettsiae. Exceptions include the *Coxiella,* which are associated with Q fever and acquired by droplet inhalation; and *Ehrlichia,* which is transmitted by tick bite, and causes fever and lymphadenopathy. It is thought that these two genera may be biologically and genomically distinct from other rickettsiae. Common to many, but not all, rickettsial infections is the development of a crusted skin lesion **(eschar),** which may appear at sites where the arthropod has bitten the human or arthropod excreta has entered abraded skin. Once in a host, rickettsiae enter host cells by what appears to be an induced endocytosis in which they are enveloped in phagosomal membranes. The rickettsiae, however, soon escape the phagosome and enter the cytosol, where they begin dividing by binary fission. Depending upon the disease, the rickettsiae may either continue to divide until the host cell ruptures, or may be actively expelled by the host cell in cytoplasmic projections. Defense of the host against the rickettsia appears to involve interferon- and T-lymphocyte-dependent immune responses. Lasting immunity can be produced by both infection and vaccination. Pathologically, rickettsial infections tend to be dominated by damage to small blood vessels, characterized by **focal vascular inflammation,** which is often associated with a **rash.** Vascular microthrombi, focal ischemia, and hemorrhage may also occur. The areas of inflammation are usually nodular, occur sparsely, and are characterized by a predominantly mononuclear infiltrate. The rickettsial diseases may be life-threatening. They usually respond promptly to appropriate wide-spectrum antibiotics, but diagnosis, particularly of isolated rather than epidemic cases, may be difficult. Rickettsia-specific serum antibody titers are highly useful in establishing a definitive diagnosis, but tend to rise relatively late (during the second week of the illness), so in practice, the diagnosis should be suspected and treated before the results from the antibody titers are available.

Typhus Fever

The typhus group of diseases is characterized by rash, vasculitis, and typhus nodules in many organs.

The **typhus group of diseases** includes epidemic typhus, Brill-Zinsser disease, flying squirrel typhus, and murine typhus. **Epidemic typhus,** caused by *Rickettsia prowazekii,* is spread by fecal contamination of skin by human head and body lice. Headache and fever develop after a 1- to 2-week incubation period and are followed several days later by a maculopapular rash that characteristically begins on the trunk and extends to the extremities and head. Many patients die during this period; in those who recover, the rash fades and the temperature subsides, usually during the third week of illness. Throughout the body, venules, arterioles, and small arteries show endothelial proliferation and swelling, perivascular inflammation, and thrombosis. Necrosis of the vessel wall is uncommon in typhus, compared with Rocky Mountain spotted fever. Characteristic **"typhus nodules"** in the brain are focal microglial proliferations that also contain other leukocytes and may be associated with the small vessel lesions. Structures resembling typhus nodules can also be observed in heart, kidney, testes, and liver.

Immunofluorescent staining for rickettsia in skin biopsy specimens may be helpful in establishing an early diagnosis. During the second week of the illness, the diagnosis can be confirmed by demonstrating elevated titers of compliment-fixing or agglutinating antibodies directed against *Rickettsia prowazekii*. An older test, the Weil-Felix reaction, is still used as a rapid test in field settings, and is based on the cross-reaction between *Proteus* antigens and specific rickettsial antigens.

Brill-Zinsser disease is another member of the typhus group and represents a recurrence of epidemic typhus that may appear many years after the initial attack; in the United States, this disease is observed most frequently in immigrants from eastern Europe. The recurrence is usually milder than epidemic typhus and is not associated with necrosis or gangrene. **Flying squirrel typhus** is observed in the southeast United States, where it causes a sporadic occurrence of typhus fever, and is caused by an agent that is indistinguishable from *Rickettsia prowazekii*. **Murine typhus** is caused by *Rickettsia typhi (mooseri)*, which is transmitted by rat fleas and is endemic throughout the world, particularly in Central and South America. Both the flying squirrel and the murine forms of typhus have a lower mortality than does the epidemic form.

Spotted Fevers

The **rickettsial spotted fevers** include Rocky Mountain spotted fever, boutonneuse fever, North Asian typhus, Queensland tick typhus, and rickettsial pox. These agents are transmitted to humans through chance encounter with ticks, with the exception of rickettsial pox, which is transmitted by mites parasitic for urban rodents. The spotted fevers are characterized by development of an eschar at the site of the tick bite, which is subsequently followed by a disseminated hemorrhagic rash. Milder cases can mimic other common febrile illnesses since the eschar and the rash may be inconspicuous. The prototype disease is **Rocky Mountain spotted fever,** which is native to the Americas. Its causative agent is *Rickettsia rickettsii,* whose hosts are several species of hard ticks. Clinical disease begins with formation of an **eschar** 2 to 12 days after a tick bite. The patient then experiences fever, headache, and muscle pain. A maculopapular **rash** begins in the distal extremities, later extends toward the trunk, and can involve the palms of the hands and the soles of the feet. The rash may be accompanied by high fever, chills, and mental apathy with occasional stupor. A severe necrotizing acute **vasculitis** may involve many organs. Deaths in Rocky Mountain spotted fever are most often due to shock, renal failure, or central nervous sys-

The rickettsial spotted fevers are characterized by eschar formation, rash, vasculitis, and shock.

tem damage; patients with glucose-6-dehydrogenase deficiency are particularly susceptible to severe disease. Antibiotic and supportive therapy can markedly improve the prognosis, but the mortality rate even in treated patients remains 3 to 10 percent, in part because the diagnosis is often delayed. Skin biopsy specimens may stain with immunofluorescence for rickettsia.

Scrub Typhus

Scrub typhus differs from other forms of typhus by having a milder rash and a higher incidence of lymphadenopathy and serosal inflammation.

Rickettsia tsutsugamushi is a mite-borne rickettsial organism that causes **scrub typhus** (tsutsugamushi fever), particularly in the Far East and Pacific rim. Scrub typhus was originally thought to be a consistently serious, often fatal disease; however, since effective serodiagnosis and early antibiotic treatment have become available, the vast majority of infections are much milder. The rash is usually macropapular and may be so mild as not to be particularly prominent. Vascular necrosis, hemorrhage, and thrombosis are uncommon. Scrub typhus otherwise resembles, grossly and microscopically, other members of the typhus group, although lymphadenopathy and serosal inflammation of the pericardium, pleura, and peritoneum are somewhat more common.

Q Fever

Q fever differs from other rickettsial diseases and is an airborne cause of pneumonia.

Q fever is caused by *Coxiella burnetii* and differs in many respects from other rickettsial diseases. *Coxiella burnetii* is harbored in infected animals, particularly sheep and cattle, and is transmitted to humans via a respiratory route rather than through the bite of a tick or mite. Respiratory involvement is often prominent and may cause death due to an interstitial pneumonia that is virtually indistinguishable from viral pneumonia or primary atypical pneumonia. Death occurs uncommonly, usually due to superimposed bacterial infection, infection of cardiac valves, or progressive liver failure. Endemic areas include Australian sheep farms and California cattle-raising areas. After the second week of the febrile illness, complement fixation tests using *Coxiella burnetii* antigen will show at least a fourfold rise in titer. *Coxiella burnetii* can also be visualized by immunofluorescent staining of biopsy material, but this is usually not necessary.

MYCOPLASMAL DISEASES

Mycoplasma organisms can cause venereal infection and pneumonia.

Mycoplasma organisms (pleuropneumonia-like organisms, Eaton agents) are small and bacterial-like; they can exist either as free-living forms or as parasites. *Mycoplasma* organisms do not form a cell wall, and they resemble the so-called L-forms of bacteria. While many *Mycoplasma* organisms exist in nature, only a small number cause human disease, notably *Mycoplasma pneumoniae, Ureaplasma urealyticum,* and *Mycoplasma hominis.* The latter two agents cause "postgonococcal" urethritis and a chronic inflammatory pelvic disease. *Mycoplasma pneumoniae* is thought to cause up to one-third of cases of primary interstitial pneumonia, particularly in adolescents and young adults. Mycoplasmal **pneumonia** resembles viral pneumonias. *Mycoplasma pneumoniae* infection can initiate (in somewhat more than one-third of infections) cold agglutinins, which are immunoglobulins that cause the agglutination of group O red cells at 4°C. This phenomenon is the basis of a test frequently used to confirm the diagnosis of mycoplasma pneumonia. *Mycoplasma pneumoniae* can also cause false-positive serologic reactions for syphilis and streptococcal infections. Mycoplasmal pneumonia typically lasts several weeks, and death is uncommon. Wide-spectrum antibiotics are effective in treatment.

STAPHYLOCOCCAL INFECTIONS

Staphylococci are common commensal organisms of the nasopharynx and skin. Only a few strains of staphylococci cause disease in healthy individuals, although severely immunosuppressed individuals may acquire a variety of staphylococcal infections. Staphylococci that produce the enzyme coagulase (e.g., *Staphylococcus aureus*) tend to be more virulent than those that do not (e.g., *Staphylococcus epidermidis*). *Staphylococcus aureus* causes many diseases. Suppurative inflammation of the skin and subcutaneous tissues can produce either a **furuncle** (boil) or the larger **carbuncle,** which can invade the deep subcutaneous fascia and may erupt in multiple adjacent skin sinuses. **Hidradenitis suppurativa** is a similar condition in which the skin containing apocrine glands, notably the axilla, develops persistent abscess formation. **Paronychia** and **felons** are, respectively, staphylococcal infections of the nail bed or the palmar side of the fingertips; these are often quite painful, and are typically initiated following trauma, including imbedded splinters. Skin and deeper **surgical wounds** can also be infected by a variety of staphylococcal strains. Both staphylococci and streptococci can also produce impetigo, in which the skin infection is confined to the horny layer of the skin; this is discussed under streptococcal infections on page 38.

A few strains of *Staphylococcus aureus* can produce **toxic epidermal necrolysis** (scalded skin syndrome), which occurs most often in children of nursery school age and causes subepidermal blistering with subsequent exfoliation due to the action of an epidermolytic toxin. Staphylococci isolated from the upper airways are often colonists, but in patients who are severely debilitated or neutropenic, a variety of **potentially life-threatening staphylococcal infections** can occur including necrotizing staphylococcal pharyngitis, tonsillitis, sinusitis, otitis, or retropharyngeal abscesses. **Suppurative sialadenitis** is an infection of salivary ducts that occurs as a consequence of bacterial spread back up the duct, usually in patients who are dehydrated. Staphylococcal **pneumonia** is a highly destructive form of bronchopneumonia, which is described in the chapter on lung.

The **toxic shock syndrome** was initially described in menstruating women using vaginal tampons, particularly highly-absorbent tampons left in for long periods, which grew staphylococcal organisms. Toxins produced by the organisms were systemically absorbed through the endometrial and vaginal mucosa, causing a rapidly developing illness in which shock was a prominent feature. Other features included fever, a diffuse macular rash, conjunctivitis, sore throat, and gastrointestinal upset. Similar conditions have been seen following surgical wound infection or a staphylococcal superinfection of viral pneumonia.

Staphylococci tend to cause suppurative infections of skin and respiratory tracts.

The clinical features of toxic shock syndrome are due to an absorbed staphylococcal toxin.

Staphylococcal food poisoning is due to enterotoxin ingestion.

Staphylococcal food poisoning follows ingestion of food (milk products, meats) contaminated by enterotoxin produced by staphylococcal organisms. The disease is only rarely fatal, begins 1 to 6 hours after ingestion, and has symptoms of nausea, vomiting, abdominal cramps, and diarrhea. No histologic changes are observed in the gastrointestinal mucosa. The diagnosis is made by culturing the food.

Certain staphylococcal species have been more commonly associated with some diseases.

Staphylococcus aureus tends to cause skin abscesses; severe suppurative bronchopneumonia; impetigo; surgical and traumatic contamination of wounds; and rarely, severe enteritis as a consequence of direct invasion of the gut. Staphylococcal toxins are involved in diarrheal food poisoning, toxic shock syndrome, and the scalded skin syndrome. *Staphylococcus epidermis* is most frequently isolated from traumatic wounds, surgical wounds, and prosthetic implants. Life-threatening infections by *Staphylococcus epidermis* are usually observed in immunocompromised or debilitated patients. *Staphylococcus saprophyticus* is a coagulase-negative organism isolated as a relatively frequent cause of lower urinary tract infection in women.

Life-threatening staphylococcal septicemia may follow rupture of a walled-off abscess.

Patients with known or suspected staphylococcal infections who suddenly develop increased body temperature should be promptly evaluated, since a previously walled-off abscess may have spread into the bloodstream or a body internal surface. Such spread carries a significant risk of subsequent development of life-threatening **staphylococcal endocarditis.** Involvement of large arteries can cause mycotic aneurysms. Patients can also die of **staphylococcal septicemia** (so-called grampositive shock), which typically arises from lesions of skin, lungs, kidneys, intestinal tracts, or bones.

STREPTOCOCCAL INFECTIONS

Streptococci can cause both suppurative inflammation and hypersensitivity diseases.

Streptococcal infections remain a major cause of human infection, particularly among underprivileged patients. Streptococcal infections can cause suppurative inflammations characterized by a thin exudate and a tendency to spread extensively. Alternatively, the streptococcal infections can cause poststreptococcal hypersensitivity diseases including rheumatic fever, immune complex glomerulonephritis, and erythema nodosum. These are discussed in the chapters on heart, kidney, and blood vessels, respectively. Streptococcal virulence factors include capsular polysaccharides, M-proteins, streptokinase, streptodornase, and streptolysin. Additionally, those strains of streptococci that are associated with the rash of scarlet fever produce erythrogenic toxin.

Streptococcal skin infections tend to cause less abscess formation than staphylococci, but are more apt to involve lymphatics.

Streptococcal skin infections, commonly caused by Lancefield **group A β-hemolytic organisms,** include pyoderma, impetigo, erysipelas, and folliculitis. Streptococcal infections are more apt than staphylococcal infections to involve adjacent lymph vessels, characteristically producing red streaks of inflammation above draining lymphatics. Focal tissue necrosis and abscess formation are observed much less frequently than with staphylococcal organisms. β-hemolytic group A streptococci also infect lungs, heart valves, and meninges, with the potential to cause death.

Patients with splenic dysfunction or absence are particularly apt to develop fulminant septicemia. Group A organisms were formerly important causes of puerpural sepsis and perinatal streptococcal disease; these conditions are now uncommon due to improvements in sterile techniques on obstetric wards. While group A infection has become less common in these settings, **group B streptococci** are still an important cause of perinatal sepsis. The enterococci and other **group D streptococci** are microaerophilic organisms that differ considerably from the more aerobic streptococci, and are clinically apt to cause diseases similar to those of the gram-negative bacilli, including urinary, gastrointestinal, and post-surgical infections, as well as endocarditis and septicemia. The wound infections may become complicated by gram-negative organism infection with associated suppuration and pus pocket formation in deep, subcutaneous, and muscle tissues (phlegmon). ***Streptococcus viridans,*** an "untypable" α-hemolytic organism, is a normal commensal of the mouth, but may cause endocarditis in people with previously damaged hearts. ***Streptococcus bovis*** is an anaerobe that has been known to cause septicemia and endocarditis. It is associated, for unknown reasons, with carcinoma of the colon.

Streptococci can cause skin, gynecologic, urinary tract, and gastrointestinal infections, as well as pneumonia, endocarditis, and septicemia.

PNEUMOCOCCAL INFECTIONS

Streptococcus pneumoniae was formerly considered to be a separate organism **(pneumococcus),** but has been reclassified as a streptococcus. Pneumococci are important causes of both lower respiratory tract infections (lobar pneumonia, bronchopneumonia, empyema) and upper respiratory tract infections (sinusitis, middle ear infections, mastoid infections). Other diseases produced by pneumococcus include meningitis, brain abscess, suppurative arthritis, endocarditis, peritonitis, and pneumococcal bacteremia. Despite their sensitivity to penicillin therapy, pneumococcal infections, notably pneumococcal pneumonia, remain a leading cause of death among aged and immunosuppressed patients.

Pneumococci can cause middle ear infections, pneumonia, meningitis, endocarditis, arthritis, and septicemia.

The virulence of pneumococci is related to the polysaccharides of the capsules. The pus produced by pneumococci resembles that of staphylococci more than of other streptococci because of its thick, viscid consistency as a consequence of failure to lyse fibrin and nuclear DNA. This manifests clinically in the great difficulty with which pneumococcal empyema can be drained. While many attempts have been made, a truly effective prophylactic pneumococcal vaccine has still not been developed.

Virulent strains of pneumococci have a polysaccharide capsule and produce a viscid pus.

MENINGOCOCCAL INFECTIONS

Meningococci (*Neisseria meningitidis*) are capable of causing life-threatening meningitis and bacteremia. The bacteremia may take a chronic recurrent form or may present fulminantly as the life-threatening **Waterhouse-Friderichsen syndrome** (see p. 364) with hemorrhagic rash, adrenal hemorrhage, and shock. Meningococcal meningitis is the most common form of invasive meningococcal infections. **Meningococcal meningitis** is sometimes observed in epidemics, and smaller versions can be observed in families or in institutions. Uncommonly, meningococci can additionally infect the lung parenchyma, joints, endocardium, pericardium, conjunctiva, and genitalia. The meningococci typically enter the body through the nasopharynx, producing trivial symptoms resembling those of a common cold.

Meningococci can cause life-threatening meningitis and Waterhouse-Friderichsen syndrome.

Neisseria meningitidis is subclassified based on serogroupings of antigens in the polysaccharide capsule. The organisms produce proteases that can cleave the IgA immunoglobulins, facilitating upper respiratory tract mucosal colonization. They also produce a lipopolysaccharide within the cell walls that is similar to endotoxin and can induce shock and disseminated intravascular coagulation. Infection and colonization do induce protective antibodies, but these are effective only against the particular infecting strains and are not protective against new strains.

GONOCOCCAL INFECTIONS

Gonococci (*Neisseria gonorrhoeae*) are gram-negative diplococci that cause the sexually transmitted disease gonorrhea. In addition to **urethritis,** gonorrhea can also present as pharyngitis or proctitis, depending upon the form of sex used. Many infections are silent. Nonsexual transmission can cause **neonatal conjunctivitis** in infants of infected mothers and gonococcal vaginitis in young girls who share linen with infected adults. The retrograde spread of the gonococci to involve the internal genitalia can produce chronic purulent inflammation of either the male or female genitalia, and **pelvic inflammatory disease.** In women, because spread through the fallopian tubes can involve the abdominal cavity, **gonococcal perihepatitis,** which is notably painful, may also occur. Additionally, gonococci can spread in both sexes through the bloodstream, producing bacteremia or **septicemia,** which may manifest with prominent skin rash, **arthritis** (either immune-mediated or purulent), **endocarditis,** or **meningitis.** In rare cases, gonococci can enter the body through a skin wound.

Gonococcal lesions tend to produce pus initially, which is followed by granulation tissue and scarring. Gonococcal exudates characteristically show host neutrophils containing *Neisseria* gonorrheal organisms. Strains of *Neisseria* gonorrhea possessing larger numbers of pili appear to be more pathogenic than are "smooth" strains. Gonococci undergo repetitive genetic variations and consequently resist effective vaccination. Extreme degrees of penicillin resistance are characteristic of some strains. Diagnosis is most effectively made by culture on sensitive media such as Thayer agar.

GRAM-NEGATIVE BACILLI

Gram-negative bacilli can cause nosocomial and opportunistic urinary tract infections, intra-abdominal infections, and some pneumonias. These organisms are often normal commensals that have acquired substantial drug resistance, usually due to exchange of plasmids and resistance factors acquired by conjugation and transduction.

Escherichia coli is an enteric organism with hundreds of serotypes, of which only a few are virulent for normal humans. *Escherichia coli* can cause gastrointestinal illness (see p. 43); uncomplicated lower and upper urinary tract infections; intra-abdominal suppurative infections (appendicitis, cholecysitis, others); perianal infections; and severe hemorrhagic bronchopneumonia in debilitated patients. In most of these settings, invasive *Escherichia coli* causes nonspecific suppurative reactions. Mixed infections that include *Escherichia coli* can become gangrenous. *Escherichia coli* sepsis can cause death. Therapy of *Escherichia coli* infections may be difficult because of marked resistance to antibiotics.

Klebsiella pneumoniae and **Enterobacter aerogenes** are closely related organisms that can cause pneumonia, urinary tract infection, and sepsis. Pneumonias due to these organisms tend to occur in patients who are at risk for inhalation or aspiration of the organisms. The pneumonia is typically a bronchopneumonia, which is distinguished from other gram-negative bacillary pneumonias by abscess formation and pleural involvement. Lobar pneumonia is sometimes observed in community-acquired infections, particularly in alcoholics. Other sites that can be infected include the urinary tract, the biliary tract (particularly with mixed infections), the sinuses and middle ears, and the meninges. *Klebsiella* can also cause a fulminating gram-negative bacteremia with septicemia that can cause death. **Proteus mirabilis** can cause diseases similar to those of *Escherichia coli* and *Klebsiella pneumoniae,* particularly pneumonia in debilitated hospitalized patients and chronic urinary tract infection. **Serratia marcescens** can cause pneumonia, upper respiratory tract infection, and a variety of other infections, generally in hospitalized, debilitated, or immunosuppressed individuals. Healthy individuals are usually resistant to infection by this organism.

Pseudomonas aeruginosa causes acute nosocomial and opportunistic infections, predominantly in the form of epidemics in nurseries, intensive care units, and burn units. Pseudomonas has a high pathogenicity, related to production of exotoxin A and a leukocidin. Pseudomonas species cause recurrent bronchopneumonia, particularly in patients with cystic fibrosis; chronic urinary tract infections; and infections of the external ear. Independent of the site of the initial pseudomonas infection, pneumonia is a frequent sequela as a consequence of bacteremia. Because of its very high **drug resistance,** pseudomonas frequently superinfects other antibiotic-treated bacterial infections. Gross features of pseudomonas infections include a bluish or greenish discoloration due to pigment production by some strains; a **"fleur-de-lis"** pattern in infected lungs caused by alternating whitish necrotic areas and darker hemorrhagic areas; and well-demarcated, oval, necrotic skin lesions following infection of burns. Characteristic microscopic features of the necrotizing inflammation include large numbers of bacteria, a scarce neutrophilic response, and vasculitis with thrombosis and hemorrhage. Pseudomonas bacteremia often causes disseminated intravascular coagulation, and may be complicated by endocarditis or meningitis. Mortality due to pseudomonas infections remains higher than desirable.

Legionella pneumophila was identified in 1976 following an epidemic of lethal pneumonia that affected the American Legion Convention in Philadelphia; since then, other Legionella pathogens have also been identified. *Legionella* are flagellated rods best visualized by immunofluorescence, Dieterle silver stain, or modified Gram stains. They are usually acquired by **inhalation** from environmental sources (water reservoirs, air-conditioners). Multiplication in macrophages has been observed, but the definitive basis of pathogenicity is still unknown. Legionnaire's disease is a severe lobular and fibrinopurulent pneumonia with a 20 percent fatality rate in inappropriately treated patients. *Legionella* can also cause Pontiac fever, which is a self-limited, systemic, febrile disease with mild symptoms.

Klebsiella pneumoniae, Enterobacter aerogenes, Proteus mirabilis, and *Serratia marcescens* cause diseases similar to *Escherichia coli.*

Pseudomonas aeruginosa is a particularly virulent pathogen with high drug resistance.

Legionella pneumophila causes a severe pneumonia that is acquired by inhalation of droplets of infected water.

Anaerobic species are frequent components of mixed infections.

The human bowel, vagina, and mouth contain a large number of gram-negative **anaerobic species,** of which only a few are human pathogens. The incidence of anaerobic bacterial infection is underestimated, since these organisms are frequent components of mixed infections, and a failure to use rigorous anaerobic methods of culture may demonstrate only the coexisting aerobic organisms. The most commonly isolated organisms include the enteric organism *Bacteroides fragilis* and the mouth commensal *Bacteroides melaninogenicus*. The *Bacteroides* organisms have a cell wall that differs from that of other gram-negative organisms and is not usually associated with sepsis. ***Bacteroides fragilis*** typically causes, or is a participant in, infections involving the abdomen, pelvis, surgical wounds, or lung. ***Bacteroides melaninogenicus*** tends to be found in abscesses involving the floor of the mouth, the retropharynx, the lung, or the brain, often associated with aerobic organisms. Reasonably healthy patients who develop *Bacteroides* infections usually do well, but debilitated hosts often die of septicemia. Drug resistance is a common problem; surgical drainage combined with appropriate antibiotics is necessary for effective therapy.

INFECTIONS OF CHILDHOOD

Haemophilus influenzae **causes meningitis, pneumonia, epiglottitis, conjunctivitis, endocarditis, urinary tract infections, and arthritis.**

Haemophilus influenzae is a coccobacillary or pleomorphic gram-negative organism harbored in the mouths of some healthy children. Vaccination, directed against the capsular B antigen, is available but is not completely effective, particularly in very young children. Meningitis due to *Haemophilus influenzae* occurs in young children, with peak incidence at 1 year. Patients develop rapidly progressive purulent **meningitis** with prominent systemic manifestations caused by release of endotoxin by the bacteria. In older children, *Haemophilus influenzae* causes severe **pneumonia,** potentially life-threatening **epiglottitis,** and systemic infections. Other infections caused by *Haemophilus influenzae* include acute purulent conjunctivitis (pink eye), septicemia, endocarditis, pyelonephritis, cholecystitis, and suppurative arthritis. *Haemophilus influenzae* infection can be suspected by the finding of gram-negative coccobacillary forms in an exudate or in spinal fluid. Rapid tests for the B antigen by ELISA, electrophoresis, and latex agglutination can also contribute to a prompt diagnosis.

Bordetella pertussis **causes whooping coughs and grows in the brush border of respiratory tract epithelia.**

Bordetella pertussis is a small, pleomorphic, gram-negative coccobacillus that causes respiratory infection that may range from mild acute bronchitis to a severe laryngotracheobronchitis characterized by violent coughing paroxysms, followed by loud, inspiratory "whoop" **(whooping cough)** and accompanied by a striking peripheral lymphocytosis. *Bordetella pertussis* grows in the brush border of the epithelium, forming colonies that become entangled in the brush border and release exotoxin, which diffuses into the body. Widespread use of diphtheria-pertussis-tetanus (DPT) vaccine has reduced the incidence of whooping cough in the United States.

Corynebacterium diphtheria **causes diphtheria, with formation of a pseudomembrane.**

Corynebacterium diphtheriae, the agent of **diphtheria,** tends to infect the respiratory tract in children ages 2 to 15 years. Symptoms range from a limited nasal diphtheria to obstructive bronchitis **(croup).** The organism produces a phage-mediated toxin that causes ulceration of the respiratory mucosa, with accompanying formation of an inflammatory membrane composed of proliferating organisms and coagulated fibrinosuppurative exudate **(diphtheria pseudomembrane).** The toxin is also capable of damaging remote organs, particularly the heart (potentially causing arrhythmias) and nerves (potentially causing a usually reversible weakness of muscles in the face, palate, and extremities). Dislodgement of the pseudomembrane can cause asphyxiation. Antitoxic serum to the diphtheria toxin is effective in preventing both cardiac and neurologic damage, but only if the antitoxin is given early in treatment before damage occurs. *Corynebacterium diphtheriae* can also cause infections of the adult human respiratory tract and skin, which may be complicated by exotoxin production. Childhood immunization has reduced the incidence of diphtheria in the United States.

ENTEROPATHOGENIC BACTERIA

Bacteria have several mechanisms of producing diarrhea, including bacterial adhesion to mucosal epithelium, which induces a hypersecretory state; enterotoxin release; and true invasion of the gut wall. True invasion of the gut wall is associated with a prominent leukocytic infiltration with exudation of leukocytes into the stool. The other forms of diarrhea production do not produce exudate or recognizable anatomic mucosal lesions, but instead induce large diarrheal fluid losses. A consequence of this distinction is that direct microscopic stool examination for leukocytes can aid in the diagnosis of bacterially induced diarrhea. Culture media specifically designed for growth of fastidious enteric organisms are also helpful. DNA and RNA analysis techniques that permit serotyping of the infecting organisms are becoming more widely available. Factors that can aggravate enteric infections include antacids, immunosuppressive drugs, and antispasmodic drugs.

Diarrhea due to invasion of the intestinal wall by bacteria produces pus, while diarrhea produced by other mechanisms does not.

Escherichia coli Enteric Infections

Escherichia coli has many strains, most of which are normal commensals of the human intestinal tract. A few cause diarrhea and dysentery in people of all ages. **Invasive *Escherichia coli,*** usually from the O group, produce crampy diarrhea with watery stools that may contain mucus flecks and neutrophilic exudate. Some members of the O-group serotype have also acquired a plasmid that codes for **enterotoxin,** whose mode of action is similar to that of cholera, and is associated with a morphologically normal mucosa and production of a very watery ("rice-water") diarrhea. A few strains of *Escherichia coli* cause an **enteroadhesive enteritis** in which plasmid-activated bacterial pili adhere to the intestinal mucosa cell membrane.

Escherichia coli strains cause diarrhea by a variety of mechanisms.

Salmonella Infections

The ***Salmonella enterititis* group** has a very large number of strains, of which the most prevalent in the United States are *Salmonella typhimurium, Salmonella paratyphi, Salmonella newport,* and *Salmonella heidelberg. Salmonella* organisms are usually acquired by ingestion of contaminated food (notably poultry and eggs) or water.

Salmonella organisms often invade the gut wall or alter mucosal brush borders.

Salmonella do not produce enterotoxins, but are invasive or alter mucosal cell brush borders. Following invasion into the gut wall, the bacteria are ingested by neutrophils and macrophages in the lamina propria, in which they are able to multiply within phagosomes. With time, the phagocytes acquire the ability to destroy the salmonellae, which triggers clinical convalescence.

Typhoid fever is caused by *Salmonella typhi*. Typhoid fever can be considered a systemic disease that is initiated by gastrointestinal infection. The salmonella organisms induce diarrhea; penetrate the gut mucosa; and subsequently cause bacteremia and are ingested by macrophages. There is a diffuse enlargement of reticuloendothelial lymphoid tissue throughout the body, particularly prominent in Peyer's patches of the terminal ileum. The mucosa over the ileal lymphoid nodules may ulcerate, causing **elongated ulcers** oriented in the direction of bowel flow. During the height of the disease, the body (particularly spleen, liver, bone marrow, and lymph nodes) contains large numbers of small, nodular aggregates (**typhoid nodules**) of bacteria-filled macrophages with smaller numbers of lymphocytes and plasma cells. A transient skin rash (**"rose spots"**) may involve the lower anterior chest and upper abdomen. Gallbladder colonization may induce a carrier state that may require cholecystectomy to eliminate bacterial shedding. Death is most common in infants, children, and elderly patients, but may occur at all ages due to intestinal perforation leading to peritonitis, massive intestinal hemorrhage, or secondary infections, particularly pneumonias.

Enteric fevers resembling typhoid fever, but causing less serious disease, are associated with *Salmonella typhimurium, Salmonella paratyphi, Salmonella choleraesuis,* and other salmonella species. A few fatalities have been observed with *Salmonella typhimurium* infection. *Salmonella* species may also cause isolated bacteremia, pyelonephritis, cholecystitis, meningitis, pericarditis, mycotic aneurysm, endocarditis, and salpingitis. For unknown reasons, patients with sickle cell anemia are particularly prone to develop salmonella bacteremias and salmonella osteomyelitis. In Egypt and Brazil, chronic salmonellosis is associated with *Schistosoma* infections of the urinary tract or gut; the bacteria apparently thrive on the helminths' tegment. The mildest form of salmonella infection is food poisoning with vomiting and diarrhea.

Bacillary Dysentery

Bacillary dysentery is a severe (up to 50 stools a day) diarrhea with abdominal cramping and tenesmus caused by *Shigella* species. These gram-negative enteric organisms traverse the colonic mucosa, multiply in the lamina propria, and are carried to regional lymph nodes. They do not cause distant infections or bacteremia. The colonic mucosa in severe dysentery shows nodular enlargement of lymphoid follicles and ulcerated, edematous colonic mucosa covered by a fibrinosuppurative pseudomembrane. The scanty, blood-stained, stools contain pus flecks and numerous neutrophils. Mild cases resemble food poisoning. Antibiotic therapy prevents transmission but may not shorten the course.

Typhoid fever is a systemic disease that begins in the gut.

Diseases resembling mild typhoid fever can be caused by many *Salmonella* species.

***Salmonella* species can infect many organ systems and cause food poisoning.**

***Shigella* species cause bacillary dysentery.**

Cholera

Vibrio species can cause **cholera** and other enteric infections. The prototype ***Vibrio cholerae*** has caused cholera pandemics that typically begin in the Ganges river basin. Recent minor outbreaks of cholera have also been reported in the southwestern United States. Spread of *Vibrio cholerae* is by the fecal–oral route, with asymptomatic carriers and long-term excretion by convalescents providing major sources of organisms. The comma-shaped organisms are confined to the gut lumen and epithelial brush border, where they may be visualized by direct microscopy or immunofluorescence. *Vibrio cholerae* **enterotoxin** activates **adenylate cyclase** in the plasma membranes of small intestinal crypt mucosal cells, causing massive secretion of isotonic fluid with **"rice-water" stools** that characteristically contain few leukocytes. Survival is almost entirely due to adequate fluid therapy, often with oral electrolyte preparations. Cholera vaccines are presently protective for only 3 to 6 months.

***Vibrio cholerae* activates mucosal adenylate cyclase to produce a severe secretory diarrhea.**

Helicobacter Enteritis

Helicobacter species are flagellated, comma-shaped, gram-negative organisms that are difficult to culture, and have only recently been recognized as pathogens. *Helicobacter* species are important causes of chronic gastritis, enterocolitis, and septicemia. ***Helicobacter pylori*** is discussed with the pathology of the stomach (see p. 237). ***Helicobacter jejuni*** is a common cause of hospital acquired diarrhea in the United States. The gastrointestinal disease ranges from subclinical infection to incapacitating dysentery with foul-smelling stools that may contain microscopic blood and exudate. Abdominal pain is often prominent. A watery diarrhea similar to cholera can be produced by *Helicobacter* strains that produce toxin. Other strains invade intestinal epithelium and cause mucosal necrosis. *Helicobacter* strains can also invade the intestinal wall by a mechanism called translocation, causing fever without frank dysentery. It is unclear whether the different disease patterns represent differences among strains of *Helicobacter jejuni,* or a shift in the expression of pathogenic properties depending on the host response. The entire intestine from jejunum to anus becomes inflamed. Crypt abscesses and ulcerations reminiscent of chronic ulcerative colitis may be present. Antibiotic therapy can shorten the symptomatic period and prevents transmission to other patients.

***Helicobacter* species can cause gastritis, enterocolitis, and septicemia.**

Yersinia Enteritis

Yersinia enterocolitica is a major cause of pediatric bacterial **enteritis,** and may also cause adult disease. The organism can invade both the upper digestive tract, causing pharyngitis or tonsillitis with cervical lymph node enlargement, and the lower digestive tract, causing diarrhea. The distal ileum and colon typically contain ulcerative intestinal lesions similar to those of typhoid fever; alternatively, a diffuse enteritis with villus shortening, crypt hyperplasia, and mucosal microabscesses may be seen. Microabscesses rimmed by activated mononuclear phagocytes may be found in mesenteric lymph nodes. *Yersinia enterocolitica* can cause severe dysentery, which may lead to death and may present as

***Yersinia enterocolitica* can cause severe pediatric diarrhea and tonsillitis.**

acute gastroenteritis, appendicitis, or chronic relapsing ileocolitis. The prolonged course can be shortened by appropriate antibiotic therapy.

CLOSTRIDIA

Clostridial species produce stable spores and cause nasty diseases.

Clostridia are gram-positive **anaerobes** that normally inhabit animal intestines and produce spores found in pastures and garden soil. While only a few species cause human disease, the clostridia are characterized by production of powerful, specific toxins that can cause life-threatening illness.

Tetanus

The clostridial toxin, tetanospasm, poisons inhibitory neurons, producing spastic muscle contractions.

Tetanus can be produced when *Clostridium tetani* spores germinate in wounds and the vegetative organisms subsequently produce the neurotoxin tetanospasm. The tetanospasm is absorbed by peripheral nerve endings; passes in the peripheral nerves to motor neurons without affecting their function; and then crosses synapses to enter spinal cord inhibitory neurons. **Clinical tetanus** is the result of inhibition of these inhibitory neurons, leading to severe spastic contractions of voluntary muscles, often with early involvement of facial muscles (**"lockjaw,"** risus sardonicus). Sympathetic inhibition is also lost, with resulting cardiovascular instability. Patients often show arching of the back and may die of asphyxiation if intubation is not used. The patient's mentation and consciousness are characteristically unaffected, as the toxin does not cross the blood–brain barrier. Morphologic changes both in the wound and nervous system tend to be minimal and nonspecific. *Clostridium tetani* can also infect fecal-soiled **umbilical cord stumps** in newborn infants. The incidence of neonatal tetanus in the United States has been reduced by the use of booster toxoid doses during pregnancy that increase maternal antibodies that cross the placenta. **Tetanus toxoid** is used for active immunization against tetanus, but the immunization needs to be renewed every 5 to 10 years, as the immunity fades. **Antitoxin** may block the development of clinical disease and is usually given in situations in which tetanus infection is possible. Formerly, clinical tetanus had a dismal prognosis, but the mortality has been lowered at experienced intensive care centers. Those patients who survive do not experience permanent sequelae.

Botulism

The botulism neurotoxin produces paralysis.

Ingestion of preformed *Clostridium botulinum* neurotoxin, often from contaminated home-prepared canned foods, causes severe paralyzing illness. Uncommonly, **botulism** can be caused either by an actual wound infection, or by growth of the organism in the intestine of infants. In the latter case, the usual source of spores is contaminated honey. **Type A exotoxin** is the most lethal form. In contrast to the very sturdy botulinum spores, the heat-sensitive toxin can be destroyed by boiling for as short as 10 minutes. Toxin absorbed from the gut into the bloodstream preferentially attaches to cholinergic nerves and causes skeletal muscle paralysis. Other features of the illness include respiratory muscle paralysis, cranial nerve palsies, ptosis, diploplia, dysphagia, voice changes, and paralytic ileus. Mentation remains normal. **Antitoxin** is effective in preventing binding of the toxin to cholinergic nerves, but once the toxin has been bound to the synaptic vesicles, it can no longer be enactivated. In these cases, intensive supportive care permits survival and ultimate complete recovery of the majority, but not all, victims. Deaths are usually secondary to respiratory infections. Botulism poisoning in both adults and infants remains very uncommon, but has been difficult to eradicate completely. Food poisoning can also be caused by *Clostridium perfringens* (*welchii*), which produces an enterotoxin that causes sudden vomiting and diarrhea.

Septic Clostridial Infections

Clostridia can invade traumatic or surgical wounds including amputation stumps, uteri following illegal abortions, and ischemic or perforated bowel. **Gas gangrene** (clostrial myonecrosis) is caused by *Clostridium perfringens* and other clostridial species. The gangrene begins in large wounds with low oxygen tension where the clostridia produce collagenases, lecithinases, and other enzymes that facilitate tissue destruction and spread of the organisms.

Bacterial gas production by fermentation reactions causes additional mechanical damage. Bacilli are present in large numbers in an often bulky serosanguinous exudate. Gas gangrene can lead to death secondary to absorption of elaborated enzymes and invasion of the bloodstream, producing sepsis. The active hemolysis observed in gas gangrene may be so severe that, by the time of death, no intact erythrocytes may remain. The disease is best prevented by adequate débridement and cleansing of extensive tissue injuries. Not all cases of *Clostridium perfringens* infection form frank gas gangrene; the milder clostridial **necrotizing cellulitis** is characterized by tissue destruction accompanied by edema and sloughing of skin. *Clostridium perfringens* can additionally cause a severe invasive form of **enteritis** in malnourished patients.

Gas gangrene is a particularly nasty wound infection that can cause death.

Pseudomembranous Colitis

Clostridium difficile is normally a minor commensal of the gut, but can occasionally proliferate sufficiently to cause symptomatic disease, particularly in patients who receive wide-spectrum antibiotic therapy. Intraluminal organisms produce enterotoxin, which causes severe **colitis** with formation of pseudomembranes composed of fibrin, necrotic material, and inflammatory cells that adhere to a diffusely hyperemic colonic mucosa. The inflammation tends to spread laterally and superficially, but does not involve deeper tissues, although thrombosis of submucosal venules can be observed.

Pseudomembranous colitis can follow wide-spectrum antibiotic therapy.

ZOONOTIC BACTERIA

Zoonotic bacteria are bacteria whose normal hosts are animals. They are transmitted to humans by direct contact, environmental contamination, insect vectors, or consumption of animal products. While the etiologic agents vary, the diseases are similar since public health measures related to the animal sources can lower disease transmission. Organisms such as salmonella and clostridia that are both harbored by animals and widely disseminated in the environment are not included among the zoonoses.

Anthrax

Anthrax occurs in cutaneous, pulmonary, and intestinal forms.

Bacillus anthracis is a large, gram-positive organism that produces spores and is found in many animal species. The spores can persist in soil for very long periods of time. Once the spores vegetate, the organism is highly pathogenic because it elaborates factors that inhibit phagocytic activity, cause edema, and are cytotoxic (lethal factor). At present, most human **anthrax** occurs through skin contact with spore-bearing soil or animal products. Cutaneous anthrax begins with a relatively painless, pus-filled pustule (**malignant pustule**) that then ruptures to form a black eschar surrounded by circumferentially expanding brawny edema; it may be accompanied by enlarged lymph nodes showing nonspecific lymphadenitis. The disease remains localized in most cases. In cases that develop bacteremia, complications may include meningitis, pneumonia, and infections in other sites. Inhalation of spores can cause hemorrhagic pneumonia (**woolsorter's disease**), which may be followed by septicemia and death. Intestinal anthrax can also occur, most recently in a Russian outbreak, and has a high mortality.

Listeriosis

Listeria monocytogenes can cause severe congenital and neonatal infection, enteritis, and leptomeningitis.

Listeria monocytogenes causes community outbreaks of **enteritis** secondary to contaminated milk products; amnionitis in fetuses; and infection of immunosuppressed adults. The organism is a gram-positive microaerophilic motile rod that forms aggregates on culture that resemble Chinese letters. Infected pregnant women characteristically have only mild infection, while damage to the fetus is profound (**granulomatosis infantiseptica**). A pyogenic **leptomeningitis** with predominantly intracellular gram-positive rods is a prominent feature in both neonatal listerial and opportunistic infections in immunosuppressed adults. Transplant patients appear to be particularly prone to develop listerial leptomeningitis; it is suspected that undetected latent *Listeria* infection may be relatively common.

Plague

Plague may cause pneumonia, septicemia, and lyphadenopathy.

Yersinia pestis, the **plague** organism, is a gram-negative bacillus that resembles a safety pin in methylene blue-stained smears. The organism produces a potent gram-negative enterotoxin and a capsular glycoprotein that inhibits phagocytosis. *Yersinia pestis* infection is endemic in many wild animal populations, in whom it is transmitted from animal to animal, either by direct contact or by arthropod bite. The human is an accidental host. Human plague can produce constitutional symptoms accompanied by mild lymphadenopathy (**"plague minor"**); prominent lymph node swelling (**bubonic plague**); **pneumonic plague;** or **septicemic plague.** The regional lymph nodes in bubonic plague swell dramatically, producing large hemorrhagic **buboes** that may either infarct or rupture through the skin. Pneumonic plague is characterized by a severe bronchopneumonia with prominent hemorrhage and necrosis, accompanied by fibrinous pleuritis. Septicemic plague is characterized by fulminating bacteremia, which induces disseminated intravascular coagulation with widespread hemorrhages and thrombi. Plague lesions are characterized by large numbers of organisms; tissue edema and necrosis; vascular thrombosis and hemorrhage; and neutrophilic infiltrates at the margins of necrotic areas. Appropriate antibiotic therapy has reduced a formerly high mortality, but the antibiotics must be given within 24 hours of onset of pneumonic or septicemic forms to be effective.

Tularemia

Francisella tularensis, the agent of **tularemia,** is a small, pleomorphic, gram-negative coccobacillus that is usually contracted from rabbits or rabbit skins. **Ulceroglandular tularemia** develops as a rupturing pustule accompanied by lymph node involvement. Other features include bacteremia, splenomegaly, rash, pneumonia, or endotoxemic shock. Local sites (meninges, heart, bones) may continue to harbor festering infection for months. Other variants of tularemia include the **oculoglandular and glandular forms,** in which the initial site of entry may be either in the conjunctiva or inapparent. A **typhoidal form** resembles *Salmonella* sepsis, and presents with fever, hepatosplenomegaly, and toxemia. The pathology of the lesions is similar in all forms. Early skin lesions show pyogenic ulceration. Later, disseminated lesions resemble tubercules. A disease that clinically closely resembles tularemia can also be produced by *Pasteurella multocida,* which is usually transmitted by the bite of a dog or cat.

Tularemia has many forms.

Brucellosis

Brucella are gram-negative aerobic cocci that are notoriously difficult to culture or visualize in infected tissue. *Brucella abortus* (from cattle) is the predominant species isolated in the United States, and *Brucella melitensis* (from goats) is probably the most frequent organism isolated globally. A **carrier state** has been demonstrated in people routinely exposed to animals or animal products. Brucellosis can also cause an **acute self-limited disease** that lasts months, resembles a viral infection, and may be complicated by pneumonia, spondylitis, orchitis, or pyelonephritis. **Chronic brucellosis** uncommonly may cause a variety of poorly defined symptoms including transient fever, abdominal and musculoskeletal pain, personality changes, and sometimes mild hepatomegaly or splenomegaly. The organisms proliferate intracellularly in macrophages and lymphocytes and colonize the lymphoreticular system following a brief bacteremic phase. This proliferation is associated with formation of granulomas that contain numerous neutrophils and may or may not have necrotic centers. Destructive local lesions resembling abscesses or focal infarctions, which may heal with focal calcification, may also be observed at many body sites. Brucellosis is responsive to antibacterial therapy.

Chronic brucellosis may produce poorly defined symptoms and induce granuloma formation.

Glanders and Meliodosis

Pseudomonas mallei is a small, gram-negative bacillus that is harbored by donkeys, mules, and horses, and is usually spread by contact with broken skin. *Pseudomonas mallei* causes **glanders,** which may take the form of either severe acute illness or a protracted infection resembling tuberculosis. The pathology tends to be nonspecific, and diagnosis is based on serologic tests. Culture is not recommended due to the risk to laboratory workers. Glanders remains endemic in South America, Asia, and Africa, but is rare elsewhere, with many cases being imported. *Pseudomonas pseudomallei* is the agent of **melioidosis,** which resembles glanders. *Pseudomonas pseudomallei* is found in southeastern Asian countries as a soil and water contaminant and in rodents, dogs, cats, horses, and other animals.

Leptospirosis and Weil's Disease

Leptospira are tightly wound spirochetes that are often shaped like a shepherd's crook; *Leptospira interrogans* is the most frequently isolated pathogen. **Mild** (anicteric) **leptospirosis** is a febrile disease that has an initial **(septicemic)** phase, during which the organism can be cultured from blood and cerebral spinal fluid. This phase is characterized by rapidly rising fever and severe muscle pain. The leptospira do not at this stage trigger any visible immune response. The fever subsequently defervesces but later returns, accompanied by signs of meningeal irritation. During this second **(immune)** phase, the organisms are found only in the urine. With time, mononuclear cell infiltrates adjacent to focal necrosis become increasingly prominent in organs such as muscle or kidney. **Weil's disease** is a severe form of leptospirosis accompanied by jaundice, bleeding, renal failure, skeletal muscle necrosis, and reticuloendothelial activation. Conjunctival hyperemia may be seen in both mild leptospirosis and Weil's disease. One variant, **"Fort Bragg fever,"** was also characterized by a pretibial skin rash at the onset of the illness. Patients typically survive mild leptospirosis without sequelae; Weil's disease formerly had a high mortality, which has been reduced with improved supportive care, including dialysis and the earlier use of antibiotics.

Relapsing Fever

Borrelia **species** are loosely wound spirochetes, which, unlike the syphilis organism, stain well with Wright-Giemsa stain, and are consequently easy to observe in blood smears or other body fluids. Both tick-borne and louse-borne forms of **relapsing fever** due to *Borrelia recurrentis* are characterized by periods of fever separated by more or less symptom-free intervals. The relapses are a consequence of preprogrammed genomic shifts by the borreliae that prevent the host from generating effective antibodies. Eventually, the severity of the attacks lessens, and a spontaneous cure occurs in many patients. Antibiotics can effectively kill borreliae, but may exacerbate the symptoms as the organisms die **(Herxheimer reaction),** possibly as the result of massive release of endotoxin. The louse-borne disease is more apt to be complicated by shock, hepatic failure, or central nervous system symptoms. Patients dying of louse-borne relapsing fever have septic foci in many organs including spleen, liver, heart, kidneys, and meninges. Disseminated intravascular coagulation and bacterial pneumonia due to superinfection are often present.

Lyme Disease

Borrelia burgdorferi is a spirochete that is transmitted from animal reservoirs to humans via the ticks of the genus *Ixodes*. It has been observed throughout Europe and in the eastern and western United States, Canada, and Australia. **Lyme disease** has only been recently described, as its many manifestations were originally thought to be separate diseases. It resembles syphilis in that it can be clinically divided into three stages, with a **primary stage** involving a skin lesion at the inoculation site; the secondary stage showing systemic dissemination; and, the tertiary stage being characterized by specific organ involvement, including heart, nervous system, and joints. The inoculation site lesion (erythema chronicum migrans, erythema migrans) consists of one or several slowly spreading skin lesions with erythemateous margins and pale centers.

Weeks to months after the rash clears, the **second stage** develops, with highly variable manifestations that may include meningoencephalitis; facial palsy; cardiac disease including atrioventricular block, left ventricular dysfunction, and pericarditis; or joint disease reminiscent of early rheumatoid arthritis. The patient usually experiences months of flare-ups alternating with remissions. Permanent joint deformities, and, less commonly, permanent cardiovascular or neural sequelae are sometimes observed. Some patients who have been followed for longer periods are now developing **tertiary neural and vascular lesions,** and cases of stillbirth have been reported. Skin and synovial biopsy specimens show a nonspecific lymphoplasmacytic infiltrate with edema and fibrin deposition. The synovium may also show an arteritis with "onion skinning" features. It is suspected that, like syphilis, *Borrelia burgdorferi* can survive in host tissue for long periods as a latent infection, but this has not yet been proved. Tetracycline or penicillin therapy during the early erythema chronicum migrans stage appears to prevent later systemic manifestations.

Lyme disease resembles syphilis but is transmitted to humans by tick bite.

Rat-Bite Fever

Rat-bite fever is actually two diseases of similar presentation that can follow a rat bite. *Spirillum minus* causes the spirillar form (**sodoku**) of rat bite fever, and *Streptobacillus moniliformis* causes the streptobacillary form (**Haverhill fever**). Both diseases tend to occur in urban slums and cause swelling with local lymphadenopathy at the bite site, which is then followed by fever and an extremity rash resembling viral infection. Infection by *Spirillum minus* tends to have a 1- to 4-week incubation period, while infection by *Streptobacillus moniliformis* has a 1- to 2-day incubation period. The spirillar form also tends to go through repeated exacerbations and remissions that may last up to 2 months. The streptobacillary infections tend to last only 1 or 2 weeks, but may be accompanied by arthralgia or inflammation of large joints of the extremities. The spirilla organism can be observed by examination of blood,

Rat-bite fever is actually two different bacterial diseases.

either with Giemsa stain smears, or under darkfield conditions. Streptobacillary infection is best documented by either blood culture or agglutinin titers.

Cat-Scratch Disease

Cat-scratch disease is a self-limited bacterial infection caused by a pleomorphic gram-negative bacterium, best visualized by silver stains or electron microscopy in primary lesions and lymph nodes. Cat-scratch disease tends to occur 1 or more weeks after a feline scratch (occasionally after a splinter or thorn injury), and most often affects children. Several weeks after the injury, patients develop localized lymphadenopathy, which may take the form of the **ocular glandular syndrome** (Parinaud syndrome) consisting of swelling of the eye, jaw, and high cervical lymph nodes. The early, nonspecific lymphadenitis is followed by the development of sarcoid-like granulomas, which subsequently coalesce to form stellate abscesses with irregularly shaped central accumulations of neutrophils surrounded by palisaded epithelial macrophages. Stellate abscesses, while distinctive, can also be observed in other diseases including lymphogranuloma venereum. Cases usually resolve without sequelae.

TREPONEMES

Syphilis

The venereal disease syphilis (lues) is caused by a corkscrew-shaped spirochete, *Treponema pallidum,* which can be transmitted venereally via sexual intercourse or transplacentally during pregnancy. In **acquired primary syphilis,** a hard chancre forms a button-like mass below eroded skin or mucosa, often on the glans penis in males and the cervix in females. The chancre contains an intense, predominantly plasmacytic infiltration, and obliterative endarteritis may be seen in the vicinity of the lesion. Silver impregnation or immunofluorescence techniques may demonstrate spirochetes in the exudate, ulcer, or regional lymph nodes. Serologic tests for syphilis or treponemal antibodies are usually negative during this early stage of syphilis. Penicillin therapy will prevent the subsequent development of secondary or tertiary syphilis.

Secondary syphilis is characterized by a disseminated mucocutaneous rash that may be accompanied by generalized adenopathy, sore throat, or bone pain. The rash involves the entire body, including mucus membranes, palms, and soles. Papular lesions involving the perianal region, penis, vulva, or lips are termed **condyloma lata.** The mucocutaneous lesions typically show obliterative endarteritis and a perivascular plasma cell infiltrate. Most patients with secondary syphilis appear relatively well; a few develop complications including subacute meningitis, iritis, hepatitis, periostitis, or nephrotic syndrome secondary to immune complex glomerulopathy. Serologic and antitreponemal tests for syphilis are almost always positive at this stage. Adequate penicillin therapy prevents progression to tertiary syphilis.

Tertiary syphilis is a severe disease that is now rare, possibly as a consequence of both specific therapy of early stages and accidental therapy of unsuspected syphilis when patients are given antibiotics for other conditions. Cardiovascular system involvement is most common. The **aorta** shows endarteritis of the vasa vasorum, leading to inflammatory scarring of the tunica media, with consequent aneurysm formation of the arch of the aorta. Aneurysm dilation that involves the root of the aorta may cause aortic incompetence and narrow coronary ostia. Less commonly, **central nervous system** involvement may cause meningovascular syphilis (neuropsychiatric symptoms), tabes dorsalis (spinal cord demyelination), and general paresis (mild paralysis). Patients who experience tabes dorsalis with related ataxia and sensory loss may undergo secondary destructive degenerative arthritis of the knee joint (Charcot's joint). Tertiary syphilis is additionally characterized by the formation of **syphilitic gummas** in the liver (hepar lobatum), bone, testes, and other sites. Small gummas may resemble tubercules or sarcoid lesions; larger gummas may form large masses of necrotic material, which characteristically has a rubbery, gummatous necrosis. Treponemes may be difficult to demonstrate in the gummas.

> **Tertiary syphilis can affect the aorta, central nervous system, joints, and internal organs.**

Transplacental infection causes **congenital syphilis.** Antibiotic therapy early in pregnancy can completely protect the baby since the spirochetes do not cross the placenta until approximately the fifth month of gestation. Syphilis may cause late **abortion,** stillbirth, death soon after delivery, or latent infection that becomes manifest only during childhood or adult life. Mucocutaneous involvement in the perinatal and infantile forms produces a diffuse **rash** that may show extensive sloughing of epithelium periorally, perianally, on palms, and on soles. Spirochetes are common in the mucocutaneous lesions. A generalized osteochondritis and periosteitis is present, which most prominently affects the nose (**saddle nose deformity**) and tibia (**saber shin**). Congenital syphilis also causes diffuse fibrosis with occasional **gumma formation** in the liver; diffuse interstitial fibrosis of the lungs; and diffuse interstitial inflammatory reactions throughout the body. Congenital syphilis can be complicated by **central nervous system meningovascular syphilis. Eye changes** can include interstitial keratitis, choroiditis, and abnormal pigment production. Small, abnormally shaped incisors (**Hutchinson's teeth**) are the result of spirochete infection during tooth development. Meningovascular involvement can lead to nerve deafness and blindness secondary to optic nerve atrophy.

> **Congenital syphilis may produce death or devastating disease that involves the skin, skeletal system, nervous system, teeth, and internal organs.**

Yaws, Bejel, and Pinta

Yaws, bejel, and pinta are spirochete diseases transmitted by nonvenereal person-to-person contact. **Bejel** is observed in desert zones, where it causes a chronic disorder that begins in childhood and has initial mucocutaneous lesions. **Yaws** is observed in the moist tropics and is characterized by an initial raised skin ulcer ("mother yaw") and gummatous involvement of the bones later; central nervous system or cardiovascular involvement are not seen. **Pinta** is a disease of rural Latin America that causes skin involvement with unsightly pigment changes, but does not appear to cause systemic disease. Yaws, bejel, and pinta appear to have some antigenic cross-reactivity with syphilis, and may cause false-positive serologic tests for syphilis.

> **Yaws, bejel, and pinta resemble syphilis but are not usually transmitted venereally.**

MYCOBACTERIA

The pathogenic **mycobacteria** are acid-fast organisms that characteristically have a cell wall containing distinctive phosphoglycolipids and waxes. Mycobacteria tend to be intracellular invaders that divide slowly and are difficult to culture. The lepra bacillus, which causes leprosy, has never been successfully cultured.

Tuberculosis

Tuberculosis characteristically produces caseating granulomas.

Human **tuberculosis** can be caused by either *Mycobacterium tuberculosis hominis* or *Mycobacterium tuberculosis bovis.* The characteristic lesion of tuberculosis is the tubercle, which is a granuloma composed of aggregated epithelioid macrophages with interspersed Langhans multinucleate giant cells. The edges of the granuloma are rimmed by fibroblasts and lymphocytes. If a central area of caseation necrosis is present, the tubercle is considered "soft" rather than "hard." Other inflammatory changes may be present in infected tissues, including purulent and fibrotic lesions. While tuberculosis is a prototype granulomatous disease, many other infectious and noninfectious conditions can also cause granulomas.

Primary tuberculosis often produces the Ghon complex, composed of a single pulmonary granuloma accompanied by prominent mediastinal lymphadenopathy.

The term **primary tuberculosis** is used for an initial infection with the tubercle bacillus. Primary pulmonary tuberculosis tends to form a single granuloma (the **Ghon focus**) in either the lower part of the upper lobes or the upper part of lower lobes, often immediately subjacent to the pleura. Since the body does not initially respond to the bacillus, tubercule bacilli are able to drain to the tracheobronchial lymph nodes, where they evoke caseating granulomas. This nodal involvement is typically on the same side of the tracheobronchial tree as the lung focus. The term **Ghon complex** is used to describe both the combination of the primary lung lesion and lymph node involvement. Usually, primary tuberculosis resolves with fibrosis, calcification, and sometimes, ossification of both the Ghon focus and the granulomas in the lymph nodes. Bacilli may persist in dormant form for years, and possibly for life, within the calcified lesions. A small percentage of primary tuberculosis, particularly in children, follows a more aggressive course with erosion into adjacent bronchi, dissemination through the lung, miliary tuberculosis, tuberculous meningitis, or airway obstruction. Tuberculosis infections of sites other than the lung (gastrointestinal tract, oropharyngeal lymphoid tissue, skin) cause primary complexes similar to those of the pulmonary form, which consist of granulomas at the infection site and also in the appropriate regional lymph nodes.

Secondary tuberculosis is more common than primary tuberculosis.

Most "tuberculosis" that is observed clinically is **secondary tuberculosis** in which a previously sensitized individual acquires infection, either through exogenous exposure to tubercle bacilli, or, more commonly, through reactivation of asymptomatic primary disease. Secondary tuberculous involvement of the lungs tends to involve the highly oxygenated apical and posterior segments of one or both upper lobes **(Simon's foci).** Unlike the Ghon complex, regional lymph nodes are characteristically not involved, possibly as a consequence of prompt phagocytosis with destruction of bacilli by activated macrophages adjacent to the granulomas. Immunosuppressed patients may be unable to mount a granulomatous response, and may have necrotic foci filled with mycobacteria with little evidence of leukocytic response. Alternatively, abundant neutrophils may be present, notably when cavities have eroded into airways, and are vulnerable to secondary infection.

Secondary tuberculosis can have a wide variety of outcomes. Fibrocalcific "arrested" tuberculosis occurs if the lesion undergoes healing with calcification. Progressive pulmonary tuberculosis may be complicated by extensive pulmonary and pleural involvement; tracheobronchial or laryngeal tuberculosis; intestinal tuberculosis following swallowing of infected sputum; **miliary dissemination** in the body or lungs; tuberculous **meningitis;** isolated cervical node involvement; adrenal involvement, which can cause **Addison's disease;** tuberculous osteomyelitis including vertebral involvement **(Pott's disease);** and genital tuberculosis.

Long-standing untreated tuberculosis may also cause systemic secondary **amyloidosis.** While acid-fast stains can be helpful, the diagnosis should not be considered definitively established until the organisms have either been cultured or seen in typical lesions. In tissues, the typical mycobacteria are more likely to be found in recent necrotic foci. In general, primary tuberculosis is frequently silent; secondary tuberculosis can also be silent. However, many patients with secondary tuberculosis have systemic symptoms including fever, night sweats, weakness, fatigability, and loss of appetite and weight. Miliary tuberculosis can present as fever of unknown origin. Atypical presentations of tuberculosis can occur in AIDS patients, in older individuals, and in patients with pre-existing major illness such as malignancy or chronic renal failure. In these settings, unexplained fever should suggest the possibility of tuberculosis. Most strains of tuberculosis remain sensitive to antibiotic therapy.

Secondary tuberculosis has many complications.

Atypical Mycobacterial Infections

Atypical mycobacteria are organisms related to *Mycobacterium tuberculosis* that cause opportunistic infections in immunocompromised patients. *Mycobacterium kansasii* and *Mycobacterium avium-intracellulare* cause **pulmonary disease,** particularly in middle-aged or older men with pre-existing lung conditions. *Mycobacterium avium-intracellulare* and *Mycobacterium scrofulaceum* also can cause **lymphadenitis,** usually in children. *Mycobacterium ulcerans* can cause **ulcerative skin lesions,** usually in Australia, Latin America, and Africa; *Mycobacterium marinum* causes similar skin lesions in patients exposed to aquariums. *Mycobacterium fortuitum* and *Mycobacterium chelonei* cause sporadic **injection abscesses.** AIDS victims and other severely immunosuppressed patients may develop life-threatening **bacteremias,** with the most common infecting organism being *Mycobacterium avium-intracellulare.* Diagnosis of a particular species of mycobacterium is by culture followed by typing by differential biochemical tests or DNA hybridization.

Atypical mycobacteria can cause pulmonary disease, adenopathy, skin lesions, and bacteremia.

Leprosy

Mycobacterium leprae is an acid-fast intracellular organism similar to *Mycobacterium tuberculosis* that only naturally infects humans and armadillos. In humans, it causes **leprosy** (Hansen's disease), which is a slowly progressive mycobacteria infection of low communicability with

Leprosy may take tuberculoid or lepromatous forms.

prominent involvement of skin and peripheral nerves. Patients who respond to the *Mycobacterium leprae* organism by mounting a vigorous T-cell-mediated immunity have granuloma formation resembling tuberculosis **(tuberculoid leprosy).** These patients usually have only a few mycobacteria; prominent peripheral nerve involvement; and atrophy of skin and extremity muscles. Patients who do not mount a vigorous immune response to the mycobacteria develop **lepromatous leprosy,** characterized by nodular facial lesions ("leonine facies") and less prominent nerve involvement. The nodules are characteristically located deep in the epidermis and are composed of lipid and bacillary-laden "lepra" cells. Intermediate cases also exist. An experimental vaccine against leprosy has been developed.

ACTINOMYCETES

Nocardia are weakly acid-fast bacteria that resemble fungi and can cause pulmonary abscess, skin infection, or disseminated disease.

The **actinomycetes** include both *Nocardia* and *Actinomyces* species. These organisms superficially resemble fungi, but are actually similar to mycobacteria. ***Nocardia*** are weakly acid-fast organisms found widely in nature that can cause life-threatening chronic necrotizing **pulmonary abscesses** and **disseminated nocardiosis** in immunocompromised hosts. *Nocardia asteroides* is the most frequently observed species. *Nocardia brasiliensis* is associated with skin infection **(mycetoma)** in patients in Central and Latin America without known predisposing conditions. The organisms in the lung lesions tend to produce discreet filaments, but can form mycelial colonies in mycetomas. Both pulmonary and disseminated nocardiosis tend to be suspected only after more common bacteria have been excluded.

Non-acid-fast *Actinomyces* resembles *Nocardia* and can cause severe, locally destructive lesions.

Actinomyces resembles *Nocardia* species, but the organisms are not acid-fast and are commensuals of the oral cavity, alimentary tract, and vagina. Actinomyces infection **(actinomycosis)** causes chronic suppurative infections in devitalized tissues, which have the tendency to spread by contiguity, and contain multiple abscesses that may drain to skin or other surfaces. These lesions also often contain mixed bacterial infection. **Cervicofacial actinomycosis** begins in the gingiva and adjacent soft tissues, which, with time, become indurated (lumpy jaw). These aggressive lesions may extend to the skin, with formation of multiple sinuses and may additionally cause periostitis and osteomyelitis. A central diffuse area of suppurative necrosis often contains a bacterial colony composed of masses of filaments (rays) that are capped by hyaline material (clubs). Granulation tissue surrounds the necrosis. Tiny yellow particles ("sulfur granules") can sometimes be observed in pus draining from the lesion. Actinomycosis with similar locally destructive lesions can also involve the **abdomen** or **thorax.** Actinomycosis should be suspected in patients who have large inflammatory masses that are forming fistulae. The disease responds to sustained antibiotic treatment.

UNCOMMON BACTERIA

Rhinoscleroma

Rhinoscleroma is a tumor-like inflammation of the nose.

Klebsiella rhinoscleromatis is an encapsulated, gram-negative bacillus related to *Klebsiella pneumoniae.* The bacteria is endemic in many parts of the world and causes the facial deformity and upper airway obstruction known as **rhinoscleroma.** *Klebsiella rhinoscleromatis* is transmitted by unknown mechanisms and responds well to treatment. The disease initially resembles an ordinary cold, but extensive chronic inflammation eventually produces a tumor-like submucosal mass. The lesions contain large numbers of foamy macrophages, some of which are multinucleate **(Mikulicz cells),** that are filled with encapsulated diplococci.

Ozena

Ozena is a rare cause of chronic rhinitis caused by the ***Klebsiella ozaenae;*** mixed cultures with other gram-negative bacilli have also been identified. The organisms cause nonspecific exudative and necrotizing inflammation with atrophy of the turbinates accompanied by foul-smelling, greenish exudate. Nasal obstruction and anosmia are observed.

Ozena is another rare nasal infection.

Granuloma Inguinale

Calymmatobacterium donovani causes the venereal disease **granuloma inguinale,** characterized by chronic mucocutaneous ulceration with granulomas. The organism is a small, intracellular bacillus, also known as a Donovan body, which is most often observed in vacuolated macrophages in active disease lesions. The distribution is worldwide, with New Guinea and India having the highest incidence, and Europe and the United States having only a few cases. The usual mode of transmission is sexual contact, with men more often affected than women. The initial lesion is a genital or perineal papule that later forms an elevated sore with a necrotic center and an indurated, raised border. The lesion heals with dense scarring that may sometimes progress to keloid formation. The disease is distinguished from lymphogranuloma venereum by the absence of lymph node involvement and rectal strictures. The bulk of the lesion consists of richly vascularized granulation tissue with macrophages containing organisms that appear as faint bluish dots in hematoxylin and eosin-stained sections. Neglected cases tend to produce disfiguring lesions, which can be prevented by appropriate chemotherapy.

Granuloma inguinale is a granulomatous venereal disease.

Chancroid

Haemophilus ducreyi is a highly infectious organism that is usually transmitted by sexual intercourse, with subsequent autoinoculation causing the formation of multiple soft, necrotic ulcers **(chancroid** or soft chancre). The disease is prevalent in the Orient, West Indies, and North Africa, and has an increasing incidence in the United States. Regional lymph nodes may be enlarged, tender, and suppurative **(bubos).** The ulcers are composed of disintegrating red and white blood cells overlying granulation tissue, with vessels showing endothelial hyperplasia and sometimes thrombosis. The deepest zone contains a chronic inflammatory reaction with fibroblastic proliferation. Diagnosis of chancroid is by culture of *Haemophilus ducreyi.* A skin test for chancroid has also been developed, and usually remains positive for several years following infection.

Chancroid is an inflammatory venereal disease.

Bartonellosis

Bartonella bacilliformis is an unusual bacteria that preferentially
infects erythrocytes, causing life-threatening hemolytic anemia,
hepatosplenomegaly, and fever (Oroya fever or **Carrión's disease**). The
organism is carried by a sandfly vector, *Phlebotomus verrucarum,* which
limits its endemic zone to the high Peruvian Andes. Patients who survive
the initial hemolytic phase develop skin lesions that contain the
Bartonella organisms and highly vascularized nodular collections of
inflammatory cells. Chloramphenicol can effectively control the infection.
Occasionally, laboratory workers in the United States have been infected
by related organisms, which cause hemolysis in animals.

SARCOIDOSIS

Sarcoidosis is a common disease of unknown etiology that is discussed
here because it is similar to other granulomatous diseases of bacterial or
fungal origin. The granulomas of sarcoidosis are noncaseating ("hard").
The diagnosis of sarcoidosis is made by exclusion, since many other diseases, including other microbacterial or fungal infections and berylliosis,
can produce similar granulomas. The most common presentation is bilateral hilar lymphadenopathy or lung involvement visible by chest radiography. Other common presentations include eye and skin lesions.
Sarcoidosis is more prevalent in women than in men. In the United
States, American blacks have a much higher incidence of sarcoidosis
than do whites; Chinese and Southeast Asians only very uncommonly
develop sarcoidosis. Sarcoidosis can involve virtually every organ in the
body. Involved nodes typically show **noncaseating granulomas** composed of an aggregate of tightly clustered epithelioid cells, which may
contain Langhans or foreign body-type giant cells. With time, the granulomas can become enclosed within fibrous rims or replaced by hyaline
fibrous scars. The sarcoid granulomas may also contain **Schaumann
bodies,** composed of laminated concretions of calcium and proteins, and
asteroid bodies, which are enclosed within giant cells.

Asteroid bodies and Schaumann bodies may also be observed in other
granulomatous diseases including berylliosis. The lungs can contain
small granulomas distributed throughout the parenchyma, often near
blood vessels, bronchi, or lymphatics; these granulomas are typically not
visible macroscopically, unless they have coalesced into small nodules.
Many of these small granulomas will heal, and varying stages of fibrosis
and hyalinization may also be found, associated with interstitial pulmonary fibrosis. The skin, spleen, liver, and bone marrow may also contain small granulomas. **Mikulicz syndrome** is sarcoidotic involvement
of the eye, uveal tracts, and salivary glands (combined uveal parotid
involvement). Patients may have either a steadily progressive course, or
may experience periods of activity and remission. Steroid therapy sometimes initiates the remissions. Many patients recover with minimal to no
residual manifestations. Patients who die most commonly have progressive pulmonary fibrosis and cor pulmonale, but may also have cardiac or
central nervous system damage.

FUNGI

Only a small number of fungal species cause human disease. Fungal infection restricted to the epidermal surface is called superficial, and is usually not a cause of serious concern. Deep fungal infections are those that invade into organs and tissues. This discussion will primarily concern deep fungal infections.

CANDIDIASIS

The most commonly isolated deep fungal organisms are *Candida* species, particularly ***Candida albicans.*** The *Candida* vegetative form is a nonbranching chain of tubular cells called pseudohyphae. The yeast forms by budding off 2- to 4-mm blastospores. Either vegetative or yeast forms (or both) can be seen in diseased tissues, and can be stained with Gram, periodic acid-Schiff (PAS), and silver stains. *Candida albicans* can be isolated from normal body cavities and surfaces including the oral cavity, gastrointestinal tract, and vagina in many individuals. Suppression of the normal bacterial microflora, as by antibiotics or pH changes, facilitates the growth of *Candida.* Patients apt to develop serious *Candida* infections include diabetics, the debilitated, burn patients, and immunosuppressed patients. Sites of involvement can include the oral cavity, esophagus, vagina, skin, fingernails, and deeper tissues. Superficial candidiasis of the oral cavity **(thrush)** or vagina produces similar patterns characterized by superficial, curdy, almost fluffy membranes that can be easily detached from the surface, leaving an irritated underlying surface. Invasive candidiasis can be caused either by spread from a superficial lesion or direct inoculation, as by a needle or catheter.

Candidal sepsis may resemble bacterial sepsis, although it tends to develop somewhat more slowly. While no organ is immune, frequent targets include the kidney, heart valves, lung, and liver. In general, deep fungal infections are characterized by the formation of microabscesses, with the yeast or pseudohyphal forms of the fungus occupying the lesion centers. *Candida* endocarditis can cause the formation of large, friable vegetations that may cause infectious emboli. ***Candida glabrata*** (*Torulopsis glabrata*) produces lesions similar to those of *Candida albicans,* but does not cause thrush or dermatitis, and can be distinguished from *Candida albicans* by the presence of 2- to 3-μm blastospores.

Candida **grow on skin and mucosal surfaces, and they may also cause invasive disease.**

MUCORMYCOSIS

Mucormycosis can cause severe rhinocerebral, pulmonary, or gastrointestinal infection in debilitated patients.

Mucormycosis (zygomycosis, phycomycosis) is an opportunistic infection that can be caused by a variety of species that are members of the **phycomycetes** including the genera *Mucor, Absidia, Rhizopus,* and *Cunninghamella.* These infections are often acquired in hospitals and are usually seen in terminally ill patients. Primary sites of invasion include the nasal sinuses, lungs, and gastrointestinal tract. Rhinocerebral mucormycosis is a feared complication, since the fungus can spread to sinuses, orbit, and brain. Lung involvement may occur either primarily or secondary to rhinocerebral disease. Gastrointestinal mucormycosis can be observed in severely malnourished children. Mucormycosis tends to have a poor prognosis, primarily because of the debilitated underlying condition of the patient. In tissue, the fungus appears as a nonseptate, irregularly wide (6- to 50-μm) hyphal form with frequent right angle branching. The organism has a predilection for invading arterial walls and can cause extensive necrosis.

ASPERGILLOSIS

***Aspergillus** can colonize bronchial mucosa or pulmonary cavities and it can also cause invasive pneumonia and disseminated disease.*

Aspergillus species, including ***Aspergillus fumigatus*** and ***Aspergillus niger,*** are important causes of invasive fungal infections, particularly in hospitals. *Aspergillus* can also cause allergic reactions by inhalation of spores, and can noninvasively proliferate in the lumen of previously damaged airways. **Allergic aspergillosis** may clinically resemble bronchial asthma, or it can produce an allergic alveolitis with type III and type IV hypersensitivity reactions. Superficial colonization of the bronchial mucosa by *Aspergillus* produces allergic bronchopulmonary aspergillosis, which can cause a progressively more severe hypersensitivity reaction that predisposes for chronic obstructive lung disease with peribronchial fibrosis and irreversible airway dilation. This colonizing form of aspergillosis can produce masses of fungal hyphae (fungus balls or **aspergillomas**) within pulmonary cavities caused by tuberculosis, bronchiectasis, old infarcts, or abscesses. **Invasive pulmonary aspergillosis** usually occurs in immunosuppressed or debilitated hosts and may subsequently disseminate through the body. The *Aspergillus* organism appears in tissues as septate filaments with relatively uniform branching at typically 40-degree angles. The lung lesions are associated with areas of necrotizing pneumonia, which usually have sharply delineated boundaries, and may contain *Aspergillus* invading blood vessels or bronchi. **Localized involvement** of tissues can occur in the eyes, perinasal sinuses, or external ear. A **rhinocerebral form** similar to that caused by phycomycetes also occurs.

CRYPTOCOCCOSIS

Crytptococcal pneumonia is observed in patients with AIDS or hematopoietic disorders.

Cryptococci cause opportunistic infection that may infect either healthy individuals following massive exposure or immunocompromised patients, particularly those with AIDS or hematopoietic disorders, with smaller exposures. The cryptococcal organisms are usually inhaled, and birds (pigeons) serve as a reservoir. In tissues, ***Cryptococcus neoformans*** occurs as a 4- to 10-μm yeast that divides by unequal budding.

Cryptococcal strains that have broad, slimy capsules that stain with mucicarmine tend to be more virulent than do strains without capsules. While the lung is the usual initial site of infection, the infection may be asymptomatic until the fungus spreads, potentially producing meningitis or widely disseminated disease. In immunosuppressed patients, no immune response may be mounted to the infecting fungi. A chronic granulomatous reaction may be produced in protracted disease and in more normal individuals. Immunosuppressed patients with cryptococcal infections, particularly meningitis, tend to have a poor prognosis; the best prognosis is for patients with isolated pulmonary infection, which can be surgically excised.

BLASTOMYCOSIS

Blastomycosis has a strong male predominance and usually occurs in North America, particularly in the Mississippi–Ohio river basins and the Middle Atlantic states; sporadic cases have been observed elsewhere. In tissues, **Blastomyces dermatitidis** occurs as a 5- to 25-μm, round to oval yeast with a thick refractile wall. The budding form is usually broad based. Blastomycosis is characterized by the production of focal, suppurative, and granulomatous lesions, usually in the lungs and skin. The most common form of **pulmonary blastomycosis** is as a solitary focus of consolidation that heals by fibrosis and is sometimes accompanied by erythema nodosum of the skin or involvement of regional nodes. Pulmonary blastomycosis uncommonly causes progressive lung disease, with either cavity formation or production of miliary abscesses throughout the lung. The inflammation may be either abscess-like or form granulomas. **Cutaneous blastomycoses** usually involves the distal extremities with an indolent, chancre-like papule that progresses to large, cancer-like ulcers. Self-limited forms of blastomycosis do not require antifungal therapy; late progressive stages tend to respond poorly and have a poor prognosis.

> Blastomycosis causes granulomatous, pulmonary, and skin disease.

PARACOCCIDIOIDOMYCOSIS

Paracoccidioidomycosis (South American blastomycosis) is endemic in South and Central America, with most cases occurring in agricultural workers in Brazil, Venezuela, and Colombia. The causative fungus is a 10- to 60-μm yeast form of *Paracoccidioides brasiliensis* that characteristically shows multiple budding around a mother cell ("ship's wheel image"). The initial indistinctive pulmonary lesion can be followed by an extrapulmonary spread that produces mucocutaneous lesions of the mouth, nose, or larynx; spreading lymph node infection; or systemic dissemination with involvement of skin, gastrointestinal tract, lungs, liver, or other organs. Histologically, either granulomatous inflammatory reactions or microabscesses can be produced.

> Paracoccidioidomycosis is another cause of granulomatous pulmonary or systemic disease.

COCCIDIOIDOMYCOSIS

Coccidioides immitis causes coccidioidomycosis, which clinically resembles acute or chronic tuberculosis. It is most prevalent in the Southwest and far West of the United States (**San Joaquin Valley**

> Coccidioidomycosis resembles tuberculosis.

fever); parts of Central and South America also contain the organism. The organism in tissue specimens is a nonbudding spherule 20- to 60-μm in diameter with a thick wall. The organism may be filled with endospores. Many initial infections are asymptomatic. Symptomatic patients with lung lesions have fever, cough, and pleuritic pains, and may additionally have erythema nodosum or erythema multiforme. Histologically, either abscesses or granulomas may form. Hilar lymphadenopathy may be present resembling the Ghon complex of tuberculosis. A small percentage of patients develop progressive coccidioidomycosis that resembles progressive tuberculosis, with a somewhat increased prevalence in black and Asian males, possibly as a failure of cell-mediated immunity. Most cases of coccidioidomycosis have a good prognosis, but systemic dissemination of the organisms, particularly with development of bone or central nervous system infection, may require long-term antifungal treatment.

HISTOPLASMOSIS

Histoplasmosis also resembles tuberculosis.

The infecting organism of **histoplasmosis** is the dimorphic fungus *Histoplasma capsulatum,* which is observed most frequently in the Ohio–Mississippi River region of the United States, but has been reported elsewhere (e.g., Argentina); *Histoplasma duboisii* causes a similar disease in central Africa. In soil, the organism grows in mycelial form, and characteristically produces sprouting conidia of two sizes (microconidia and macroconidia). In mammalian tissue, the organism grows as a 2- to 5-μm yeast form with a thin cell wall, but no true capsule (despite the name), that best stains with methamine silver. The yeast forms are not infectious, either in tissue sections or by the patient. The clinical presentation is similar to tuberculosis and coccidioidomycosis. Latent or asymptomatic histoplasmosis is common, and may be discovered long after infection by the finding of fibrocalcific residues in lungs or hilar lymph nodes. The diagnosis is confirmed by a positive histoplasmin skin test.

UNUSUAL DEEP FUNGAL INFECTIONS

The feet are particularly vulnerable to deep fungal infections.

Other deep fungal infections are typically either rare or observed in tropical countries. Fungal infections, particularly of the foot, may be associated with multiple draining sinuses **(mycetomas)** and can be caused by a variety of species including *Nocardia brasiliensis* (Central and North America) and some of the actinomycetes species. **Chromomycosis** produces skin lesions in Mexico and Puerto Rico.

SUPERFICIAL FUNGI

Superficial fungal infections of the epidermis, hair, or nails are discussed with the skin (see p. 112). These lesions are, in general, more a cause of cosmetic discomfort than of life-threatening illness. The causative fungi can usually be seen in skin scrapings and hair shafts.

PARASITES

PROTOZOAL DISEASES

Parasitic protozoal diseases remain prevalent in industrial countries and are an important cause of disease and death in developing countries. These eukaryotic parasites tend to have complex life cycles and pathogenetic mechanisms. Many parasitic protozoa have life cycles that alternate between a specific mammalian host and a specific, usually insect, vector or external environmental niche. Human infections can be broadly grouped as those occurring on epithelial surfaces (luminal); within the bloodstream (hemic); or within cells (intracellular).

Parasitic protozoa often have complex life cycles.

LUMINAL PROTOZOA

Amebiasis

Entamoeba histolytica, the usual cause of **amebiasis,** is a 15- to 40-μm diameter amoeba that may contain ingested erythrocytes and has a small nucleus with a distinctive tiny central karyosome and aggregated RNA–DNA against the nuclear membrane. An infectious quadrinucleate cyst form is produced in unfavorable conditions. The cyst is converted in the gut to the motile trophozoite following gastric digestion of the cyst wall. Disease manifestations can be widely variable. Entirely asymptomatic carriers are common. Gastrointestinal symptoms produced can range from mild chronic diarrhea to severe purging dysentery. The large colon, particularly the cecum and ascending colon, may have flask-shaped amebic ulcers that occasionally cause bowel perforation or induce formation of constricted lesions (amebomas). In a substantial percentage of symptomatic cases, the amoeba may spread to the liver to produce a usually solitary amoebic abscess up to 10 cm or greater in diameter. Amoebic liver abscesses can be secondarily infected by bacteria that may dominate the clinical picture. Amoebic abscesses can also develop in many other sites as a consequence of either embolization or direct extension. While *Entamoeba histolytica* is the most common cause of amebic dysentery in humans, **Balantidium coli,** a large ciliate intestinal parasite, can also occasionally cause similar disease.

Entamoeba histolytica **can cause colonic ulcers and liver abscesses.**

Amebic Meningoencephalitis

Several amoeba are known to cause meningitis, the most important of which are free-living **Naegleria fowleri** and **Acanthamoeba.** The former organism is particularly important because it can be present in stagnant water, and is able to kill a healthy child or adolescent within a few

Naegleria causes meningitis in healthy swimmers, while Acanthamoeba causes meningitis in immunosuppressed patients.

days despite aggressive medical therapy. In contrast, *Acanthamoeba* causes rare cases in immunosuppressed patients. *Naegleria fowleri* can closely resemble human cells in cerebrospinal fluids, smears, and tissue sections. A helpful feature is the presence of marked motility in fresh preparations. Olfactory nerves and brain are most commonly involved. The meninges show clouding with focal hemorrhage, which is accompanied by extensive fibrinoid necrosis and thrombosis of blood vessels. *Acanthamoeba* has also been identified as a cause of chronic keratitis of the eye, related to chronic use of soft contact lenses.

Giardiasis

Giardia can cause diarrhea and intestinal malabsorption.

Giardia lamblia is a very common human pathogenic small intestinal protozoan that can cause both asymptomatic and symptomatic infections. Infective cysts are intermittently shed into stools, and may subsequently be ingested in contaminated drinking water. A few patients develop prolonged diarrhea or intestinal malabsorption. Severe giardiasis can be associated with host factors such as low serum IgA or low overall immunoglobulin levels. In smears, *Giardia lamblia* trophozoites have a distinctive pear-shaped appearance that appears to have a "face." In cross sections in biopsies of routinely stained material, the organisms are often found adjacent to the epithelial brush border and appear crescent-shaped. An ELISA test for *Giardia* antigens in stool may replace duodenal aspiration for demonstrating the infection. Intestinal biopsy specimens may show either normal morphology or changes including clubbing or absence of villi.

Cryptosporidial and Isosporal Enteritis

Cryptosporidium and Isospora are additional causes of diarrhea.

Cryptosporidium can cause transient diarrhea or dysentery in normal children. In AIDS patients, cryptosporidiosis causes severe chronic malabsorption and diarrhea that can lead to death. Cryptosporidial cysts can be identified in feces by use of a modified acid-fast staining technique. *Isospora belli* is another uncommon cause of diarrhea, and has also been observed in nonintestinal infections in AIDS patients.

Trichomoniasis

Trichomonas causes an often asymptomatic venereal infection.

Trichomonas vaginalis is a 15- to 18-μm long flagellate that roughly resembles a turnip in shape. It has a single nucleus, three to four anterior flagellae, and a single posterior flagellum with a characteristic undulating membrane with an axostyle. *Trichomonas vaginalis* causes frequent, often asymptomatic, **venereal infection** with long-term colonization in the vaginas of postpubertal women. Severe genital inflammatory lesions are usually due to a combination of *Trichomonas vaginalis* and bacterial pathogens. Both men and women can experience burning, itching, and discharge, particularly around micturition. The affected mucosa may develop small blisters or granules (**"strawberry mucosa"**). The organisms are notoriously difficult to recognize on Papanicolaou smears because they stain only faintly and can be easily missed; they are best observed in fresh preparations (where they are very motile) or Giemsa-stained smears.

Pneumocystis pneumonia

Pneumocystis carinii is an opportunistic parasite that may be more closely related to fungi than to protozoa. Nearly all normal children have acquired antibodies to pneumocystis by their second birthday. Individuals who develop clinical infection include children with protein calorie malnutrition and immunosuppressed adults. The presence of pneumocystis in AIDS patients is so common that it has been included as a diagnostic criterion for clinical AIDS. Human infection may result from activation of latent infection. The **trophozoites** of *Pneumocystis carinii* are visible in thin sections and by electron microscopy and have long filopodia and a size of up to 6 μm. They are typically attached to, but have not invaded into, alveolar epithelial cells. The trophozoites produce cup-shaped or boat-shaped **cysts** with sharply outlined cell walls that are usually used for diagnosis when stained with silver methenamine. The cysts are characteristically found in intra-alveolar spaces in an amphophilic, foamy, amorphous material that contains both the parasites and cell debris. The combination of early treatment and prophylactic drug therapy for patients at risk has decreased the finding of classic widespread pneumocystosis at autopsy of AIDS patients. Pneumocystis infection can also be demonstrated in nonpulmonary sites.

Pneumocystis **pneumonia is particularly prevalent in AIDS patients.**

BLOOD AND TISSUE PROTOZOA

Malaria

Human **malaria** can be caused by *Plasmodium vivax, Plasmodium ovale, Plasmodium falciparum,* and *Plasmodium malariae.* These protozoa produce similar diseases that are observed worldwide, most commonly in Africa and Asia. Transmission to humans is via the bite of the *Anopheles* **mosquito,** whose saliva contains the sporozoite form of the parasite. Transmission by transfusion among drug addicts has also been observed. The organisms spread from the skin to the liver, where they undergo an **exoerythrocytic cycle** leading to production of merozoites. The merozoites re-enter the bloodstream, where they are capable of invading erythrocytes. The merozoites produce trophozoites, which later divide to form numerous schizonts, which are released by rupture of the erythrocyte. It is this **intraerythrocyte asexual cycle** that is associated with most of the anatomic and clinical features of malaria. The free schizonts can enter other red cells, beginning a new cycle. A few red cells develop intraerythrocyte gametocytes that correspond to male and female offspring, the only forms capable of initiating the insect cycle when taken up by mosquitos.

Clinical differences between infections caused by *Plasmodium* species are due primarily to patterns in the timing of the asexual intraerythrocyte cycle. *Plasmodium vivax* and *Plasmodium ovale* characteristically produce fever spikes at roughly 48 hours (**benign tertian malaria**); in contrast, *Plasmodium malariae* causes fever spikes at 72-hour intervals (**benign quartan malaria**). These species are only rarely fatal, and *Plasmodium malariae* is associated with long latent periods. In contrast, *Plasmodium falciparum* causes more serious disease and has an irregular periodicity, but often the fever appears at 48-hour intervals (**malignant tertian malaria**).

Plasmodia have a complex life cycle with stages both within and outside erythrocytes.

Different malarial organisms cause slightly different clinical patterns.

Anemia is observed in all forms of malaria. Malarial pigment produced by digestion of heme by the parasite stains spleen, liver, and bone marrow. Splenomegaly and hepatomegaly are common. *Plasmodium falciparum* has a higher morbidity and mortality as a consequence of a number of factors, the most important of which may be that the organism indiscriminately parasitizes red cells of all ages, rather than selectively preferring either young or old red cells, as do the other strains. *Plasmodium falciparum* historically produced **blackwater fever** (possibly due to coexisting drug or alcohol toxicity), with hemoglobinuria and renal failure. Malignant *Plasmodium falciparum* malaria may additionally show extreme congestion of brain vessels, which can cause parenchymal hypoxia. Pulmonary edema and shock with disseminated intravascular coagulation can occur. Diagnosis of malaria is based on the identification of parasites in the blood smear. Sickle cell trait and glucose-6-phosphate dehydrogenase deficiency may be partially protective against malaria.

Babesiasis

Babesia are related to plasmodia and grow in erythrocytes. ***Babesia microti*** causes sporadic infections in Eastern seaboard sites of the United States. Infection is usually transmitted by the bite of the nymphal form of the tick *Ixodes dammini* and has also occasionally been transmitted by transfusions. Humans are usually accidental hosts. Recognized symptomatic cases are relatively uncommon, and usually occur in persons older than 40 years, particularly asplenic individuals, who may die. The organism invades red blood cells, and may be mistaken for *Plasmodium falciparum*. Clinically, babesiasis is characterized by roughly 1 week of fever, headache, chills, and fatigue, which is followed by a slow but spontaneous recovery. Severely debilitated and splenectomized patients may have severe disease characterized by prolonged or recurrent symptoms accompanied by vomiting, hemolysis, jaundice, hemoglobinuria, renal failure, and even coma. The parasitemia may involve up to 30 percent of red cells. Fatal cases are usually due to shock and hypoxia. Diagnosis is by Giemsa-stained blood smears. Occasional cases due to ***Babesia bovis*** have a higher lethality.

African Trypanosomiasis

Trypanosoma rhodesiense (East African savannah) and ***Trypanosoma gambiense*** (West African bush) can cause several clinical conditions including acute fever with purpura and **disseminated intravascular coagulation;** a chronic condition characterized by repeated episodes of fever accompanied by **lymph node swelling** and splenomegaly; and chronic progressive neurologic dysfunction, leading to cachexia and death (**"sleeping sickness"**). Some patients experience all three stages, while in others, only the latter two chronic stages are clinically apparent. The African trypanosomes are transmitted by the saliva of the tsetse fly (*Glossina* vector) from wild animal reservoirs. While the infections are similar, *Trypanosoma rhodesiense* infections tend to present with an acute virulent disease, while *Trypanosoma gambiense* infection is more apt to cause chronic disease. The trypanosomes proliferate at the bite site, sometimes causing formation of a large **chancre,** and then enter the lymphatic and vascular systems. In the bloodstream, the trypanosomes (trypomastigotes) are motile protozoa with a fusiform, flagellate shape characterized by an undulating membrane along the length of the organism. Much of the pathogenicity of the trypanosomes appears to be caused by their ability to generate a large number of variations of surface antigens. The persistent bouts of fever appear to be due to repeated attempts by the host to mount an immune (polyclonal IgM) response to the organisms. Trypanosomes damage tissue by unknown mechanisms, possibly related to antigen–antibody complexes triggering host responses. Trypanosomes are most easily visualized with "overstained" Giemsa-stained sections, particularly of the choroid plexus and glomeruli, where they are found concentrated in capillary loops.

INTRACELLULAR PROTOZOA

Chagas Disease

Trypanosoma cruzi causes **Chagas disease** (American trypanosomiasis) in Central America, South America, and occasionally Texas. Many acute cases are asymptomatic; some patients develop acute **myocarditis** with fever. Chronic Chagas disease is an important cause of **cardiac failure** leading to death in some Latin American countries. For reasons that are not clear, in Brazil alone, Chagas disease is also associated with **megaesophagus** and **megacolon.** The organism is a fusiform hemoflagellate with an undulating membrane that multiplies in tissue cells and is acquired by the nocturnal bite of the housing parasite *Triatominae* ("kissing bug"). In individual cells, such as myocardial fibers, the organism multiplies in a leishmanial form in pseudocysts. With disease progression, the number of parasites in the blood decreases, but the tissue forms remain.

Chagas disease can cause cardiac failure, megaesophagus, and megacolon.

Leishmaniasis

Leishmania are parasites similar to trypanosomes whose parasitic stage is a tiny (less than 3 μm), nonflagellated, intracellular mastigote. In tissue section, the organism is recognizable as basophilic dots that correspond to the nucleus and a modified mitochondrial structure called the kinetoblast. Sandflies (diverse flablotamus species in the Old World, and leutzomiaea in the New World) are the vectors for the leishmanial species. Different leishmanial organisms cause quite different disease manifestations. **Visceral leishmaniasis** (kala-azar) is caused by *Leishmania donovani,* which invades the mononuclear phagocytic system, causing hepatosplenomegaly, lymphadenopathy, pancytopenia, fever, weight loss, and elevated serum IgG. Treated survivors may develop disfiguring lesions reminiscent of leprosy. **Mucocutaneous leishmaniasis** (espundia), due to *Leishmania brasiliensis* and other species, is observed in South America, particularly Brazil. An initial chronic skin ulcer is followed by leishmania-containing lesions located at mucocutaneous junctions that slowly progress to granulomas. **Cutaneous leishmaniasis** (tropical sore), associated with *Leishmania major* and *Leishmania mexicana,* is observed in both the Old and New Worlds, and it often involves the ear. **Diffuse cutaneous leishmaniasis** is found in Ethiopia, Venezuela, Brazil, and Mexico. This is the least common form of dermal infection and begins as a single skin nodule. It then

Leishmania **cause several forms of chronic skin and visceral diseases.**

spreads to involve nearly all of the body with bizarre nodular lesions composed of aggregates of leishmanial stuffed macrophages.

Toxoplasmosis

Toxoplasma gondii is an intracellular parasite that is usually acquired by ingestion of oocysts from cat feces and less commonly by ingestion of tissue forms in poorly cooked meat. *Toxoplasma gondii* tachyzoites are bow-shaped organisms approximately 3 x 6 μm found outside host cells. The intracellular form of the organism is the bradyzoite, which is found in large numbers within cysts. Infection in immunocompetent persons usually causes mild, self-terminating infection. In contrast, vulnerable individuals (**fetuses, babies, and immunosuppressed patients**) can experience devastating toxoplasmosis characterized by severe central nervous system damage, blindness, or both. Pregnant women are advised to avoid infected or potentially infected cats and to abstain from eating uncooked meat. *Toxoplasma gondii* enters via the gastrointestinal tract, spreads in the form of **tachyzoites,** and can penetrate virtually any type of host cell to form **cysts** filled with bradyzoites. The parasites can be identified in large numbers in newborns and immunosuppressed patients, where they are visible as tiny single dots. Small numbers of cysts containing large numbers (hundreds) of bradyzoites can also occasionally be found, and are quite distinctive. Neonatal toxoplasmosis is characterized by the formation of destructive lesions throughout the body, particularly the brain. A severe form of acute adult toxoplasmosis resembles neonatal toxoplasmosis, but tends to be somewhat less destructive. *Toxoplasma* chorioretinitis is associated with a granulomatous reaction in the choroid and sclera to tachyzoite proliferation with subsequent destruction of the retina.

HELMINTHIC DISEASES

Helminths (worms) are highly evolved endoparasites. Individual worms persist for long periods of time within the host. The worms typically produce eggs or larvae, which are then cycled to the environment and through intermediate hosts before they can infect humans again. In general, helminths have strict host specificities, and achieve only stunted development in unsuitable hosts. Worldwide, millions of people are infected with helminths. Normally, only heavily infected patients become ill.

INTESTINAL ROUNDWORMS

Ascariasis

Ascaris lumbricoides is the most common and largest (up to 35 cm) of the intestinal roundworms. It has a worldwide distribution and is spread between humans by fecal–oral contamination. *Ascaris lumbricoides* inhabits the gut lumen, often without producing disease. Ascaris eggs are fecally excreted with release of the larvae when the eggs reach the stomach of a new host. These larvae migrate systemically, and re-enter the gut via the lung, larynx, and trachea. After this second re-entering of the gut, the worms remain within the gut lumen and mature to adults. Ascariasis is occasionally complicated by gut obstruction, intestinal perforation, bacterial infection, peritonitis, cholangitis, sepsis, or allergic respiratory symptoms.

Ascariasis occasionally causes gut obstruction, cholangitis, peritonitis, sepsis, or allergic respiratory symptoms.

Trichuriasis

Trichuris trichuria (whipworm) is a small (5 cm or less) intestinal roundworm with an attenuated anterior "whip." This common worldwide parasite is transmitted by fecal contamination and does not usually cause symptomatic disease. Occasionally, mentally retarded patients or poor children, usually in the tropics, may acquire large numbers of worms, which may cause eosinophilia, tenesmus, persistent diarrhea, and occasionally intestinal obstruction, intussusception, or rectal prolapse.

Whipworm infection occasionally causes intestinal obstruction or rectal prolapse.

Enterobiasis

Enterobius vermicularis (pinworm) is a small (less than about 1.3 cm) roundworm with prominent lateral ridges (alae) that inhabits the distal gut. Female worms migrate nightly to the perianal skin to lay eggs, causing intense pruritis, insomnia, and irritability. These eggs can be passed to siblings and sometimes adults. Diagnosis is usually made either by inspection of the anus for worms, or by placing a piece of Scotch tape over the anus to pick up eggs, which can be visualized by microscopy.

Female pinworms lay eggs on perianal skin.

Hookworm Disease

Necator americanus and *Ancylostoma duodenale* are distinctive intestinal roundworms (hookworms) that feed on blood rather than gut lumenal contents. These roundworms have sharp mouthplates that penetrate duodenal and jejunal mucosa. The worms are not particularly efficient at ingesting the released blood, much of which is wastefully excreted into the intestinal lumen. Iron deficiency anemia is seen in heavy infections, typically when hookworm disease coexists with other potential causes of iron deficiency anemia. The parasites penetrate unshod skin of human feet; migrate systemically through the body to reach the lungs; and then re-enter the gut by being expectorated and swallowed. Larval migration through the lung is usually clinically silent. The larvae then mature in the human gastrointestinal tract, and obtain lengths of up to about 1 m. Hookworm infection tends to be most serious in children who inhabit areas, such as the tropics, where fecal soil contamination is heavy. Heavily infected malnourished individuals may develop anemia, hypoalbuminemia, and intestinal malabsorption.

Hookworms attach to intestinal mucosa and feed on blood.

Strongyloidiasis

Strongyloides stercoralis is a parthenogenic roundworm that is only 1 mm in length when mature; it can be buried entirely in an intestinal crypt of the duodenum or upper jejunum, where the worms live. This predilection for inhabiting intestinal crypts tends to damage the absorptive surface of the gut, leading to malabsorption syndrome and chronic enteritis. Larvae produced within the lumen by *Strongyloides stercoralis*

***Strongyloides* hyperinfection is potentially fatal.**

can be passed in an infective state to the soil, or they can be reingested, or can penetrate the host intestine itself. This latter ability permits the development of *Strongyloides* "**hyperinfection**" with progressive, potentially lethal accumulations of worms and migratory larvae. *Strongyloides* hyperinfection is more apt to be observed in malnourished and immunosuppressed individuals. The larvae usually initially enter the body by penetrating skin, migrate to the lung, and then are expectorated and swallowed. The chronic intestinal phase of the infection may either be asymptomatic, or may be associated with intermittent bouts of diarrhea. A small percentage of patients exhibit a spruelike syndrome with weight loss, fatty stools, and a protein-losing enteropathy. Fatal infections may have worms throughout the body. The roundworm *Capillaria philippinensis* can cause a similar syndrome in the Philippines and Northeast Thailand.

TISSUE ROUNDWORMS

Visceral Larva Migrans

Visceral larva migrans is due to larval migration in humans of dog or cat parasites.

The human is an accidental host for the *Toxocara* parasites that normally infect puppies (**Toxocara cani**) and kittens (**Toxocara cati**). Infection in humans is acquired by ingestion of eggs excreted in canine or feline fecal material. Following ingestion, the **larvae** are liberated, enter the circulatory system, and then can reach any organ (liver, lung, heart, nervous system, eye) of the body. Worm development can only progress to the larval stage, but can cause significant tissue destruction and hypersensitivity reactions. The larvae provoke lesions with central necrosis surrounded by eosinophil-rich inflammatory foci that may contain Charcot-Leyden crystals. The usual clinical presentation includes fever, hepatosplenomegaly, and sometimes prominent gastrointestinal, respiratory, or visual symptoms. Diagnosis is established by serologic tests or identification of larvae in tissue samples. Human infection tends to be self-terminating, but the course can be alleviated, and possibly prevented, by treatment.

Guinea Worm Infection

The long guinea worm migrates subcutaneously and discharges larvae through broken skin blisters.

Dracunculus medinensis (guinea worm) is a very long (over 1 m) thin tissue helminth that burrows into human subcutaneous tissue, causing painful inflammatory swellings of the skin. The worm is acquired by ingestion of drinking water containing the freshwater **cyclops,** which serves as the intermediary host. The adult worm discharges larvae into skin blisters (often on the outer malleous of the foot) that subsequently rupture in water and are vulnerable to bacterial superinfection.

Trichinosis

Trichinella **larvae encyst in striated muscle cells.**

Trichinella spiralis is a parasite whose larvae are transmitted by ingestion of larvae encysted in muscle. The human is an accidental host. The parasite can be present in many carnivores including pig, bear, and wild game. Regulations pertaining to pork handling have reduced the incidence of trichinosis in the United States. The larvae encysted in improperly cooked meat are released in the stomach by proteolytic digestion. They mature to adult worms in the duodenum, causing transitory enteritis. The adult worm copulates and produces large numbers of larvae that penetrate into the lacteals to reach the bloodstream. The adult worms subsequently die and are expelled. The larvae travel through the body and can produce tissue damage at many sites including lung, heart, and brain. When they reach striated skeletal muscle cells, they penetrate the muscle cells and become enclosed within a membrane produced by the host. They then persist in this state without death of either the muscle cell (**"nurse cell"**) or the larvae for periods of years. Death of the larvae and the host's skeletal muscle cell induces a marked inflammatory reaction composed of lymphocytes and eosinophils. The larval site may eventually calcify. The larvae have a predilection for parasitization of the most active muscles of the body, including diaphragm, extraocular eye muscles, laryngeal muscles, deltoid, gastrocnemius, and intercostal muscles. While the larvae survive only encysted in skeletal muscle, their entry into cells in other tissues can cause disease, including myocarditis, that may lead to cardiac failure, pulmonary edema or hemorrhage, and leptomeningitis.

Filariasis

Filariae are long, string-like nematodes introduced into the body by the bite of an insect vector in the form of third-stage larvae. The larvae subsequently migrate from the biting site to their definitive habitat in the human body. After several months of maturation, mating occurs, and the fertilized females release tiny filariae into lymph, blood, or skin, where they are available to be taken up by biting insects, completing the cycle. While only a few cases are observed in the United States, filarial disease infects many millions of people in the world.

Filariasis is an important cause of disease worldwide.

Lymphatic filariasis (elephantiasis) can be caused either by *Wuchereria bancrofti* or *Brugia malayi. Wuchereria bancrofti* has a worldwide tropical distribution; can measure up to 10 cm in length; and has no known animal reservoir. *Brugia malayi* is a smaller filariae measuring up to 2.5 cm; is limited to Southeast Asia; and can use monkeys and cats as potential reservoir hosts. The specific insect vector varies with the species and is usually a mosquito. The urban form of *Wuchereria bancrofti* filariasis tends to be milder than the rural form. Newcomers to endemic areas may develop fever, scrotal swelling, urticarial rashes, or tender lymphadenopathy. Chronically, the filariae have a predilection for lymphatic invasion with secondary persistent severe edema (lymphedema) that can involve the scrotum, penis, leg, vulva, breast, or arm. The lymphedema is associated with subcutaneous fibrosis and epithelial hyperkeratosis (elephantiasis). Disintegrating worms tend to cause the worst inflammation. With time, the acute inflammation becomes replaced by granulomas resembling tubercules in which a diligent search may reveal the parasite's cuticular remnants.

Elephantiasis is due to filariae in lymphatics.

Onchocerciasis is caused by the largest (up to 50 cm) of the human filariae, *Onchocerca volvulus.* This filariae is transmitted by the *Simulium* species of blackflies. The adult worms nest in subcutaneous tissue rather than in lymphatics. Microfilariae are discharged into the interstitium of the skin. Severe infections can cause chronic dermatitis and blindness, with large numbers of microfilariae accumulated in skin and eye chambers. Onchocerciasis is endemic in Africa, Yemen, and Central America.

***Onchocerca* filariae are found in subcutaneous tissues.**

Loa loa ("eye worm") migrates under the skin, particularly the conjunctiva, and causes transient skin swellings. ***Dipetalonema streptocerca*** causes skin nodules that may resemble leprosy or onchocerciasis. Both of these microfilarial diseases induce eosinophilia, and sometimes fever, but rarely cause incapacitating illness.

Zoonotic filariasis can cause human disease. In general, the zoonotic filariases do not cause common or serious illness, but may present diagnostic puzzles. ***Dirofilaria immitis*** is the dog heartworm, and is capable of developing into the larval stage in humans. The larvae inhabit cardiac chambers, and may cause small pulmonary infarctions when they embolize into a pulmonary artery branch. A raccoon worm, ***Dirofilaria tenuis,*** can cause inflammatory subcutaneous nodules resembling granulomas or dermatofibromas; these worms are also found in the conjunctiva. A parasite of raccoons and other wild animals along the Eastern seaboard of the United States causes **North American Brugia,** which typically presents as a swollen lymph node on the neck or thorax. Excision of the lymph node is curative.

CESTODES

The **platyhelminthes** (cestodes) are flatworms that have a small head or scolex, and a body composed of rectangular proglottids that produce eggs. Human tapeworms can cause infection either through attaching of the mature tapeworm to the intestinal wall or invasion of organs of the body by larval forms.

Intestinal Tapeworm Infections

Tapeworms causing intestinal disease in humans include ***Taenia saginata*** (beef), ***Taenia solium*** (pork), ***Hymenolepis nana*** (dwarf), and ***Diphyllobothrium latum*** (fish). These tapeworms are usually acquired by ingestion of undercooked meat or fish, and have a worldwide distribution. The undercooked meat or fish contains encysted larvae that mature in the human intestinal tract. Adult tapeworms have a **scolex** that bears hooks and sucker plates, which permits their attachment to the bowel wall, where they remain throughout their life. These worms may become very long (up to 6 m), and in some cases, the presence of even a single worm, notably *Taenia solium,* may prevent the acquisition of additional infections. In patients with only a small tapeworm load, the worms may cause no symptomatic disease. The principal clinical manifestations observed when systematic disease is produced are intestinal obstruction due to the mass of worms, and megaloblastic anemia due to ingestion by the worms of vitamin B_{12}. Diagnosis is by finding of proglottids or eggs in stools, or contrast media radiography to show the outlines of large tapeworms. Worms removed with vermifuges should be examined to be sure that the scolex has been expelled, since the worms are capable of regenerating.

Cysticercosis

Taenia solium can cause both intestinal tapeworm infection when the adult tapeworm is ingested in uncooked pork, or **cysticercosis** when the *Taenia* eggs are ingested on fecally contaminated vegetables, or by self-contamination with eggs from a human *Taenia solium* intestinal infection. Cysticercosis is a more serious condition than is intestinal tapeworm. The ingested eggs give rise to an embryo that penetrates the gut to enter the circulatory system, where it develops into a larva (cysticercus). These larvae can be disseminated throughout the body to any site, including central nervous system and heart. Disease manifestations vary with the number and location of the cysticerci. The encysted larval form produces a cyst with a thick (greater than 100 μm) cyst wall rich in glycoproteins, which contains an invaginated scolex bathed in clear cyst fluid. These cysts can range up to 1.5 cm in size. Intact cysts invoke little host response, and may remain dormant for many years. Eventually, they degenerate and can induce granuloma formation, focal scarring, and calcification, which may be visible on radiographs as round, opaque densities. Degenerate forms of cysticerci are recognizable, because the tiny shark-tooth-shaped hooklets remain long after the death of the organism.

Larval *Taenia solium* (cysticerci) can encyst through the body.

Echinococcosis

The *Echinococcus* genus contains tapeworms whose definitive host for the adult worms is the dog. The human is an accidental intermediary host who acquires infection by ingesting the eggs, which subsequently hatch in the duodenum. The released embryos cross the small intestinal mucosa to enter branches of the portal venous system. The infection is initially silent. The embryos form slowly growing parasitic cysts called hydatids in the liver and other organs. The cysts may eventually compress vital structures, release markedly allergenic cyst fluid, or form large numbers of "daughter cysts." Cysts are also vulnerable to bacterial superinfection with abscess formation. The **European strain of** *Echinococcus granulosus* is observed throughout the world where sheep of European ancestry are present, forms a unilocular hydatid cyst, and has a life cycle involving both dogs and sheep. A **northern strain of** *Echinococcus granulosus* less commonly causes disease because the cycle involves wolves and deer. The northern strain is associated with particularly severe disease. *Echinococcus multilocularis* and *Echinococcus vogeli* are two additional species that cause multilocular hydatid cysts, which can invade the liver, much like a tumor. Diagnosis can be made with serologic tests for *Echinococcus granulosus* antigen and antibodies; computed tomography has also facilitated diagnosis. Drug therapy can sterilize cysts; surgery may be necessary to remove larger cysts or cysts located in key locations.

Echinococcus causes hepatic hydatid cysts.

TREMATODES

Fascioliasis

Fasciola hepatica is a hermaphroditic flatworm (trematode or fluke) for which humans are an accidental host. Human fascioliasis is acquired by eating watercress contaminated with the metacercarial form of the parasite, which is released into the water by sheep and cattle feces. In humans, the ingested metacercarial forms migrate from the gut into the tissues, causing fever and abdominal pains. The flukes have a predilection for growing in the gallbladder and bile ducts, and chronically may

Fasciola can cause biliary obstruction.

cause biliary obstruction. *Fasciola hepatica* is found throughout the world in both temperate and tropical zones including Puerto Rico; ***Fasciola gigantica*** causes similar disease in Hawaii. The adult *Fasciola hepatica* parasites have a leaf shape that can be up to several centimeters long. *Fasciola* eggs are present in usually small numbers in the feces, and have a distinctive, operculated morphology. Uncommonly, ectopic migration of worms in subcutaneous tissue can produce painful nodules.

Clonorchiasis and Opisthorchiasis

Clonorchis and *Opisthorchis* are associated with chronic cholangitis, gallstones, and cholangiae carcinoma.

Clonorchis sinensis and ***Opisthorchis viverrini*** are small liver flukes that are acquired by eating raw freshwater fish or crayfish containing metacercariae. *Clonorchis sinensis* is found in inner China and other areas of the Far East; *Opisthorchis viverrini* is found in Thailand and Laos; ***Opisthorchis felineus*** is found in Poland and the Soviet Union. In general, these organisms can infect humans, dogs, and cats and are often present in large numbers. In contrast to *Fasciola hepatica,* they often produce prominent chronic cholangitis with extensive liver damage and intrahepatic gallstones as a consequence of colonization of the small and large intrahepatic bile ducts. These liver flukes are also associated with an increased incidence of cholangiocarcinoma. The tiny (30 μm), thick-walled, operculated eggs of these liver fluke species can be found in the stools and are diagnostic.

Fasciolopsiasis

Fasciolopsis buski is an intestinal fluke.

Fasciolopsis buski is a large intestinal fluke that can be up to centimeters long. The flukes have a complex life cycle involving humans or other animals (pigs), snails, and free-living forms. After ingestion of cysts on water plants, the larval forms emerge in the human upper gastrointestinal tract, where they mature into adult worms and attach to the small bowel mucosa by suckers. The sucker attachment locally causes an initially nonspecific hemorrhagic inflammation containing principally eosinophils, which may progress to actual formation of mucosal abscesses with destruction of intestinal mucosa. *Fasciolopsis buski* infection is found principally in China and countries abutting the Indian Ocean. Patients often experience abdominal pain and diarrhea; in the presence of heavy fluke burdens, they may have fever accompanied by facial and periorbital edema. Uncommonly, acute intestinal obstruction may follow tangling of masses of worms in the gut lumen. The diagnosis is usually made by identification of characteristic eggs in fecal material.

Paragonimiasis

Paragonimus flukes can infect lung, brain, and abdominal organs.

The *Paragonimus* flukes are small flatworms (1.2-cm long) that are ingested in metacercarial form from uncooked crabs and crayfish; they cause cystic and inflammatory lesions in the **lung** and, less commonly, the brain and abdominal organs. These flukes usually have many definitive hosts including dogs, cats, and humans. Human pulmonic involvement is characterized by chronic cough, bronchiectasis, and hemoptysis. Paragonimiasis was initially thought to be due only to ***Paragonimus***

westermani, which is localized in the Far East and the Philippines but it has since been established that other species found in tropical countries and other sites can cause the condition. The ingested flukes cross the gut wall, peritoneum, and diaphragm to migrate to the lung. This migration does not usually cause significant lesions or symptoms, unless the parasites die in ectopic locations (gut wall, pancreas, brain), where focal abscesses can occur. Once the parasites reach the lung, they incite an inflammatory host reaction and exist in multiple cysts. The wall around the cysts is formed by the host and begins as an encapsulated inflammatory reaction rich in eosinophils that progresses to formation of a fibrous capsule, which may contain granulomas. Often present are abscesslike collections of eosinophils mixed with Charcot-Leyden crystals. The cysts eventually rupture into bronchioles, and the eggs, exudate, and blood are expectorated or swallowed. Those eggs that reach bodies of water are available for release of miracidia, which enter several snail species. Long-standing paragonimiasis can resemble tuberculosis. Diagnosis is dependent on identification of thick-shelled, operculated eggs in sputum or feces. Depending on the degree of infection, symptoms may be mild, or lethal disease may be produced.

Schistosomiasis

Schistosomes are a trematode species that reproduce sexually in venous blood. In general, the adult parasites do not produce much pathology. The eggs can cause hypersensitivity granulomas whose site varies with the infecting species. The most important human schistosomal species are **Schistosoma mansoni** (Africa, Latin America, Near East), **Schistosoma japonicum** (Far East), and **Schistosoma haematobium** (Africa, Near East). *Schistosoma haematobium* tends to infest the pelvic vena caval tributaries; other schistosoma species preferentially seek the portal vein branches.

Human schistosomiasis is typically acquired when **free-swimming cercariae** in contaminated water burrow through the human epidermis and convert to the young worm form **(schistosomula).** The worms migrate to the lung and then liver via the bloodstream. The worms then descend into mesenteric or pelvic venules where they begin mating and laying large numbers of **eggs.** The females preferentially seek venules near the gut or urinary lumen, and expulsion of the eggs can cause the excretion into feces or urine. Other eggs are either caught in the blood vessels, or swept back into the bloodstream into the liver or lung. This acute phase may be either asymptomatic, or patients may have nonspecific symptoms. With time, the often millions of eggs release soluble antigens that incite host cellular immunity and hypersensitivity, causing formations of perivascular granulomas, which are often rich in eosinophils. Following the death of the egg, the individual granulomas heal, sometimes with fibrous scarring. However, since the adults continue to produce eggs, new crops continue to appear. In patients containing large numbers of worms with **heavy egg burdens,** severe fibrotic lesions will eventually develop. Light *Schistosoma mansoni* or *Schistosoma japonicum* infections are characterized by scattered eggs with pinhead-sized granulomas involving the gut, liver, and lung; they occur sporadically elsewhere. Severe schistosomiasis mansoni or japonica can produce

Schistosomes are blood flukes that lay eggs in the portal vein branches or pelvic vena caval tributaries.

Millions of eggs may be produced.

Schistosoma haematobium **usually involves the bladder rather than the gut.**

colonic pseudopolyps, fibrous portal enlargement in the liver (**pipe stem fibrosis),** granulomatous **pulmonary arteritis,** and **renal glomerular disease.**

Schistosoma haematobium infection differs from *Schistosoma mansoni* or *Schistosoma japonicum* in that the predominant involvement is in the **bladder.** An early massed egg deposition can cause bladder inflammation, which later develops sandy or fibrous patches. The entire bladder mucosa may eventually develop a radiologically visible calcified layer. Multiple ureteral stenoses due to inflammation and fibrosis secondary to egg deposition may cause hydronephrosis. Renal failure and death can occur. Patients with a history of *Schistosoma haematobium* are predisposed for developing squamous cell carcinoma of the bladder.

6

Hematopoietic System

ERYTHROCYTES AND HEMORRHAGIC DIATHESES

ANEMIAS OF BLOOD LOSS

Shift of fluid from the interstitial space into the vascular space after **acute blood loss** helps to restore blood pressure, but also causes a decrease in hematocrit that reaches a minimum 2 to 3 days after the hemorrhage. Mobilization of platelets and neutrophils from marginal pools causes thrombocytosis and leukocytosis. The reticulocyte count may increase to 10 to 15 percent of the total erythrocyte count by 1 week after a significant hemorrhage. Mild **chronic blood loss** does not usually cause anemia, unless it is superimposed on other causes, such as depleted iron resources, that limit the regenerative capacity of the erythroid precursors. Iron deficiency anemia may also develop if significant external hemorrhage has occurred.

The body handles acute and mild chronic blood loss differently.

HEMOLYTIC ANEMIAS

Hemolytic anemias of diverse etiologies show many similar features. Increased erythrocyte destruction shortens the erythrocyte life span and increases erythropoiesis. The products of erythrocyte catabolism, notably hemoglobin, may also accumulate. **Intravascular hemolysis** can cause hemoglobinemia, methemalbuminea, hemoglobinuria, hemosiderinuria, and jaundice secondary to increased unconjugated bilirubin. In **extravascular hemolysis,** which most often occurs in the spleen, hemoglobinemia and hemoglobinuria are not prominent, but jaundice and anemia still occur. The marrow responds in both types of hemolysis with markedly increased numbers of normoblasts that produce a prominent reticulocytosis in the peripheral blood. Expansion of bone marrow in severe cases may cause pressure atrophy of the inner table of cortical

Hemolytic anemias of many etiologies are clinically similar.

77

bone in ribs, facial bones, and calvaria. Increased bilirubin may induce pigment gallstone cholelithiasis. Hemosiderin may be deposited in tissues, usually within reticular-endothelial cells.

HEREDITARY HEMOLYTIC ANEMIAS

Hereditary hemolytic anemias can be due to disorders of the erythrocyte plasma membrane, enzymes, or hemoglobin synthesis.

The hereditary hemolytic anemias are associated with intrinsic abnormalities of erythrocytes that typically cause principally extravascular hemolysis due to phagocytic ingestion of erythrocytes in the splenic sinusoids. The major hereditary hemolytic anemias can be subclassified as disorders of the red cell membrane, red cell enzymes, and hemoglobin synthesis.

Red Cell Membrane Disorders

Hereditary spherocytosis is a red cell membrane cytoskeleton disorder.

Hereditary spherocytosis is the most important intrinsic red cell membrane disorder and is observed in people of Northern European descent. It is characterized by spheroidal erythrocytes; moderate splenic congestion and enlargement; and other changes typical of extravascular hemolytic anemias. The altered erythrocyte geometry is often due to deficiency of the cytoskeleton protein spectrin. Affected newborns may exhibit marked jaundice and require exchange transfusion. Older patients typically have a stable clinical course that is interrupted by anemic crises due to massive active hemolysis or temporary failure of erythropoiesis. Splenectomy usually ameliorates the anemia, although the spherocytes persist. Less common hereditary red cell membrane disorders include the cytoskeleton disorder elliptocytosis and disorders of lipid synthesis that produce a selective increase in membrane lecithin.

TRAUMATIC HEMOLYTIC ANEMIA

Erythrocytes are fragmented by passing through abnormal vessels in microangiopathic hemolytic anemia.

In **microangiopathic hemolytic anemia,** narrowed or obstructed arterioles and capillaries traumatize erythrocytes, causing fragmentation with significant intravascular hemolysis. Microangiopathic hemolytic anemia can occur in malignant hypertension, disseminated intravascular coagulation, thrombotic thrombocytopenic purpura, systemic lupus erythematosus, renal disease, and metastatic cancer. The peripheral smear shows many erythrocyte abnormalities, including fragmented erythrocytes (schistocytes), burr cells, and helmet cells. Traumatic hemolytic anemia can also be produced by the shear stresses of turbulent flow around prosthetic heart valves. Traumatic hemolytic anemias are usually mild, and the patient's clinical course is dominated by the underlying disease.

ANEMIAS OF DIMINISHED ERYTHROPOIESIS

Anemia due to diminished erythropoiesis can be the result of either a deficiency of an essential nutrient (iron, vitamin B_{12}, or folate) or marrow stem cell failure (aplastic anemia, pure red cell aplasia, or anemia of renal failure).

Megaloblastic Anemias

The peripheral blood in **megaloblastic anemias** is characterized by erythrocyte anisocytosis with many macrocytic, oval-shaped cells with mean corpuscular volumes over 100 mm^3. The peripheral blood additionally shows a reduced reticulocyte count, nucleated erythrocytes, and hypersegmented neutrophils. Both the abnormal erythrocytes and the abnormal neutrophils appear to form as the result of delayed DNA synthesis compared with synthesis of other cell constituents. Despite the decreased production of mature erythrocytes, the **bone marrow** in megaloblastic anemias is characteristically hypercellular and usually has an increased erythroid to myeloid ratio. Megakaryocytes may be enlarged and have multilobate nuclei. The observed anemia is a consequence of both **ineffective erythropoiesis** and **hemolysis** of the abnormal erythrocytes. Leukopenia and thrombocytopenia may occur, in part because granulocyte and platelet precursors are also vulnerable to lysis. With time, patients tend to develop hemosiderosis secondary to the hemolysis.

Vitamin B$_{12}$ and folic acid deficiency are the most common causes of megaloblastic anemia. Deficiencies of vitamin B$_{12}$ or folate can be due to increased requirement (pregnancy, metastatic cancer, increased hematopoiesis) or deficient intake (poor diet, many malabsorption states). Vitamin B$_{12}$ deficiency is also associated with intestinal bacterial overgrowth, tapeworms, or intrinsic factor deficiency due to gastrectomy or pernicious anemia. Folic acid deficiency can additionally be due to impaired absorption due to oral contraceptives or anticonvulsants; increased loss by hemodialysis; or impaired utilization because of folic acid antagonists. Megaloblastic anemias that are not responsive to vitamin B$_{12}$ or folic acid therapy also occur and can be due to drugs (mercaptopurines, fluorouracil, cytosine); as part of acute erythroleukemia; and as pyridoxine- and thiamine-responsive megaloblastic anemia. In vitamin B$_{12}$ deficiency, but not folate deficiency, neurologic changes (subacute combined degeneration of the spinal cord) are also observed.

Pernicious anemia, a form of megaloblastic anemia, occurs as a consequence of chronic atrophic gastritis with profound loss of gastric parietal cells, which normally synthesize intrinsic factor. The resulting lack of gut lumenal intrinsic factor limits absorption of vitamin B$_{12}$, which is normally absorbed bound to intrinsic factor. Pernicious anemia was formerly an intractable form of chronic anemia that is now treated by parenteral B$_{12}$. Nonanemic features of pernicious anemia include atrophic glossitis; chronic atrophic gastritis; myelin degeneration of the dorsal and lateral tracts of the spinal cord; and widespread nonspecific alterations secondary to generalized tissue hypoxia. The initial cause of pernicious anemia appears to be autoantibodies directed against gastric parietal cells or B$_{12}$–intrinsic factor complexes. Pernicious anemia may coexist with autoimmune thyroid and adrenal diseases. **Juvenile pernicious anemia** is similar to the adult form, but is not associated with chronic gastric atrophy and may be due to hereditary defects in the synthesis or absorption of intrinsic factor.

IRON DEFICIENCY ANEMIA

Iron deficiency anemia is common throughout the world. Iron deficiency can be caused by low dietary intake or malabsorption that may be either generalized (sprue, celiac disease) or follow gastrectomy, which

The abnormal cells in megaloblastic anemias appear to form as the result of delayed DNA synthesis.

The most common causes of megaloblastic anemia are folate and vitamin B$_{12}$ deficiency.

In pernicious anemia, chronic atrophic gastritis causes vitamin B$_{12}$ deficiency.

increases duodenal transit time by decreasing acidity. Chronic blood loss, typically from the gastrointestinal tract (ulcers, cancer, intestinal parasites, hemorrhoids) or female genital tract (menstruation, cancer), is the most common cause in the western world. Iron deficiency anemia is also encountered in states associated with increased iron demand such as infancy and pregnancy. Iron deficiency of all causes produces a hypochromic microcytic anemia. The bone marrow may show increased erythropoiesis in the form of increased normoblasts, but sideroblasts are diminished or absent, and iron cannot be stained in the marrow reticuloendothelial cells. **Plummer-Vinson syndrome** is the cluster of microcytic hypochromic anemia, esophageal webs, and atrophic glossitis; the pathologic significance of this cluster of findings has been questioned since they may simply represent a coexistence of several common diseases. The diagnosis of iron deficiency anemia can be substantiated by demonstrating increased iron-binding capacity and below normal values for serum iron and serum ferritin.

APLASTIC ANEMIA

Aplastic anemia is actually a pancytopenia characterized by failure of multipotent myeloid stem cells leading to anemia, neutropenia, and thrombocytopenia. In contrast to iron deficiency and megaloblastic anemias, the **bone marrow** is almost always markedly hypocellular, with reduced numbers in all cell lines. Aplastic anemia occurs in hereditary **(Fanconi's anemia)** and, more commonly, acquired forms. Acquired aplastic anemia has many causes, including idiopathic stem cell defects; idiopathic immune-mediated anemia; drugs with dose-related aplastic anemia (antineoplastic agents, benzene, chloramphenicol, arsenicals); drugs that produce idiosyncratic anemia (chloramphenicol, phenylbutazone, arsenicals, hydantoins, streptomycin, chlorpromazine, insecticides); physical agents (radiation); and viral infections (cytomegalovirus, Epstein-Barr virus, non-A and non-B hepatitis, herpes varicella-zoster). The peripheral smear usually shows erythrocytes with normal morphology or slight macrocytosis. A distinctive feature is a nearly complete absence of reticulocytes. Splenomegaly is characteristically absent. Aplastic anemia must be distinguished from other causes of pancytopenia such as **"aleukemic" leukemia** and myelodysplastic syndromes. The prognosis for aplastic anemia varies with etiology. Removal of a toxic drug sometimes permits marrow recovery. In idiopathic cases, the prognosis is poor, but bone marrow transplantation or antithymocyte globulin may be effective.

PURE RED CELL APLASIA

Pure red cell aplasia may be considered a variant of aplastic anemia in which only the erythrocyte line is aplastic. Acute aplastic "crises" can occur as a complication of hemolytic anemia, drug therapy, or infection. Chronic pure red cell aplasia tends to develop insidiously, and many affected patients have a coexisting thymoma whose removal may ameliorate the red cell aplasia. Immunosuppressive therapy may be helpful in patients with autoantibodies directed against erythroid precursors.

OTHER FORMS OF
MARROW FAILURE

Other causes of marrow failure include space-occupying lesions, severe liver or renal disease, and some infections and chronic inflammatory states.

POLYCYTHEMIA

An increased concentration of peripheral red cells is called **poly-cythemia** (erythrocytosis). **Relative polycythemia** occurs when red cells become concentrated due to reduction of plasma volume by processes such as dehydration, vomiting, diarrhea, or diuresis. **Primary absolute polycythemia** (polycythemia vera, see also p. 98) is the result of an intrinsic abnormality that causes proliferation of myeloid stem cells and appears to be similar to other myeloproliferative disorders. **Secondary absolute polycythemias** are usually due to increased erythropoietin levels, which may be either physiologically appropriately due to stimuli such as lung disease or cyanotic heart disease, or an inappropriate result of secretion by tumors (renal cell carcinoma, cerebellar hemangioblastoma, hepatoma).

Polycythemia may be relative or absolute; absolute polycythemia occurs in primary and secondary forms.

PAROXYSMAL NOCTURNAL
HEMOGLOBINURIA

Paroxysmal nocturnal hemoglobinuria is an acquired intrinsic disorder of erythrocytes characterized by chronic intravascular hemolysis. Paroxysmal nocturnal hemoglobinuria appears to be due to deficiency of a membrane glycoprotein, decay accelerating factor. The deficiency causes the erythrocytes to be unusually sensitive to complement-mediated lysis. These patients are also vulnerable to intravascular thromboses and infections. The deficiency of decay accelerating factor may be caused by proliferation of an abnormal clone of multipotent myeloid stem cells. Occasional patients with paroxysmal nocturnal hemoglobinuria later develop other stem cell disorders, including aplastic anemia and acute leukemia. Despite the name, most patients experience chronic hemolysis without dramatic hemoglobinuria. These patients have a median survival of 10 years, with death commonly being related to infection or venous thrombosis, particularly in hepatic, portal, or cerebral veins.

The erythrocytes in paroxysmal nocturnal hemoglobinuria are unusually sensitive to complement-mediated lysis.

AUTOIMMUNE HEMOLYTIC
ANEMIAS

The **autoimmune hemolytic** (immunohemolytic) **anemias** are characterized by hemolysis related to the appearance of antierythrocyte antibodies. All of these diseases produce a **positive Coombs antiglobulin test.** In this test, the invo coating of the patient's erythrocytes by autoimmune antibodies causes erythrocytes to agglutinate when animal antibodies to human globulins are added. The autoimmune hemolytic anemias can be classified based upon the characteristics of the autoimmune antibody.

Autoimmune hemolytic anemias are due to antierythrocyte antibodies.

Warm Antibody Autoimmune Hemolytic Anemia

Warm antibody hemolytic anemia is usually due to IgG.

Warm antibody autoimmune anemia is typically caused by **IgG antibodies** that are active at normal body temperature and do not fix complement. They may occur idiopathically or secondary to neoplastic diseases (lymphomas, leukemias), autoimmune disorders (systemic lupus erythematosus), and drugs. Since the IgG autoantibodies do not activate complement, the hemolysis is characteristically extravascular and occurs in the spleen, which develops moderate to severe splenomegaly. Drug-induced warm autoantibodies are most clearly understood. The drugs can induce antibody formation by a variety of mechanisms that include acting as a hapten bound to the red cell membrane (penicillin, cephalosporins); acting as a hapten bound to serum proteins with subsequent formation of an immune complex that binds to the red cell (quinidine, phenacetin); and initiating autoantibodies directed against intrinsic red cell antigens, typically Rh blood group antigens (methyldopa).

Cold Agglutinin Autoimmune Hemolytic Anemia

IgM antibodies are associated with cold agglutinin autoimmune hemolytic anemia.

Cold agglutinin autoimmune hemolytic anemia is typically caused by IgM antibodies that usually agglutinate erythrocytes and fix complement only in the peripheral cool parts of the body. Acute cold agglutinin antibodies are usually observed during the recovery phase of infections including mycoplasmal pneumonia and infectious mononucleosis. These antibodies usually do not cause hemolysis, and their production is self-limited. In contrast, chronic cold agglutinin antibodies can be either idiopathic or associated with lymphoproliferative disorders (lymphomas). The chronic autoantibodies are often monoclonal and act by fixing the complement factor C3b to erythrocyte surfaces. The coated cells are then susceptible to phagocytosis, which, for unknown reasons, usually occurs in the liver rather than the sinusoids of the spleen. Patients also experience Raynaud's phenomenon and cyanosis of exposed body parts secondary to vascular obstruction by agglutinated erythrocytes.

Cold Hemolysin Autoimmune Hemolytic Anemia

IgG antibodies are associated with cold hemolysin autoimmune hemolytic anemia.

Cold hemolysin autoimmune hemolytic anemia is characteristically due to IgG autoantibodies that can bind to erythrocytes at low temperatures. This particular type of IgG antibody appears most often to be directed against **P blood group antigen;** can fix complement; and can cause intravascular hemolysis. Patients experience paroxysmal cold hemoglobinuria, characterized by massive hemolysis following cold exposure. Patients may also experience hemoglobinuria, fever, and muscle pain. Most cases of paroxysmal cold hemoglobinuria follow **infection** (mycoplasmal pneumonia, measles, mumps, "flu" syndromes). Syphilis was formerly an important cause, and the autoantibodies were called **Donath-Landsteiner antibodies.** An **idiopathic form** of cold hemolysin autoimmune hemolytic anemia also occurs, which tends to have a prolonged benign course punctuated by intermittent hemolysis.

RED CELL ENZYME DEFICIENCY

Glucose-6-phosphate dehydrogenase deficiency is the most important red cell enzyme deficiency that produces intermittent extravascular hemolytic anemia. Glucose-6-phosphate dehydrogenase is an enzyme in the hexose monophosphate shunt pathway whose deficiency impairs the regeneration of reduced glutathione. Reduced glutathione normally protects erythrocytes from oxidant injury. Affected erythrocytes are vulnerable to damage by infection and oxidant drugs (primaquine, quinacrine, sulfonamides, nitrofurans, and others). **Decreased erythrocyte deformability,** leading to increased splenic destruction, is caused by attachment of precipitated hemoglobin **(Heinz bodies)** to the erythrocyte membrane. Some erythrocytes are "repaired" by splenic phagocytic cells that pluck out the damaged membrane and adjacent Heinz bodies in a process called "pitting."

X-linked glucose-6-phosphate dehydrogenase deficiency is divided into the **severe Mediterranean** and the **milder A-variants,** observed, respectively, predominantly in the Middle East and in blacks in America and Africa. In both variants, the hemolysis tends to peak 2 to 3 days after the initial oxidant injury, and recovery is heralded by reticulocytosis. Other less common red cell enzyme deficiencies that can cause extravascular hemolytic anemias include deficiencies of **glutathione synthetase, pyruvate kinase,** and **hexokinase.**

> **Glucose-6-phosphate dehydrogenase deficiency causes drug-induced hemolytic anemia.**

DISORDERS OF STRUCTURALLY ABNORMAL HEMOGLOBIN SYNTHESIS

Sickle cell disease is the most important hereditary hemoglobinopathy. The biochemical defect is a substitution of hydrophobic **valine** for hydrophilic glutamic acid in the sixth amino acid of the β-**chain of hemoglobin.** The resulting hemoglobin S (HbS) becomes "sticky" when deoxygenated and tends to aggregate and polymerize, causing deformation of erythrocytes to sickle and holly-leaf shapes, which may occlude small vessels. Increased splenic destruction of abnormal erythrocytes causes an **extravascular hemolytic anemia.** Sickle cell disease shows the features discussed previously that are associated with hemolytic anemias in general. Painful ischemic damage including infarction can involve bones, brain, kidney, liver, retina, and lungs. Other features include fatty change in heart, liver, and kidneys; cor pulmonale secondary to pulmonary vascular stasis; and leg ulcers secondary to subcutaneous vascular stasis. The spleen is initially enlarged and congested, but repeated infarction causes **"autosplenectomy."** Patients usually experience a protracted course with repeated "crises" including **vaso-occlusive** (painful) **crises** following ischemic damage to bones or organs; **aplastic crises** following interrupted erythropoiesis; and **sequestration crises** in children when massive splenic sequestration induces hypovolemia and shock. The splenic damage renders patients vulnerable to serious bacterial infection, particularly of encapsulated organisms such as *Streptococcus pneumoniae* and *Haemophilus influenzae.* For unknown reasons, *Salmonella* osteomyelitis also frequently occurs.

> **Sickle cell disease is due to "sticky" hemoglobin that tends to precipitate.**

Other red cell disease may modify the expression of sickle cell anemia.

Thalassemias are character-ized by the decreased produc-tion of normal hemoglobin.

β-Thalassemias may be due to a variety of genetic mutations.

α-Thalassemia has a wider range of expression than β-thalassemia because the α-chain has four gene copies.

The tendency of HbS to precipitate is based in large part on the concentration within the erythrocyte of HbS. Heterozygotes for sickle cell hemoglobin (**sickle cell trait**) have mild disease, since only about 40 percent of the hemoglobin is HbS, the remainder being almost all HbA. Other coexisting conditions (**HbC, HbD, thalassemias, infancy**) that decrease the HbS concentration also produce mild disease. It has been postulated that sickle cell trait may confer modest protection against falciparum malaria.

THALASSEMIAS

The **thalassemias** are a group of inherited disorders characterized by decreased production of structurally normal hemoglobin. Hemoglobin A is composed of two α- and two β-chains. **β-thalassemia** is the result of insufficient β-chain synthesis; **α-thalassemia** is the result of insufficient α-chain synthesis. In both types, there is a relative excess of the chain that is synthesized in normal amounts. This contributes to the anemia by intraerythrocyte precipitation of the excess chain, leading to premature destruction of maturing erythroblasts (ineffective erythropoiesis) and splenic destruction of erythrocytes (hemolysis).

β-Thalassemia

The **β-thalassemias** are due to two broad categories of genetic mutations that cause either a complete absence (β^0-thalassemias) or very small amounts (β^+-thalassemias) of β-chain synthesis in the homozygous state. Mutations in the β-chain gene tend to cause β^0-thalassemia, while mutations in the promotor region tend to cause β^+-thalassemia. Homozygotes for either type have severe, transfusion-dependent anemia, known as **thalassemia major,** which is characterized by a severe hemolytic anemia that manifests 6 to 9 months after birth when synthesis of HbF declines. Heterozygosity is more common, and produces milder, often asymptomatic, hypochromic and microcytic anemia known as **thalassemia minor.** A few patients with intermediate manifestation are said to have **thalassemia intermedia.** The β-thalassemias are observed most frequently in Mediterranean countries and parts of Africa and Southeast Asia. Thalassemia trait may be partially protective against falciparum malaria. Active research is directed toward early prenatal diagnosis; long-term research into genetic manipulation may eventually provide effective therapy.

α-Thalassemias

The **α-thalassemias** are due to deficient synthesis of hemoglobin α-chains. Unlike the β-globin genes, four copies of the α-globin gene are present in the human genome. Clinical syndromes associated with the α-thalassemias vary markedly in severity, depending upon the number of affected genes. A **silent carrier state** is characterized by abnormalities (often deletion) of one gene, with only a barely detectable decrease in α-chain synthesis. Abnormalities of two genes produce **α-thalassemia trait,** which clinically resembles β-thalassemia minor and is seen most often in Asian and African populations. Abnormalities of three genes produce **hemoglobin H disease,** which is seen more commonly in Asian than African populations, because the former are more apt to have two abnormal genes on a single chromosome than the latter. Hemoglobin H disease is characterized by symptoms that resemble β-thalassemia intermedia, since the excess β-chains are more soluble than the excess α-chains. HbH precipitates can be demonstrated in vitro by incubation of red cells with brilliant cresyl blue. Abnormalities of all four α-chain genes cause death in utero from **hydrops fetalis,** which resembles erythroblastosis fetalis caused by Rh incompatibility and is characterized by fetal pallor, edema, and massive hepatosplenomegaly.

DISSEMINATED INTRAVASCULAR COAGULATION

Disseminated intravascular coagulation is characterized by the intravascular (often intracapillary) formation, and often subsequent lysis, of microthrombi composed of platelets, fibrin, and coagulative factors. The microthrombi can be either localized to a specific organ or tissue, or, more commonly, erratically distributed throughout the body, particularly in the brain, heart, lungs, kidneys, adrenals, spleen, and liver. Disseminated intravascular coagulation can consequently present with symptoms related to the **thrombosis** and subsequent tissue hypoxia. True infarction can also occur, usually when very large numbers of microthrombi are formed. The formation of microthrombi can also consume most of the body's supply of platelets and coagulation factors, predisposing for a hemorrhagic disorder **(consumption coagulopathy),** which is aggravated by the activation of the fibrinolytic mechanism to lyse microthrombi. This hemorrhagic diathesis may be the most prominent clinical manifestation, and is similar to other coagulopathies. The presentation of disseminated intravascular coagulation may consequently be highly variable, and may include respiratory symptoms, neurologic symptoms, oliguria, and shock. Disseminated intravascular coagulation is a feared complication of a variety of disorders, including many obstetric complications; sepsis and other severe infections; malignancies; massive tissue injury; and many other miscellaneous conditions. In general, trauma, surgery, burns, and obstetric complications tend to produce disseminated intravascular coagulation with prominent bleeding complications. More slowly developing disseminated intravascular coagulation, such as that observed in cancer patients, tends to produce prominent thrombotic complications. The management of disseminated intravascular coagulation is difficult (and, unfortunately, often unsuccessful) because blocking the thrombotic tendency with anticoagulants tends to worsen the hemorrhagic tendency, and administering coagulants, such as plasma and platelets, may worsen the thrombotic tendency.

Rapidly developing disseminated intravascular coagulation tends to present as a thrombotic diathesis, while slowly developing disease tends to present as a consumption coagulopathy.

HEMORRHAGIC DIATHESES

The **hemorrhagic diatheses** are bleeding disorders that tend to cause both spontaneous bleeding and prolonged bleeding following trauma, including surgery. It is convenient to discuss hemorrhagic diatheses in terms of their causes: vessel fragility, platelet abnormalities, coagulation defects, and mixed disorders.

Fragile Vessels

Hemorrhagic diatheses related to increased vascular fragility are sometimes called **nonthrombocytopenic purpuras.** These disorders tend to cause petechiae and purpura in the skin and mucous membranes, but only uncommonly cause significant hemorrhage in other sites. Platelet count and bleeding time are typically normal. In a few cases, decreased or abnormal platelets may contribute to an underlying vascular fragility. Infections (meningococcemia, severe measles, rickettsial disease) can cause petechiae and purpura, probably either by vasculitis or disseminated intravascular coagulation. Drug reactions can induce hypersensitivity (leukocytoclastic) vasculitis, either via autoantibody formation or immune complex deposition. Impaired collagen formation or collagen atrophy causes vascular fragility in scurvy, Ehlers-Danlos syndrome, Cushing syndrome, and in the very elderly. Henoch-Schönlein purpura causes a generalized hypersensitivity vasculitis that clinically produces purpura, acute glomerulonephritis, polyarthralgia, and abdominal pain (see also p. 206).

Thrombocytopenia

Peripheral blood platelet counts less than about 20,000 platelets/mm^3 are a common cause of generalized bleeding. Spontaneous bleeding in **thrombocytopenia** is typically from small vessels in the skin (petechiae, ecchymoses), gastrointestinal tract, and genitourinary tract. Less commonly, but dangerously, intracranial bleeding can also occur. Thrombocytopenia due to **decreased production** of platelets can be caused by generalized diseases of bone marrow such as aplastic anemia or marrow replacement by tumor; selective impairment of platelet production by drugs (alcohol, thiazides, antineoplastic agents) or infections (rubella); and ineffective megakaryopoiesis (megaloblastic anemias, Wiskott-Aldrich syndrome). Thrombocytopenia due to **decreased platelet survival** can be due to increased consumption (disseminated intravascular coagulation, microangiopathic hemolytic anemias, thrombotic thrombocytopenic purpura, giant hemangiomas) or to immunologic destruction (systemic lupus erythematosus, idiopathic thrombocytopenic purpura, infectious mononucleosis, acquired immunodeficiency syndrome [AIDS], transfusions, quinidine, heparin). **Hypersplenism** can cause sequestration of platelets. Repeated transfusions can cause a dilutional thrombocytopenia.

Severe thrombocytopenia can be encountered in neonatal and post-transfusion (isoimmune) thrombocytopenia, idiopathic thrombocytopenic purpura, and thrombotic thrombocytopenia purpura. **Neonatal thrombocytopenia** occurs by a mechanism analogous to the hemolysis that occurs in Rh$^+$ babies of Rh$^-$ mothers, but involves the platelet antigen PL^{A1}. In **post-transfusion thrombocytopenia,** a previously sensitized PL^{A1}-negative patient receives PL^{A1}-positive blood, which destroys both the transfused platelets, and, for unknown reasons, those of the patient. In rare **thrombotic thrombocytopenic purpura,** platelets and fibrin form dense intravascular aggregates (hyaline microthrombi) that occlude arterioles and capillaries throughout the body, producing thrombocytopenia, microangiopathic hemolytic anemia, fever, transient neurologic defects, and renal failure. The formerly dismal prognosis has been modified by therapy with corticosteroids, platelet aggregation inhibitors, or exchange transfusions. In **idiopathic** (autoimmune) **thrombocytopenic purpura,** platelets are destroyed by autoimmune mechanisms that appear to involve phagocytosis of opsonized platelets. The bone marrow may show increased numbers of megakaryocytes with some immature megakaryocytes with single nuclei. Acute idiopathic thrombocytopenic purpura tends to follow viral infection (rubella, infectious mononucleosis, viral hepatitis, cytomegalovirus infection); is most common in children; and usually resolves spontaneously. In contrast, chronic idiopathic thrombocytopenic purpura is a disease of adults, often women who may have other immunologic disorders such as lupus erythematosus or hemolytic anemia. Chronic idiopathic thrombocytopenic purpura tends to have a prolonged course that is often ameliorated by steroid therapy or splenectomy.

DEFECTIVE PLATELET FUNCTION

Hemorrhagic diatheses can also be produced by defective platelet function that may be either congenital or acquired. In autosomal recessive **Bernard-Soulier syndrome,** platelets do not adhere to subendothelial collagen because of a deficiency of platelet membrane glycoprotein GPIb. In autosomal **thrombasthenia,** a possible deficiency in two other membrane glycoproteins, GPIIb and GPIIIa, prevents platelets from aggregating when triggered by adenosine diphosphate (ADP), collagen, epinephrine, or thrombin. Genetic disorders of platelet secretion also exist in which platelet aggregation can occur but the aggregated platelets do not release prostaglandins or ADP. Uremia and aspirin ingestion are the most common causes of **acquired platelet dysfunction**, and can increase bleeding time, bruisability, and blood "oozing" during surgery.

Deficiency of platelet membrane glycoproteins produces Bernard-Soulier syndrome and thrombasthenia.

CLOTTING FACTOR ABNORMALITIES

Many acquired and hereditary **clotting abnormalities** have been described. **Hereditary disorders** tend to cause deficiency of a single clotting factor, while **acquired disorders** tend to have multiple clotting abnormalities. Clotting factor abnormalities usually manifest clinically with prolonged bleeding after trauma, which may cause large ecchymoses or hematomas. Spontaneous petechiae and purpura are not usually seen. The large joints, gastrointestinal tract, and urinary tract are particularly vulnerable to bleeding. Acquired disorders of clotting factors can be caused by vitamin K deficiency, severe liver disease, and disseminated intravascular coagulation. Hereditary deficiencies of each of the clotting factors have been described, the most important of which are classic hemophilia, von Willebrand's disease, and hemophilia B.

Classic hemophilia and **von Willebrand's disease** are related conditions that involve the factor VIII–von Willebrand complex, which is necessary for activation of factor X in the intrinsic coagulation pathway. The two components are coded by separate genes. Deficiency of factor

Hereditary clotting disorders tend to cause deficiency of a single clotting factor, while acquired disorders often exhibit multiple clotting abnormalities.

VIII produces the sex-linked recessive disorder classic hemophilia (hemophilia A). Deficiency of the much larger protein to which factor VIII binds, von Willebrand factor, produces von Willebrand's disease.

Since **classic hemophilia** is X-linked recessive, excessive bleeding is most frequently observed in males and homozygous females. Rare heterozygous females also have excessive bleeding, presumably as the result of random inactivation of the normal X chromosome ("unfavorable lyonization"). Milder deficiencies tend to be asymptomatic or only cause moderately prolonged post-traumatic bleeding. Several variants of classic hemophilia exist, and factor VIII may be absent, severely diminished, or abnormal. Classic hemophilia manifests clinically with massive bleeding following trauma. "Spontaneous" bleeding also occurs into commonly traumatized body parts, particularly joints where painful and crippling hemarthroses are produced. Coagulation time is characteristically prolonged, but bleeding time is normal. The formerly poor prognosis for classic hemophilia has been improved by therapy with factor VIII concentrates, but unfortunately many hemophiliacs treated before the mid-1980s have developed AIDS as a result of receiving human immunodeficiency virus (HIV)-contaminated concentrates.

von Willebrand's disease is characterized by prolonged bleeding time, which manifests as menorrhagia, spontaneous bleeding from mucous membranes, and excessive bleeding following trauma. von Willebrand's disease has several genetic variants, the most common (type I) of which is an autosomal dominant reduced quantity of circulating von Willebrand factor as a consequence of a failure to release normally synthesized multimers of the factor. Less commonly (type II), the assembly of the more active multimers is impaired, and the large aggregates are consequently absent from the blood. For unknown reasons, patients with von Willebrand's disease also have somewhat reduced serum factor VIII levels. von Willebrand factor also has an important role in facilitating platelet aggregation and adhesion to collagen. Clinically, patients experience more symptoms related to platelet dysfunction (prolonged bleeding time, spontaneous bleeding from mucous membranes) than symptoms related to factor VIII deficiency, such as hemarthroses.

Factor IX deficiency (Christmas disease, hemophilia B) is transmitted as an X-linked recessive trait and is clinically indistinguishable from classic hemophilia. The diagnosis is made by assay of factor levels.

Classic hemophilia and von Willebrand's disease both involve the factor VIII–von Willebrand's complex, but have quite different clinical presentations. Classic hemophilia causes massive bleeding after trauma, and "spontaneous" bleeding into joints is common.

Patients with von Willebrand's disease tend to have symptoms related to platelet dysfunction such as spontaneous bleeding from mucous membranes.

Factor IX deficiency clinically resembles classic hemophilia.

GRANULOCYTES AND LYMPHOCYTES

LEUKOPENIA

An abnormally low white cell count (**leukopenia**) is usually due to a deficiency in neutrophils (**neutropenia,** granulocytopenia). Deficiencies in lymphocytes (**lymphopenias**) are less common, tend to occur in specific clinical settings (Hodgkin's disease, nonlymphocytic leukemias, congenital immunodeficiency diseases), and will not be discussed here.

Leukopenia is usually due to neutropenia.

Neutropenia

Since circulating neutrophils survive only 6 to 7 hours, a **failure of granulocytopoiesis** will rapidly produce a decrease in their number. Such inadequate or ineffective granulopoiesis may be due to suppression of the myeloid stem cells (aplastic anemia, leukemias, lymphomas); suppression of the committed precursors for the neutrophils (drugs); or nutritional deficiencies (vitamin B_{12}, folate). Alternatively, neutropenia can be produced by accelerated removal or **destruction of neutrophils** (infections, splenic sequestration) or as an autoimmune process (idiopathic, Felty syndrome). Drugs producing generalized marrow suppression include alkylating agents and antimetabolites. A very large number of drugs can also cause idiosyncratic agranulocytosis (aminopyrine, chloramphenicol, chlorpromazine, thiouracil, phenylbutazone, sulfonamides). The changes produced in bone marrow vary with the etiology of the neutropenia. Hypercellular marrow is associated with ineffective granulopoiesis and excessive destruction of mature neutrophils. Hypocellular marrow is associated with stem cell or committed precursor suppression. Patients with severe agranulocytosis with a virtual absence of neutrophils may experience overwhelming infections that rapidly produce death. Less severely affected patients often develop repeated and persistent minor infections.

Inadequate granulopoiesis rapidly leads to neutropenia since circulating neutrophils survive only 6 to 7 hours. Excessive destruction of neutrophils can also produce neutropenia.

REACTIVE PROLIFERATIONS OF WHITE CELLS AND NODES

Leukocytosis

Leukocytosis is an increase in numbers of circulating white cells. **Neutrophilic leukocytosis** is most often observed in acute inflammation, particularly pyogenic infections, but may also be seen in nonmicrobial settings including burns and myocardial infarction. In patients with severe infections, the neutrophils have coarser than normal granules

Leukocytosis can be due to increased numbers of neutrophils, eosinophils, monocytes, or lymphocytes.

(toxic granules), pale blue inclusions (Döhle bodies), and cytoplasmic vacuoles. **Eosinophilic leukocytosis** is observed in conditions with an allergic basis (bronchial asthma, hay fever, parasitic infections) and in some, probably immunologically mediated, diseases of the skin (pemphigus, eczema, dermatitis herpetiformis). Allergic drug reactions are probably the most common cause of eosinophilia in hospitalized patients. **Monocytic leukocytosis** is observed in many conditions with a prominent immunologic component including severe chronic infections (tuberculosis, bacterial endocarditis, brucellosis, rickettsiosis, malaria) and systemic immunologic disorders (systemic lupus erythematosus, rheumatoid arthritis, ulcerative colitis, Crohn's disease). **Lymphocytosis** is also observed in chronic inflammatory states (brucellosis, tuberculosis) and reflects a sustained immune response. Acute viral infections (viral hepatitis, cytomegalovirus, infectious mononucleosis) also cause lymphocytosis. **Reactive leukocytosis** is usually distinguished from leukemias by the lack of immature cells in the blood. This distinction may be blurred in some inflammatory states that tend to produce the so-called **leukemoid reaction** characterized by the presence of many immature white cells in the peripheral blood.

Acute Nonspecific Lymphadenitis

Lymph nodes challenged by microbial agents develop acute nonspecific lymphadenitis.

Acute nonspecific lymphadenitis is the term used for the reactive changes observed in lymph nodes challenged by microbial agents or their toxic products. These changes are also observed when cell debris is introduced into wounds or the circulation, as in drug addiction. Acutely inflamed nodes tend to be enlarged, edematous, tender to the touch, and, if necrosis is present, fluctuant. The overlying skin may be inflamed or contain draining sinuses. The affected nodes have **prominent germinal centers** and lymphoid follicles. Spread of the infection to adjacent tissues may lead to inflammatory changes in the perinodal tissues. Neutrophils, areas of necrosis, and hypertrophy of lymphoid sinuses may also be present in severely inflamed nodes. Acute nonspecific lymphadenitis may either resolve completely or may scar lymph nodes.

Chronic Nonspecific Lymphadenitis

Patterns of chronic nonspecific lymphadenitis include follicular hyperplasia, parafollicular hyperplasia, and sinus histiocytosis.

Chronic nonspecific inflammation of lymph nodes usually produces follicular hyperplasia, paracortical lymphoid hyperplasia, or sinus histiocytosis. **Follicular hyperplasia** is characterized by enlarged germinal centers containing phagocytic cells, blast forms, and B lymphocytes. Follicular hyperplasia can be produced by chronic infections, rheumatoid arthritis, toxoplasmosis, and AIDS. **Parafollicular hyperplasia** (paracortical lymphoid hyperplasia) is produced by microbiologic agents that stimulate T cells (smallpox vaccination) and by drugs (Dilantin). The T-cell regions between germinal follicles become hyperplastic and may contain blast forms. **Sinus histiocytosis** is encountered most frequently in regional nodes draining cancer and is characterized by marked hypertrophy of endothelial cells lining the sinuses, which may also contain large numbers of histiocytes. In practice, combinations of the above reactions are frequently encountered. Chronically infected nodes are not usually under increased pressure and are consequently not tender. The inguinal and axillary nodes are particularly apt to show chronic changes, and are consequently not considered appropriate specimens for the study of hematologic and lymphomatous disorders.

MALIGNANT LYMPHOMAS

Cells native to the lymphoid tissues include lymphocytes, histiocytes, their precursors, and their derivatives. The term **lymphoma** is used for malignant proliferations of any of these cell lines. In general, lymphomas are of monoclonal origin, which can be documented by isoenzyme markers and clonal gene rearrangements. Malignant lymphomas are historically divided into two large groups, Hodgkin's disease and lymphocytic lymphomas.

LYMPHOCYTIC LYMPHOMAS

Two-thirds of the **lymphocytic** (non-Hodgkin's) **lymphomas** arise as a localized or generalized lymphadenopathy. The remainder arise in lymphoid tissues found in the oropharynx, gut, bone marrow, skin, and other sites. The often markedly enlarged involved nodes are usually nontender. Lymphomas can spread from an origin in a single node or chain of nodes to other nodes with eventual dissemination to spleen, liver, bone marrow, blood, and other tissues. This dissemination blurs the distinction between a primary lymphoma with marrow involvement and a primary leukemia with nodal involvement.

The subclassification of non-Hodgkin's lymphomas is complex. Presented here is a Working Formulation in clinical use. Previously used classification schemes include the Rappaport classification, based on cytologic appearance and growth pattern, and the Lukes-Collins classification, based on the T- or B-cell origin and degree of maturation. The Working Formulation represents an attempt to integrate these two patterns of classification. Non-Hodgkin's lymphomas are classified based on prognosis into low-grade, intermediate-grade, high-grade, and miscellaneous categories. Diffuse lymphomas tend to behave more aggressively than follicular lymphomas. Some patients with follicular lymphomas will eventually develop diffuse lymphomas.

Low-Grade Lymphomas

The low-grade lymphomas include small lymphocytic lymphoma, predominantly small cleaved cell lymphoma, and the mixed small cleaved and large cell lymphoma. **Small lymphocytic lymphoma** is a diffuse lymphoma with little or no cytologic atypia, and only rare mitotic figures. Small lymphocytic lymphoma tends to affect older patients; closely resembles chronic leukocytic leukemia; and often has hepatic, splenic, bone marrow, and blood involvement. Some patients have **Waldenström's macroglobulinemia** due to production of monoclonal IgM by plasma cells or "plasmacytoid lymphocytes" found in affected lymph nodes in addition to the well-differentiated lymphocytes.

Both the **small cleaved follicular lymphomas** and the **mixed small and large cell follicular lymphomas** tend to occur in older individuals. These lymphomas frequently have tumor cells containing a characteristic T(14;18) translocation. Patients have a median survival of

Lymphocytic lymphomas can arise either in lymph nodes or lymphoid tissues in other sites.

The working formulation subclassifies lymphomas as low-grade, intermediate-grade, high-grade, and miscellaneous.

The low-grade lymphomas include small lymphocytic lymphoma, predominantly small cleaved cell lymphoma, and the mixed small cleaved and large cell lymphoma.

7 to 9 years, which is unmodified by treatment. Emergence of an aggressive subclone of neoplastic B cells can cause transformation of some of these lymphomas to a higher grade histiologic type.

Intermediate-Grade Lymphomas

The only follicular tumor in the intermediate-grade lymphomas is the **predominantly large cell follicular lymphoma.** These lymphomas have a tendency to evolve later into diffuse lymphomas. Diffuse lymphomas within the intermediate-grade category include the **diffuse small cleaved cell lymphoma, diffuse mixed small and large cell lymphoma,** and **diffuse large cell lymphoma.** The lymphomas in the intermediate-grade category tend to affect older adults and have an intermediate prognosis.

High-Grade Lymphomas

High-grade lymphomas include large cell immunoblastic lymphoma, lymphoblastic lymphoma, and small noncleaved lymphomas (Burkitt's lymphoma and related B-cell neoplasms).

Large cell immunoblastic lymphoma tends to be an aggressive and rapidly fatal (if untreated) tumor of older adults, but fortunately often responds with partial or complete remission to chemotherapy.

Lymphoblastic lymphoma is a T-cell lymphoma composed of tumor cells that resemble intrathymic T cells and appear to be closely related to those observed in T-cell acute lymphoblastic leukemia. Lymphoblastic lymphoma typically contains large numbers of mitoses and has a "starry sky" histologic pattern related to the presence of interspersed, benign macrophages. Lymphoblastic lymphomas are tumors of childhood and adolescent patients with a male predominance. While this tumor is very aggressive, some clinical protocols are producing encouraging results.

The **small** (compared with the large noncleaved cell) **noncleaved cell lymphoma** includes both Burkitt's lymphoma and related tumors seen outside Africa. Burkitt's lymphoma is related to infection by the Epstein-Barr virus. The lymphoma cells tend to form monotonous masses in which are interspersed occasional larger, benign macrophages that create a "starry sky" histologic pattern. Both African and non-African cases tend to be found in children to young adults. The African Burkitt's lymphoma tends to involve primarily the maxilla or mandible, while the non-African cases tend to involve the abdomen (bowel, retroperitoneum, ovaries).

Miscellaneous Lymphomas

The miscellaneous category of the Working Formulation includes a variety of tumors, of which the most important are the mycosis fungoides and the adult T-cell leukemia/lymphoma. The **mycosis fungoides** and related tumors are cutaneous T-cell lymphomas. These diseases are discussed with the dermatologic disorders (see p. 120). The **adult T-cell leukemia/lymphoma** is an uncommon T-cell neoplasm, which has recently become more clinically important because it is associated with human T-cell leukemia virus-I, which shows some similarities to the HIV-1 virus. Adult T-cell leukemia/lymphoma tends to have a very aggressive course with median survival after diagnosis of about 8 months.

HODGKIN'S DISEASE

Hodgkin's disease is a common form of malignancy in young adults (mean age at diagnosis is 32 years) that is now aggressively and successfully treated in most cases. Hodgkin's disease is actually a cluster of lymphomas characterized by distinctive neoplastic giant cells **(Reed-Sternberg cells)** admixed with a variable amount of inflammatory infiltrate. The cell of origin of the Reed-Sternberg neoplastic cell is still not identified with certainty. The Reed-Sternberg cell is a large cell that in its most characteristic form contains a bilobed mirror-image nucleus that may contain prominent "owl-eyes" nucleoli surrounded by a clear halo. Other tumor cell variants also exist, but are not considered diagnostic of Hodgkin's disease. Since cells similar to Reed-Sternberg cells have been found in other conditions (infectious mononucleosis, cancers, mycosis fungoides, lymphomas), the diagnosis of Hodgkin's lymphoma should be made by the combination of Reed-Sternberg cells and a histologic pattern following one of the known types for Hodgkin's disease.

The **lymphocyte-predominant** form of Hodgkin's disease is characterized by a usually diffuse (sometimes slightly nodular) infiltrate of mature lymphocytes that contain interspersed Reed-Sternberg cells, histiocytes, and small numbers of other inflammatory cells. The Reed-Sternberg cells are characteristically few in number, and it may require an extensive search to identify them definitively. Necrosis and fibrosis are usually not present. The typical patient is male, less than 35 years of age, and has limited disease with an excellent prognosis.

Mixed cellularity Hodgkin's disease is characterized by plentiful Reed-Sternberg cells in a heterogeneous cellular infiltrate that may include eosinophils, plasma cells, benign histiocytes, and a moderate number of lymphocytes. Small areas of necrosis and fibrosis may be present. A male predominance is also characteristic of this form of Hodgkin's disease, and patients have an intermediate prognosis.

Lymphocyte depletion Hodgkin's disease is characterized by comparatively abundant Reed-Sternberg cells or their pleomorphic variants, which are surrounded by relatively small numbers of lymphocytes. One morphologic form of lymphocyte depletion Hodgkin's disease is characterized by diffuse fibrosis with a hypocellular node that is largely replaced by proteinaceous material. A second morphologic variant is the reticular variant, which tends to be more cellular and contains large pleomorphic cells resembling Reed-Sternberg cells; typical Reed-Sternberg cells are only occasionally recognized. Patients with lymphocyte depletion Hodgkin's disease tend to be older, have more dissemination, present with systemic manifestations, and have aggressive disease.

Nodular sclerosing Hodgkin's disease is quite different histologically and clinically from the other forms. A distinctive histologic feature is a variant of the Reed-Sternberg cell, the **lacunar cell,** which is characterized by a single hyperlobated nucleus that contains multiple small nucleoli and is surrounded by abundant pale cytoplasm with well-defined borders. The cells often shrink differentially in formalin-fixed

The origin of the neoplastic cell in Hodgkin's disease, the Reed-Sternberg cell, is still disputed.

The lymphocyte-predominant form of Hodgkin's disease has an excellent prognosis.

The mixed cellularity form of Hodgkin's disease has an intermediate prognosis.

The lymphocyte depletion form of Hodgkin's disease has a poor prognosis.

The nodular sclerosing form of Hodgkin's disease has an excellent prognosis.

tissue, giving rise to a cleft around them (lacunae). A second distinctive feature of nodular sclerosing Hodgkin's disease is the presence of narrow to broad collagen bands that divide the lymphoid tissue into nodules. The lymphoid tissue may contain a cellular infiltrate with varying proportions of lymphocytes and lacunar cells. Classic Reed-Sternberg cells are only rarely identified. The patients tend to be young women who have an excellent prognosis.

LEUKEMIAS AND MYELOPROLIFERATIVE DISEASES

Leukemias are primarily diseases of bone marrow rather than blood.

Diffuse replacement of bone marrow by neoplastic hematopoietic cells produces **leukemias.** The leukemic cells often, but not always, spill over into the blood, where they may be seen in large numbers. These cells may also be observed throughout the body, particularly in lymph nodes, liver, and spleen. Occasional patients with diffusely infiltrated bone marrow may present with leukopenia (**"aleukemic" leukemia**) instead of leukocytosis. Leukemias can be classified by cell type and maturity, producing four broad patterns of leukemia: acute lymphoblastic leukemia, chronic lymphocytic leukemia, acute myelocytic leukemia, and chronic myelocytic leukemia. Both **acute lymphoblastic** and **acute myelocytic leukemia** tend to have a rapidly fatal course in untreated patients. Prominent clinical features (anemia, infections, hemorrhage) are related to replacement of normal marrow elements by proliferating "blast cells" that do not undergo maturation. **Chronic lymphocytic leukemias** and **chronic myelogenous leukemias** have different clinical courses. Further, chronic myelogenous leukemia, polycythemia vera, essential thrombocythemia, and myeloid metaplasia may be similar clonal neoplastic proliferations of the multipotent myeloid stem cells. In these diseases, one cell line tends to dominate, but interconversions and overlaps between some members of the group are well described. The chronic lymphoproliferative disorders include chronic lymphocytic leukemia and hairy cell leukemia; these diseases are also related to the non-Hodgkin's small lymphocytic lymphomas.

ACUTE LEUKEMIAS

Acute Lymphoblastic Leukemia

Acute lymphoblastic leukemia is a common childhood acute leukemia.

Acute lymphoblastic leukemia is the most common of the childhood acute leukemias (peak age, 4 years). Acute lymphoblastic leukemia can be subclassified by immunohistotyping or on the basis of cell size and morphology (French-British-American classification). The most favorable clinical outcome is associated with B-cell acute lymphoblastic leukemia, composed of early precursor cells; this is fortunately the most common immunophenotype. Poor prognosis is associated with the B-cell acute lymphoblastic leukemia that represents the leukemic phase of Burkitt's lymphoma. Intermediate prognosis is associated with T-cell and pre-B-cell acute lymphoblastic leukemia. Karyotypic abnormalities are common in the leukemic cells of patients with acute lymphoblastic leukemia.

Acute Myeloblastic Leukemia

Acute myeloblastic leukemias affect both children and adults and have a peak incidence between the ages of 15 and 39 years. The defect producing a leukemia can occur in the multipotent myeloid stem cells (producing cytogenic abnormalities in both granulocytic and erythroid precursors); in the common granulocyte monocyte precursor (producing myelomonocytic disease); or in particular lines of differentiation. The French-American-British classification for acute myelocytic leukemias is based on morphologic features and histochemical findings. **Acute myelocytic leukemia without differentiation** (class Ml) contains a predominance of myeloblasts that are positive for myeloperoxidase and contain distinct nucleoli and few granules or Auer rods. **Acute myelocytic leukemia with differentiation** (M2) is characterized by myeloblasts and promyeloblasts that may contain Auer rods. **Acute promyelocytic leukemia** (M3) is characterized by hypergranular promyelocytes that may contain many Auer rods per cell and may have bilobed or reniform nuclei. **Acute myelomonocytic leukemia** (M4) is characterized morphologically by myelocytic and monocytic differentiation with myeloid elements resembling those in class M2 and peripheral monocytosis. **Acute monocytic leukemia** (M5) is characterized by promonocytes or undifferentiated blasts and is positive for nonspecific esterase. **Acute erythroleukemia** (M6) is characterized by bizarre, multinucleated, large erythroblasts, and occasional myeloblasts. **Acute megakaryocytic leukemia** (M7) is characterized by pleomorphic undifferentiated blasts with myelofibrosis or increased bone marrow reticulin, and the blasts react with antiplatelet antibodies. Types M1, M2, and M4 are the most common. Special staining techniques that may be helpful in establishing the leukemic class include myeloperoxidase (M1 to M6), nonspecific esterase (M4, M5), periodic acid-Schiff (PAS) (M6), and platelet peroxidase (M7). Approximately 90 percent of acute myeloblastic leukemia patients have karyotypic abnormalities, many of which can be detected by standard cytogenic techniques.

Acute myeloblastic leukemia has many morphologic forms, depending on the particular cell line of differentiation.

Clinical Presentation and Treatment of Acute Leukemias

Clinically, acute lymphoblastic and acute myeloblastic leukemias tend to present abruptly with symptoms related to **depression of normal marrow function,** including fatigue (anemia), fever (infection), and bleeding (thrombocytopenia). Other findings include generalized lymphadenopathy, splenomegaly, and hepatomegaly as a consequence of leukemic infiltration of the organs. **Leukemic infiltration** of organs tends to be more characteristic of acute lymphocytic leukemia than of acute myelocytic leukemia. Central nervous system manifestations may be due to both leukemic infiltration and intracerebral or subarachnoid hemorrhage. **Disseminated intravascular coagulation** occurs particularly in promyelocytic (M3) leukemia and can be triggered by chemotherapy causing cell lysis with release of thromboplastic substances from the granules. **Bone marrow** involvement by acute leukemias can cause subperiosteal bone infiltration and bone reabsorption with bone pain and tenderness. Involvement of the **thymus** can

Symptoms related to depression of normal bone marrow function are prominent in acute leukemias.

produce a mediastinal mass, particularly in T-cell acute lymphocytic leukemia. Leukemic cells can be found in almost any extramedullary site, with particularly common involvement of the testes in acute lymphocytic leukemia, and soft tissues and bones (chlormas) in acute myelocytic leukemias, particularly in M1 and M2. M4 and M5 acute myelocytic leukemias tend to produce infiltration of the gums.

Laboratory findings typically include anemia, which is usually accompanied by depressed platelet count and may be part of a pancytopenic process. Alternatively, the white cell count may be markedly elevated, and blast forms may be found among the immature white cells in both blood and marrow. When pancytopenia is present, the leukemia is referred to as aleukemic leukemia and can be differentiated from aplastic anemia by marrow examination. The treatment of acute lymphocytic leukemia, particularly in children, can almost always successfully achieve remission and sometimes apparent cures. In acute myelocytic leukemia, the prognosis is poorer, although most patients have chemotherapy-induced remissions that last 1 to 1 $^1\!/_2$ years.

Myelodysplastic Syndromes

Myelodysplastic syndromes are stem cell disorders that lead to ineffective hematopoiesis.

Myelodysplastic syndromes are stem cell disorders characterized by ineffective hematopoiesis as a consequence of maturation defects. These myelodysplastic syndromes have an increased risk of transformation into acute myeloblastic leukemias. Patients with myelodysplasia tend to be elderly (with peak at 60 to 70 years of age), with a male predominance, and present with symptoms related to pancytopenia including weakness, infections, and hemorrhage. Patients may also be found incidentally during blood tests. Roughly one-third of patients later develop frank acute myelocytic leukemia, while the others experience symptoms related to recurrent infections and hemorrhage. Survival varies with the specific form of the myelodysplasia and the karyotypic abnormalities, and tends to range from 1 to 5 years.

CHRONIC LEUKEMIAS

Chronic Myeloid Leukemia

Cells in chronic myeloid leukemia often have an acquired chromosomal translocation known as the Philadelphia chromosome.

Chronic myeloid leukemia is a disease primarily of adults aged 25 to 60 years (peak, fourth and fifth decades), with a slight male predominance. The Philadelphia (Ph^1) chromosome is found in up to 90 percent of patients with chronic myeloid leukemia, and is usually due to a reciprocal chromosome 22 to 9 translocation. The Philadelphia chromosome is also occasionally seen in acute lymphocytic leukemia, and it is thought that a variety of stem cell lines can be affected. Chronic myeloid leukemia tends to present with slowly developing **anemia,** weakness, weight loss, and anorexia. Extreme **splenomegaly** may cause abdominal complaints. The peripheral leukocytes may exceed 100,000 cells per mm^3, with the most prominent cells being neutrophils and metamyelocytes. Patients also often have **thrombocytosis** early in their course, reflecting the myeloid stem cell origin of the tumor. The granulocytes in chronic myeloid leukemia characteristically contain almost no **alkaline phosphatase,** which helps to differentiate myeloid leukemia from reactive leukocytosis. Chronic myeloid leukemia tends to progress slowly. At about 3 years after diagnosis, many patients develop an **"accelerated phase,"** with increasing anemia and thrombocytopenia that often terminates as a **"blast crisis"** resembling acute leukemia. In other patients, the blast crisis can occur abruptly without an intermediate accelerated phase. The blasts frequently, but not always, resemble myeloblasts; in some cases, the blasts can resemble primitive lymphoid cells. This observation suggests that the transformed cell may be the pluripotent stem cell, capable of both myeloid and lymphoid differentiation. The treatment of chronic myeloid leukemia tends to be characterized by the induction of remissions by chemotherapy without alteration of median survival. Once a blast crisis develops, all forms of treatment tend to become ineffective.

Chronic myeloid leukemia tends to progress slowly but often terminates in a blast crisis.

CHRONIC LYMPHOCYTIC LEUKEMIA

Chronic lymphocytic leukemia shows a considerable similarity to small lymphocytic lymphoma and appears to be a neoplastic disorder of B cells, with rare cases being due to T-cell neoplasia. Roughly one-half of patients with chronic lymphocytic leukemia have recognizable abnormal karyotypes in the neoplastic cells. Chronic lymphocytic leukemia develops indolently, and many patients are asymptomatic or have only nonspecific symptoms such as fatigability, weight loss, and anorexia. Generalized **lymphadenopathy** and **hepatosplenomegaly** may be present. The peripheral **lymphocytosis** may be either slight or as marked as 200,000 cells/mm^3. Lymphocytes with crushed nuclei (smudge cells) are often seen in the peripheral smears. Most of the peripheral lymphocytes are small and mature-appearing, with occasional larger lymphocytes whose nuclei may contain nucleoli. Despite the very large numbers of leukemic cells, these patients tend to have **hypogammaglobulinemia** and increased susceptibility to bacterial infections as a consequence of the nonfunctional state of the leukemic B cells. **Autoimmune hemolytic anemias** and **thrombocytopenias** occur in some patients, apparently as a consequence of autoantibodies directed against red cells and platelets. Blast transformation does not usually occur.

Chronic lymphocytic leukemia is very similar to small lymphocytic lymphomas.

HAIRY CELL LEUKEMIA

Hairy cell leukemia is a distinct form of chronic leukemia in which the neoplastic cells are covered with fine, hairlike projections. The cells appear to be of the B-cell lineage, but may also express surface markers of T cells and monocytes. The cells can be cytochemically identified by the presence of tartrate-resistant acid phosphatase. Hairy cell leukemia is a disease of older men that produces infiltration of liver, bone marrow, and spleen, resulting in hepatocytomegaly and pancytopenia.

The cells in hairy cell leukemia have hairlike projections and express markers for several cell lines.

MORPHOLOGY OF LEUKEMIAS

Leukemias tend to produce similar morphologic pictures related to the tissue changes caused by infiltration of leukemic cells. Grossly, the **bone marrow** tends to develop a muddy, red-brown to grayish color as the

Leukemias of different types may have similar clinical presentations and organ involvement.

normal marrow is replaced by masses of leukemic cells. **Splenic enlargement** is often present and may be moderate (acute leukemias, chronic lymphocytic leukemia) to massive (chronic myelocytic leukemia, hairy cell leukemia). Some **lymph node enlargement** is present in all forms of leukemia and may be extreme in lymphocytic leukemias. Involved nodes tend to form discrete, rubbery masses. Leukemic cells may efface the lymph node architecture and spill into surrounding tissues. The **liver** may also be enlarged. Lymphocytic infiltrates tend to involve the portal areas; myelogenous infiltrates tend to involve the sinusoids. Focal infiltrates can also be found in many other organs. Nervous system involvement is most common in acute lymphocytic leukemia and is clinically important since the cells may be protected from chemotherapy by the blood–brain barrier.

The **pancytopenia** that is a consequence of almost all forms of leukemia characteristically produces sometimes severe anemia and thrombocytopenia with bleeding diathesis. Additionally, while the total white blood cell count may be markedly elevated, the leukemic cells do not function normally, and patients may be markedly susceptible to bacterial infections, with common sites of involvement including the oral cavity, skin, lungs, kidneys, urinary bladder, and colon. Opportunistic infections are often present, caused by organisms such as fungi, *Pseudomonas,* and commensal organisms.

MYELOPROLIFERATIVE DISORDERS

Myeloproliferative disorders are proliferations of multipotent myeloid stem cells.

The **myeloproliferative disorders** are neoplastic proliferation of clones of multipotent myeloid stem cells, and include chronic myeloid leukemia (see p. 96), polycythemia vera, myeloid metaplasia with myelofibrosis, and rare essential thrombocythemia, which will not be discussed here.

Polycythemia Vera

Polycythemia vera is an excessive production of all marrow elements that is most marked in the erythrocyte line.

In **polycythemia vera** (see also p. 81), there is excessive production of all marrow elements, which is most marked in the erythrocyte line. Polycythemia vera may be the consequence of a clonal proliferation of stem cells that are very sensitive to erythropoietin. The proliferation produces an absolute increase in red cell mass. Polycythemia vera consequently differs from relative polycythemia, which is the result of hemoconcentration. Also, polycythemia vera differs from secondary polycythemias in that serum erythropoietin levels are lower than normal. The increase in blood volume and viscosity associated with the erythrocytosis causes vascular congestion leading to hepatosplenomegaly; thrombosis and infarction; and hemorrhages. Extramedullary hematopoiesis can often be observed in the spleen and sometimes the liver. The bone marrow is usually markedly hypercellular with hyperplasia of erythroid, granulocytic, and megakaryocytic elements. With disease progression, bone marrow reticulin increases, and the marrow becomes progressively fibrotic (myelofibrosis) or may be replaced by blasts (leukemic transformation). Polycythemia vera occurs in older middle-aged individuals and has a slight male predominance. Untreated patients have a poor prognosis, but repeated phlebotomy to maintain red cell mass at near normal levels can lead to median survival of 10 years. In treated patients who survive the initial phase, a "spent phase" with transfusion-dependent anemia may gradually develop as myelofibrosis forces hematopoiesis out of the bone and into the spleen, which markedly enlarges. A few patients develop terminal **myeloblastic leukemia,** possibly related to chemotherapy or radiotherapy.

Myeloid Metaplasia with Myelofibrosis

Myeloid metaplasia with myelofibrosis is a chronic myeloproliferative disorder characterized by a fibrotic, hypocellular marrow (**myelofibrosis**) and proliferation of neoplastic myeloid stem cells in extramedullary sites (**myeloid metaplasia**), particularly in the spleen, which consequently becomes massively enlarged. Myeloid metaplasia with myelofibrosis may arise idiopathically or may be observed following "burn out" of either polycythemia vera or, less commonly, chronic myeloid leukemia. The myelofibrosis appears to be due to stimulation of non-neoplastic marrow fibroblasts. The proliferation of neoplastic stem cells is known to begin within the marrow, and subsequently causes seeding of other organs, particularly the spleen and sometimes the liver. Splenic and other foci of **extramedullary hematopoiesis** usually show relatively normal proportions of normoblasts, granulocytic precursors, and megakaryocytes. Patients with myeloid metaplasia are usually over 50 years of age, and may come to clinical attention either because of progressive anemia or marked splenic enlargement, or because of preceding polycythemia vera or chronic myeloid leukemia. The peripheral blood smear shows a moderate to severe normochromic normocytic anemia with marked variation in erythrocyte size and shape including characteristic teardrop-shaped erythrocytes (**poikilocytes).** The peripheral blood also contains normoblasts and basophilic stippled red cells. With time, thrombocytopenia with giant forms of platelets or other morphologic abnormalities develops. **Leukocyte alkaline phosphatase** levels are elevated or normal in myeloid metaplasia, while they are low to absent in chronic myeloid leukemia. Also, the Ph[1] chromosome is absent in those cases of myeloid metaplasia that do not follow chronic myeloid leukemia. Careful history taking may be required to exclude the possibility of a myelophthisic anemia secondary to an identifiable cause of marrow injury, such as cancer. Some patients survive for years if appropriately transfused. Other patients experience splenic infarctions; secondary gout as a complication of rapid turnover of blood cells; life-threatening infections; life-threatening thrombotic or bleeding episodes related to platelet abnormalities; or transformation to acute leukemia.

> **Myeloid metaplasia is characterized by marrow fibrosis and extramedullary proliferation of neoplastic stem cells.**

PLASMA CELL DYSCRASIAS AND RELATED DISORDERS

Expansion of a single clone of immunoglobulin-secreting cells produces a **plasma cell dyscrasia.** Many plasma cell dyscrasias are characterized

Plasma cell dyscrasias and related disorders include multiple myeloma, plasmacytoma, Waldenström's macroglobulinemia, heavy chain disease, and monoclonal gammopathy of undetermined significance.

Multiple myeloma is a multifocal plasma cell cancer that often causes lytic bone lesions and typically produces monoclonal immunoglobulin fragments.

by increased serum levels of a homogenous immunoglobulin or its fragments. Typically, the plasma cell dyscrasias behave like neoplastic diseases, although occasionally otherwise normal elderly individuals may be asymptomatic except for elevation of a monoclonal immunoglobulin. These immunoglobulin-secreting cells are derived from B-cell lymphocytes, and are consequently related to the non-Hodgkin's B-cell lymphomas.

Multiple Myeloma

Multiple myeloma is the most common of these syndromes and is a multifocal plasma cell cancer of the osteosystem. The immunoglobin produced is usually **IgG,** or, somewhat less commonly, IgA, IgM, IgE, and IgD. When the complete immunoglobulin is produced, serum electrophoresis shows a well-defined spike (**M component**) in the gamma globulin area. Some myelomas produce only immunoglobulin fragments, typically light chains, that are often excreted in urine as **Bence Jones proteins,** which can be identified as a sharp protein spike by urine electrophoresis. Multiple myelomas often have chromosomal abnormalities in the affected clonal B cells that usually involve chromosome 14 band q32. Prolonged antigenic stimulation also appears to predispose for multiple myeloma. The neoplastic cells usually resemble mature plasma cells, but less mature and **binucleate forms** can also be identified. Protein aggregates composed of immunoglobulin may form homogeneous cytoplasmic inclusions (**Russell bodies**), which can also be observed in reactive plasma cells that are actively synthesizing immunoglobulins. Activation of osteoclasts produces multifocal destructive lesions (**"punched-out defects"** by x-ray) that can occur throughout the skeletal system. Late in the disease, other organs may become infiltrated by plasma cells. Multiple myeloma can also produce renal involvement (**myeloma nephrosis);** a distinctive component is protein casts surrounded by multinucleate giant cells in the distal convoluted and collecting tubules. Other complications can include neuropathy (due either to myeloma involvement of nerve or trauma from fractured vertebrae), infection, blood hyperviscosity (particularly when IgA is produced), hypercalcemia, and amyloidosis. Hemolytic anemia and coagulation defects are occasionally observed when the M components possess antibody activity against red cells or clotting factors. Death is most often due to either infection or renal insufficiency. Median survival remains only 2 to 3 years.

Solitary Myeloma (Plasmacytoma)

A lesion that resembles multiple myeloma can occur in solitary form in either bone or soft tissue (lungs, nasopharynx, nasal sinuses). The lesions may cause a modest monoclonal spike by electrophoresis of serum or urine. If the **solitary myeloma** occurs in bone, classic multiple myeloma may eventually (up to 10 to 20 years) develop; if it occurs in extraosseous sites, multiple myeloma rarely develops, and local resection is usually curative.

Plasmacytoma is a solitary plasma cell proliferation resembling those of multiple myeloma. Osseous plasmacytomas may eventually progress to true multiple myeloma.

Waldenström's Macroglobulinemia

Waldenström's macroglobulinemia is characterized by diffuse, rather than focal, infiltration of the bone marrow by lymphocytes, plasma cells, and hybrid forms. This infiltration can also occur in extraosseous sites and is associated with a monoclonal IgM immunoglobulin production, which causes **macroglobulinemia.** Waldenström's macroglobulinemia can be considered to be an intermediate form between multiple myeloma and small lymphocytic lymphoma. While the neoplastic B cells produce monoclonal immunoglobulin, the tumor spreads in a pattern that resembles lymphoma more than it does multiple myeloma. Waldenström's macroglobulinemia tends to present in the sixth to seventh decade. Blood hyperviscosity is a consequence of aggregations of the abnormal protein. Bleeding may be a problem due to both inhibition of clotting factors and interference with platelet function. Patients may experience neurologic symptoms that may include deafness or visual impairment. Symptoms resembling those of cryoglobulinemia (cold urticaria, Raynaud's phenomenon) can be observed in those cases in which abnormal globulins precipitate at low temperature. Renal damage tends to be less severe than that in multiple myeloma. The median survival is 2 to 5 years in treated patients.

The infiltration in Waldenström's macroglobulinemia tends to be diffuse and contain both lymphocytes and plasma cells. The IgM produced increases blood viscosity.

Heavy Chain Disease

Rarely, a neoplastic clone of plasma cells or leukocytes may produce the heavy chains associated with different classes of immunoglobulins. In patients whose monoclonal gammopathies elaborate the γ-chain of IgG (**γ-chain disease**), the disease is most commonly encountered in elderly patients, in whom it resembles malignant lymphoma more than it resembles multiple myeloma. The most common form is **α-chain** (IgA heavy chain) **disease,** which usually occurs in young adults, particularly from the Mediterranean area. α-Chain disease causes diarrhea and hypocalcemia with massive infiltration of abdominal lymph nodes and the lamina propria of the intestine by lymphocytes, plasma cells, and histiocytes. The rarest of the monoclonal gammopathies is **μ-chain disease** (IgM heavy chain), which may be associated with lymphocytic leukemia, and a characteristic form of vacuolated plasma cells may be encountered in the marrow.

Heavy chain disease occurs when a neoplastic clone of plasma cells or leukocytes produces heavy chain immunoglobulin fragments.

Monoclonal Gammopathy of Undetermined Significance

Elderly patients occasionally have elevated levels of IgG, IgM, or IgA, without appearing to have any of the well-defined immunoglobulin-producing diseases. These patients are considered to have a **monoclonal gammopathy of undetermined significance.** Over a period of years, roughly one-fifth of these patients eventually develop some form of well-defined monoclonal gammopathy (myeloma, macroglobulinemia, amyloidosis, or lymphoma). The remainder do not develop overt disease, but may have a slow increase in the amount of the serum monoclonal protein.

Some elderly patients have a relatively stable monoclonal gammopathy that may or may not progress to another, better defined gammopathy.

HISTIOCYTOSES

The **histiocytoses** are proliferations of histiocytes or macrophages and include both reactive and neoplastic disorders, as well as a few diseases whose classification is less clear. Clearly neoplastic histiocytoses include the monocytic leukemias and rare histiocytic lymphomas. Clearly reactive histiocytoses include those produced by tuberculosis and other infec-

Histiocytoses are both reactive and neoplastic proliferations of histiocytes or macrophages.

tious granulomas. Histiocytoses whose classifications are less clear include Letterer-Siwe disease, Hand-Schüller-Christian disease, and eosinophilic granuloma. These latter disorders are composed of large, histiocytelike cells containing ultrastructural granules (histiocytosis X bodies) that resemble by electron microscopy the "tennis-racket"-shaped Birbeck granules of the Langerhans cells of the epidermis.

Acute Disseminated Langerhans Cell Histiocytosis (Letterer-Siwe Disease)

Letterer-Siwe disease is a progressive proliferation of mature and immature histiocytes throughout the body.

Letterer-Siwe disease affects infants and children under 3 years of age and may be present from birth; rare reports suggest that a similar disorder may be found in adults. The disease is characterized by an acute or subacute progressive proliferation of mature and immature histiocytes, which can be found throughout the body. Clinical features include lytic bone lesions, pancytopenia, fever, rash, hepatosplenomegaly, and lymphadenopathy. The formerly dismal prognosis has been modified by intensive chemotherapy.

Unifocal and Multifocal Langerhans Cell Histiocytoses

The Langerhans histiocytoses are accumulations of histiocytes within bone marrow that erode the adjacent bone.

The **Langerhans histiocytoses** are characterized by accumulation of histiocytes within medullary cavities in either a unifocal or multifocal pattern, with subsequent erosion of the adjacent bone and displacement of normal marrow. The accumulations sometimes resemble granulomas, in that they may contain central areas of necrosis and may be rimmed by a more intense infiltration of neutrophils, which may contain multinucleated histiocytes. The number of eosinophils in these lesions is highly variable and can range from scattered mature eosinophils to sheetlike masses of cells. Histiocytes present in the lesions may contain histiocytosis X bodies. The tumors can be found throughout the skeletal system; particularly favored locations include the skull, ribs, and femurs. Lesions resembling the bone lesions are sometimes found in other sites including skin, lungs, and stomach. The **unifocal form** of Langerhans histiocytosis (eosinophilic granuloma) tends to occur in children and young adults, with a male predominance. The solitary lesions do not usually cause systemic manifestations and may either be asymptomatic, or cause local pain and tenderness as the lesion erodes bone. Some cases heal by spontaneous fibrosis within 1 or 2 years of diagnosis; others are cured by excision or local irradiation. **Multifocal** Langerhans cell histiocytosis is a much more aggressive disease that can involve lymph nodes, bone marrow, liver, spleen, lung, orbits, and pituitary. Patients typically present in early childhood with fever, scaly rash, and frequent localized infections (otitis media, mastoiditis, upper respiratory infections, gingival inflammations). The **Hand-Schüller-Christian triad** consists of calvarial bone defects, diabetes insipidus, and exophthalmos; while this is the classic form of the disease, only a minority of patients actually have all three findings. Multifocal Langerhans cell histiocytosis may be a variant of acute disseminated histiocytosis with good prognosis.

SPLEEN

SPLENOMEGALY

Splenomegaly is observed in a variety of situations including infections (granulomatous diseases, parasitic diseases, some viral diseases), congestive states related to portal hypertension (hepatic cirrhosis), lymphohematogenous disorders (lymphoma, leukemia, hemolytic anemias), immunologic-inflammatory conditions (rheumatoid arthritis, Felty syndrome, systemic lupus erythematosus), storage diseases (Gaucher's disease, Niemann-Pick disease, mucopolysaccharidoses), and miscellaneous diseases (amyloidosis, primary and secondary neoplasms). In a minority of patients with splenomegaly, **hypersplenism** is seen. This condition is characterized by one or more of anemia, leukopenia, or thrombocytopenia. Hypersplenism is associated with hyperplasia of the marrow and is corrected by splenectomy. Hypersplenism appears to be due to increased sequestration of the involved blood cells, with a consequent increased likelihood that splenic macrophages will phagocytize the involved cells.

Splenomegaly is a relatively nonspecific finding observed in a wide variety of conditions.

CONGENITAL ANOMALIES

The spleen can be affected by a variety of congenital anomalies, of which the most common are **accessory spleens** and **abnormal lobulations.** Accessory spleens tend to be situated in the gastrosplenic ligament or the tail of the pancreas, although other locations may be found including the omentum and the mesenteries of the small and large intestine. Most accessory spleens are small and of little clinical significance. When large (and missed), they occasionally limit the benefit of splenectomy. **Complete absence of the spleen** is only rarely observed and is usually associated with other congenital, particularly cardiac, abnormalities.

Accessory spleens and abnormal lobulations are the most common congenital anomalies of the spleen.

NONSPECIFIC ACUTE SPLENITIS

Following almost any blood-borne infection, the spleen may **nonspecifically enlarge.** In the enlarged spleen, the white pulp is usually obscured, and the cut surface of the spleen appears grayish red to deep red. The major histologic change is **acute congestion** that preferentially involves the red pulp and may even efface the lymphoid follicles. Closer examination of the sinusoids may show **reticuloendothelial hyperplasia** and numerous macrophages, which may be filled with disintegrating bacteria and amorphous debris. Neutrophils, plasma cells, and occasional eosinophils may also be encountered. Focal necrosis or

Nonspecific acute splenitis may follow almost any blood-borne infection and is characterized by acute congestion of the red pulp that may efface the lymphoid follicles.

abscess formation is occasionally seen, as are bland or septic infarcts. Features that may suggest a particular etiology include acute necrosis of the centers of the splenic follicles (hemolytic streptococcal infection); bland or septic infarcts (infective endocarditis); striking reticuloendothelial hyperplasia and erythrophagocytosis (typhoid fever); and atypical lymphocytes (infectious mononucleosis). In most cases, the causative agent cannot be identified. Acute splenitis is also observed following non-microbial inflammatory disease.

REACTIVE HYPERPLASIA OF SPLEEN

Reactive hyperplasia of the spleen, characterized histologically by prominent splenic follicles, can be seen in viral infections and diseases with autoimmune components.

Reactive hyperplasia causes enlargement of the spleen in many inflammatory conditions, including rheumatoid arthritis, Felty syndrome, bacterial endocarditis, systemic lupus erythematosus, infectious mononucleosis, herpes simplex, and graft rejection. In contrast to the spleen in nonspecific acute splenitis, the splenic follicles are often prominent and contain large **germinal centers.** The red pulp may be congested and show marked reticuloendothelial hyperplasia with phagocytic cells within the sinusoids. Macrophages, eosinophils, and plasma cells can often be found throughout the spleen. Control of the underlying disease usually causes the spleen to return to normal.

CONGESTIVE SPLENOMEGALY

Congestive splenomegaly, which may contain small scarred areas (Gandy-Gamma nodules), is observed in hepatic cirrhosis and other conditions that impede blood flow through the splenic vein.

Congestive splenomegaly is produced when the venous drainage of the spleen through the splenic vein is impeded. The most common cause is **hepatic cirrhosis;** other causes include cardiac decompensation and portal vein thrombosis.

The spleen in long-standing congestive splenomegaly is typically enlarged, firm, and has a thickened fibrous capsule. The malpighian corpuscles are indistinct, and the pulp contains small, gray-to-brown, firm nodules **(Gandy-Gamma nodules).** The nodules are composed of foci of fibrosis containing hemosiderin and calcium deposition, which are the consequence of organization of old hemorrhages. Early in congestive splenomegaly, the red pulp becomes effused with cells; with time, the increased portal pressure leads to fibrosis and rigidity of the sinusoid walls. **Hypersplenism** can occur secondary to phagocytosis of red cells by sinusoidal macrophages. In spleens affected by long-standing splenic congestion, occasional foci of hematopoiesis may appear.

SPLENIC INFARCTS

Triangular splenic infarcts may be caused by bland or septic emboli.

The spleen is vulnerable to **infarction,** which is usually caused by occlusion of the major splenic artery or its branches by emboli arising in the heart. The infarcts may be of any size and tend to be of the bland, anemic type; infective endocarditis can cause septic infarcts. Splenic infarction is also uncommonly caused by local thromboses (myeloproliferative syndromes, sickle cell anemia, polyarteritis nodosa, Hodgkin's disease, bacteremic diseases). Splenic infarcts are characteristically pale and triangular, with bases at the periphery. Septic infarcts may develop abscesses that heal with large, depressed scars. The infarcts present with sudden onset of left upper quadrant abdominal pain and usually resolve without sequelae. They are clinically significant primarily because they must be differentiated from other causes of intra-abdominal pain.

SPLENIC NEOPLASMS

Primary tumors of the spleen are rare and include a variety of **benign tumors** (fibroma, osteomas, chondromas, lymphangiomas, hemangiomas), of which the most common are lymphangiomas and cavernous hemangiomas. **Malignant primary tumors** that can involve the spleen include non-Hodgkin's lymphomas, Hodgkin's disease, and hemangiosarcomas. Involvement of the spleen by secondary tumors is much more common. **Secondary involvement** can be from Hodgkin's disease or disseminated non-Hodgkin's lymphomas. Metastases from other tumors also occur, although these are usually very small and only occur when the primary lesion has disseminated widely.

Primary splenic neoplasms are much less common than secondary involvement by lymphomas or other malignancies.

RUPTURE

Rupture of a normal spleen is usually only observed following severe **crushing injury** (automobile accident) or a severe blow. Enlarged spleens are much more vulnerable to trauma, and **"spontaneous" rupture** can be encountered in a variety of conditions causing splenomegaly (infectious mononucleosis, malaria, typhoid fever, leukemia, other acute forms of splenitis). Splenic rupture is a life-threatening surgical emergency because of the potential for a massive intraperitoneal hemorrhage. Long-term follow-up of some survivors of splenic rupture has demonstrated that splenic tissue can subsequently be found growing in either localized areas or scattered throughout the peritoneum cavity, apparently due to seeding during the rupture.

Splenic rupture is a life-threatening surgical emergency.

7
Connective Tissue

SKIN

ACUTE INFLAMMATORY DERMATOSES

Urticaria

Urticaria (hives) are pruritic wheals caused by localized degranulation of mast cells, usually as a consequence of antigen-induced sensitization by IgE antibodies. Such **IgE-dependent degranulation** can be triggered by a wide variety of antigens in pollens, drugs, foods, or insect venoms. **IgE-independent urticaria** can also occur, and is caused by either direct degranulation of mast cells (drugs including opiates, some antibiotics, radiographic contrast media) or by mediation through mechanisms involving prostaglandin synthesis (aspirin or other chemicals), or activation of the complement system (necrotizing vasculitis, serum sickness). Urticaria occur most often in young adults, although all ages can be affected. Histologically, the lesions are only subtly different from normal skin, with widely spaced collagen bundles and dilated superficial lymphatic channels as a consequence of dermal edema. While degranulation of mast cells has occurred, their numbers are usually not increased. Most urticaria resolve within 1 to several days. Persistent urticaria suggests either a failure to remove the causative antigen or systemic disease such as Hodgkin's disease or collagen–vascular disorders. **Angioedema** is similar to urticaria, but the edema involves both the dermis and the subcutaneous fat. **Hereditary angioneurotic edema** is a rare form of angioedema characterized by an inherited deficiency of C1 esterase inhibitor (C1 activator) that causes inappropriate activation of the complement system.

> Hives are pruritic, edematous, wheals that may or may not be triggered by IgE-dependent mechanisms.

Acute Eczematous Dermatitis

Acute eczematous dermatitis (eczema, spongiotic dermatitis) refers to a broad group of skin disorders characterized by oozing, crusted papules and vesicles that may, if the condition becomes chronic, progress to scaling plaques. Eczema is subclassified based on the etiology: atopic dermatitis, drug-related eczema, photoeczematous dermatitis, or contact

> Eczema is characterized histologically by epidermal edema.

107

dermatitis. Different forms of eczema have a similar histologic appearance characterized by edema within the epidermis that causes the keratinocytes to be slightly separated by edema fluid (**spongiosis).** The desmosome intercellular attachment sites consequently become vulnerable to mechanical stresses, and intraepithelial vesicles may form. With many forms of eczema, mast cells are degranulated, and a lymphocytic infiltrate is observed around papillary dermal vessels. Eosinophils are often additionally present in the infiltrate in drug-related eczema. The pathophysiology of many types of eczema appears to involve trapping of antigens by epidermal Langerhans cells, which then present the antigen to T-helper lymphocytes. These sensitized T lymphocytes, together with mast cell degranulation, can then induce the changes in permeability of capillaries and venules that lead to the epidermal edema.

Erythema Multiforme

The "multiform" lesions of erythema multiforme show extensive epithelial cell degeneration and a lymphocytic infiltrate.

In contrast to eczema, in which the skin damage is done by accumulation of edema fluid, **erythema multiforme** is characterized by extensive epithelial cell degeneration and death. This cytotoxic reaction pattern produces **"multiform"** lesions that may include macules, papules, and blisters. Often, a red macule or papule has a pale necrotic or vesicular center, producing a **"target lesion"** characteristic of erythema multiforme. Histologically, erythema multiforme is characterized by a perivascular **lymphocytic infiltrate** that extends to the dermoepidermal junction, where the lymphocytes are found closely associated with degenerating keratinocytes. **Blister formation** occurs as the zones of degeneration become confluent. The pathophysiology of erythema multiforme appears to involve epithelial damage by suppressor-cytotoxic lymphocytes. Erythema multiforme is usually self-limited and has been associated with a variety of conditions including infections (herpes, mycoplasma, histoplasmosis, leprosy, typhoid and others); drugs including antibiotics (sulfonamides, penicillin, antimalarial agents), salicylates, barbiturates, and others; carcinomas and lymphomas; and collagen-vascular diseases including lupus erythematosus, dermatomyositis, and polyarteritis nodosa. **Stevens-Johnson syndrome** is a severe variant that is observed most frequently in children in which the erythema multiforme involves most of the body surface and may extend to the oral mucosa, genitalia, and conjunctiva. Patients with Stevens-Johnson syndrome are vulnerable to life-threatening sepsis following infection of involved areas. **Toxic epidermal necrolysis** is another dangerous variant characterized by extensive sloughing of skin and mucous membranes. Erythema multiforme may be accompanied by marked vascular injury, suggesting that it is related to hypersensitivity vasculitis.

Stevens-Johnson syndrome and toxic epidermal necrolysis are severe forms of erythema multiformes.

Erythema Nodosum and Erythema Induratum

Erythema nodosum is a nodular panniculitis. Erythema induratum is a panniculitis that appears to evolve from a vasculitis.

Both erythema nodosum and erythema induratum are inflammations of the subcutaneous adipose tissue (panniculitis). **Erythema nodosum** produces poorly defined tender nodules, often on the lower legs. Erythema nodosum can progress to subacute or chronic disease. Histologically, the inflammation involves predominantly the septae between fat lobules. Early lesions show acute inflammation; more chronic lesions may have fibrosis and granulomatous inflammation with multinucleated giant cells. While many cases are idiopathic, erythema nodosum has been associated with a variety of conditions including infections (streptococcal infections, tuberculosis, and systemic fungal infections), pharmacotherapy (oral contraceptives, sulfonamides), systemic diseases (sarcoidosis, inflammatory bowel disease, malignancies). **Erythema induratum** is an uncommon panniculitis that appears to evolve from a primary vasculitis. Erythema induratum is most often observed in adolescents and menopausal women who do not have associated underlying disease. The lesion causes an erythematous nodule that often ulcerates. Other forms of panniculitis also exist, including Weber-Christian disease, characterized by crops of erythematous plaques; factitial panniculitis caused by self-inflicted injury; deep-seated fungal infections; and systemic diseases such as lupus erythematosus.

CHRONIC INFLAMMATORY DERMATOSES

Psoriasis

Psoriasis is a common chronic skin inflammation that can affect any age but is most commonly seen in young adults who may have an associated disease such as acquired immunodeficiency syndrome (AIDS), arthritis, or myopathy. Established lesions in psoriasis typically consist of well-defined salmon-pink plaques covered by silvery adherent scales, although many variations exist. The lesions are most often found on the knees, elbows, scalp, genitalia, and lower back and are frequently accompanied by abnormal finger- or toenails. The lesions characteristically bleed from multiple points when the scales are peeled (Auspitz sign). Histologically, established psoriatic lesions show a thinned stratum granulosum; an extensive parakeratotic scale; marked epidermal thickening (acanthosis); elongation of rete ridges; increased epidermal mitotic activity; and dilated papillary blood vessels. Clusters of neutrophils may be found in the superficial epidermis (spongiform pustules) or parakeratotic stratum corneum (Munro's microabscesses). One variant of psoriasis, **pustular psoriasis**, is characterized by small pustules in erythematous plaques that may be either generalized or localized to the hands and feet. These pustules consist histologically of neutrophil accumulations resembling abscesses within the epidermis or stratum corneum. Psoriasis occasionally causes total body erythema with scaling (**erythroderma).** The pathogenesis of psoriasis is still obscure, but may involve a complement-mediated reaction in the stratum corneum.

The plaques of psoriasis show an abnormal, thickened epidermis and dilated papillary vessels.

Lichen Planus

Lichen planus is a self-limited disease of unknown (possibly autoimmune) etiology characterized by flat-topped, pruritic, purple papules that often contain white dots or lines (**Wickham striae**). The lesions usually resolve within several years, but may leave hyperpigmented postinflammatory zones. The lesions tend to be symmetrically distributed and occur on the extremities, glans penis, or mouth. Lichen planus that specifically involves hair-bearing skin is called **lichen planopilaris.** A dense band of lymphocytes infiltrates the upper dermis and dermoepidermal junction ("lichenoid" inflammation). Degenerating basal keratinocytes associated with the lymphocytes resemble cells in the stra-

The papules of lichen planus show a dense band of lymphocytes in the upper dermis and dermoepidermal junction.

tum spinosum (squamatization). The dermoepidermal junction is modified as a consequence of the degenerating basal cells and may develop clefts and a sharply angulated ("saw-tooth") contour. Keratinized, necrotic basal cells without nuclei (colloid or Civatte bodies) are sometimes found in the papillary dermis. The epidermis is hyperplastic, with thickening of the stratum corneum (hyperkeratosis) and granular cell layer (hypergranulosis).

Lupus Erythematosus

The most distinctive feature of the skin involvement of lupus erythematosus is a granular band of complement and immunoglobulin at the dermal-epidermal junction.

Cutaneous manifestations of lupus erythematosus can occur either as part of the systemic disease or in a localized, cutaneous form (discoid lupus erythematosus). The most common lesion observed in **systemic lupus erythematosus** is a poorly defined erythema over the malar prominences of the cheeks. The characteristic lesion of **discoid lupus erythematosus** is a large, erythematous scaling plaque with sharply defined ("discoid") margins. However, lupus erythematosus cannot always be distinguished from discoid lupus erythematosus by clinical and histologic evaluation of skin lesions, since lesions resembling discoid lupus erythematosus are sometimes encountered in patients with systemic lupus erythematosus. The skin lesions of lupus erythematosus are believed to be the result of both humoral and cell-mediated mechanisms leading to the destruction of basal cells, probably involving immune complex and complement deposition in the basement membrane of the epithelium. The **discoid lesions** are characterized histologically by lymphocytic infiltration at the dermal-epidermal or dermal–follicular epithelial junction and around blood vessels and skin appendages (e.g., sweat glands); diffuse vacuolization of the pigment-containing basal cell layer; atrophied epidermis with loss of normal rete ridges and epithelial atrophy of hair follicles; and variable hyperkeratosis of the epidermis. A distinctive feature of the lesions is a granular band of complement and immunoglobulin observed by direct immunofluorescence along the junctions between the dermis and the epidermis of follicular epithelium ("lupus-band test"). This band can also sometimes be seen in apparently "normal" skin of patients with systemic lupus erythematosus. A rare cutaneous manifestation of lupus erythematosus, **lupus profundus,** is characterized by a chronic inflammation or subcutaneous fat (panniculitis) with significant epidermal changes.

Acne Vulgaris

Acne vulgaris is a chronic inflammation of the hair follicle and adjacent skin.

Acne vulgaris is a chronic inflammation of the hair follicle and adjacent skin that is observed most often in teens of both sexes, possibly as the result of the hormonal changes observed in adolescence. The severity of acne appears to be influenced by heredity and, questionably, diet. Bacterial lipases produced by **Propionibacterium acnes** may also be involved in the pathogenesis of acne. Acne can also be induced or exacerbated by a wide variety of systemic drugs (sex steroids, corticosteroids, gonadotropins, trimethadone, iodine or bromine-containing compounds); contact with chemicals (coal, tar, chlorinated hydrocarbons); or physical conditions causing the skin to be warm and moist (tropical climates, heavy clothing). Acne is subclassified into noninflammatory and inflammatory types. Two forms of noninflammatory lesions are observed. **Open comedones** (singular, comedo) are papules that form around a hair follicle occluded by a keratin plug that appears black as a consequence of oxidation of melanin pigment. **Closed comedones** are similar to open comedones but do not have a visible central plug because the keratin is trapped deeper within the follicle. Closed comedones may undergo follicular rupture with resulting inflammation. Such inflammatory acne may produce erythematous papules, nodules, and pustules, and, in more severe forms **(acne conglobeta),** cause significant scarring. Histologically, open and closed comedones are masses of lipid and keratin that dilate the follicles and induce atrophy of follicular epithelium and sebaceous glands. In open comedones, the follicular orifice is dilated, while in closed comedones, it is narrow. The microscopic appearance of inflammatory acne additionally includes perifollicular acute and chronic inflammation, sometimes with abscess formation.

SKIN INFECTIONS AND INFESTATIONS

Among the common skin infections are verrucae, molluscum contagiosum, impetigo, and superficial fungal infections.

Verrucae

Verrucae (warts) are epidermal hyperplasias caused by DNA-containing papillomaviruses. Most warts spontaneously regress after 6 or more months. Verrucae are classified by morphology and location. **Verruca vulgaris** (common wart) is a rough-surfaced tan papule found most commonly on the thin skin of the hands, usually on the dorsal surface or periungal region. **Verruca plana** (flat wart) is a smooth surfaced papule found most commonly on the face or the thin skin of the hands. **Verruca palmaris** and **verruca plantaris** are rough-surfaced, often large (up to 2 cm in diameter) warts found on the palms or soles, respectively. **Condyloma acuminatum** (venereal wart) is a cauliflower-like mass (up to several centimeters in diameter) found on the skin of the male and female genital and perianal areas. The histologic appearance of the different types of warts is similar. The epidermis has an often undulant hyperplasia (verrucous or **papillomatous epidermal hyperplasia**) that can produce papillary projections in rough-surfaced warts. Individual cells, particularly in the more superficial epidermal layers, can show **koilocytosis** (cytoplasmic vacuolization) in which nuclei containing viral particles (as seen by electron microscopy) are surrounded by clear-appearing cytoplasm. Many strains of papillomavirus have been identified; some are associated with particular types of warts and lesions found on the uterine cervix. Anogenital warts are caused most often by types 6, 11, 16, and 18 (see p. 331). Types 16 and 18 have been isolated from uterine cervical carcinoma (see p. 333); type 16 has also been isolated from in situ squamous cell carcinoma of the genitalia. Types 5 and 8 have been isolated from the squamous cell carcinomas that occur in a form of familial flat warts, known as **epidermodysplasia verruciformis**.

> Warts are tumorlike epidermal hyperplasias caused by papillomaviruses.

Molluscum Contagiosum

Molluscum contagiosum is a verrucous epidermal hyperplasia caused by a DNA-containing pox virus that can cause multiple papules on the skin and mucous membranes. Cheeselike material can often be expressed from the lesions. The distinctive histologic appearance is characterized by a **"volcano"** of epidermal hyperplasia with a core of keratinized debris. Cells in the stratum granulosum and stratum corneum contain characteristic cytoplasmic inclusions known as **molluscum bodies,** which are large (up to 30 or more μm), eosinophilic, homogenous ellipsoids containing numerous virions when observed by electron microscopy. Molluscum contagiosum is a common viral skin infection of children and young adults that is most often spread by direct contact and will usually spontaneously regress.

Impetigo

Erythematous macules and small pustules can be caused by superficial bacterial skin infection, producing **impetigo.** The most common infecting organisms are coagulase-positive staphylococci and group A β-hemolytic streptococci. The lesions are found on exposed skin, often of the hands or face, and the pustules tend to break and become crusted with yellowish dried serum. Microscopically, neutrophils accumulate beneath the stratum corneum, sometimes with the formation of small subcorneal pustules. Bacteria can be demonstrated with Gram stain in these foci.

Superficial Fungal Infections

Fungal infections confined to the stratum corneum are considered **superficial infections** and usually produce mild, self-limited infections. The lesions are classified by site of infection. **Tinea capitis** affects the scalp of children, in whom it causes erythema, scaling, and patchy hair loss. **Tinea barbae** affects the beards of adult men. **Tinea corporis** produces an expanding erythematous plaque with a raised border on the body surface of children and adults. **Tinea cruris** produces moist, red patches in the groin. **Tinea pedis** (athlete's foot) causes diffuse erythema and scaling that typically begins in the web spaces. Involvement of the nails is called **onychomycosis. Tinea versicolor** is a distinctive fungal infection caused by *Malassezia furfur,* which produces macules that may be either lighter or darker than the adjacent skin. In all of these superficial fungal infections, fungal cell walls can be identified with PAS stain in the anucleate cornified layer of affected skin or hair. The underlying skin may show reactive epidermal changes. Culture of hair or skin scrapings can identify the infecting organism.

BLISTERING DISEASES

A **blister** is a fluid-filled separation between adjacent skin layers. Blisters smaller than 5 mm are called **vesicles;** large blisters are called **bullae.** While blisters can occur as a secondary phenomenon in many unrelated conditions (burns, herpesvirus infections), blisters are the primary feature of a smaller group of diseases known as bullous diseases. These diseases are distinguished primarily by the level of the skin at which the blister forms.

Pemphigus

Pemphigus is characterized by blister formation in the epidermis at approximately one cell layer above the dermal epidermal junction. The result is a suprabasal acantholytic blister that forms as a result of an autoimmune dissolution of intercellular epithelium. Pemphigus is a rare autoimmune disease characterized by **IgG antibodies** directed against the intercellular cement substance of skin and mucous membranes. This IgG is deposited within the epidermis as a netlike pattern of intercellular deposits localized to sites of acantholysis. Pemphigus has several subtypes. **Pemphigus vulgaris** is the most common form and is characterized by superficial vesicles and bullae that rupture easily to form shallow erosions crusted with dried serum. The blisters can be found on oral mucosa and skin of the head and trunk. **Pemphigus vegetans** is distinguished by considerable overlying epidermal hyperplasia, so that the gross appearance of the lesions resembles a wart rather than a blister. **Pemphigus foliaceus** resembles pemphigus vulgaris, but mucous membranes are only rarely affected. Pemphigus foliaceus can occur in either sporadic or epidemic forms (usually in South America). At physical examination, most or all of the very superficial bullae have usually ruptured, leaving erythematous, crusted skin. The lesions are found on the head and trunk. **Pemphigus erythematosus** can be considered a mild form of pemphigus foliaceus that selectively involves the malar area of the face.

Pemphigus is characterized by blister formation one cell layer above the dermal epidermal junction.

Bullous Pemphigoid

Bullous pemphigoid, in contrast to pemphigus, is characterized by blister formation in the dermis immediately below the epidermis. Because of this deep location, the vesicles and bullae of bullous pemphigoid do not rupture easily and may reach diameters of 4 to 8 cm. The bullae are usually found on moist surfaces such as the inner thighs, axilla, groin, or flexor surface of the arms. Antibody is characteristically deposited in a linear pattern along the basement membrane between the epidermis and dermis. The blister wall can be infiltrated by lymphocytes, eosinophils, and occasional neutrophils.

Bullous pemphigoid is characterized by blister formation in the dermis immediately below the epidermis.

Dermatitis Herpetiformis

Dermatitis herpetiformis forms very pruritic plaques and vesicles. The characteristic histologic lesions are microabscesses, composed of fibrin and neutrophils, located in zones of dermoepidermal separation (**microscopic blisters**) at the tips of the dermal papillae. Granular deposits of IgA can be identified in the tips of the dermal papillae. Dermatitis herpetiformis is most common in men in the third and fourth decades of life. The disease is associated with **celiac disease** and improves with the removal of gluten from the diet. The vesicles and pruritic plaques preferentially form groups of herpetiform lesions that involve elbows, knees, back, and buttocks.

Dermatitis herpetiformis is characterized by formation of microscopic blisters at the tips of the dermal papillae.

Noninflammatory Blistering Diseases

Noninflammatory blistering diseases also occur. **Porphyria** is a group of uncommon metabolic diseases (both genetic and acquired) character-

Porphyria and epidermolysis bullosa are uncommon causes of noninflammatory blister formation.

ized by abnormal metabolism of the porphyrin pigments found in hemoglobin, myoglobin, and cytochromes. These systemic diseases can cause sun-sensitive skin with urticaria and vesicles. **Epidermolysis bullosa** is a group of unrelated diseases characterized by formation of blisters at sites of pressure or trauma. The blisters characteristically develop at or soon after birth.

BENIGN EPITHELIAL TUMORS

Benign epithelial tumors are common and are typically only cosmetically significant.

Seborrheic Keratoses

Seborrheic keratoses are common benign lesions characterized by hyperkeratosis and horn cysts of the superficial epidermis.

Seborrheic keratoses (senile keratoses; dermatosis papulosa nigra on dark-skinned individuals) are sharply demarcated, flat, round, plaques that may be up to several centimeters in diameter. A thickened area of epidermis is composed of orderly proliferations of cells resembling the basal cells of normal epidermis. These cells produce large amounts of keratin (hyperkeratosis), whose accumulation may form small cysts (**horn cysts**) and downgrowths (pseudohorn cysts) within the superficial epidermis. The basaloid cells can contain melanin pigment, which causes the brown color of the lesion. In some cases, the tumor grows downward because the epithelium of the hair follicles is involved, producing **inverted follicular keratoses.** Seborrheic keratoses are usually clinically insignificant lesions that can be easily removed by curettage. Large numbers of seborrheic keratoses occasionally occur as a paraneoplastic syndrome.

Acanthosis Nigricans

Acanthosis nigricans is a darkly pigmented hyperplasia of the stratum spinosum of the epidermis.

Acanthosis nigricans is a darkly pigmented hyperplasia of the stratum spinosum of the epidermis that tends to occur in the flexural areas (axilla, groin). Acanthosis nigricans may be observed in a variety of benign and malignant conditions, including obesity, diabetes or other endocrine disorders, several rare congenital conditions, and cancers, particularly adenocarcinoma. The epidermis characteristically shows variable hyperplasia in the form of sharp peaks and valleys. The basal cell layer may be slightly hyperpigmented, and excess keratin (hyperkeratosis) may be present.

Fibroepithelial Polyps

Fibroepithelial polyps are soft, baglike tumors with a fibrovascular core covered by squamous epithelium.

Fibroepithelial polyps (skin tags, acrochordon, squamous papilloma) are common, inconsequential, cutaneous lesions that form soft, baglike tumors attached by a slender stalk to the skin. Microscopically, fibroepithelial polyps have fibrovascular cores covered by normal-appearing squamous epithelium. Fibroepithelial polyps may increase in number during pregnancy and have occasionally been associated with diabetes and intestinal polyposis.

Epithelial Cysts

Epithelial cysts (wens) are a common cystic, keratin-lined expansion of a downward growth of epidermis or of the epithelium surrounding a hair follicle. Several subtypes can occur. **Epidermal inclusion cysts** are lined with epithelium closely resembling the epidermis and filled with keratin strands. **Tricholemmal** (pilar) **cysts** are lined by an epithelium without a granular cell layer that resembles the epithelium of the hair follicle and contains a homogenous mass of keratin and lipid. **Dermoid cysts** resemble epidermal inclusion cysts but also contain skin adnexal structures, such as hair follicles, in the cyst wall. **Steatocystoma multiplex** are cysts with a wall resembling sebaceous gland ducts that may occur in a familial form.

Epithelial cysts are keratin-containing expansions of a downward growth of epidermis.

Keratoacanthomas

Keratoacanthomas are a benign proliferation of epithelial cells that form a rapidly growing **"volcano"** with a keratin-filled center. Keratoacanthomas may strongly resemble well-differentiated squamous cell carcinomas but are clinically benign and may even heal spontaneously. Some investigators suspect that keratoacanthomas and well-differentiated squamous cell carcinomas may actually involve the same pathologic process, except that the host response is more effective in patients with keratoacanthomas.

Keratoacanthomas are clinically benign lesions that resemble well-differentiated squamous cell carcinoma.

Adnexal Tumors

Adnexal tumors comprise a large variety of neoplasms that arise from skin adnexal structures. The more significant benign tumors are described below. **Eccrine poromas** arise from eccrine sweat glands, usually on the palms or soles. **Cylindromas** show differentiation resembling that of apocrine sweat glands with islands of basaloid cells in a fibrous dermal matrix. Cylindromas are most commonly observed on the forehead or scalp, and may eventually form a turbanlike growth (turban tumor). **Syringomas** are papules usually found near the lower eyelid that contain ducts, islands, and strands of epithelium resembling that of eccrine ducts. **Trichoepitheliomas** form hair-follicle-like structures. **Trichilemmomas** contain glassy cells resembling the most superficial portion (infundibulum) of the hair follicle. Malignant adnexal tumors are uncommon, but can occur and may produce sebaceous, eccrine, or apocrine carcinomas.

Adnexal tumors arise from skin adnexal structures and show a variety of histologic patterns.

PREMALIGNANT AND MALIGNANT EPIDERMAL TUMORS

Actinic Keratoses

Chronic exposure to sunlight, ionizing radiation, hydrocarbons, or arsenicals can produce dysplastic skin lesions known as **actinic keratoses.** These lesions typically are small (less than 1 cm diameter) and have a rough consistency with a color that may be tan, red, or skin-colored. Histologically, the actinic keratoses are characterized by atypical basal cells with eosinophilic cytoplasm. These atypical basal cells, unlike the cells in basal cell carcinomas, still have intercellular bridges, which can be seen by light microscopy. The stratum corneum usually contains nuclei (parakeratosis) and may be markedly thickened; the remainder of the epidermis may be thinned. The underlying dermis usually shows changes caused by sun damage, including blue-gray elastic fibers (solar

Actinic keratoses are dysplastic skin lesions with atypical basal cells and an often markedly thickened stratum corneum.

elastosis). Actinic keratoses are considered premalignant lesions and can be treated by curettage, cryosurgery, or topical antineoplastic agents.

Squamous Cell Carcinoma

Squamous cell carcinomas of the skin and mucous membranes resemble squamous cell carcinoma arising in other sites.

Squamous cell carcinoma can arise in skin and occurs most often in older individuals on sun-exposed areas. Risk factors include chronic sun exposure; tars and oils; ionizing radiation; severe chronic immunosuppression and chronic inflammation associated with ulcers; draining osteomyelitis; and old burn scars. **Xeroderma pigmentosum** is an hereditary condition characterized by a high incidence of squamous cell carcinoma. Squamous cell carcinomas of the skin and mucous membranes resemble squamous cell carcinomas arising in other sites. **In situ carcinoma** is the term used for squamous cell carcinoma confined to the epidermis above the basement membrane of the dermoepidermal junction. **Invasive squamous cell carcinomas** can vary from well- to poorly-differentiated. Well-differentiated squamous cell carcinomas can strongly resemble keratoacanthomas; often contain zones of keratinization (keratin pearls); and are composed of polygonal squamous cells. Poorly differentiated tumors are often composed of round, highly anaplastic cells that may undergo focal necrosis. Keratin pearls are rare or absent, although individual cells may undergo keratinization (dyskeratosis). Electron microscopy and immunohistochemical techniques can be helpful in establishing the squamous cell nature of very poorly differentiated carcinomas. Squamous cell carcinomas of the skin are usually recognized when the tumor is still small, and the prognosis following resection is excellent.

Basal Cell Carcinoma

Basal cell carcinomas can cause extensive destruction of adjacent structures.

Basal cell carcinomas of the skin are composed of cells resembling the basal cells of the epidermis. Basal cell carcinomas tend to occur in sun-exposed skin, often on the face. Other risk factors include chronic **immunosuppression** and the inherited diseases **xeroderma pigmentosum** and **basal cell nevus syndrome.** Basal cell carcinomas tend to form pearly papules with dilated subepidermal vessels. In the past, the term "rodent ulcer" was used, as neglected tumors sometimes caused extensive destruction of adjacent structures (bone, facial sinuses). Histologically, the tumor is composed of cords and islands of basophilic cells with hyperchromatic nuclei resembling normal basal cells of the epidermis. Cells at the periphery of the islands are often arranged in a radial (palisading) fashion. On a larger scale, two patterns of growth are seen. **Nodular lesions** grow deeply into the dermis. The individual islands are often embedded in a mucinous matrix and surrounded by lymphocytes and fibroblasts. Clefts between the islands and stroma can form during tissue processing, and are helpful in distinguishing nodular basal cell carcinomas from benign proliferations of basal cells, such as are observed in some adnexal tumors. A **multifocal growth pattern** is confined to the more superficial levels of the skin. This pattern suggests that the carcinoma arises in a field of dysplastic cells and is clinically significant because an apparently complete excision around a lesion may actually leave residual tumor. Basal cell carcinomas tend to grow slowly, possibly because the prominent lymphocytic infiltrate limits expansion into adjacent tissue.

Merkel Cell Carcinoma

The Merkel cells of the epidermis are neuroendocrine cells derived from the neural crest; they appear to have a role in tactile sensation in some animals. Rarely, Merkel cells can undergo neoplastic change, producing **Merkel cell carcinoma,** which most often affects elderly individuals and tends to form solitary nodules on the extremities, head, or neck. These tumors behave aggressively and have often metastasized before diagnosis. The tumors are composed histologically of nests of small round cells that by light microscopy resemble oat cell carcinoma metastatic to the skin. By electron microscopy, the cells contain granules similar to those in normal Merkel cells. Immunohistochemical studies show both neuroendocrine and epithelial cell markers.

Merkel cell carcinoma is a neuroendocrine tumor that histologically resembles oat cell carcinoma but whose cells can be demonstrated by electron microscopy to contain distinctive granules.

DISORDERS OF SKIN PIGMENTATION

Localized areas of skin may be either paler or darker than adjacent areas. **Vitiligo** is a patchy light skin most visible in people with either naturally dark or tanned skin. The lesion is associated with a partial or complete loss of melanocytes. The involved skin is usually otherwise normal, but is particularly vulnerable to sunburn since the protective pigmentation is lost. Vitiligo is associated with many autoimmune diseases (pernicious anemia, Addison's disease, thyroiditis) and appears to have an autoimmune basis. In contrast to vitiligo, the number of melanocytes in the genetic disease **albinism** is normal, but the melanocytes are not able to synthesize melanin. **Freckles** (ephelis) are ubiquitous tan to brown macules that appear after sun exposure and are characterized histologically by basal cells containing increased amounts of melanin pigment. The melanocytes may be slightly enlarged but usually are present in normal numbers. **Melasma** (mask of pregnancy) presents, usually in pregnancy, as poorly defined macules on the cheeks, forehead, and temples. Histologically, increased melanin deposition is observed in either the basal layers of the epidermis (epidermal type) or in macrophages in the papillary dermis (dermal type). **Lentigo** is a small, brown macule that, unlike freckles, does not darken after exposure to sunlight. The dark pigmentation is due to melanocytic hyperplasia with a resulting hyperpigmentation of the basal cell layer of the epidermis. In addition to the disorders of pigmentation described above, there are hyperpigmented skin elevations that range from benign nevi to dysplastic nevi to melanoma.

Skin hypopigmentation may take the form of vitiligo or albinism; hyperpigmentation can be caused by freckles, lentigos, or melasma.

NEVI

Nevocellular Nevus

A **nevocellular nevus** (mole, pigmented nevus) is a benign neoplasm of melanocytes. The nevus cells are transformed melanocytes that become round to oval in shape. Nevocellular nevi occur in several forms. The **common acquired nevus** is a small, evenly pigmented (usually dark brown) papule with well-defined rounded borders. The common acquired nevus has several subtypes. In a **junctional nevus,** the nevus cells are

Moles are melanocytic neoplasms classified by location and morphology of the nevus cells.

found at the dermoepidermal junction. In a **compound nevus,** the nevus cells are found at both the dermoepidermal junction and growing downward into the dermis. In a **dermal nevus,** the junctional cells are lost, and only nevus cells in the deeper dermis remain. Nevus cells at the dermoepidermal junction tend to be pigmented and arranged in a layer next to the junction. Nevus cells in the superficial dermis tend to be non-pigmented and arranged in cords. Nevus cells in the deep dermis tend to be nonpigmented, spindle-shaped, and arranged in clusters. These changes are helpful for distinguishing some benign nevi from malignant melanoma.

Congenital nevocellular nevi are present at birth and may become more prominent with time. Larger lesions may involve large segments of the body surface. The nevus cells may be found in the lower dermis and even subcutaneous fat. Malignant melanoma may develop within a congenital nevus. **Blue nevi** contain unusual nevus cells that are highly pigmented and have a dendritic rather than rounded shape. These cells are usually located in the middle to deep dermis, causing the mole to appear blue clinically due to the overlying epidermis and superficial dermis. The **compound nevi of Spitz** are easily confused with malignant melanoma because the spindle-shaped and plump epithelium-like ("epithelioid") nevus cells show sometimes striking nuclear pleomorphism. **Halo nevi** have a surrounding zone of hypopigmentation that is associated with lymphocytic infiltration, possibly representing an immune reaction directed against the nevus cells, despite the nevi's biologically benign behavior.

Dysplastic Nevi

When compared with common acquired nevi, dysplastic nevi tend to be larger, to have more irregular contours, and to contain more cells with nuclear atypia.

Dysplastic nevi are a subgroup of nevocellular nevi that have a higher risk of progressing to malignant melanoma than do the nevi described above. Clinically, dysplastic nevi tend to be larger (greater than 6 mm) and may be present in large numbers. Compared with common acquired nevi, the dysplastic nevi show greater variation in pigmentation and a more irregular contour. Histologically, the dysplastic nevi are usually compound, and the nevus cells nest within the epidermis and are larger than in nondysplastic nevi. The normal basal cell layer along the dermoepidermal junction begins to be replaced with single nevus cells **(lentiginous hyperplasia).** The nevus cells tend to be more fusiform than round and may show nuclear atypia characterized by angulated nuclear contours and hyperchromasia. A familial syndrome associated with a susceptibility gene on chromosome 1 carries a strong probability that one or more dysplastic nevi will eventually develop melanoma (**heritable melanoma syndrome**).

Malignant Melanoma

Malignant melanomas with radial growth patterns are more often cured by surgical excision than are those with a vertical growth pattern.

Malignant melanoma is a malignancy of nevus cells that often develops near a pre-existing dysplastic nevus. Sunlight also appears to be a predisposing factor, since lightly pigmented individuals have a higher incidence of malignant melanoma than do darkly pigmented individuals. Exposure to unidentified carcinogens may also be a risk factor. In contrast to the common acquired nevi, melanomas tend to have **variegated color** (black, brown, red, gray, blue, white) and irregular, notched borders. In addition to sites on skin, melanomas are sometimes found in a wide variety of other sites including scalp, mouth, anus, nail beds, eyes, gastrointestinal tract, and leptomeninges. The pattern of growth of the melanoma has prognostic value. Melanomas that grow parallel to the epidermis (radial growth) have a better prognosis than those that are growing deep into the dermis (vertical growth), possibly because the vertical growth has a greater probability of involving a dermal lymphatic, causing metastasis. In most melanomas, the radial growth pattern occurs before the vertical one. Melanomas with a radial growth pattern can often be cured by wide surgical excision; those with a vertical growth pattern may additionally require chemotherapy, which is often of limited effectiveness. Compared with benign nevus cells, melanoma cells are usually larger and have pleomorphic nuclei with prominent nucleoli. In the epidermis, the cells grow as individual cells or poorly formed nests that may be seen at any level of the epidermis. In the dermis, the melanoma cells form large nodules.

TUMORS OF THE DERMIS

The dermis is a complex tissue composed of many elements (smooth muscle, vessels, fibroblasts, nerve), any of which may undergo benign or malignant neoplasia. Many of these tumors are similar to soft tissue tumors observed at other sites, and this section will discuss only those dermal tumors that have distinctive features.

BENIGN FIBROUS HISTIOCYTOMA

A heterogeneous family of benign neoplasms of fibroblasts and histiocytes is called **benign fibrous histiocytoma.** These tumors form tan to brown papules that occur most often on the legs of young to middle-aged women. Unlike nodular melanoma, the nodules often dimple inward when compressed laterally. **Dermatofibroma** is the most common variant of benign fibrous histiocytoma, and is composed of a nonencapsulated mass of spindle-shaped fibroblasts, sometimes with rare foamy histiocytes. Dermatofibromas are typically located in the mid-dermis but may extend into the subcutaneous fat. The overlying epidermis is often hyperplastic and has elongated, hyperpigmented rete ridges. Other types of benign fibrous histiocytomas contain proportionally more foamy histiocytes and fewer fibroblasts. Some variants contain prominent blood vessels (**sclerosing hemangiomas**).

Benign fibrous histiocytomas are neoplasms of fibroblasts and histiocytes.

Dermatofibrosarcoma Protuberans

Dermatofibrosarcoma protuberans is the malignant counterpart of dermatofibroma and is composed of a proliferation of fibroblasts that may be arranged in radial patterns resembling a pinwheel (**storiform pattern**). The tumors tend to occur on the trunk and form solid nodules that may aggregate into a "protuberant" plaque. Extension into the subcutaneous fat may make surgical excision more difficult.

Dermatofibrosarcoma protuberans is a malignant proliferation of fibroblasts.

Xanthomas

Xanthomas are tumor-like dermal collections of foamy histiocytes, often with multinucleate giant cells that may have clustered nuclei and foamy cytoplasm **(Touton giant cells).** The foamy cytoplasm contains cholesterol, phospholipids, and triglycerides. Xanthomas may be observed idiopathically or in association with hyperlipidemia or lymphoproliferative malignancies. Xanthomas have been divided into subtypes based on clinical appearances; these subtypes have been associated with different types of hyperlipoproteinemias. **Eruptive xanthomas** are yellow papules found on buttocks, thighs, knees, and elbows; tend to occur in showers that appear and disappear with changing plasma triglyceride levels; and occur in many types (I, IIB, III, IV, V) of hyperlipoproteinemia. **Tuberous xanthomas** are yellow nodules observed in patients with hyperlipoproteinemia, most often of types II and III. **Tendonous xanthomas** are similar to tuberous xanthomas but occur on tendons such as the Achilles tendon and extensor tendons of the fingers. **Plane xanthomas** occur in skin folds, notably palmar creases, as linear yellow lesions and are associated with types III and IIA hyperlipoproteinemias. **Xanthelasma** are soft, yellow plaques usually found on eyelids that may occur idiopathically or in association with types II and III hyperlipoproteinemias.

Kaposi's Sarcoma

Hemangioma, vascular malformations ("port wine stain"), and angiosarcomas can occur in the skin and are discussed elsewhere (see p. 207). **Kaposi's sarcoma** is a malignant vascular tumor that usually arises in skin and is of increasing importance because it is common in patients with AIDS. Kaposi's sarcoma forms red-purple macules, papules, and plaques composed of irregular and angulated spaces in a stroma composed of collagen bundles containing bland-appearing spindle cells. The spaces are lined by elongated endothelial tumor cells, whose origin is still unclear but appears to be either from blood vessels or lymphatic endothelium. The relationship of Kaposi's sarcoma to AIDS is also still unclear. In addition to Kaposi's sarcoma associated with AIDS, an aggressive form of Kaposi's sarcoma is observed in Africa, and a relatively mild form is observed in middle-aged and older men of Mediterranean origin.

OTHER TUMORS

Cutaneous Lymphomas

Lymphomas of T-cell lines can arise in the skin, producing several clinicopathologic patterns. **Mycosis fungoides** is a malignant proliferation of T-helper cells (CD4 antigen-positive) known as **Sézary-Lutzner cells.** These cells have highly convoluted ("cerebriform") nuclei and are found predominantly in the superficial dermis, where they form bandlike aggregates. Single cells and small clusters of Sézary-Lutzner cells **(Pautrier's microabscesses)** also invade the epidermis. Clinically, patients with mycosis fungoides have skin lesions that initially are red-brown patches resembling eczema, but may later progress to raised scaling plaques that resemble psoriasis. Mycosis fungoides is most common after age 40 and may either remain localized to the skin or progress to systemic T-cell lymphoma. **Sézary syndrome** occurs in a few individuals when the development of systemic lymphoma is accompanied by erythema and scaling involving all the body skin (erythroderma). **Mycosis fungoides d'emblée** is a variant of mycosis fungoides, characterized by a nodular pattern of skin eruptions in which the Sézary-Lutzner cells grow in nodules in the deep dermis and do not usually involve the epidermis. An **adult T-cell leukemia or lymphoma** can also involve the skin and often has a rapidly progressive downhill course. When the T-cell lymphomas are limited to the skin, therapy may involve topical corticosteroids, ultraviolet light, or topical chemotherapeutic agents. When the disease progresses to systemic involvement, aggressive systemic chemotherapeutic regimens are usually used.

Mastocytosis

Rarely, mast cells may proliferate in the skin or other organs. Whether these proliferations occur in response to local stimuli or are true neoplasms is still disputed. **Urticaria pigmentosa** affects children and is the most common form of mast cell proliferation. Urticaria pigmentosa is localized to the skin, where it usually causes multiple, widely distributed round to oval papules and plaques. **Solitary mastocytomas** and **mastocytosis with systemic manifestations** can also occur. Histologically, mastocytosis in all of its forms is characterized by increased numbers of spindle-shaped or stellate mast cells, often located either around superficial dermal blood vessels, or, if the mastocytosis is marked, in large groups of tightly packed cells in the dermis. If extensive degranulation has occurred, the mast cells may be difficult to distinguish from lymphocytes, and electron microscopy may be helpful in establishing the diagnosis. Degranulation of mast cells with subsequent release of histamine and other substances can cause pruritis, flushing, or formation of hives. Triggers for degranulation vary from patient to patient and may include alcohol, drugs (aspirin, narcotic analgesics), or specific foods. Localized rubbing of the skin can produce a wheal **(Darier's sign); dermatographism** refers to the linear hive produced by stroking the skin with a pointed instrument. In addition to the skin changes, degranulation of mastocytes can cause systemic symptoms including rhinorrhea, bone pain, and, rarely, gastrointestinal bleeding.

Cutaneous mast cell proliferations may take the forms of urticaria pigmentosa, solitary mastocytomas, or mastocytosis with systemic manifestations.

SOFT TISSUE TUMORS AND TUMORLIKE CONDITIONS

SOFT TISSUE TUMORS

Immunohistochemical techniques may help in establishing the histologic type of poorly differentiated soft tissue tumors.

The soft tissue tumors discussed in this section include those of skeletal muscle, fat, and fibrous tissue. While benign tumors and well-differentiated sarcomas of different histologic types tend to appear clearly different, more poorly differentiated sarcomas can be difficult to distinguish. In these cases, immunohistochemistry to stain the filaments produced by the cells may be helpful in establishing a diagnosis. Grading of soft tissue sarcomas tends to be based on extent of necrosis, pleomorphism, cellularity, and number of mitoses. A variety of staging systems for soft tissue tumors have been developed. One of the most commonly used is based on tumor grade, size, and presence or absence of regional or distant metastases. Low-grade sarcomas that are adequately excised have an excellent long-term prognosis; high-grade sarcomas have a poor prognosis. Male sex is associated with worse prognosis.

Granular Cell Tumors

Granular cell tumors are composed of cells with abundant eosinophilic cytoplasm that contains prominent PAS-positive, diastase-resistant, cytoplasmic granules.

Granular cell tumors are small (usually less than 3 cm), firm, poorly encapsulated (but usually benign) nodules that are most often found on the tongue or in subcutaneous tissues of young to middle-aged adults. Their histogenesis is disputed; the tumors may arise from precursors of Schwann cells. The tumor cells are round to polygonal cells with centrally located, small, dark nuclei; abundant eosinophilic cytoplasm; and distinct cell borders. The tumor cells tend to grow in nests or sheets and exhibit only minimal mitotic activity, nuclear pleomorphism, or multinucleation. A distinctive feature of the cells are prominent periodic acid-Schiff (PAS)-positive, diastase-resistant, **cytoplasmic granules** of varying size that can be shown by electron microscopy to be membrane-bound phagolysosomes containing amorphous material that probably represents disintegrating cellular organelles. Granular cell tumors located near squamous epithelium may induce pseudoepitheliomatous hyperplasia of the epithelium, which may be mistaken for squamous cell carcinoma. Malignant granular cell tumors occur uncommonly. They tend to be larger (over 8 cm), more rapidly growing, more anaplastic, and more obviously infiltrative than their benign counterparts.

Benign and Malignant Fibrous Histiocytoma

Both benign and malignant **fibrous histiocytomas** are composed of a variety of immature cells that can include primitive mesenchymal cells, fibroblasts, myofibroblasts, histiocytes, and cells with mixed features. Other histologic features include varying numbers of giant cells, lipid-containing xanthomatous cells, and prominent vascularization. In the past, many different names (dermatofibromas, fibroxanthomas, histiocytomas, xanthogranulomas, sclerosing hemangiomas, giant cell tumors of tendon sheath) were based on the predominant growth patterns, but modern usage tends to classify these tumors simply as fibrous histiocytomas based on their histogenesis from pluripotent primitive mesenchymal cells. Benign fibrous histiocytomas often involve the skin (see p. 119).

Malignant fibrous histiocytomas are a common form of soft tissue sarcoma and are found in soft tissues and occasionally bone. The malignant fibrous histiocytomas tend to affect elderly individuals with a modest male predominance, but can occur at any age. Common sites of origin include the extremities and abdomen including the retroperitoneum. Most malignant fibrous histiocytomas arise near skeletal muscle, with other sites (deep fascia, subcutaneous tissue) occurring less commonly. Malignant fibrous histiocytomas arising in bone tend to occur around the knee, with less common sites including other regions of the pelvis and extremities. Malignant fibrous histiocytomas of soft tissue are usually multilobulated, gray-white masses that appear deceptively well circumscribed but are actually unencapsulated. Areas of hemorrhage and necrosis are common. Malignant fibrous histiocytoma has been subclassified into five histologic types, of which the first two, storiform-pleomorphic and myxoid forms, are most common. **Storiform-pleomorphic** malignant fibrous histiocytomas contain histiocytoid cells with characteristic filopodial cytoplasmic extensions seen on electron microscopy; spindle cells (both fibroblasts and myofibroblasts) that are often arranged in a cartwheel (storiform) pattern around small, slitlike blood vessels; and small, nonspecialized mesenchymal cells. The **myxoid** variant has a somewhat better prognosis than other variants and is characterized by areas of loose myxoid stroma rich in acid mycopolysaccharides and containing spindle or stellate mesenchymal cells. In between these myxoid areas are regions of the tumor that resemble the storiform–pleomorphic variant. Less common variants of malignant fibrous histiocytoma include giant cell, inflammatory, and angiomatoid. These variants are characterized, respectively, by prominent giant cells, lymphocytes, and blood vessels within a tumor matrix.

Lipoma and Liposarcoma

Tumorous collections of fatty tissue are common and can be subdivided into lipomas, non-neoplastic lipomatous masses, and liposarcomas. **Lipomas** are very common, benign tumors. They often arise in subcutaneous tissues (although other sites do occur, often on the back, shoulder, or neck) and are most prevalent in older adulthood. A small percentage of patients have multiple lipomas, sometimes as part of a familial pattern. Histologically, lipomas are composed of mature adipose tissue surrounded by a delicate fibrous capsule. They may contain areas of fibrous tissue (**fibrolipoma**), proliferating vessels (**angiolipoma**), or bone marrow elements (**myelolipoma**). Resection is curative. **Non-neoplastic lipomatous masses** differ histologically from lipomas by the absence of a well-defined fibrous capsule. They can be found in many deep tissue sites, including within the spermatic

Fibrous histiocytomas may be either benign or malignant. They are composed of a variety of immature cells because they arise from pluripotent primitive mesenchymal cells.

The most common types of malignant fibrous histiocytomas are the storiform–pleomorphic and myxoid variants.

Lipomas and liposarcomas are tumorous collections of fatty tissue. Lipomas tend to arise in subcutaneous tissues.

cord, or adjacent to muscle, tendon, or nerve. They usually have no clinical significance.

Liposarcomas are uncommon tumors arising from primitive mesenchymal cells that differentiate along lipocyte lines. The tumors can be difficult to resect because they appear well circumscribed, but actually frequently have projections into adjacent structures. Some liposarcomas are massive (up to 40 kg), in part because they tend to arise deep within the abdomen or thigh, where they may not produce symptoms until very late in the course. Four histological types of liposarcoma have been characterized. **Well-differentiated** liposarcomas can be difficult to distinguish from lipomas. Histologic features that may be helpful in establishing the diagnosis of well-differentiated liposarcoma include a discernible rim of cytoplasm around the fat droplet; slightly "scalloped" nuclei; and occasional lipoblasts with abundant cytoplasm and one or more small lipid droplets. The well-differentiated liposarcomas may also, but do not always, contain mitoses, tumor giant cells, myxomatous tissue, or small areas resembling malignant fibrous histiocytoma. **Myxoid** liposarcomas are the most common variant. They have a loose, myxoid stroma containing abundant mucopolysaccharide ground substance in which are located tumor cells with varying degrees of maturation, ranging from primitive mesenchymal cells, to pleomorphic stellate cells with minute vacuoles, to adult-appearing fat cells. Vascularization is often prominent, sometimes in a branching "chicken-wire" pattern of capillary channels. A few tumor giant cells and mitoses may be present. **Round cell** liposarcoma is composed of small round cells that resemble those of malignant lymphomas or Ewing's sarcoma. The diagnosis is established by finding occasional lipoblasts with small, fatty vacuoles. **Pleomorphic** liposarcoma is a highly anaplastic lesion that resembles other highly undifferentiated soft tissue sarcomas. The diagnosis is established by identifying scattered lipoblasts. Giant tumor cells with multivacuolated cytoplasm, possibly derived from lipoblasts, can also sometimes be observed.

Rhabdomyoma and Rhabdomyosarcoma

Benign and malignant tumors of striated muscle are called, respectively, rhabdomyomas and rhabdomyosarcomas. **Cardiac rhabdomyomas** are probably hamartomas rather than true neoplastic proliferations. Many patients with cardiac rhabdomyomas also have the hamartomatous condition tuberous sclerosis. **Extracardiac rhabdomyomas,** which may contain either adult or fetal striated muscle tissue, are probably true neoplasms but are extremely rare.

Rhabdomyosarcomas are common soft tissue sarcomas that most often affect children in the head, neck, and urogenital region. Only one-quarter of cases arise in muscle; the remainder arise throughout the body. Four histologic subtypes occur. The **embryonal subtype** is the most common. Embryonal rhabdomyosarcoma characteristically contains cells with varying degrees of differentiation, including primitive round or oval cells with hyperchromatic nuclei; slightly more differentiated cells with more cytoplasm that may be binucleated and occasionally contain cytoplasmic cross striations; distinctive elongated, straplike cells that may be multinucleate and that often have prominent cross striations;

Liposarcomas are sometimes massive at the time of diagnosis.

The relatively common cardiac rhabdomyoma is probably a hamartoma rather than a true neoplastic proliferation.

Rhabdomyosarcomas are subclassified into embryonal, botryoid, alveolar, and pleomorphic types.

distinctive "racquet-shaped" cells with a thin rim of cytoplasm around the nucleus and a prominent cytoplasmic extension that forms the "handle of the racquet"; and distinctive "spider cells," which are tumor giant cells with multiple prominent glycogen-containing vacuoles that split the cytoplasm of the cell into thin strands ("spider legs"). The proportions of these cells vary from tumor to tumor. Immunohistochemical staining for desmin, actin, myosin, and myoglobin may help to establish the diagnosis. **Botryoid rhabdomyosarcoma** can be considered a variant of the embryonal pattern that is characterized by a distinct gross morphology resembling a cluster of grapes. Botryoid rhabdomyosarcoma is usually found projecting into an open space such as the vagina or urinary bladder. The histology is similar to that of embryonal rhabdomyosarcoma. **Alveolar rhabdomyosarcoma** is characterized by clusters of small, undifferentiated tumor cells within a honeycomb of fibrovascular stroma. Histologically, this honeycomb pattern loosely resembles pulmonary alveoli, since the centers of the cell clusters have often necrosed, leaving thin fibrovascular alveolar walls to which tumor cells are loosely adherent. Mitoses, spindle cells, and multinucleate giant cells can often be seen. **Pleomorphic rhabdomyosarcoma** is the most poorly differentiated form of rhabdomyosarcoma. The appearance is similar to embryonal rhabdomyosarcoma, but the better differentiated elongated strap cells are rare, and cross striations may be completely absent. The diagnosis is usually established by immunohistochemical or ultrastructural studies that may show thick and thin filaments. Many cases formerly considered to be pleomorphic rhabdomyosarcoma are now classified as malignant fibrous histiocytomas. Rhabdomyosarcomas are highly malignant tumors that are characteristically difficult to excise completely, particularly when they occur in the head and neck.

Leiomyoma and Leiomyosarcoma

Leiomyoma and **leiomyosarcoma** are, respectively, benign and malignant proliferations of cells with smooth muscle differentiation. These tumors are common in the female genital tract and are discussed in detail in that section (see p. 338). Leiomyosarcomas are also found in the retroperitoneum, gastrointestinal tract, and subcutaneous tissue.

Leiomyoma and leiomyosarcoma are proliferations of cells with smooth muscle differentiation.

Fibroma and Fibrosarcoma

Despite the tissue's prevalence, true neoplastic proliferations of connective tissue are uncommon. **Fibromas** are benign neoplasms composed of spindle-shaped fibroblasts, which, in contrast to smooth muscle cells, have elongated, pointed nuclei. The cells may be arranged either randomly or in broad ribbons. The amount of collagen between the cells may be either scant ("cellular fibromas") or abundant. True fibromas occur most commonly along nerve trunks (neurofibroma) or in the ovaries. Many lesions formerly thought to be fibromas are now classified as non-neoplastic fibromatosis (see p. 127). **Fibrosarcomas** are rare, but may arise throughout the body, with common sites including retroperitoneum, thigh, knee, and distal extremities. Grossly, the tumors are "fish-flesh" unencapsulated masses that often show focal hemorrhage

Fibromas and fibrosarcomas are surprisingly uncommon.

and necrosis. The cells in well-differentiated fibrosarcomas sometimes grow in a "herringbone" pattern. Some well-differentiated fibrosarcomas can be difficult to distinguish from fibromas. Distinguishing leiomyosarcomas from fibrosarcomas may also be difficult. Immunohistochemistry can be helpful since most leiomyosarcomas stain for desmin and muscle actin, while fibrosarcomas either do not or only stain weakly.

Synovial Sarcoma

Synovial sarcomas are found near joints and apparently arise from multipotential mesenchymal cells.

Synovial sarcomas are uncommon soft tissue tumors most commonly observed in young adults with a modest male predominance. They apparently arise from multipotential mesenchymal cells that differentiate along synoviocyte lines. These tumors are all malignant, although some grow slowly. They are almost never found in joint cavities, but instead occur near joints adjacent to tendon sheaths, joint capsules, or bursae. Rarely, synovial sarcomas can arise in the abdominal wall or near the pharynx. The tumors have a distinctive histologic biphasic pattern of growth, with both epithelial cells and proliferating spindle cells.

Neuroblastoma and Ganglioneuroma

Neuroblastomas and ganglioneuromas are childhood cancers that arise from neural crest cells.

Neuroblastoma (see also p. 195) is one of the principal forms of cancer in children, with most of the tumors occurring below the age of 5 years and many below 2 years. Neuroblastomas arise from neural crest cells and are most often found in the adrenal medulla, but can also be found in the posterior mediastinum, pelvis, neck, lower abdominal sympathetic chain, or other sites. **Ganglioneuromas** (see p. 195) are a related tumor that may be considered a well-differentiated variant of neuroblastoma.

Neuroblastomas tend to form lobular, soft, red-gray masses that may contain hemorrhage, necrosis, cysts, and calcification. Neuroblastomas are composed of small cells with hyperchromatic nuclei that are usually arranged in sheets with occasional Homer-Wright pseudorosettes in which tumor cells are located along the periphery of a circle whose center contains young nerve fibers that arise from the tumor cells. In ganglioneuroma, the tumors completely differentiate to form ganglion cells embedded in a stroma background that contains many fibro-cytes and Schwann cells. Rare tumors with differentiation between that of neuroblastomas and ganglioneuromas are sometimes called **ganglioneuroblastomas**.

Metastases of neuroblastomas tend to develop rapidly and may be extensive at the time of tumor diagnosis.

Hutchinson-type neuroblastoma refers to the presence of extensive bony metastases of the skull and orbit that cause exophthalmos. **Pepper-type syndrome** refers to the presence of massive metastasis to liver.

Neuroblastomas are aggressive tumors; ganglioneuromas have a better prognosis.

Neuroblastomas are aggressive tumors that frequently kill within 2 years. The better differentiated ganglioneuromas and ganglioneuroblastomas have a better prognosis. Staging of neuroblastomas is based on extension outside the original organ, crossing of the body midline, and presence of metastatic disease. Patients with only microscopic evidence of metastatic disease have a better prognosis than patients with bulk metastatic disease. Aggressive tumor behavior also appears to be related to the number of copies of the *N-myc* **oncogenes** that are present in the tumor cells. Cytogenic studies have also shown that many neuroblastomas contain **double, minute chromosomes.** Neuroblastomas can also produce catecholamines, although the amounts elaborated are usually much less than those produced by pheochromocytomas, and hypertension is rare.

Neurofibroma and **neurilemmoma** are tumors composed of mature glial (or possibly fibrous) elements that are discussed with peripheral nerve disease (see also p. 198).

TUMORLIKE CONDITIONS

Non-neoplastic processes can mimic soft tissue tumors.

Fibromatosis

Fibromatoses are aggregates of moderately mature fibroblasts dispersed in a dense collagen matrix that tend to form either nodular or poorly defined masses. Their etiology is unclear. Fibromatoses are classified on the basis of site: palmar, plantar, and penile fibromatoses (**Peyronie's disease).** In each of these sites, the mass of connective tissue impairs mobility and may eventually produce deformity.

Fibromatoses are non-neoplastic aggregates of fibroblasts that are subclassified by site.

Desmoid

Desmoids (aggressive fibromatoses) are exuberant proliferations of fibroconnective tissue that often form large, infiltrative masses that may recur after excision but do not metastasize. The desmoids tend to infiltrate surrounding structures such as muscles. Cells at the center of the lesion tend to appear more mature than those at the periphery. The cells at the periphery may also show mild anaplasia, increasing the desmoid's resemblance to a low-grade fibrosarcoma. Intra-abdominal desmoids are frequently associated with **Gardner syndrome** and occur most often in the mesentery and pelvic walls. Abdominal desmoids are often associated with pregnancy and involve the anterior abdominal wall. Extra-abdominal desmoids are observed in both sexes and tend to involve the musculature of the trunk and proximal regions of the extremities.

Desmoids are exuberant proliferations of fibroconnective tissue that may histologically and clinically resemble low-grade fibrosarcoma.

Nodular Fasciitis

Nodular (pseudosarcomatous) **fasciitis** is a reactive fibroproliferative lesion that affects young to middle-aged adults of both sexes, and has the reputation of being one of the most common non-neoplastic conditions to be mistaken for a malignant tumor. Nodular fasciitis typically produces nodules or masses on the extremities that attach to underlying fascia and appear to be invasive. Nodular fasciitis is subdivided into three forms based upon the location of the nodules. The **subcutaneous form** is characteristically well circumscribed but not encapsulated and extends from superficial fascia to the subcutis. The **fascial form** spreads along fascial planes. The **intramuscular form** extends from superficial fascia into adjacent skeletal muscle.

Histologically, the tumor is composed of fibroblasts similar to those found in granulation tissue. Mitotic figures are frequent, and the fibroblasts often have large, irregularly shaped nuclei and prominent

Nodular fasciitis is a reactive fibroproliferative lesion that attaches to fascia and may be mistaken for a malignancy.

nucleoli. These features leave the mistaken impression that this benign lesion is a sarcoma. A helpful histologic feature is that abnormal mitoses are absent. Nodular fasciitis tends to progress through three histologic stages as the fibrous tissue matures. The **myxoid stage** is characterized by irregular aggregates of fibroblasts in a myxoid stroma with prominent neovascularization. The **cellular stage** is characterized by closely packed fibroblasts. The **fibrosing stage** is characterized by thick collagenous bundles containing a few residual fibroblasts. These stages can be considered analogous to the changes granulation tissue progresses through as it becomes mature scar tissue.

Traumatic Myositis Ossificans

Traumatic myositis ossificans is a tumorlike lesion that can be observed either in skeletal muscle or subcutaneous fat. Despite the name, the condition is not inflammatory and does not always ossify. The lesion appears to form by fibrous replacement and often ossification of a **hematoma.** The patient often recalls an initiating incident of soft tissue trauma. Traumatic myositic ossificans forms a well-circumscribed mass that may be up to 5 to 8 cm in diameter and that often has a gritty consistency. The periphery of the mass often has bone spicules surrounded by fibroblasts. More centrally, the mass is composed of less densely packed fibroblasts and immature osteoid. The calcification of the mass, which is often attached to or adjacent to the skeleton, may cause it to be mistaken radiographically for a bone tumor.

Traumatic myositis ossificans appears to form by fibrous replacement and ossification of a hematoma.

JOINT, TENDON, AND MUSCLE

DEGENERATIVE JOINT DISEASE

Degenerative joint disease (**osteoarthritis**) is the most common form of arthritis. This form of joint disease is characterized by a progressive destruction of articular cartilage accompanied by subchondral bony thickening and bony outgrowths (osteophytes or "spurs") around the joint margins. **Primary degenerative joint disease** primarily affects the elderly, although a few individuals (mostly men) develop significant disease by later middle age. **Secondary degenerative joint disease** occurs in previously damaged or congenitally abnormal joints and can affect any age. Degenerative joint disease of both primary and secondary forms can be considered a "wear and tear" process. In the primary form, the joints most severely affected tend to be those subjected to the most stresses, such as the elbows of tennis players or the metatarsophalangeal joints of dancers. The damaged cartilage develops pits and vertical clefts that may extend to the subchondral bone. With time, pieces of cartilage may break off, and areas of cartilage may become completely eroded, leaving only bone as the articular surface. The subchondral bone responds to the stresses by becoming vascularized and thickened. The joint motion may polish the bone surface (**eburnation**). Other areas of bone may show loss of bone mass, with microcyst formation or microfractures. These changes tend to modify the contours of the ends of the bones, which may become mushroom-shaped or flattened. **Osteophytes** (spurs) may form at the margins of the joints, either by ossification of cartilaginous outgrowths or osseous metaplasia of connective tissue. When the osteophytes occur at the margins of the distal interphalangeal joints, they are called **Heberden's nodes.** "**Joint mice**" form when free pieces of cartilage or osteophytes become trapped in the joints. Many cases of degenerative joint disease are nearly asymptomatic. Advanced disease tends to cause greater pain and greater restriction of joint motion. No definitive therapy for degenerative joint disease is known. Analgesics can control the pain. Surgical replacement of a severely affected joint can restore mobility.

Osteoarthritis is due to "wear and tear" damage to joints and is characterized by progressive destruction of articular cartilage accompanied by subchondral bony thickening.

RHEUMATOID ARTHRITIS

Rheumatoid arthritis is a chronic systemic disease with prominent joint manifestations. Women are affected more often than men, and the peak prevalence for the disease is in middle age. Rheumatoid arthritis

Rheumatoid arthritis is a systemic autoimmune disease with prominent joint manifestations.

Joint involvement by rheumatoid arthritis eventually produces a thick pannus that limits joint mobility.

Rheumatoid arthritis also produces rheumatoid nodules that may involve skin or internal organs.

appears to be an autoimmune disease, and many patients have HLA-DR4 or HLA-DR1 antigens. Approximately four-fifths of patients have a circulating antibody, rheumatoid factor, which is directed against the fixed portion of their own IgG. The rheumatoid factor itself is usually IgM, but may alternatively be IgG, IgA, or IgE. Patients may also have other autoantibodies that can be directed against collagen, nuclear antibodies, or cytoskeletal proteins. Cell-mediated immunity also appears to be activated in the joints of patients with rheumatoid arthritis. The factors initiating these changes and their role in the pathogenesis of rheumatoid arthritis remain an active area of research.

Rheumatoid arthritis has its most prominent effects in the musculoskeletal system, but skin, blood vessels, and other organ systems are also affected. In the **musculoskeletal system,** the joint involvement in rheumatoid arthritis is usually symmetrical, and typically involves the distal extremities, notably the proximal interphalangeal and metacarpophalangeal joints. With progression, wrists, elbows, ankles, and knees may become involved. In early disease, the synovium of affected joints becomes thickened by edema and nonspecific inflammatory changes. Turbid synovial fluid accumulates that contains neutrophils with cytoplasmic inclusions of phagocytized immune complexes. These **RA cells** can help to establish the diagnosis of rheumatoid arthritis. Later, exuberant inflammation of the synovium produces a **pannus,** which is characterized by villous projections composed of markedly thickened, edematous synovium that projects into the joint space. With time, joint mobility can be limited as the pannus fills the joint space and the adjacent cartilage becomes irregularly eroded as a consequence of both mechanical damage and release of enzymes by the inflamed synovium. The subchondral bone may also be damaged. The periarticular soft tissue becomes edematous and inflamed, producing the soft tissue swelling characteristic of an actively inflamed rheumatoid joint. Later, the pannus undergoes organization, and bridging bands of fibrosis **(fibrous ankylosis)** may form between opposed villous projection. The fibrous ankylosis may then ossify, producing **bony ankylosis.** These changes deform the joint and destroy its remaining function. In addition to the joint changes just described, the musculoskeletal system also can have focal chronic inflammation of tendon, muscles, and periarticular connective tissue at sites either near to or distant from involved joints.

In many patients with rapidly progressive rheumatoid arthritis, the **skin** develops subcutaneous rheumatoid nodules that typically involve areas subjected to pressure, such as the elbows, backs of the forearms, or back of the skull. The nodules have a central core of fibrinoid necrosis, which is surrounded by palisading epitheloid cells that are in turn surrounded by chronic inflammatory cells including lymphocytes, plasma cells, and macrophages. While the nodules are most common in skin, rheumatoid nodules may also be found in many other organs, including lungs, spleen, pericardium, myocardium, heart valves, and aorta. Patients with severe rheumatoid arthritis can have high titers of circulating immune complexes, which appear to be the cause of an **acute vasculitis** that may range in severity from a venulitis involving primary skin to systemic arteritis similar to polyarteritis nodosa. The vessels of the kidneys are characteristically spared.

Rheumatoid arthritis has a variable clinical course. Some patients develop only mild symptoms that resolve without sequelae; others may progress slowly or rapidly to crippling disease. In many patients, the disease peaks in severity 4 or 5 years after diagnosis. Nonspecific systemic symptoms such as malaise, low-grade fever, or diffuse musculoskeletal pain are common and may precede the development of obvious arthritis. Laboratory studies may show increased erythrocyte sedimentation rate, mild anemia, and, in many but not all patients, the presence of rheumatoid factor. The diagnosis may be supported by synovial fluid analysis of involved joints, which may demonstrate RA cells. Extra-articular manifestations, such as subcutaneous rheumatoid nodules, pleuropulmonary disease, or vasculitis may occasionally be the presenting complaint.

The prognosis of rheumatoid arthritis is variable.

VARIANTS OF RHEUMATOID ARTHRITIS

The rheumatoid arthritis described in the preceding section is the classic form of adult-onset rheumatoid arthritis. Other variants are described below. **Juvenile rheumatoid arthritis** (Still's disease) differs from classic rheumatoid arthritis in the following respects. Most patients are less than 16 years of age at onset of the disease. A low-grade fever commonly precedes joint manifestations by weeks to months. The knees and ankles are often affected early in the disease; hand involvement is less common; and some patients have arthritis of only one or few joints. Rheumatoid factor is usually not present. The joint changes are indistinguishable grossly and microscopically from those in classic rheumatoid arthritis. Some pathologists reserve the term **Still's disease** for what appears to be juvenile rheumatoid arthritis presenting in adult life. **Felty syndrome** is the term used to describe the constellation of polyarticular rheumatoid arthritis, leg ulcers, and splenomegaly. **Ankylosing spondylitis** (rheumatoid spondylitis, Marie-Strümpell disease) is an inflammatory arthritis that principally involves the sacroiliac joints, with sometimes additional involvement of hip or shoulder joints. Ankylosing spondylitis has a strong male predominance and has been strongly associated with HLA-B27. Some patients with ankylosing spondylitis have other inflammatory diseases including inflammatory bowel disease, Reiter syndrome, or uveitis. The arthritis begins with inflammation of the ligamentous insertions on the vertebrae and later progresses to fibrous and bony ankylosis that impairs mobility, and in severe cases causes fusion of vertebral bodies.

Variants of rheumatoid arthritis include juvenile rheumatoid arthritis, Felty syndrome, and ankylosing spondylitis.

SUPPURATIVE ARTHRITIS

Bacterial invasion of a joint space can induce **acute suppurative arthritis.** While any joint can be infected, involvement of large joints (hips, knees, elbows, shoulders) is more common. Usually only one joint is involved. The usual route of spread is by hematogenous dissemination from a distant infected site. Direct spread from adjacent tissues can occur, particularly during trauma or surgery. **Drug addicts** and debilitated or **immunocompromised adults** tend to be infected by staphylococci or gram-negative organisms. Gonococcal infections are most common in women with neglected **venereal infections. Children** tend to be infected by *Haemophilus influenzae* or by spread from adjacent

Acute suppurative arthritis can be caused by staphylococci, gonococci, and gram-negative organisms.

osteomyelitis. Patients with **sickle cell anemia** tend to develop *Salmonella* infections. The involved joint usually shows a nonspecific suppurative infection. With virulent organisms (staphylococci) and chronic infection, ulceration of the synovium and destruction of underlying articular cartilage can occur, causing permanent joint damage. This damage can be exacerbated if the lesion heals with fibrous or osseous bridging. Prompt therapy, with antibiotics and sometimes surgical drainage, can minimize permanent joint damage.

LYME DISEASE

Lyme disease resembles syphilis and may have prominent joint involvement in its third stage.

Lyme disease (see also p. 51) is a multisystem disease caused by the spirochete *Borrelia burgdorferi,* which infests humans via the bite of infected ticks including *Ixodes dammini.* Lyme disease is more prevalent in the northeastern United States, where the tick infests field mice and whitetail deer. The arthritis observed in Lyme disease occurs in the third stage of the infection, following a **skin** lesion (first stage), and involvement of the **cardiac and nervous systems** (second stage). An initial migratory **polyarthritis** may be transiently observed during the second stage of the infection, but this usually passes without sequelae. Months to years later, a chronic, symmetric polyarthritis affects about one-tenth of patients. One or both knees are most commonly affected; small joint involvement can also be seen. The arthritis is histologically similar to rheumatoid arthritis, but in about one-quarter of cases, the spirochete can be visualized with silver stains. A second distinctive histologic feature is "onion-skin" thickening of arteriolar walls, similar to that observed in syphilis. Like rheumatoid arthritis, joint function may be lost by the inflammatory and reparative changes in the joint.

GOUT

Gout is induced by the deposition of urate crystals in joints.

Hyperuricemia from a variety of causes can cause intermittent episodes of acute arthritis triggered by crystallization of urates in joints; it also causes the formation of tophi by aggregation of urates, which, when they involve joints, can cause chronic and sometimes crippling arthritis. **Gout** is the term used to describe both the acute and chronic changes described above that occur as a consequence of hyperuricemia. Uric acid is produced principally through the catabolism of the purines of acids. Hyperuricemia can be produced either through overproduction or undersecretion of uric acid. Hyperuricemia is subclassified based on its cause. When the principal manifestation of the disease causing the hyperuricemia is gout, the gout is considered to be primary (90 percent of cases). **Idiopathic primary gout** with undefined enzymatic defects is the most common form and has multifactorial inheritance. Idiopathic gout may be due to either normal production of uric acid with underexcretion or overproduction with normal or increased excretion. **Partial hypoxanthine–guanine phosphoribosyltransferase deficiency** has X-linked genetics and is characterized by inadequate function of purine salvage pathways driving de novo purine synthesis, which leads to overproduction of uric acid. **5-phosphoribosyl-1-pyrophosphate synthetase variants** with increased activity have X-linked genetics and cause overproduction of purines and, consequently, uric acid.

Idiopathic primary gout may be due to either overproduction or underexcretion of uric acid.

Secondary gout comprises those forms of gout in which the underlying disease has prominent nongout manifestations. Secondary gout associated with increased nucleic acid turnover causes overproduction of uric acid. Examples include leukemia, lymphoma, polycythemia, and chronic granulomatous diseases. Secondary gout associated with severe hypoxanthine–guanine phosphoribosyltransferase deficiency has X-linked genetics, produces Lesch-Nyhan syndrome, and is characterized by overproduction of uric acid. Secondary gout associated with decreased excretion of uric acid is due to renal changes such as reduced renal functional mass, inhibited tubular secretion, or enhanced reabsorption of uric acid. Secondary gout is also associated with drugs or intoxications that cause overproduction or undersecretion of uric acid. In general, patients with overproduction and consequently increased excretion of uric acid are more vulnerable to urate nephropathy than are those with decreased excretion.

In **acute arthritis** formation of needle-shaped birefringent microcrystals of urates in a joint effusion causes acute inflammation of the synovium, which is accompanied by large numbers of neutrophils and macrophages in the synovial fluid. Usually only one or two joints become inflamed. In most patients, the great toe is affected; other sites include the instep, ankle, heel, knee, and wrist. The area of the involved joint becomes exquisitely painful, inflamed, and warm. The drug **colchicine** acts to interrupt an acute attack of gout, probably by inhibiting leukocyte function. Even without colchicine, the attacks of acute gout are self-limited, possibly because the local rise in temperature caused by the inflammation permits the urate crystals to dissolve. Eventually, the repeated precipitation of urates into the joint space, where they may encrust the articular surfaces, produces **chronic arthritis.** The synovium proliferates, with production of a thick pannus, and the underlying articular cartilage and sometimes bone can be damaged. Proliferation of marginal bone and formation of fibrous or bony ankylosis may also occur, destroying joint function. Urate-containing **tophi** may develop in adjacent soft tissues. The center of a tophus is composed of a mass of crystalline or amorphous urates. This mass is surrounded by an intense inflammatory reaction containing macrophages, lymphocytes, and fibroblasts. A distinctive feature of the inflammatory reaction is the giant cells that partially circle the urate with cytoplasmic processes. The tophi produce soft, nontender, palpable lesions. Tophi can be found in many sites, with common sites including the external ears, bursae of the olecranon and patella, ligaments, and renal medulla or pyramids. The central nervous system is usually protected from tophi because uric acid does not readily cross the blood–brain barrier. Since urate is soluble in water, tissue to be histologically examined for tophi should ideally be fixed in nonaqueous fixatives such as absolute alcohol.

Many patients with chronic gouty arthritis develop one of several forms of renal involvement. **Acute uric acid nephropathy** refers to the precipitation of free uric acid crystals in renal tubules, which can cause acute obstruction. Acute uric acid nephropathy is typically observed following chemotherapy for a lymphoproliferative disorder, which can cause the catabolism of large quantities of nucleic acids from lysed cells. **Uric acid nephrolithiasis** refers to the formation of uric acid stones in the renal collecting systems. Uric acid nephrolithiasis tends to occur when the urine is concentrated secondary to volume depletion. **Chronic urate nephropathy** refers to the presence of inter-

Secondary gout may also be due to either overproduction or underexcretion of uric acid.

Acute gouty arthritis is characterized by formation of needle-shaped urate crystals in a puslike joint effusion.

Chronic gouty arthritis is characterized by pannus formation within the joint and urate-containing tophi in adjacent soft tissues.

Gout can damage the kidney.

stitial urate deposits, and sometimes tophi, in the renal medulla. Since primary renal disease can also cause hyperuricemia, it is sometimes difficult to decide which features of the patient's renal disease cause and which are caused by the hyperuricemia.

CALCIUM CRYSTAL DEPOSITION ARTHRITIS

Arthritis similar to gout can be caused by deposition of calcium pyrophosphate or basic calcium phosphates.

Acute and chronic arthritis analogous to gout can be produced by calcium pyrophosphate or basic calcium phosphates (hydroxyapatite) deposited within joints. Both forms of crystal deposition are usually encountered in the elderly. **Pseudogout** (chondrocalcinosis), caused by calcium pyrophosphate deposition, tends to affect primarily knees but can also affect other joints of the extremities and spine. The crystals in affected joints are distinctive, short rhomboids that cause chalky deposits in the joint and adjacent structures. Pseudogout occurs idiopathically, in a hereditary form, and associated with metabolic disease, trauma, or surgery. Metabolic diseases associated with pseudogout include hyperparathyroidism, hemochromatosis, gout, ochronosis, hypothyroidism, and Wilson's disease. **Hydroxyapatite arthropathy,** caused by deposition of basic calcium phosphates, characteristically affects knees and shoulders ("Milwalkee shoulder syndrome").

OTHER FORMS OF ARTHRITIS

Arthritis is also observed in association with extra-articular disorders.

Arthritis is associated with a number of extra-articular disorders. **Reiter syndrome** develops following either nongonococcal urethritis or bacillary dysentery and is characterized by the triad of urethritis, conjunctivitis, and arthritis. Mucocutaneous lesions can also involve the soles, palms, glans penis, and mouth. Young men are most commonly affected; the majority are HLA-B27 positive. The arthritis that is produced, particularly if it becomes chronic, histologically resembles rheumatoid arthritis but rheumatoid factor and antinuclear antibodies are negative.

In somewhat over one-tenth of cases of **inflammatory bowel disease,** an arthritis of the vertebral column (**spondylitis**) or large, peripheral joints is observed. The spondylitis is indistinguishable from ankylosing spondylitis. The large joint changes consist of nonspecific acute inflammation of the synovium that does not progress to pannus formation and resolves in weeks to months without damaging the joint. Roughly 1 in 20 patients with **psoriasis** have joint involvement that resembles rheumatoid arthritis, but rheumatoid factor is almost never present. Alternatively, some patients develop a spondylitis that closely resembles ankylosing spondylitis; these patients are usually HLA-B27 positive.

Migratory polyarthritis is a principal manifestation of **acute rheumatic fever.** The polyarthritis usually heals without residual changes. **Tuberculous arthritis** can arise in both children and adults, either as a complication of tuberculous osteomyelitis or as hematogenous spread from a pulmonary or other focus.

MISCELLANEOUS LESIONS

Synovial membranes also proliferate in joints and tendon sheaths in pigmented villonodular synovitis and nodular tenosynovitis (giant cell tumor of tendon sheath). It remains an area of controversy whether these conditions represent neoplastic or inflammatory synovial proliferations. **Pigmented villonodular synovitis** is characterized grossly by darkly pigmented synovium in an exuberant, villous growth that covers most or all of the synovial surface of a joint. Usually only one joint, often the knee or hip, is affected. Histologically, the villous projections are composed of inflamed synovium covered by proliferating surface synoviocytes. The pigmentation observed grossly is associated with numerous histiocytes containing hemosiderin and, less often, lipid. A few multinucleate giant cells and a nonspecific chronic inflammatory infiltrate may also be present. Clinically, pigmented villonodular synovitis can be mistaken for rheumatoid or infectious arthritis since it causes pain, swelling, and limitation of motion. **Nodular tenosynovitis** refers to a sharply localized, well-encapsulated nodule within a tendon sheath, often in a finger, although the lesions can also be found in other sites. Histologically, the nodule is composed of rounded or polygonal cells. Scattered in these sheets are macrophages, giant cells, and hemosiderin-containing round or spindle cells. When the giant cells are very numerous, the lesion is called giant cell tumor of the tendon sheath. Excision is curative.

Proliferations of synovial membranes in joints and tendon sheaths cause, respectively, pigmented villonodular synovitis and nodular tenosynovitis.

OTHER FORMS OF TENOSYNOVITIS

Tenosynovitis can also be associated with other causes. **Traumatic tenosynovitis** is attributed to excessive stress, often due to a repetitive motion on particular tendons and their sheaths. Traumatic tenosynovitis is observed in the wrists of stenographers and upper extremities of manual laborers. **Suppurative tenosynovitis** is observed most frequently when a penetrating injury, such as an accidental needle puncture in a hospital staff member, introduces skin pathogens into the tendon. The infection can usually be cured by antibiotics; surgical drainage is occasionally required. **Tuberculous tenosynovitis,** now rare in developed countries, can occur by hematogenous spread of tuberculosis from other sites.

Tenosynovitis can also be due to trauma or infections, including tuberculosis.

BURSITIS

Inflammation of bursa (**bursitis**) is observed more commonly in men than women. The inflammations most often involve the subdeltoid bursa, the prepatellar bursa, the olecranon bursa, or the radiohumeral bursa. Trauma secondary to excessive use has been demonstrated to be important in tennis elbow and may play a role in bursitis at other sites, although the evidence is less clear. Often, no cause is identified. Bursitis is characterized in early stages by distention of the bursa by watery or mucoid fluid. Later, chronic bursitis can develop, characterized by filling of the bursa space by altered blood that contains basophilic calcium deposits. The bursa wall is composed of chronically inflamed, dense fibrous tissue lined by granulation tissue or precipitated fibrin.

Bursitis is often idiopathic but may be related to excessive use.

Neovascularization of the wall may produce collections of capillaries that resemble hemangioma. The pain of bursitis can often be relieved by local installation of corticosteroids. Surgical excision may be necessary if calcification is extensive.

GANGLION AND BAKER'S CYST

Ganglions are benign cystic lesions that arise from myxoid degeneration of connective tissue.

Small cystic lesions, termed **ganglions,** are sometimes found in the collagenous connective tissue of the joint capsule or tendon sheath. Clinically, ganglions usually present as firm, pea-shaped subcutaneous nodules, often in the wrist. The cysts appear to arise from myxoid degeneration followed by cystic softening of connective tissue. **Baker's cysts** are herniations of the knee joint into the popliteal space. Baker's cysts tend to occur in knees affected by rheumatoid or suppurative arthritis, where there may be a marked increase in intra-articular fluid. Herniations of other joint spaces occur less commonly.

BASIC PATHOLOGIC REACTIONS OF MUSCLE

Muscle fibers can atrophy, degenerate, regenerate, or undergo a variety of nonspecific myopathic changes.

Muscle fibers have a limited number of ways of responding to disease. **Atrophy** of muscle fibers occurs following denervation, disuse, or chronic ischemia. On cross section, atrophic fibers appear small, angulated, and have clumped nuclei. **Degeneration** of muscle fibers is observed in many diseases. The degenerating fibers initially lose their striations and become more eosinophilic. With time, macrophages and other inflammatory cells digest the necrotic area. **Regenerating** muscle fibers are formed by activation and multiplication of myoblasts. The myoblasts are small, spindle-shaped cells found within normal muscle. A regenerating muscle fiber can be recognized by a basophilic tint (due to large numbers of ribosomes) and large, centrally located nuclei that may contain prominent nucleoli. A variety of **myopathic,** but generally nonspecific, changes can be seen, most often in primary muscle disease. **Ring fibers,** which are seen in myotonic dystrophy, have disordered myofilaments that are arranged circumferentially around a central, longitudinal core of myofilaments. **Fiber splitting** may actually be due to defective regeneration rather than splitting of mature muscle fibers. Increased **variation in myofiber diameter** is observed in both neurogenic and myopathic disease. Increased numbers of **centrally located nuclei** are a nonspecific change seen in many muscle diseases. Localized **hypercontraction** of myofibers produces visible contraction bands and may be either an artifact or, if present to large degree, the result of muscular pathology such as Duchenne muscular dystrophy. Endomysial and perimysial **fibrosis,** which may be accompanied by fatty infiltration, is a nonspecific marker for previous muscle atrophy or inflammation.

NEUROGENIC MUSCLE DISEASE

Abnormal or deficient innervation can produce syndromes, known as myasthenic syndromes, characterized by muscular weakness and fatigability.

Myasthenia Gravis

Myasthenia gravis is the most common of the myasthenic syndromes. The disease is the result of autoantibodies directed against the acetylcholine receptor in the postsynaptic membrane of the neuromuscular junction. Transmission of a nerve impulse across the junction is hampered or blocked when antibody binds to the receptor. The morphologic changes produced are best observed by electron microscopy, which shows the postsynaptic membrane of the neuromuscular junction to have markedly reduced size and number of junctional folds. Immunologic techniques have demonstrated antibody (usually IgG) binding to the motor end plate. Patients are typically young women aged 20 to 40 years who may have coexisting **thymic hyperplasia** (see p. 367) or **thymoma** (see p. 368). Patients experience muscle weakness that is aggravated by repeated use. Eye muscles and other muscles with small motor units tend to be affected first. Patients may have mild to fatal disease.

The weakness observed in myasthenia gravis is due to antibodies directed against acetylcholine receptor.

Eaton-Lambert Syndrome

The **Eaton-Lambert syndrome** is a muscle weakness caused by impaired release of acetylcholine that is observed in patients with cancer, typically oat cell carcinoma of the lung. Eaton-Lambert syndrome differs from myasthenia gravis in that repetitive stimulation improves the muscle weakness.

Eaton-Lambert syndrome is a paraneoplastic condition.

Denervation Atrophy

When the nerve supplying a muscle is lost, the muscle will atrophy. In contrast, demyelination of a nerve slows conduction but does not cause muscle atrophy. Many neurologic syndromes (e.g., amyotrophic lateral sclerosis) can cause denervation of one or more groups of muscles. Histologically, denervated muscle is initially characterized by the production of small, angulated, atrophic fibers. If the nerve damage is not too severe, the atrophied muscle fibers may be reinnervated by **collateral sprouts** from an adjacent nerve fiber. The reinnervation restores the muscle fiber size. However, since the biochemical type of the muscle fiber is determined by its innervation, the formerly atrophic fiber will have the biochemical type coded by the new axon that innervates it. This can be observed in histochemical studies as **type grouping** of muscle fibers into bundles of type 1 and type 2 fibers. This histochemical pattern is characteristic of recovery from denervation and is quite different from the normally random distribution of type 1 and type 2 fibers. With continued nerve damage, **group atrophy** may be seen as axons innervating bundles of fibers die. Clinically, relatively rapid denervation of muscle, such as is seen in amyotrophic lateral sclerosis, tends to produce muscle fasciculations as a consequence of denervation hypersensitivity. The involved muscle becomes weak and loses bulk. With continued nerve damage, paralysis occurs.

Denervation can lead to muscle atrophy.

MYOPATHIC DISEASE

Myopathies are primary muscle diseases.

Muscular Dystrophies

Muscular dystrophies are genetically determined primary muscle diseases.

Duchenne muscular dystrophy is X-linked recessive and also causes reduced intelligence and cardiac involvement.

Myotonic dystrophy is an autosomal dominant disease that affects many organ systems in addition to muscle.

Less common forms of muscular dystrophy include fascioscapulohumeral dystrophy, limb-girdle muscular dystrophy, and ocular myopathy.

Muscular dystrophies are a heterogenous group of progressive, genetically determined myopathies. The major forms are described below, of which the most common are the Duchenne, Becker, and myotonic types. **Duchenne muscular dystrophy,** the most common and severe of the muscular dystrophies, is an X-linked recessive disease that presents in male children in early childhood with progressive weakness that destroys the patient's ability to walk by puberty. About one-third of cases are thought to be due to new mutations. Duchenne muscular dystrophy produces a characteristic pattern of progressive, symmetrical weakness that begins in muscles around the hips and later progresses to the lower legs, shoulders, and trunk. Duchenne muscular dystrophy also produces reduced intelligence and cardiac involvement. Death, secondary to the weakness, usually occurs by age 20. The biochemical defect in Duchenne muscular dystrophy is a gene deletion that leads to an inability to synthesize **dystrophin,** a protein of unknown function, possibly a structural protein in myocyte membranes. Pathologically, individual muscle fibers show necrosis and attempted regeneration. The necrotic muscle tissue becomes replaced by fibrofatty tissues. Grossly, this fibrofatty replacement produces "pseudohypertrophy" of the calves. Other microscopic findings early in the disease include wider than normal variation in muscle fiber diameter; centrally located nuclei; contraction bands; and fiber splitting. End-stage disease is characterized by almost complete replacement of the muscle by fibrofatty tissue containing only scattered muscle fibers. **Becker muscular dystrophy** can be considered a milder variant of Duchenne muscular dystrophy. Becker muscular dystrophy also has X-linked genetics, but partially functional dystrophin is produced, and the disease only becomes symptomatic in the second decade and impairs the ability to walk in adulthood.

Myotonic dystrophy is an autosomal dominant disease that has a widely variable age of onset (infancy to middle adult life). Myotonic dystrophy is the result of a mutation on chromosome 19 that affects many organ systems, and causes muscular dystrophy, cataracts, testicular atrophy, heart disease, dementia, and baldness. The patient's lifespan is normal. The myotonic dystrophy is characterized by weakness and difficulty in relaxation (**myotonia**) that is most pronounced in the muscles of the hands and feet. Microscopically, muscles involved by myotonic dystrophy show features including increased numbers of centrally located nuclei; chains of nuclei; disorganized sarcoplasmic masses without normal striations; prominent ring fibers; and atrophy of type 1 fibers. **Fascioscapulohumeral dystrophy** is an autosomal dominant form of muscular dystrophy that can present from childhood to adult life and does not shorten life. The weakness usually begins in the face, and progresses to the shoulder and arm. **Limb-girdle muscular dystrophy** is an autosomal recessive disease that can present from childhood to adult life and does not shorten life. The weakness may involve either the shoulder or the hip. Disability usually develops within 20 years. **Ocular myopathy** is probably an autosomal dominant disease, is characterized by variable age of onset, and is rarely progressive. Ocular myopathy appears to be a group of syndromes with the common characteristic of early extraocular muscle weakness. The face, neck, or limbs may also be involved.

OTHER MUSCLE DISEASES

Many **enzyme deficiencies** can affect muscle. Disorders of glycolysis and related pathways include myophosphorylase deficiency (McArdle's disease), acid maltase deficiency, and phosphofructokinase deficiency. Disorders of carnitine metabolism produce mitochondrial defects in substrate transport and include carnitine deficiency and carnitine palmitoyltransferase deficiency. Mitochondrial ATPase deficiency limits mitochondrial energy conservation. Cytochrome deficiencies in the mitochondrial respiratory chain also occur. **Congenital myopathies** are a heterogenous group of diseases that tend to produce "floppy infants" with symmetric weakness. These syndromes tend to be associated with other congenital defects. **Central core disease** is an autosomal dominant syndrome characterized by abnormal (mostly type 1) myocytes that contain an amorphous and dysfunctional central core. **Nemaline** (rod body) **myopathy** has variable (usually autosomal dominant) genetics and is characterized by muscle fibers containing rod-shaped masses of Z-band material. **Centronuclear** (myotubular) **myopathy** has variable inheritance and is characterized by centrally located nuclei and numerous mitochondria and glycogen vacuoles. **Congenital fiber-type disproportion** has variable inheritance and may have either type 1 or type 2 fiber predominance. The fibers may be normal or abnormal.

Myopathies can also be caused by **endocrine disorders** and **toxins**. Hypothyroidism, hyperthyroidism, and steroids (usually iatrogenic) can cause myopathies characterized by diffuse weakness and sometimes wasting. The diagnosis is usually one of exclusion, since the morphologic changes are not distinctive. Toxins that can cause myopathies include alcohol, which can cause acute rhabdomyolysis with risk of renal damage; the antifibrinolytic agent epsilonaminocaproic acid, which can also cause acute rhabdomyolysis; chloroquine, which causes vacuolar degeneration of muscle fibers; and penicillamine and procainamide, which can cause vasculitis involving muscle. Primary muscle tumors are considered with other soft tissue tumors.

Enzyme deficiencies that can affect muscle may involve glycolysis, carnitine metabolism, or mitochondrial enzymes.

Congenital myopathies often have distinctive muscle fibers and tend to be associated with other congenital defects.

A variety of endocrine disorders and toxins can also damage muscle.

BONE

BONE INFECTIONS

Important bone infections include pyogenic osteomyelitis, tuberculosis, and syphilis.

Pyogenic Osteomyelitis

Bacteria or, rarely, fungi can cause suppurative infection of bone.

Pyogenic osteomyelitis is a suppurative infection of the bone or marrow caused by bacteria or (rarely) fungi. Routes of infection include the bloodstream, spread from contiguous infections, and trauma (including surgery). In adults, vertebrae are most often involved, and common etiologic agents include *Staphylococcus aureus, Escherichia coli, Pseudomonas,* and *Klebsiella.* Postsurgical and postfracture osteomyelitis are often caused by mixed or anaerobic organisms. Neonatal osteomyelitis is often caused by *Haemophilus influenzae* or group B streptococci. Patients with sickle cell disease are vulnerable to *Salmonella* osteomyelitis; drug addicts tend to develop *Pseudomonas* osteomyelitis. In many cases of osteomyelitis, no organism is isolated, possibly because of prior antibiotic therapy or inadequate culture techniques.

Blood-born osteomyelitis tends to affect the ends of long bones.

Osteomyelitis that develops by a blood-borne route tends to affect the ends of long bones, possibly because of the slow capillary blood flow of the metaphyseal marrow. The accumulation of pus within the confined marrow may then compromise blood flow there, leading to ischemic tissue damage and favoring the spread of the infection. Infection can also spread through the haversian and lacunar systems of the cortical bone, causing sinus tract formation, or eventually reaching the periosteum, where periostitis or a **subperiosteal abscess** develops. In some cases, bone necrosis can cause a fragment of devitalized bone (**sequestrum**) to break off. Such sequestra may be resorbed or occasionally dissect through the skin. In infants, the normal vascularization of the epiphyseal plate can permit infection to spread to the joint, causing suppurative arthritis. **Suppurative arthritis** is less common in adults because the cartilage resists bacterial invasion, but can occur in severe infections via spread through adjacent soft tissues. Such suppurative arthritis can destroy a joint, causing permanent disability. In the spine, osteomyelitis can spread from one vertebrae to another via involvement of the contiguous intervertebral discs. In some cases of acute osteomyelitis, the infection heals by walling off a localized abscess, which may remain infected (**Brodie's abscess**). Smoldering infection can irritate the periosteum, stimulating osteoblastic activity to form subperiosteal bone (involucrum) that surrounds the infected site. When such neo-osteogenesis is prolonged, the process is called **Garré sclerosing osteomyelitis.**

Histologically, osteomyelitis is characterized by suppurative inflammation, ischemic necrosis, and fibrous and bony repair. Clinically, osteomyelitis can present either indolently with fever as its only obvious manifestation, or more acutely with both fever and sometimes intense pain localized to the involved bone. Radiography can be helpful in establishing the diagnosis, but may not show any changes in the first 2 weeks of infection. Osteomyelitis can be complicated by spontaneous fracture of the involved bone and by distant abscesses (including bacterial endocarditis) initiated by hematogeous spread of organisms from osteomyelitic sites. Chronic osteomyelitis can also be complicated by amyloidosis.

Osteomyelitis is characterized histologically by suppurative inflammation, ischemic necrosis, and fibrous and bony repair.

Tuberculosis

Tuberculous infection of bone (**tuberculous osteomyelitis**; see also p. 55) is presently rare in developed countries, but remains common in the third world. Most cases of tuberculous osteomyelitis in developed countries are observed in patients with advanced age, diabetes, AIDS, or other reasons for immune compromise. In developing countries, adolescents and young adults are commonly affected. Compared with pyogenic osteomyelitis, **tuberculous osteomyelitis** (Pott's disease) tends to develop insidiously; tends to be more difficult to control with antibiotics; and tends to be much more destructive. Pott's disease is also characteristically complicated by spread of tuberculous exudation along the paravertebral muscles, sometimes producing a psoas abscess. The long bones of the extremities are another favored site for tuberculous osteomyelitis. In the long bones, the infection can spread for long distances in the medullary cavity and cause destruction of adjacent cortical bone. Infection of adjacent soft tissues can cause formation of large sinus tracts, some of which may drain through the skin.

Tuberculous osteomyelitis remains common in the third world.

Syphilis

Syphilis osteomyelitis (see also p. 53) is uncommon in developed countries. It occurs in congenital and acquired forms. **Congenital syphilis** tends to involve either the periosteum (periostitis), particularly of long bones, or the junction between the metaphysis and the epiphysis (osteochondritis). The irritation associated with the periostitis can cause a ragged new bone formation (**"crew haircut"** appearance) on the surface of the cortical bone. When such bone thickening involves the tibia, **"saber shin"** may be produced. Histologically, the inflamed tissues show obliterative endarteritis; perivascular infiltrates composed principally of plasma cells; and reactive bone formation.

Congenital syphilis produces prominent reactive bone formation.

FRACTURES

Several terms are used to describe fractures. **Complete fractures** are breaks that leave at least two bone fragments. **Incomplete** (greenstick) **fractures** are breaks in which the fracture does not separate the bone into fragments. **Spiral fractures** of long bones are a common form of incomplete fracture. **Comminuted fractures** produce splintering of the bone into many fragments. In **closed** (simple) **fractures,** the overlying soft tissues are intact. In **compound** (open) **fractures,** the skin and

Fractures are classified by the type of break.

Fractures heal by sequential formation of a procallous, fibrocartilaginous callus, and then osseous callus.

soft tissue adjacent to the fracture are damaged, facilitating bacterial infection. In general, comminuted and compound fractures heal more slowly and are more prone to complications than other types. Closed, incomplete fractures tend to heal most rapidly. Healing of a fracture, while actually a continuous process, can be considered to occur in three stages. A soft **procallus** (provisional callus) composed of newly formed cartilage and bone matrix develops during the first weeks as the hematoma of the fracture site organizes, with ingrowth of fibroblasts and new capillary buds. The procallus is usually much larger than the original bone, fusiform in shape, and serves as a splint for the fracture. The weak procallus is subsequently converted to a stronger **fibrocartilaginous callus.** Eventually, the fibrocartilaginous callus is replaced by **osseous callus,** which undergoes remodeling directed by muscle and weight-bearing stresses on the bone. This remodeling slowly (over months to years) changes the shape of the callus from a fusiform mass to a sometimes near perfect reconstruction that may make it impossible to find the fracture site on X-rays taken years later. Healing of a fracture can be impeded or prevented by a variety of complications including disorders impeding callus formation (malalignment, comminution of the bone, inadequate mobilization), infection, systemic derangements (calcium or phosphorus deficiency, vitamin deficiency, systemic infections, ischemia), and bone disease (osteomalacia, osteoporosis).

OSTEOPOROSIS

Loss of otherwise normal bone produces osteoporosis.

Osteoporosis is characterized by a loss of otherwise normal bone as a consequence of increased osteoclastic compared with osteoblastic activity, which leaves the skeleton vulnerable to fracture. Osteoporosis is observed in the following clinical settings. **Primary osteoporosis** of the elderly is very common. **Idiopathic osteoporosis** is also sometimes encountered in young adults and children. **Secondary osteoporosis** is seen in diverse settings. Hormonal disorders that can cause osteoporosis include prolonged exposure to thyroid hormone, endogenous glucocorticoids, or exogenous glucocorticoids; deficiencies of pituitary hormones or androgens; and pregnancy. A variety of other conditions can also cause secondary osteoporosis including malabsorption, malnutrition, chronic heparin administration, or the weightlessness of space. Osteoporosis, particularly of the elderly, may be difficult to distinguish from the normal bone loss associated with aging. The pathogenesis of osteoporosis is still obscure, with proposed causal mechanisms including genetic factors, reduced physical activity, estrogen or androgen deficiency, and impaired parathyroid hormone, calcitonin, or vitamin D metabolism. While the bone loss occurs throughout the skeleton, some sites tend to be affected more than others, including vertebrae, femoral necks, metacarpals, the distal radius, the proximal humerus, the proximal tibia, and the pelvis. Affected bones show cortical thinning, enlargement of the medullary cavity, and conversion of trabecular plates to thin bone spicules. Histologically, the remaining bone has a normal matrix and mineral content. Osteoclasts are often increased in number and may have bizarre shapes; osteoblasts are usually normal in number.

PAGET'S DISEASE OF BONE

Paget's disease (osteitis deformans) is a disease of unknown etiology, possibly related to infection by a slow virus (paramyxovirus, respiratory syncytial virus, or measles virus), characterized by vigorous osteoclastic activity and disordered new bone formation. The disease begins with an **initial osteolytic stage** characterized histologically by patchwork areas of bone resorption by large numbers of bizarre, enlarged osteoclasts that may contain as many as 100 nuclei. In the second stage, a **secondary osteoblastic activity** causes new bone formation to balance the osteoclastic activity, but the new bone matrix is formed in a disordered manner, with delayed mineralization. The result is the mosaic pattern of bone spicules with prominent osteoid seams that is pathognomic of Paget's disease. The adjacent marrow spaces often become fibrosed and contain many small blood vessels. Late in the disease, the third stage is reached as osteoclastic activity diminishes ("burns out"), but osteoblastic activity remains active. In this stage, the bones become more dense and osteosclerotic due to excessive bone formation. However, the new bone is poorly formed and poorly mineralized and is consequently vulnerable to fractures and deformations.

> **Paget's disease is a complex bone disease characterized by vigorous osteoclastic activity and disorderd new bone formation.**

Clinical features of Paget's disease include coarsening of facial features with skull enlargement, bowing of femur and tibia, and kyphosis secondary to vertebral changes. Pain is often prominent and occurs as a consequence of nerve compression by narrowed foramina, microfractures, and secondary osteoarthritis. Shunting of blood through hypervascularized bone occasionally causes high-output cardiac failure. In about 1 percent of patients, Paget's disease is complicated by the development of sarcoma that is usually osteogenic, but may also be another form such as fibrosarcoma. The sarcomas tend to arise in the jaw, pelvis, or femur.

SECONDARY BONE DISEASES

Rickets and Osteomalacia

Deficiency of vitamin D produces **rickets** in children and **osteomalacia** in adults. The deficiency can be the result of inadequate dietary intake, inadequate sun exposure for endogenous synthesis, lipid malabsorption, and chronic renal disease leading to inadequate synthesis of active forms of vitamin D metabolism. Independent of cause, vitamin D deficiency produces a failure of bone matrix to mineralize, which can be recognized histologically by abnormally wide osteoid seams and larger than normal amounts of unmineralized matrix. In children, the growing bones can be deformed by rickets. In adults, osteomalacia is characterized by relatively radiolucent bones that tend to fracture easily.

> **Vitamin D deficiency produces a failure of bone matrix to mineralize.**

Hyperparathyroid-Induced Skeletal Changes

Excess parathormone, whether due to primary or secondary chronic **hyperparathyroidism,** can produce the following sequence of skeletal changes. **Demineralization** is the earliest change observed and produces an excess of unmineralized osteoid similar to that observed in vitamin D-related osteomalacia. **Osteitis fibrosa** is characterized by increased osteoclastic activity by somewhat bizarre shaped osteoclasts and is accompanied by fibrosis that begins around the trabeculae. Radiographic changes include thinning of cortex and trabeculae so that the bones appear "moth-eaten." Microfractures and microhemorrhages are common at this stage, and the marrow may contain large numbers of

> **Excess parathormone causes bone demineralization, fibrosis, and cyst formation.**

hemosiderin-laden macrophages within the delicate fibrous tissue. **Osteitis fibrosis cystica** (von Recklinghausen's disease of bone) is the final stage and is characterized by formation of micro- to macrocysts in the setting of still more marked bone resorption, microhemorrhages, and fibrosis. Some foci of hemorrhage undergo organization with accumulation of hemosiderin-laden macrophages, fibroblasts, and multinucleate giant cells, producing **reparative giant cell granulomas** (misnamed "brown tumors"). Primary hyperparathyroidism tends to produce more severe disease than does secondary hyperparathyroidism.

At present, improved awareness of hyperparathyroidism has led to earlier diagnosis and treatment, with the result that severe bone changes (e.g., osteitis fibrosa cystica) have become uncommon. The clinical manifestations of hyperparathyroid-induced skeletal changes (fractures, joint pains) are usually overshadowed by other manifestations of hyperparathyroidism and will often resolve with treatment of the hyperparathyroidism.

Renal Osteodystrophy

Chronic renal disease produces a pattern of bony change characterized by osteitis fibrosa cystica admixed with osteomalacia.

Patients with **chronic renal disease,** particularly when on long-term hemodialysis, can develop complex bone changes. The pathogenesis of the bone changes is complex and involves phosphate retention by the failing kidney, which then triggers secondary hyperparathyroidism with resulting hypocalcemia; failure of the kidney to convert vitamin D to its active metabolite 1,25 dihydroxy D, with resultant decreased absorption by intestine of calcium; and possibly aluminum toxicity in patients on chronic hemodialysis with resulting impairment of mineralization of bone matrix. The secondary hyperparathyroidism tends to produce osteitis fibrosa cystica. The lower levels of the active form of vitamin D, hypocalcemia, and aluminum toxicity tend to produce osteomalacia. The result is a pattern of bony change characterized by **osteitis fibrosa cystica** admixed with **osteomalacia.** Areas of osteosclerosis are also sometimes present.

Hypertrophic Osteoarthropathy

Subperiosteal new bone formation produces the finger clubbing in chronic lung disease, intrathoracic cancers, and chronic liver disease.

Finger clubbing is observed in some patients with chronic lung disease, intrathoracic cancers, and chronic liver disease. This finger clubbing is associated with **hypertrophic osteoarthropathy,** which is characterized by formation of new bone beneath the periosteum of long bones. The fingers become clubbed as a consequence of edematous fibrovascular overgrowth around the tips. Patients with hypertrophic osteoarthropathy often also experience wrist arthralgias, which are related to a nonspecific mild chronic inflammation of synovium. The relationship of the hypertrophic osteoarthropathy, arthritis, and clubbing to the underlying systemic disease is still unclear, but may involve changes in neurovascular physiology.

DEFECTS IN BONE MATURATION

Fibrous Dysplasia

Fibrous dysplasia is a benign disorder of bone characterized by localized defects composed of whorled connective tissue, which may resemble a fibroma, with irregular trabeculae of bone. The pathogenesis appears to involve a localized failure of maturation of bone that produces immature woven bone. Three clinical patterns are described. **Monostotic fibrous dysplasia** involves a single bone and is the most common form. Monostotic fibrous dysplasia tends to arise in childhood and may be arrested at puberty. Almost any bone can be affected, with common sites in descending order of frequency including ribs, femur, tibia, maxilla and mandible. **Polyostotic fibrous dysplasia** without endocrine dysfunction affects several to many (but not all) bones, appears in childhood, and continues to progress into middle age. Involvement of craniofacial bones is more common than in the monostotic form. The shoulder and pelvic girdles are also commonly involved, and crippling deformities are sometimes produced. Spontaneous fractures are common. **Polyostotic fibrous dysplasia in association with endocrinopathies** is an uncommon form of fibrous dysplasia. **Albright (McCune-Albright) syndrome** refers to polyostotic fibrous dysplasia accompanied by precocious sexual development and skin pigmentation that classically occurs as large macules with irregular margins. Polyostatic fibrous dysplasia can also be associated with excesses of glucocorticoids, thyroid hormone, growth hormone, parathormone, and adenomas of a variety of endocrine glands. The basis of the relationship of the hormonal disease to fibrous dysplasia is still unknown.

> **Fibrous dysplasia is characterized by irregular bone trabeculae within whorled connective tissue.**

Fibrous Cortical Defects

Fibrous cortical defects (nonossifying fibromas) are common developmental aberrations (not tumors) that cause lobular, radiolucent defects in the cortex of long bones (femur, tibia, fibula), chiefly in children. The lesions are common and are usually asymptomatic but can cause pain and predispose for fracture. Many of the lesions eventually disappear spontaneously. Histologically, the defects are composed of whorled fibroblasts, sometimes with scattered macrophages and multinucleate cells. Bone formation and anaplasia are absent.

> **Nonossifying fibromas are developmental aberrations that are clinically important because they produce radiolucent bone defects.**

HEREDITARY DISORDERS OF BONE

Osteogenesis Imperfecta

Osteogenesis imperfecta is a group of genetic diseases characterized by "**brittle bones**" as a result of abnormal synthesis of the type 1 collagen that is a major constituent of bone matrix. Type 1 collagen is also found in sclera, joints, ligaments, teeth, and skin. Patients with osteogenesis imperfecta often have, in addition to very fragile bones, **blue sclera;** hearing loss secondary to damage to the bones of the inner ear; and small, blue, mishapen teeth. Several variants of osteogenesis imperfecta have been described. **Type I** is a relatively mild, autosomal dominant form of the disease characterized clinically by postnatal fractures, blue sclera, normal stature, hearing impairment, and dentinogenesis imperfecta. **Type II** is lethal in utero or within days of birth. The disease can have autosomal recessive or autosomal dominant inheritance and is associated with blue sclera and skeletal deformities secondary to in

> **Osteogenesis imperfecta is a group of genetic collagen abnormalities that produce "brittle bones."**

utero fractures. **Type III** is a moderately severe form with variable inheritance patterns that is compatible with survival and produces growth retardation, progressive kyphoscoliosis, multiple fractures, hearing impairment, and dentinogenesis imperfecta. The sclera are initially blue and later become white. **Type IV** is a relatively mild, autosomal form compatible with survival and associated with moderate skeletal fragility, short stature, and some dentinogenesis imperfecta. The sclera are white. The collagen defects in the different types of osteogenesis imperfecta vary, but tend to involve synthesis of insufficient or abnormal pro-α 1 (1) or pro-α 2 (1) chains, which often lead to formation of unstable collagen triple helix.

Osteopetrosis

Impaired osteoclast function in osteopetrosis leads to reduced bone resorption, producing characteristically dense, but brittle, bone.

Osteopetrosis (Albers-Schönberg disease, "marble bones") is a group of hereditary diseases characterized by impaired osteoclast function, which leads to reduced bone resorption. The osteoclasts tend to be large and have bizarre shapes. The resulting bone becomes overgrown, but is brittle and fractures easily. Since the bone medullary cavity often becomes narrowed or obliterated, anemia and neutropenia may be features. Two subtypes have been described. Early death, usually secondary to infections, can be caused by a **malignant, autosomal recessive pattern** that presents in utero or in infancy. This form is characterized by extreme bone density; profound anemia and neutropenia; and extramedullary hematopoiesis with hepatosplenomegaly. Hydrocephalus may also be present, and narrowing of the foramen can cause nerve damage to cranial nerves. A relatively benign, autosomal dominant, **adult pattern** is characterized by relatively mild anemia. At present, no treatment is available for osteopetrosis, but animal model studies suggest that bone marrow transplantation is potentially curative.

Achondroplasia

Achondroplastic dwarfs have abnormally short limbs.

Achondroplasia is an autosomal dominant cause of congenital dwarfism. The defect is a deficiency of growing cartilaginous spicules whose later calcification causes endochondral bone formation. The skull and spine, which form by intramembranous growth, are of normal size but appear large compared with the abnormally short long bones of the limbs. Individuals who are heterozygous for this trait have abnormal skeletons, but normal longevity, mental development, and sexual development. Homozygous individuals usually die shortly after birth.

Exostoses

Misdirected epiphyseal bone growth produces an exostosis, in which a bony projection is capped by cartilage.

An **exostosis** (osteochondroma) is a cartilage-capped bone projection that occurs as a developmental aberration secondary to misdirected epiphyseal bone growth. Most patients with exostoses have sporadic, solitary lesions. An autosomal dominant form (**hereditary multiple exostoses,** osteochondromatosis) is characterized by large numbers of exostoses. Osteochondromatosis occurs (rarely) as a part of Gardner syndrome, characterized by multiple colonic polyps. Exostoses are usually asymptomatic but occasionally compress an adjacent nerve or vessel. Exostoses are observed in men more frequently than women. Common sites include the long bones of the extremities on the lateral contours of the shafts near the epiphyseal region. Less common sites include the ribs, scapula, and pelvis; the small bones of hands and feet are rarely involved. Exostoses tend to be mushroom-shaped, with a fat, cartilage-covered head and a narrow neck. Histologically, mature cartilage with a smooth surface resembling that of a joint overlies well-formed bone. The bone characteristically has a medullary cavity that communicates with the medullary cavity of the bone of origin. Chondrosarcomas occasionally arise in exostoses.

TUMORS OF THE SKELETAL SYSTEM

Bone tumors are uncommon, but are of clinical significance because some types are highly malignant. In children, benign bone tumors are more common than malignant ones; in adults, malignant tumors are more common.

Osteoblastic Tumors

Bone-forming (osteoblastic) tumors can be either benign or malignant. **Osteomas** are benign, sessile tumors made of well-formed bone composed of mature, broad, bony trabeculae separated by fibrous tissue that may be highly vascularized or contain foci of hematopoiesis. Osteomas can occur at any age and have a slight male predominance. Osteomas are most common on the bones of the skull and face, where they tend to form bosselated tumors that project into the air sinuses. **Osteoid osteoma** is a small, often painful, benign bone tumor that produces a characteristic radiologic picture. The tumor contains a small radiolucent focus (the nidus) composed histologically of delicate osteoid trabeculae surrounded by osteoblasts in a vascularized spindle cell tumor. The nidus is surrounded by dense, sclerotic bone that appears to form as a subperiosteal reaction to the nidus. Osteoid osteomas have a male predominance and are most common in children, adolescents, and young adults. The tumors are most commonly located near the ends of the tibia and femur, but can occur in almost any bone.

Osteoblastomas (giant osteoid osteomas) are similar to osteoid osteomas but are larger and have a greater chance of recurrence after resection. A small percentage convert to osteosarcomas. Osteoblasts are composed of tissue similar to that in the nidus of osteoid osteomas, but do not induce adjacent densely sclerotic bone. Osteoblastomas tend to be located in vertebrae and long bones and do not cause pain.

Osteosarcomas ("osteogenic" sarcoma) are the most common form of primary bone cancer. The tumor is best considered to be a malignant proliferation of mesenchymal cells that have the capacity to form osteoid or bone. The characteristic histologic feature of osteosarcoma is the presence of anaplastic tumor cells within the lacunae of osteoid matrix. Osteosarcomas vary in the amount of osteoid, cartilaginous, and vascular components. Primary osteosarcomas are most common in individuals less than age 20, have a male preponderance, and tend to occur in long bones before the epiphyses have closed. The majority of primary osteosarcomas that arise in jaws are observed in adults. Secondary osteosarcomas are less common than primary osteomas. They are usually observed in older adults who may have any of many predisposing conditions, including Paget's disease, multiple enchondromas or osteochon-

Benign bone-forming tumors include osteomas and osteoid osteomas. Osteoblastomas are prone to local recurrence. Osteosarcomas are frankly malignant.

dromas, fractures, osteomyelitis, or fibrous dysplasia. Clinically, osteosarcomas tend to present with pain and swelling. The formerly dismal prognosis of these aggressive tumors has been somewhat modified by combined treatment with surgery, radiation, and chemotherapy.

Chondromatous Tumors

Bones may develop a wide variety of cartilage-containing tumors.

Exostoses are cartilage-capped bony outgrowths that are discussed elsewhere (see p. 146), as they are probably disorders of development rather than tumors. **Chondromas** are benign, tumorous proliferations of mature cartilage that appear to arise from developmental remnants of epiphyseal cartilage. An **enchondroma** is a chondroma found in a bone interior. Solitary lesions can arise at any age and in both sexes, most commonly in the small bones of the hands or feet. **Enchondromatosis (Ollier's disease)** is a hereditary disorder characterized by multiple chondromas or enchondromas, which typically appear in childhood and can arise throughout the skeletal system. **Maffuci syndrome** is a form of enchondromatosis that is accompanied by hemangiomas of the skin. Sarcomatous transformation is common (in up to one-half of patients) in enchondromatosis syndromes, but rare in solitary chondromas and enchondromas. Histologically, chondromas of all types are composed of masses or islands of mature hyaline cartilage. The adjacent fibrous stroma is typically highly vascularized. While foci of calcification or ossification may be present, the cells in the lacunae, unlike osteosarcomas, are not anaplastic.

Chondromyxoid fibroma and chrondroblastoma may histologically resemble malignant tumors but are usually clinically benign.

Chondromyxoid fibroma is an uncommon benign neoplasm that is usually found in adolescents and younger adults and has a male predominance. Chondromyxoid fibroma forms a small, lobulated mass that is a metaphysis of femur and tibia, particularly adjacent to the knee, but can be found throughout the skeletal system. Chondromyxoid fibroma is characterized histologically by varying proportions of chondroid, fibrous, and myxoid tissues. The lesion may also contain small foci of bone. Dysplastic, sometimes multinucleate, cells can also be present, but do not imply malignant transformation since these tumors rarely, if ever, behave malignantly. **Chondroblastoma** is an uncommon, usually small, tumor that tends to arise in the epiphyses of long bones of adolescents and has a male predominance. The tumor is composed of small immature chondrocytes (chondroblasts) with interspersed occasional multinucleated giant cells and islands of chondroid matrix. Despite the presence of giant cells, which have benign-appearing nuclei, chondroblastoma is almost always a benign tumor.

Chondrosarcoma is the second most common primary bone cancer.

Chondrosarcoma is the second most common (after osteosarcoma) primary bone cancer. Chondrosarcomas tend to have a slower clinical evolution and a better prognosis than osteosarcomas. **Primary chondrosarcomas** tend to arise in the central skeleton or around the knee of middle-aged or older adults with a slight male predominance. Most primary chondrosarcomas arise centrally in bone, although a few arise subperiostially. **Secondary chondrosarcomas** are less common than primary chondrosarcomas and arise in pre-existing cartilaginous tumors and exostoses. Chondrosarcomas are composed of anaplastic chondrocytes within lacunae in cartilage. Well-differentiated chondrosarcomas may be difficult to distinguish from chondromas. Chondrosarcomas may have foci of ossification, but, unlike osteosarcomas, the sites of ossification tend to be within cartilage rather than arising directly from the matrix. The **clear cell variant** of chondrosarcoma tends to arise in the epiphysis of femur and humerus and usually has a better prognosis than other chondrosarcomas.

Skeletal Tumors of Unknown Origin

Ewing's sarcoma and giant cell tumors arise from undetermined cells in the skeletal system. **Ewing's sarcoma** is an aggressive malignant tumor that occurs predominantly in male adolescents. Any bone may be affected, with common sites including long tubular bones and the pelvis. The tumor is composed of small cells without distinctive cytologic features whose origin is still disputed, but may be neuroendocrine. These cells resemble those of other small cell tumors, including lymphomas, neuroblastomas, and other undifferentiated carcinomas. The cells tend to grow in sheets and may produce "pseudorosettes" in which the tumor cells rim a central clearing. Radiographically, the tumor tends to produce a radiolucent (lytic) lesion that may involve large areas of a medullary cavity. Subperiosteal new (nontumorous) bone may widen the bone shaft in a characteristic pattern ("onion skin" layering) adjacent to the tumor. Histochemical studies may demonstrate glycogen or neuron-specific enolase. Chromosome analysis of tumor cells may demonstrate a characteristic reciprocal translocation between the long arms of chromosome 11 and 22, which is also found in neuroectodermal neoplasms. Occasionally tumors resembling Ewing's sarcoma are found outside of bone, where they are called extrosseous Ewing's sarcoma. The prognosis for Ewing's sarcoma was formerly dismal but has been somewhat improved by combined surgery, chemotherapy, and sometimes radiotherapy.

Ewing's sarcoma is an aggressive tumor composed of small, possibly neuroendocrine, cells.

Giant cell tumors (inappropriately also called osteoclastomas) are peculiar neoplasms of still-disputed (possibly mesenchymal) histogenesis composed of large numbers of multinucleate cells. Giant cell tumors usually arise in epiphyses, often around the knee, although almost any other bone may be involved. Most giant cell tumors are clinically benign, but somewhat less than one-tenth are malignant. Unfortunately, effective histologic markers for malignancy have not been identified, since some histologically "benign" tumors have pulmonary metastases. Conservative surgical resection is curative in many cases, but local recurrences are common; many of them show frankly sarcomatous change.

Giant cell tumors are benign, or less commonly malignant, tumors containing large numbers of multinucleate giant cells.

8

Head and Neck

EAR

External Ear

Any dermatologic condition can affect the skin or the ear. Additionally, developmental anomalies are relatively common and usually innocuous. **Cauliflower ear** is an acquired deformity of the external ear that is commonly observed in boxers and wrestlers. Trauma-induced cartilage degeneration (chondromalacia) causes replacement of cartilage by a homogeneous matrix accompanied by perichondral and intrachondral fibrosis. **Chondrodermatitis nodularis helicis** ("painful nodule of the ear") is a small, crusted, nodular lesion that can grossly resemble basal cell or squamous carcinoma. This benign lesion is composed of degenerating collagen with accompanying chronic inflammation and hyperplastic epithelium. It often involves the helix of middle-aged or older patients and can be cured by excision. **Relapsing polychondritis** is a rare disease with usually bilateral perichondral acute inflammatory cell infiltrates adjacent to focal degeneration and vascularization of cartilage. Older inactive lesions show chronic inflammatory cells and fibrous replacement of cartilage. This rare chronic disease is of unknown etiology, but may be associated with systemic connective tissue disease. **Malignant external otitis** is a necrotizing external ear infection caused by *Pseudomonas aeruginosa* and observed most frequently in older diabetic patients. The infection may be complicated by bone involvement, meningitis, or brain abscess.

   Tumors and tumorlike conditions that can affect the external ear include epidermal inclusion cysts, squamous cell papillomas, nevi, basal cell carcinomas, squamous cell carcinomas, malignant melanomas, and neoplasms rising from cerumen-secreting sweat glands. These latter adenomas and adenocarcinomas resemble hidradenomas (sweat gland adenomas) and adenocarcinomas of skin appendages. Pleomorphic adenoma and adenoid cystic carcinomas, similar to those observed in salivary glands, have also been described.

The external ear can be affected by trauma, inflammation, and tumor.

151

Middle Ear

The middle ear can develop otitis media and tumors.

The middle ear is vulnerable to both otitis media and tumor formation. **Acute suppurative otitis media** is associated with accumulation of fluid in the middle ear, which causes bulging of the tympanic membrane accompanied by ear pain and tenderness. The most frequently isolated organisms are *Streptococcus pneumoniae* and *Haemophilus influenzae*. **Chronic otitis media** can cause conductive hearing loss secondary to persistent bacterial inflammation leading to bone resorption or formation of polyploid granulation tissue. Diseases causing granulomatous infections, such as tuberculosis and fungi, can also cause chronic otitis media. **Serous otitis media** is frequently associated with eustachian tube obstruction and is the accumulation of nonsuppurative fluid in the middle ear.

Tumors affect the middle ear uncommonly; the most frequent is the postinflammatory, non-neoplastic condition known as **cholesteatoma.** Cholesteatomas are cystic structures, lined with epidermis and containing keratin debris, that are possibly the result of ingrowth of squamous epithelium through a perforated eardrum. Large cholesteatomas can erode adjacent structures and produce hearing impairment. Treatment is by surgical removal. Paraganglioma and squamous cell carcinoma rarely occur in the middle ear.

Inner Ear

Lesions of the inner ear can cause hearing impairment and dizziness.

Lesions of the inner ear often cause hearing impairment and dizziness as a consequence of impairment of cochlear and vestibular function. **Otosclerosis** is the most common cause of hearing loss in young adults, and is an autosomal dominant disease with variable penetrance that causes bony deposition in the annulus around the stapes, leading to conductive hearing loss. **Menière's disease** is a hydropic dilation of the endolymphatic system of the cochlea, which may cause rupture of Reissner's membrane and is associated with symptoms of vertigo, nystagmus, nausea tinnitus, and hearing loss. **Labyrinthitis** can cause vestibular and cochlear dysfunction secondary to inflammation of the labyrinth, and it may be caused directly by viral infection (mumps, cytomegalovirus, rubella). Alternatively, a postinfectious form that lasts for several weeks follows upper respiratory viral infection and produces symptoms resembling Menière's disease that eventually resolve spontaneously. **Acoustic neuroma** is a neoplastic proliferation of Schwann cells that can involve the vestibular nerve, with resulting deafness.

NASAL CAVITIES AND ACCESSORY AIR SINUSES

Inflammations

Both the nasal cavities and sinuses can become inflamed.

Rhinitis is inflammation of the nasal cavity. **Acute rhinitis** is usually caused by one of the many viruses now associated with the "common cold." Many of the viruses causing acute rhinitis are adenoviruses, which can cause nasopharyngitis, pharyngotonsillitis, and many other clinical variants. The nasal mucosa is characteristically thickened, edematous, and red; a copious catarrhal discharge is typically present. **Allergic rhinitis** (hay fever) is an IgE-mediated immune response that can be triggered by many allergens, with plant pollen being a common stimulus. Mast cell degranulation and release of mediators is followed by a mixed leukocytic infiltration. **"Nasal polyps"** are inflammatory hypertrophic swellings that occur secondary to focal enlargement of the mucosa in recurrent allergic rhinitis. The polyps contain an edematous stroma with scattered mixed inflammatory cells.

Sinusitis is inflammation of the air sinuses that usually follows acute inflammation of the nasal cavities. Mucosal edema may obstruct drainage from the sinus, leading to production of a mucus-filled sinus (mucocele). Secondary infection of a mucocele by bacteria or fungi causes empyema, which may be complicated by osteomyelitis of the adjacent bone and the development of intracranial infections. **Kartagener syndrome,** caused by a defect in ciliary action, is the cluster of chronic sinusitis, bronchiectasis, and situs inversus.

Necrotizing granulomatous sinusitis includes Wegener's granulomatosis (see p. 204), mucormycosis (see p. 60), and polymorphic reticulosis (lethal midline granuloma). Polymorphic reticulosis is an ulcerating mucosal lesion of the upper respiratory tract that can cause extensive tissue necrosis and destruction of cartilage. The lesion characteristically contains a dense lymphoid infiltrate and may be a variant of peripheral T-cell lymphoma.

TUMORS OF THE NOSE, SINUSES, AND NASOPHARYNX

Isolated **plasmacytomas** are polypoid growths in sinus cavities that contain cells resembling those of malignant plasmacytomas. Olfactory **neuroblastomas** are highly malignant but radiosensitive tumors composed of small, round cells of neural crest origin that arise from olfactory mucosa. Nasopharyngeal **angiofibromas** are benign vascular tumors of adolescent males that may bleed profusely during surgery. Inverted **papillomas** are locally aggressive neoplasms that involve the nose and paranasal sinuses. They have a high rate of recurrence following excision, with potential of invasion into the orbitocranial vault, and occasionally develop into frank carcinoma. **Lymphoepithelioma** has an association with Epstein-Barr virus and is composed of epithelial growths containing abundant lymphoid infiltrate within a fibrous stroma. Other tumors that can involve the nose, sinus, and nasopharynx include keratinizing and nonkeratinizing squamous cell carcinomas, as well as transitional cell carcinomas.

Many tumors can involve the nose and adjacent structures.

LARYNX

The larynx is vulnerable to inflammations and tumors. **Laryngitis** can be observed in heavy smokers; patients with systemic diseases including tuberculosis and diphtheria; and patients with inflammations beginning in the oral cavity (streptococcal sore throat, moniliasis, and nonspecific bacterial disorders). Severe acute epiglottis caused by *Haemophilus influenzae* or β-hemolytic streptococci may cause airway obstruction requiring tracheotomy in infants and children.

Benign **polyps,** composed of squamous epithelium covering loose to dense collagenous tissue, can cause hoarseness in heavy smokers, singers ("singer's nodes"), and other individuals who vocalize extensive-

The larynx is vulnerable to inflammation and tumors.

ly. **Papillomas** are friable excrescences or nodules composed of multiple fingerlike projections of fibrous tissue covered with stratified squamous epithelium. Papillomas may grossly resemble carcinomas and have been associated with human papillomavirus type II in children with multiple juvenile papillomas.

Laryngeal carcinomas are subdivided into those that arise within the larynx itself (intrinsic) and those that extend or arise outside (extrinsic). The carcinomas are usually keratinizing or nonkeratinizing squamous cell carcinomas that begin as in situ lesions that may later fungate, ulcerate, or extend centrifugally. The cancers can produce progressive hoarseness, difficulty in swallowing, hemoptysis, and respiratory distress. The formerly dismal prognosis has been improved by combined surgery and radiotherapy.

ORAL CAVITY

Congenital Anomalies

Cleft lip and cleft palate are common oral congenital anomalies.

Congenital anomalies are common in the oral cavity. Cleft upper lip (harelip) may be accompanied by cleft palate. Cleft palate can also be associated with chromosomal disorders including trisomy 13 and 4p- syndromes. Less common congenital anomalies include macroglossia, microglossia, and ankyloglossia (tongue-tie). Branchial cleft cysts occur in the anterolateral aspect of the neck.

Inflammations

Aphthous ulcers are shallow oral ulcers of unknown etiology.

The oral mucosa is relatively resistant to infection by the many organisms that inhabit it. **Aphthous ulcers** (canker sores) are common shallow ulcerations of unknown etiology. Vulnerable patients may experience repeated crops of ulcers, particularly during the first 2 decades of life. The ulcers are also observed in patients with inflammatory bowel disease and Behçet syndrome.

Herpes causes vesiculo-inflammatory involvement of the lips and oral mucosa.

Herpes simplex type I (less commonly, type II) causes **herpetic stomatitis.** The severity of the lesions may range from small labial cold sores to gingivostomatitis, in which large areas of the oral mucosa and lips are involved in a vesiculoinflammatory eruption. Herpes simplex infection may also cause keratoconjunctivitis and disseminated disease, particularly in immunosuppressed adults and neonates. Most adults have been previously infected by herpes simplex virus. The virus remains latent in regional (often trigeminal) ganglia, but can later be reactivated to produce disease. Herpes labialis (cold sore, fever blister) is a vesicular lesion, characterized by ballooning degeneration and separation of epidermal cells (acantholysis), that is usually located on the lips or near the nares. Intranuclear inclusions composed of live and dead virions can be identified in some epidermal cells at the margins of the vesicle. Fusion of cells can produce giant cells in smears of the blister fluid (Tzanck preparations). **Primary herpetic gingivostomatitis** can be considered an extreme form of herpes labialis that occurs in immunocompromised hosts. It causes extensive oral ulceration that may be complicated by systemic dissemination.

Oral candidiasis (moniliasis, thrush) is usually caused by *Candida albicans* infection of the oral cavity. The fungus is a normal inhabitant in much of the population. Candidiasis develops in patients who have impaired immunity due to diabetes mellitus, xerostomia, AIDS, severe debilitation, or other diseases. Thrush produces a superficial, curdy, white membrane that overlies an erythematous inflammatory base. Severe infections may cause mucosal ulceration, spread to the esophagus, invade deeper tissues of the oral cavity, or disseminate through the bloodstream.

Candida **can infect the oral cavity of immunosuppressed patients.**

EYE

Neoplasms of the Eye

The eye can develop both benign **nevi** and **malignant melanomas.** The melanomas are found most often in the choroid, iris, or ciliary body. **Retinoblastoma** is the most common intraocular tumor of childhood, and typically causes opaque masses in the vitreous composed of large neuroblastic cells that may form rosettes. The tumor develops congenitally, occurs relatively commonly in both eyes, and sometimes has a genetic basis. Retinoblastoma confined to the eye can usually be cured by enucleation and radiation; obvious tumor extension to adjacent structures carries a dismal prognosis. **Angiomas** may occur in solitary form in the uveal tract; in the form of retinal telangiectasias (Coats disease); or diffusely as a component of von Hippel-Lindau disease. The eye is also vulnerable to **metastatic tumors,** notably from lung and breast, and to tumors of the lacrimal glands, which often resemble salivary gland tumors.

Diseases of the Eyelid

The skin of the eyelid is vulnerable to lesions and tumors of other hair-bearing skin. Accumulated lipid secretions due to chronic obstruction of the meiboian glands causes a **chalazion,** characterized by chronic inflammation with foreign body granuloma formation. A **stye** is an acute suppurative inflammation (often staphylococcal) of the tissues surrounding an eyelash. **Xanthelasmas** are yellow cutaneous nodules, usually observed in patients with hyperlipidemia, that are composed of lipid-containing histiocytes.

Conjunctival and Corneal Diseases

Acute conjunctivitis is associated with pain, photophobia, corneal inflammation, and sometimes temporarily impaired vision secondary to infiltration by inflammatory cells. Acute conjunctivitis can be induced by chemical, bacterial, and allergic agents. Neonatal conjunctival infections can be due to gonorrhea, *Branhamella catarrhalis,* or *Chlamydia trachomatis.* Childhood bacterial conjunctivitis is most frequently due to *Streptococcus, Haemophilus, Pneumococcus,* or *Staphylococcus.* **Chronic inflammation** of the conjunctiva and cornea can lead to blindness secondary to corneal opacification. The chronic inflammation can produce ingrowth of vascularized connective tissue into the cornea (pannus formation); proliferation of lymphoid nodules (follicular hyperplasia) in conjunctiva; or formation by proliferating granulation tissue of papillae and

Acute conjunctivitis can be induced by many agents.

Chronic conjunctivitis can cause corneal opacification leading to blindness.

Other conditions affecting conjunctiva include pinguecula, pterygium, and epidermidalization.

cryptlike spaces (papillary hyperplasia) beneath the conjunctiva. Conjunctival and corneal disease associated with *Chlamydia trachomatis* are particularly important causes of conjunctival and corneal disease, and are discussed in the chapter on bacteria (see p. 33). Solar damage to the conjunctiva can cause formation of a yellow plaque (**pinguecula**) composed of damaged collagen. Growth of vascularized connective tissue from the limbus into the corneal center produces a **pterygium**, which may impair vision. Under conditions of vitamin A deficiency or abnormally dry eyes (e.g., Sjögren syndrome or conditions impairing eyelid closure), the normal nonkeratinized conjunctival epithelium may be replaced by a thick, keratinized, opaque layer (**epidermidalization**).

Inflammatory Diseases of the Orbit

Inflammations of the orbit have many causes.

Inflammation of the uvea (**uveitis**) has many causes, including nongranulomatous infection (toxoplasmosis, herpes viruses, bacterial purulent inflammation following trauma), granulomatous infections (tuberculosis, histoplasmosis, syphilis, sarcoid), and noninfectious causes (surgery). **Sympathetic ophthalmia** is a granulomatous uveitis, thought to be mediated by an autoimmune mechanism, that occurs in a few patients following injury or surgery of the opposite eye.

Inflammation of the iris (**iridocyclitis**) or sclera (**scleritis**) is usually seen in ankylosing spondylitis or other rheumatoid conditions. Inflammation of the scleral periphery (**episcleritis**) has many autoimmune, granulomatous, and toxic etiologies. Inflammation of the inner eye (**endophthalmitis**) is usually due to either infection introduced by penetrating wounds (including surgery) or hematogenous spread (usually in immunosuppressed patients) of opportunistic organisms (*Candida, Aspergillus, Toxoplasma, Cryptococcus,* cytomegalovirus). **Ocular trauma** may cause acute or chronic inflammation; in extreme cases, the globe may atrophy with or without shrinkage.

Retrolental Fibroplasia

Fibrosis of the vitreous is obscured in premature infants exposed to high oxygen levels.

Premature infants therapeutically exposed to high oxygen tension during therapy of neonatal respiratory distress syndrome may develop **retrolental fibroplasia.** This condition is associated with vascular proliferation into the vitreous, which is followed by gliosis and fibrosis of the vitreous, leading to severe visual impairment.

Glaucoma

Glaucoma is elevated intraocular pressure.

Elevated intraocular pressure is called **glaucoma,** and may, in longstanding cases, impair vision by causing atrophy of retinal nerve fibers and degeneration of the ganglion cell layer of the retina. **Primary angle closure glaucoma** is usually due to a congenitally narrowed anterior choroid angle that narrows even further with aging. Contact with the iris consequently partially obstructs the canal of Schlemm and the trabecular meshwork. Patients experience acute attacks of edema that may cause necrosis of the iris. Sclerosis of unknown etiology involving the trabeculae can narrow the canal of Schlemm, causing slowly developing **pri-**

mary open-angle glaucoma, which is usually observed in elderly individuals. **Congenital glaucoma** is associated with the abnormal insertion of ciliary muscle fibers on trabecular bands. **Secondary glaucoma** can be due to trauma, tumor, and acute or chronic inflammation of the iris, anterior chamber, or uvea.

Cataracts

Alterations in the structure, epithelium, or capsule of the lens may cause opacification, known as a **cataract.** Most commonly, cataracts are due to aging of cortical lens cells characterized initially by focal opacities due to protein coagulation and later by liquification of portions of the cortex. Displacement of the involved lens into the anterior chamber may cause glaucoma. Uncommon causes of cataracts include injury and toxic damage.

Cataracts are opacifications of the lens.

Papilledema

Swelling of the head of the optic nerve **(papilledema)** is visible by ophthalmoscopy, and can be due to either increased intraorbital or increased intracranial pressure. Acute papilledema is associated with a usually reversible interstitial edema of the nerve head. Chronic papilledema may permanently impair vision and produces vascular varicosities, glial proliferation, and shrinkage of the nerve head.

Papilledema can be due to either increased intraorbital or increased intracranial pressure.

Retinal Detachment

The retinal neural structures can be separated from the underlying pigment epithelium **(retinal detachment)** by fluid accumulation or by traction from postinflammatory or posthemorrhagic fibrous bands. If the detached portion of the retina is not reattached (e.g., by laser therapy), cystic degeneration followed by glial replacement will occur several months later.

Detached areas of retina degenerate unless reattached.

Retinopathies

Occlusion of the retinal vein usually causes hemorrhage and development of collateral circulation. Occlusion of the retinal artery causes ischemic infarction. Acute **hypertension** produces arteriolar spasm, flame-shaped hemorrhages, edema, and exudates. Chronic hypertension produces arteriolar sclerosis, hemorrhage, retinal atrophy, and retinal edema. Malignant hypertension produces papilledema, exaggerated changes of acute hypertension, and focal ischemic necrosis (cotton-wool patches). The retinopathy of **diabetes** is a leading cause of blindness and includes venule aneurysm formation, exudates, macular edema, proliferative retinopathy, and scarring about the nerve head. **Retinitis pigmentosa** is an often hereditary pigmentary degeneration of the retinal epithelium; it causes progressive visual impairment that begins with night blindness.

Retinal damage can occur by many mechanisms.

9
Respiratory System

CONGENITAL ANOMALIES

One or both lungs can be vulnerable to agenesis, hypoplasia, and anomalous development of trachea, bronchi, or vasculature. Anomalous development of the trachea or bronchi is frequently associated with anomalous development of the esophagus. When a segment or lobe of lung tissue does not connect normally to the airway system, **bronchopulmonary sequestration** is said to have occurred. Extralobar sequestration occurs outside the pleura covering and may produce mass lesions anywhere in the thorax or mediastinum. In contrast, sequestrations within the pleura are termed intralobar and tend to become clinically significant as sites of recurrent infection or bronchiectasis. The blood supply of both intralobar and extralobar sequestration is typically from the aorta or its branches rather than from the pulmonary arteries. **Bronchogenic cysts** are single or multiple cystic structures arising from the primitive foregut, lined by bronchial-type epithelium, with walls occasionally containing cartilage or mucus glands, and mucus or air-filled cyst cavities. Bronchogenic cysts are vulnerable to rupture into an adjacent bronchus causing hemorrhage and hemoptsis; rupture into the pleura causing pneumothorax; infection causing lung abscess; and metaplasia of the cyst lining.

Congenital anomalies can affect the trachea, bronchi, or vasculature.

ATELECTASIS

Atelectasis is characterized by relatively airless pulmonary parenchyma and occurs when a portion of the lung is collapsed or fails to expand. Lung tissue may fail to expand at birth because of inadequate surfactant production by immature lungs or because a portion of the airways is obstructed, as by a developmental anomaly or foreign body. In adults, acquired atelectasis can occur by several mechanisms. Obstruction of an airway can be followed by absorption of trapped air. Following significant obstruction, the mediastinum tends to shift toward the atelectic lung. Compression, as by blood, tumor, pleural fluid, or air, can push air

Atelectasis can occur either when a portion of lung fails to expand or when it collapses.

159

out of the involved lung. In contrast to obstruction, the mediastinum tends to shift away from the atelectic lung. Contraction, as by localized fibrosis, can also force air out of the involved lung. Loss of pulmonary surfactant, as occurs in both fetal and adult respiratory distress syndrome, can cause a patchy atelectasis. In general, atelectasis is a reversible condition that becomes clinically significant only either when so much lung tissue is involved that respiratory function is compromised or when infection of the atelectic lung supervenes.

PULMONARY DISEASES OF VASCULAR ORIGIN

Pulmonary Congestion and Edema

> **Pulmonary edema usually develops either as a consequence of hemodynamic derangements or of microvascular injury.**

The accumulation of fluid in lung parenchyma and alveoli is termed **pulmonary edema** and is usually accompanied by congestion of pulmonary vessels, including the alveolar capillary bed. Pulmonary edema usually develops either as a consequence of hemodynamic derangements or of microvascular injury. **Hemodynamic pulmonary edema** occurs in settings that favor shift of fluid from the vascular space to the interstitium. These settings include increased hydrostatic pressure in the vessels (left heart failure, mitral stenosis, volume overload, pulmonary vein obstruction); decreased oncotic pressure (hypoalbuminemia due to nephrotic syndrome, liver disease, or protein-losing enteropathies); and lymphatic obstruction (tumor, granulomatous diseases). In practice, the physiologic derangements must be severe since the normal pulmonary lymphatic system can absorb a tenfold increase in lymph flow before edema develops. The lungs in pulmonary congestion are characteristically wet and heavy, with more fluid accumulation in dependent locations. The microscopic appearance is of engorged alveolar capillaries and a proteinaceous, granular, precipitate within alveoli. Microhemorrhages and hemosiderin-laden macrophages (heart failure cells) may also be present in the alveoli.

Microvascular injury causes edema by direct injury to alveolocapillary membranes, which can markedly lower the hydrostatic pressure at which fluid flows from the vascular space to the interstitium. Agents capable of directly damaging the alveolar capillary bed include infectious agents (viruses, mycoplasm); gases (smoke, nitrogen dioxide, sulfur dioxide); aspirated liquids (gastric contents, drowning); drugs and toxins (bleomycin, amphotericin, colchicine, gold, heroin, kerosene, paraquat); shock (trauma, sepsis, pancreatitis); and miscellaneous causes (radiation, heat, uremia, fat or air embolism, cardiopulmonary bypass). In contrast to the diffuse edema seen in hemodynamic pulmonary edema, microvascular injury can be localized and produce a patchy edema. When microvascular injury is diffuse, the adult respiratory distress syndrome may be produced.

Newborn Respiratory Distress Syndrome

Respiratory distress syndrome of the newborn (hyaline membrane disease) is a form of collapsed lung with high mortality observed in neonates. Risk factors include prematurity, cesarean section, and maternal diabetes. The infant initially has apparently normal respiration, but within minutes to hours develops respiratory failure with nearly complete collapse of the lungs. The basic lesion is an immaturity of lung alveoli with **reduced surfactant** production by type II pneumocytes. The alveoli are consequently difficult to maintain open because they have a high surface tension. As the infant fatigues, more alveoli close, and the baby experiences hypoxia. The problem is exacerbated by hypoxic damage to alveoli leading to exudation of plasma proteins, irritation and necrosis of pneumocytes, and formation of hyaline membranes. Microscopically, the affected lung shows atelectasis and hyaline membrane formation. These babies require high oxygen pressures, which can damage the eyes if they are not protected. Surfactant therapy in aerosol form, particularly when given early, can ameliorate the condition.

Reduced surfactant production causes a near complete collapse of the lungs in newborn respiratory distress syndrome.

Adult Respiratory Distress Syndrome

Adult respiratory distress syndrome is a final common pathway observed after diffuse alveolar capillary damage. It is characterized by the rapid onset of life-threatening respiratory insufficiency accompanied by the sequela of severe arterial hypoxemia, including cyanosis, tachycardia, and diffuse hypoxic damage to many organ systems. Many mediators of injury to the alveolar capillary endothelium have been implicated, including neutrophils, free radicals, activated complement factors, and vasoactive products derived from platelets. The clinical conditions in which adult respiratory distress syndrome can occur are the same as those that can cause microvascular injury leading to pulmonary edema. The acute stage of adult respiratory distress syndrome is characterized by firm lungs that microscopically show congestion, focal hemorrhage, edema, fibrin deposition, patchy atelectasis, and formation of waxy hyaline membranes from necrosis of epithelial cells. Bronchopneumonia may also be present. In patients who survive the acute stage, the chronic stage shows regeneration of the alveolar lining by type II pneumocytes and fibrosis of alveolar lumina and walls. Patients who develop adult respiratory distress syndrome are usually hospitalized for one of the predisposing conditions and may not have significant underlying pulmonary disease. As the adult respiratory distress syndrome develops, the patients experience increasing dyspnea and tachypnea that rapidly progresses to respiratory failure. Despite aggressive supportive therapy directed toward correcting hypoxia and acidosis, many patients die, usually of multiorgan failure.

Diffuse alveolar capillary damage of many etiologies can cause adult respiratory distress syndrome.

Pulmonary Embolism, Hemorrhage, and Infarction

Emboli, usually derived from thromboses of the deep leg veins, can pass through the right side of the heart and lodge in the pulmonary arterial circulation. Small pulmonary emboli are probably common and may not cause significant disease. The pathology produced by pulmonary emboli can have several forms. Large pulmonary emboli are one of the few causes of death in a few minutes or less. Such **sudden death** can be produced if a large embolus lodges in the main pulmonary artery or its major branches, often at a site of arterial bifurcation ("saddle embolus").

Clinically significant pulmonary emboli are often derived from deep leg vein thromboses.

The mechanism of death in such cases is usually obstruction of pulmonary blood flow or acute dilation of the right heart (acute cor pulmonale). Characteristically, no pathologic changes related to the embolus are seen in the lung parenchyma distal to the obstruction.

Pulmonary hemorrhage, in which the normal structure of the lung is preserved but the alveoli are suffused with blood, occurs when a pulmonary artery is occluded by an embolus but the circulation through the bronchial system is adequate to preserve the parenchyma. Pulmonary hemorrhage can resolve without sequelae as the blood is resorbed.

True **pulmonary infarction** is seen much less commonly than pulmonary hemorrhage and occurs when a pulmonary embolus lodges in a portion of the lung where the bronchial circulation is inadequate to allow the pulmonary parenchymal cells to survive, typically because of coexistent cardiovascular or pulmonary disease. As a consequence of the anatomic distribution of the pulmonary arterial system, pulmonary infarcts characteristically have a roughly conical geometry (wedgelike on chest radiograph) in which the apex points toward the hilum and roughly defines the site of arterial obstruction. Histologically, a pulmonary infarction resembles pulmonary hemorrhage in that the alveoli are suffused with blood, but it additionally shows ischemic necrosis with loss of cell nuclei in the lung parenchyma, including alveolar walls, bronchioles, and blood vessels. If the infarct was caused by a **septic embolus,** an intense neutrophilic response may be present.

Diffuse Pulmonary Hemorrhage

Significant **pulmonary hemorrhage** with hemoptysis can be produced by several interstitial lung diseases. **Goodpasture syndrome** is the consequence of autoantibodies directed against antigens in the renal glomerular and pulmonary basement membranes. The resulting damage to the kidneys causes a proliferative, rapidly progressive glomerulonephritis. Damage to the lungs causes a necrotizing hemorrhagic interstitial pneumonitis with linear deposits of immunoglobulin along the septal basement membranes. Goodpasture syndrome formerly rapidly progressed to death, usually by renal failure, but now can be markedly slowed by intensive use of plasma exchange. **Vasculitis-associated pulmonary hemorrhage** can follow blood vessel damage by conditions such as Wegener's granulomatosis, hypersensitivity angiitis, and lupus erythematosus. **Idiopathic pulmonary hemosiderosis** is an uncommon pulmonary disease of younger adults and children that resembles Goodpasture syndrome, but antibodies to glomerular or alveolar basement membranes cannot be demonstrated. The clinical course is variable: some patients have only intermittent episodes with no shortening of lifespan, while others die of pulmonary hemorrhage or develop progressive pulmonary fibrosis with accompanying cor pulmonale and cardiac failure.

Pulmonary Alveolar Proteinosis

Pulmonary alveolar proteinosis is an uncommon, idiopathic disease characterized by flooding of alveoli by a turbid fluid that on histologic section forms a granular precipitate. The precipitated material appears to be chemically similar to surfactant, but does not reduce alveolar sur-

Pulmonary hemorrhage is observed when embolic occlusion of a pulmonary artery is not quite sufficient to cause infarction.

Goodpasture syndrome and vasculitis are important causes of diffuse pulmonary hemorrhage.

face tension. The alveoli septae may show pneumocyte hyperplasia with focal necrosis but no inflammation. The patient develops nonspecific respiratory difficulty accompanied by cough productive of sputum containing gelatinous material. The chest radiograph is similar to those produced by diffuse infiltrative pulmonary diseases. The prognosis is variable, with resolution of disease in some patients and progressive respiratory insufficiency in others.

Pulmonary alveolar protein-osis is an idiopathic disease in which alveoli become flooded by turbid fluid.

Pulmonary Hypertension and Vascular Sclerosis

The normal pulmonary blood pressure is much less than the normal systemic blood pressure. Pulmonary hypertension occurs most commonly as a secondary process but can occur in a primary, idiopathic form. **Primary pulmonary hypertension** is seen most often in children around the age of 5 and women aged 20 to 40 years. It remains of undetermined etiology, possibly the result of chronic vasoconstriction secondary to a neurohormonal vascular hyper-reactivity.

Pulmonary hypertension usually occurs in a primary, idiopathic form.

Secondary pulmonary hypertension can be seen at any age as a consequence of either primary cardiac diseases (left heart failure) or primary pulmonary disease (multiple pulmonary emboli, obstructive pulmonary disease, restrictive pulmonary disease). A variety of vascular lesions can be seen in both primary and secondary forms of pulmonary hypertension. Atheromatous plaques, resembling those seen in systemic arteries in systemic hypertension, can be found in the main elastic arteries. Changes ranging from intimal thickening and fibrosis with mild adventitial fibrosis to medial hypertrophy are observed in medium-sized muscular arteries. Thickening and reduplication of the internal and external elastic membranes is seen in both medium and small-sized arteries. Marked thickening of the media, sometimes accompanied by near occlusive luminal narrowing, can affect arterioles and small arteries up to about 300 μm in diameter. A severe variant of intimal narrowing, known as **plexogenic pulmonary arteriopathy,** can be seen in some thin-walled, small arteries in which the vessel lumen is occluded by intima that contains a tuft of cellular capillary formations resembling a vascular plexus. Pulmonary hypertension, whether primary or secondary, predisposes for right ventricular hypertrophy with risk of decompensated cor pulmonale and death.

Vascular changes are common in pulmonary hypertension.

CHRONIC OBSTRUCTIVE PULMONARY DISEASE

Measurements of pulmonary function by pulmonary physiologists have led to the concepts of obstructive and restrictive lung disease. **Restrictive lung disease** is characterized by lungs that expand less than normal amounts as the inflation pressure is increased; **obstructive lung disease** is characterized by more than normal expansion under similar conditions. While this distinction between obstructive and restrictive lung disease is clinically useful, many pulmonary diseases are more complex than is implied by this simple dichotomy. Despite this limitation, diseases conventionally classified as chronic obstructive pulmonary diseases include emphysema, chronic bronchitis, bronchial

Chronic obstructive pulmonary disease includes emphysema, chronic bronchitis, asthma, and bronchiectasis.

asthma, and bronchiectasis. These diseases often coexist, and they are major causes of restricted activity, including bed confinement, in the United States.

Emphysema

Environmental pathogens tend to cause centriacinar emphysema, while α₁-antitrypsin deficiency causes panacinar emphysema.

Narrowly defined, **emphysema** refers to an abnormal permanent enlargement of respiratory acini with destruction of portions of the septae. **Centriacinar (centrilobular) emphysema** is characterized by distention of the centrally located respiratory bronchioles with relative sparing of the alveolar ducts and alveoli. This form of emphysema is typically more severe in the upper lobes and appears to be associated with environmental pathogens such as smoking and coal dust. **Panacinar (panlobular) emphysema** is characterized by uniform enlargement of the entire acinus distal to the terminal bronchiole. Panacinar emphysema is associated with α_1-antitrypsin deficiency and tends to be more severe in the lower portions of the lobes. **Paraseptal (distal acinar) emphysema** is characterized by relative preservation of the proximal parts of the acinus and emphysematous dilation of the alveoli, most prominently in the subpleural locations.

The term emphysema is sometimes used in a broader context than alveolar destruction.

The term emphysema is sometimes used in a broader context than that illustrated above. **Senile emphysema** (senile hyperinflation) refers to the voluminous lungs seen in elderly individuals caused by dilations of the alveolar ducts accompanied by reduction in size of alveoli. **Compensatory emphysema** refers to hyperinflation of the remaining lung tissue observed after loss of other chest contents (e.g., following lobectomy). **Obstructive overinflation** occurs when air is trapped in a portion of the lung by an obstructive process that permits air to flow into the lung more easily than it flows out. Obstructive overinflation can be caused by a movable mass (tumor, foreign body) within an airway that acts as a ball valve. Alternatively, the pulmonary alveoli distal to a complete obstruction of the airways can fill during inspiration through collateral air paths such as the pores of Kohn and then fail to empty during expiration. Obstructive overinflation can become life-threatening as overinflated tissue compresses adjacent, previously normal lung. **Congenital lobar overinflation** is seen in infants and may be the result of hypoplasia of bronchial cartilage. **Bullous emphysema** refers to the presence of large (more than 1 cm) hollow blebs or bullae, which are typically located in the subpleura and are consequently vulnerable to rupture, potentially causing pneumothorax. The blebs represent localized accentuations of any of the emphysematous processes described in the beginning of this section.

Interstitial emphysema refers to the sometimes massive quantities of air introduced into connective tissues in the mediastinum, subcutaneous tissues, or lung hilum by processes such as rupture of air spaces (violent coughing) or penetrating wounds (including thoracotomy tubes) to the chest. The trapped air tends to dissect along tissue planes and is usually of no clinical significance, although the patient's appearance can be alarming, as the neck and upper extremities "balloon" with air. Once the source of the leak is repaired, the trapped air usually resorbs spontaneously.

Chronic Bronchitis

Chronic bronchitis is a clinically defined syndrome in which chronic cough with copious sputum production has been present for 3 or more months in 2 or more consecutive years. If no evidence of obstruction to the airways is present, the bronchitis is called **simple chronic bronchitis;** the presence of an obstructive component defines **obstructive chronic bronchitis.** Chronic bronchitis is usually associated with chronic irritation by inhaled substances, notably smoking, but also smog. It can be exacerbated by pulmonary infections. The earliest feature of chronic bronchitis is excessive mucus production with hypertrophy of submucosal glands. Squamous metaplasia and dysplasia may be present. The bronchioles and small (less than 3 mm) bronchi may show goblet cell metaplasia, with consequent increased mucus production that may plug small airways. These changes are accompanied by bronchiolitis with infiltration of small airways by increased numbers of pigmented alveolar macrophages. With time, the bronchiolar walls become fibrosed, with obliteration of lumina **(bronchiolitis fibrosa obliterans)** in severe cases. Severe airway obstruction is usually the result of an accompanying emphysema, for which smoking is also a principal risk factor. Early chronic bronchitis is characterized clinically only by persistent cough with copious sputum production. Late chronic bronchitis, particularly when significant emphysema is also present, can be accompanied by dyspnea on exertion, cor pulmonale with possible progression to cardiac failure, and significantly impaired respiratory function.

> Chronic bronchitis is a clinically defined syndrome that histologically often shows hypertrophy of submucosal glands, excessive mucus production, and epithelial changes.

Bronchial Asthma

Asthma is a disease characterized by paroxysmal constriction of the bronchial airways. It is convenient to classify asthma by dominant precipitating factors. **Atopic** (allergic or reagin-mediated) **asthma** is triggered by specific allergies (pollens, house dust, etc.) and appears to be mediated by an IgE (type I) immune reaction. The patient may also have allergic rhinitis, urticaria, or eczema. Bronchopulmonary aspergillosis with the resulting exposure to spores can produce a variant of atopic asthma that appears to be mediated by both types I and II immune reactions. **Nonreaginic asthma** is triggered by respiratory infections by an unknown mechanism that does not appear to involve IgE. **Pharmacologic asthma** is triggered by drugs, notably aspirin, by a mechanism that appears to involve increased bronchoconstrictor tone as a consequence of decreased prostaglandin and increased leukotriene production. This type of asthma is associated with recurrent rhinitis and nasal polyps. **Occupational asthma** is triggered by chemical exposures (epoxy resins, plastics, wood, cotton, platinum, toluene, formaldehyde) and appears to be mediated by an IgE immune mechanism. The asthma usually develops after repeated exposure to the offending chemical and can subsequently be triggered by minute exposures. All of the above-listed types of asthma are characterized by hyper-reactive airways and may be precipitated by other agents, including cold, exercise, and stress.

> Asthma is classified by dominant precipitating factors.

Patients with severe asthma have **copious mucus production** that can plug bronchi and bronchioles. The mucus may contain shed epithelium (Curschmann's spirals), eosinophils, or crystalloids derived from eosinophil membrane protein (Charcot-Leyden crystals); these features may be observed in sputum samples. Other pathologic features of severe asthma include enlarged submucosal glands, thickened basement membranes, hypertrophied bronchial muscle, and an eosinophilic infiltrate in the bronchial wall.

Most patients with bronchial asthma have intermittent asthmatic attacks, characterized by bronchospasm and impaired ventilation, which persist for up to several hours. The attacks are followed by pronounced coughing, which tends to raise the often copious mucus secretion.

> Mucus production can be copious.

Status asthmaticus is a life-threatening emergency.

Between attacks, patients may be asymptomatic or experience chronic, low-level respiratory symptoms. A few patients develop **status asthmaticus,** in which severe paroxysms persist for days to weeks and may lead to severe cyanosis and death. Patients with asthma are vulnerable to superimposed bacterial infections, which may contribute to coexisting chronic bronchitis, bronchiectasis, or pneumonia. Cor pulmonale and heart failure develop in a few patients.

Bronchiectasis

Bronchiectasis is often related to cystic fibrosis and other conditions that predispose to obstruction or infection.

Bronchiectasis is an irreversible dilation of bronchi and bronchioles. It is associated with pulmonary conditions that predispose for obstruction or infection, including cystic fibrosis (see p. 278), tumor, chronic bronchitis (see p. 164), asthma, intralobar sequestration (see p. 159), and some pneumonias. Bronchiectasis characteristically affects the lower lobes more severely than the upper lobes, with particularly marked involvement of those air passages that are most nearly vertical. The bronchi can often be followed to the lung periphery. The shape of dilation may be cylindroid, fusiform, or saccular. Severe cases have acute and chronic inflammation of walls of bronchi and bronchioles, sometimes accompanied by ulceration or abscess formation. Squamous metaplasia or pseudostratification of the columnar cells of the lining epithelium may be present. Abscesses may heal with fibrosis of bronchial and bronchiolar walls. Bronchiectasis manifests clinically with chronic paroxysmal cough productive of foul-smelling sputum.

RESTRICTIVE LUNG DISEASES

Idiopathic Pulmonary Fibrosis

Idiopathic pulmonary fibrosis is characterized by inflammation and fibrosis of alveolar walls.

Idiopathic pulmonary fibrosis is one of many terms (usual interstitial pneumonitis, chronic interstitial pneumonitis, cryptogenic fibrosing alveolitis, Hamman-Rich syndrome) used to designate a poorly understood pulmonary disorder characterized by inflammation and fibrosis of the pulmonary interstitium, particularly the alveolar walls. Idiopathic pulmonary fibrosis can affect both sexes at any age, but is most frequently seen in middle-aged men. The disorder is probably a stereotyped inflammatory response to a variety of alveolar wall injuries. The early stages are characterized by firm lungs that histologically show pulmonary edema with mononuclear cell infiltration of the alveolar septae. Hyaline membranes and type II pneumocyte hyperplasia may be present. Later, the alveolitic process resolves in some areas of the lung and progresses to interstitial fibrosis in others. In the end stages, the lung becomes **"honeycombed"** by many small cysts with fibrotic walls lined by cuboidal to columnar epithelium. In the typical case, death occurs within 2 years, often as the combined result of respiratory difficulties and cor pulmonale that progresses to cardiac failure.

Desquamative Interstitial Pneumonitis

Desquamative interstitial pneumonitis is a disease of unknown etiology that may be a variant or early stage of idiopathic interstitial fibrosis. Desquamative interstitial pneumonitis is characterized by interstitial pneumonitis, hyperplasia of type II pneumocytes, and accumulation in alveoli of large numbers of macrophages. The macrophages contain lipid, periodic acid-Schiff (PAS)-positive granules, and lamellar bodies (surfactant) that are presumably derived from desquamated type II pneumocytes. Some cases of desquamative interstitial pneumonitis resolve spontaneously or with steroid therapy; others progress to significant interstitial fibrosis.

Desquamative interstitial pneumonitis may be a variant or early stage of idiopathic interstitial fibrosis.

Hypersensitivity Pneumonitis

Immunologically mediated pneumonitis can be caused by exposure to many antigens. **Farmer's lung** is provoked by exposure to dust from hay containing *Actinomyces* spores. **Pigeon breeder's lung** (bird fancier's disease) is caused by exposure to bird proteins in feathers and excretion. Humidifier or **air conditioner lung** is provoked by bacteria growing in warm water. **Byssinosis** is observed in textile workers who inhale fibers from natural fabrics. Hypersensitivity pneumonitis initially presents with acute attacks of fever, dyspnea, and cough in sensitized patients who inhale antigenic dust. With continual exposure, chronic disease develops that is characterized clinically by progressive respiratory failure, dyspnea, and cyanosis. Lung biopsies from chronic cases (acute cases are usually not biopsied) show an interstitial infiltrate (lymphocytes, plasma cells, macrophages), interstitial fibrosis, obliterative bronchiolitis, granuloma formation, and, in some patients, an intra-alveolar infiltrate. Byssinosis presents a pathologic picture somewhat different from other forms of hypersensitivity pneumonitis and is characterized by chronic bronchitis, emphysema, and formation of interstitial granulomas.

Hypersensitivity pneumonitis can be triggered by a variety of antigens.

Pulmonary Infiltration with Eosinophilia

A prominent eosinophilic infiltration of the pulmonary parenchyma (usually accompanied by eosinophilia in the blood) can be caused by several pathologic processes. **Löffler syndrome,** or simple pulmonary eosinophilia, is a benign disease characterized by transient pulmonary lesions, which can produce on chest x-ray sometimes striking, irregularly shaped, intrapulmonary densities of varying sizes. Histologically, the alveolar septae show focal epithelial hyperplasia and an infiltrate composed of eosinophils and occasional giant cells. Characteristically, no vasculitis, fibrosis, or necrosis is seen. **Secondary chronic pulmonary eosinophilia** can be seen following a variety of diseases including hypersensitivity pneumonitis; bacterial and fungal infections including bronchopulmonary aspergillosis; parasitic infections including pulmonary microfilariae (tropical eosinophilia); drug allergies; asthma; and polyarteritis nodosa. **Chronic eosinophilic pneumonia** is a rare, idiopathic consolidation of the pulmonary parenchyma accompanied by a dense infiltration of lymphocytes and eosinophils. The pneumonia is characterized clinically by high fever, night sweats, and dyspnea; these symptoms resolve with corticosteroid therapy.

A prominent eosinophilic infiltration is observed in Löffler syndrome, secondary chronic pulmonary eosinophilia, and chronic eosinophilic pneumonia.

PULMONARY INFECTIONS

Bronchopneumonia and Lobar Pneumonia

Acute bacterial infection of the lung can produce two gross patterns of distribution, bronchopneumonia and lobar pneumonia.

Bronchopneumonia is characterized grossly by multiple lesions distributed throughout one (or more commonly) multiple lobes. Well-developed lesions are usually centered on a bronchi or bronchiole and appear as red-gray to yellow, poorly defined areas of consolidation 3 to 4 cm in size. **Lobar pneumonia** is characterized grossly by diffuse involvement of most to all of a (usually single) lobe of lung. The involved consolidated lung has a firm consistency and a red or gray color. Intermediate cases also exist. In both bronchopneumonia and lobar pneumonia, the infection is usually established by entry of the pathogen through the airways.

The basic lesion of both bronchopneumonia and lobar pneumonia is similar. Alveoli are filled by an acute inflammatory exudate composed of neutrophils (which may contain engulfed bacteria), fibrin, and extravasated erythrocytes. As the lesion progresses, fibrin continues to accumulate; the neutrophils and erythrocytes progressively disintegrate; and the color of the lesion grossly shifts from red to gray. Healing, in the more common fortunate cases, involves enzymatic digestion of the exudate with complete restoration of the normal alveolar structure. In complicated cases, areas of extensive fibrin deposition may be replaced by fibrosis. Other complications observed in bronchopneumonia and lobar pneumonia include abscess formation with frank tissue destruction in either the lung or in other organs reached by hematogenous spread; pleuritis with or without empyema; and suppurative pericarditis.

While bronchopneumonia and lobar pneumonia have many similarities, some differences appear in many cases. The lesions of bronchopneumonia are characteristically centered on bronchi and bronchioles, which are filled with inflammatory exudate similar to that seen in adjacent alveoli. As a general rule, lobar pneumonia is associated with more virulent pathogens and heavier bacterial exposures than is bronchopneumonia. Over 90 percent of lobar pneumonias are caused by pneumococci (*Streptococcus pneumoniae*), particularly strains 1, 3 (most virulent), 7, and 2; other pathogens less commonly encountered in lobar pneumonias include *Klebsiella pneumoniae, Haemophilus influenzae,* staphylococci, streptococci, and antibiotic-resistant gram-negative organisms such as *Pseudomonas* and *Proteus* species. Bronchopneumonia can be caused by any of the above pathogens, as well as by many other bacterial pathogens, including the coliform bacteria, in immunologically vulnerable hosts. Predisposing factors that either decrease host resistance or increase the risk of exposure to pathogens are more commonly identified in patients with bronchopneumonia than in patients with lobar pneumonia. Examples of such predisposing factors include infancy, old age, severe heart disease, cancer, chemotherapy, and a tendency to aspirate food or gastric contents secondary to neurologic or gastrointestinal disease.

Patients who are immunosuppressed as a consequence of disease (notably AIDS), chemotherapy, antirejection medication, or irradiation are particularly vulnerable to life-threatening pneumonia. These patients are often infected by organisms of normally low virulence. A diffuse pulmonary infiltrate in these patients is commonly produced by cytomegalovirus and *Pneumocystis carinii,* and less commonly by other bacteria, *Aspergillus,* or *Cryptococcus.* Focal infiltrates are commonly produced by gram-negative rods, *Staphylococcus aureus, Aspergillus,* and *Candida,* and are less commonly produced by *Cryptococcus, Mucor, Pneumocystis carinii,* and *Legionella pneumophila.*

Interstitial Pneumonitis

Viral and mycoplasmal organisms can cause an atypical form of pneumonia, known as **interstitial pneumonitis,** that differs from bronchopneumonia and lobar pneumonia by the absence of a prominent intra-alveolar inflammatory exudate. Interstitial pneumonitis may be patchy or may involve entire lobes, sometimes bilaterally. The inflammation is primarily interstitial and is composed of lymphocytes, histiocytes, and occasional plasma cells. Neutrophils can also be present in acute cases. Depending upon the severity of the pneumonitis, the alveoli may be free of exudate or may contain a cellular proteinaceous material or cellular debris. Prominent hyaline membranes composed of desquamated pneumocytes may be present that resemble those seen in infant and adult respiratory distress syndromes. Many etiologic agents can cause interstitial pneumonitis, including *Mycoplasma pneumoniae* (the most common etiologic agent); viruses (influenza virus types A and B, respiratory syncytial viruses, adenoviruses, rhinoviruses, rubeola and varicella); and *Chlamydia* (psittacosis) and *Coxiella burnetii* (Q fever). In infants, bacterial infection with the low-grade pathogens *Escherichia coli* and β-hemolytic streptococci can produce a form of bronchopneumonia that histologically closely resembles the interstitial pneumonitis produced by mycoplasma and viruses. The identification of the causative organism for interstitial pneumonitis can be difficult and usually requires fastidious technical methods. Most interstitial pneumonitis occurs sporadically and produces mild infection that resolves completely. The pneumonitis presents with fever, headache, malaise, and sometimes a nonproductive cough. Interstitial pneumonitis occasionally occurs in virulent epidemics, notably the highly fatal pandemics of 1915 and 1918 caused by influenza virus, with morbidity often related to secondary bacterial infection by streptococci or staphylococci.

> Viral and mycoplasmal organisms tend to produce interstitial pneumonitis, which may resemble respiratory distress syndromes.

Pulmonary Abscess

Lung abscesses are localized lesions characterized by necrosis of lung tissue accompanied by a suppurative exudate. Predisposing factors for lung abscess formation include aspiration of infected material, particularly gastric contents; preceding bronchiectasis or bacterial pneumonia, particularly due to type 3 pneumococcus, *Staphylococcus aureus, Klebsiella pneumoniae,* or fungi; septic embolism from bacterial endocarditis or thrombophlebitis; cancer; and miscellaneous causes such as thoracic trauma or spread of infection from adjacent chest or abdominal organs. In some cases, a predisposing factor is not identified, and the abscess is termed a **"primary cryptogenic lung abscess."** Depending on the nature of the predisposing factors, lung abscesses may be single or multiple. The abscess cavities are caused by destruction of the pulmonary parenchyma and can be as large as 5 to 6 cm. The cavities can be either filled with suppurative debris, or empty, if the cavity communicated with air passages permitting the foul-smelling purulent material to be removed by coughing and/or postural drainage. The cavity walls show acute and chronic inflammatory changes, and may additionally show extensive fibroblastic proliferation if the abscess is long-standing. The necrotic material in the abscess cavity can become superinfected by saprophytes. Most pulmonary abscesses resolve with antibiotic therapy

> Pulmonary abscesses can form large cavities that heal by fibrosis of the walls.

without permanent sequelae except for loss of the involved lung tissue. Complications are usually related to direct extension or hematogenous spread of the infection to other sites (notably brain abscesses and meningitis). The presence of a lung abscess in a patient without obvious risk factors should suggest a search for carcinoma, which may be present.

LUNG TUMORS

The lungs are vulnerable to many benign and, more commonly, malignant tumors.

Bronchogenic Carcinomas

Histologic forms of bronchogenic carcinoma include squamous cell carcinoma, adenocarcinoma, bronchoalveolar carcinoma, small cell carcinoma, and large cell carcinoma.

Carcinoma arising in the bronchi or bronchioles may have many histologic forms. **Squamous cell (epidermoid) carcinoma,** the most common form, usually arises in bronchial epithelium that has previously undergone squamous metaplasia or cytologic atypia. In well-differentiated cases, keratin and intracellular bridges are present. In less well-differentiated cases, the carcinoma may resemble large cell carcinoma, described below. **Adenocarcinoma,** the second most common form, can arise in bronchial epithelium, the mucus glands associated with bronchi, or in bronchiolar epithelium. Bronchial-derived adenocarcinomas may have a histologic pattern that ranges from obvious gland formation to papillary lesions or solid masses containing occasional mucin-producing cells. **Bronchioloalveolar carcinoma** is a distinctive subtype of adenocarcinoma that arises in the terminal bronchoalveolar regions in the lung periphery. It is characterized histologically by a papillary growth pattern in which tall columnar to cuboidal cells, which are often mucin producing, line the alveolar septae and project into the alveoli. Ultrastructural studies suggest that these cells are bronchiolar cells, Clara cells, and rare type II pneumocytes. Carcinomas exhibiting both squamoid and glandular differentiation (**adenosquamous carcinomas**) can also be encountered. **Small cell carcinoma** is a highly malignant tumor characterized histologically by clusters of small cells with little cytoplasm and no evidence of glandular or squamous organization. In the classic "oat cell" form of small cell carcinoma, the cells are round to oval; other variants have spindle-shaped or polygonal cells. The cells in small cell carcinoma may contain neurosecretory granules (polypeptide hormones, neuron-specific enolase, parathormone-like substance), and these tumors can produce ectopic hormones.

Large cell carcinoma is an anaplastic form of carcinoma, possibly representing undifferentiated squamous carcinoma or adenocarcinoma, characterized by large polygonal cells with vesicular nuclei that may contain intracellular mucin but do not form recognizable glands or squamous structures. Variants of large cell carcinoma can contain multinucleate cells (giant cell carcinoma), cells with clear cytoplasm (clear cell carcinoma), or cells with elongated nuclei (spindle cell carcinoma).

Lung cancers of different types tend to be clinically similar.

Lung cancers of the histologic types described above show many common characteristics. Lung cancer is a disease of older adults with a formerly male predominance that is now diminishing, probably as a consequence of increased smoking by women. Risk factors include tobacco smoking, which is less strongly associated with squamous and oat cell carcinomas than other lung carcinomas; radiation; environmental exposures including asbestos (also associated with mesotheliomas and gastrointestinal cancers), coal, and metals (nickel, chromates, arsenic, beryllium, iron); and air pollution. There appears to be a strongly synergistic effect between smoking and most other risk factors.

Bronchogenic carcinoma can have multiple complications. Focal emphysema is produced by partial obstruction of a bronchus by tumor; atelectasis is produced by total obstruction. Severe suppurative (ulcerative) bronchitis, bronchiectasis, and pulmonary abscesses can follow impaired drainage of the airway. The superior vena cava syndrome, caused by compression or invasion of the superior vena cava, is associated with marked venous congestion. Pericarditis or pleuritis, often with significant effusion, can follow extension of the tumor to the pericardial or pleural spaces. Tumor involvement of the neural structures around the trachea (Pancoast's tumor) can compromise the cervical sympathetic plexus, producing Horner syndrome with symptoms of exophthalmos, ptosis, miosis, and anhidrosis. Lung cancers also produce paraneoplastic syndromes as a consequence of secretion of hormonally active substances. Paraneoplastic syndromes that can be produced include hyponatremia (antidiuretic hormone secretion); Cushing syndrome (adrenocorticotropic hormone [ACTH]); hypercalcemia (parathormone); hypocalcemia (calcitonin); gynecomastia (gonadotropins); carcinoid syndrome (serotonin); myopathy characterized by muscle weakness; a peripheral (usually sensory) neuropathy; acanthosis nigricans and other dermatologic abnormalities; leukemoid reactions and other hematologic abnormalities; and clubbing of the fingers (hypertrophic pulmonary osteoarthropathy).

> **Bronchogenic carcinoma can cause many complications owing to both compression or invasion of mediastinal structures and production of hormonally active substances.**

Bronchial Carcinoid

Bronchial carcinoid is an uncommon tumor composed of nests, cords, and masses of cells of neuroendocrine differentiation (Kulchitsky cells) embedded in a delicate fibrous stroma. These tumors tend to be locally invasive and do not usually metastasize until late in their clinical course, permitting resection to be curative in most cases. Because of their neuroendocrine differentiation, some of the tumors can intermittently secrete serotonin and similar substances, producing carcinoid syndrome with intermittent diarrhea accompanied by flushing and cyanosis. Other clinical manifestations (persistent cough, hemoptysis, pulmonary infections, bronchiectasis, emphysema, atelectasis) are related primarily to carcinoid growth into the bronchus lumen.

> **Bronchial carcinoid is a neuroendocrine tumor.**

Miscellaneous Tumors

The lung contains a variety of connective tissues, and benign and malignant mesenchymal tumors (fibroma, fibrosarcoma, leiomyoma, leiomysarcoma, lipoma, hemangioma, hemangiopericytoma, chondroma) are occasionally encountered. Lymphomas and benign lymphoproliferative disorders can also be seen. While not formally a tumor, the developmental defect known as a **pulmonary hamartoma** can produce a mass that can appear as a "coin lesion" by x-ray; it is composed of varying amounts of hyaline cartilage, respiratory epithelium, fibrous tissue, and blood vessels. Additionally, mediastinal tumors can compress the lungs or invade them by direct extension.

> **Many other tumors also occur occasionally in the lungs.**

Metastatic Tumors

Metastatic tumors affect the lung more often than do primary tumors.

Metastatic tumors, both carcinomas and sarcomas, affect the lung more often than do primary neoplasms. Tumor spread to the lungs can be through blood vessels, through lymphatics, or by direct extension. Metastatic tumor within the lungs tends to occur in several patterns, including scattered, multiple, discrete nodules within the pulmonary parenchyma; metastatic growths confined to the peribronchiolar and perivascular tissue spaces, presumably related to lymphatic spread; and metastatic tumor that is not obvious on gross examination but is found on histologic examination as a diffuse intralymphatic dissemination adjacent to bronchial and vascular channels. Lymphangitis carcinomatosa is an outlining of the subpleural lymphatics by metastatic tumor. The presence of lesions in the lung periphery tends to suggest metastatic tumor to the lung, while tumor predominantly located in more central locations suggests primary bronchogenic carcinoma.

MEDIASTINAL AND PLEURAL DISEASE

Mediastinal Tumors

The mediastinum can contain a large variety of tumors.

A large variety of tumors have been identified in the mediastinum; they are discussed in more detail in the appropriate chapters elsewhere in this book. The superior mediastinum can contain thymoma (see p. 368), teratoma, lymphoma (see p. 91), thyroid and parathyroid lesions (see p. 348), and metastatic tumor. The anterior mediastinum can contain thymoma, teratoma, lymphoma, and thyroid and parathyroid tumors. The posterior mediastinum can contain neurogenic tumors (see pp. 195), lymphoma, and gastroesophageal hernia (see p. 231). The middle mediastinum can contain bronchogenic cysts (see p. 159), pericardial cysts, and lymphoma.

Pleural Tumors

The pleura may be involved by metastatic tumors, benign mesotheliomas, and malignant mesotheliomas.

Metastatic tumor involvement of the pleura (typically from lung, breast, or ovarian carcinomas) is far more common than are primary tumors. **Benign mesotheliomas** (pleural fibromas) are localized growths (occasionally very large) that are often attached by a pedicle to the pleural surface. Benign mesotheliomas are composed of spindle cells resembling fibroblasts that are separated by whorls of dense reticulin and collagen fibers. The risk of developing benign mesotheliomas is not increased by exposure to asbestos. **Malignant mesotheliomas** are rare pleural tumors found most commonly among people with a history of heavy exposures to asbestos 25 to 45 years previously. Malignant mesothelioma is a diffuse lesion that tends to encase the affected lung and thoracic cavity with a thick layer of soft tumor tissue. In the sarcomatoid type of malignant mesothelioma, the cells resemble spindle-shaped mesenchymal stromal cells. In the epithelial type of malignant mesothelioma, the cells are columnar, cuboidal, or flattened and may form tubular or papillary structures that may closely resemble adenocarcinoma. The diagnosis of malignant mesothelioma is favored by positive staining for hyaluronidase-resistant acid mucopolysaccharide and strong staining for keratin proteins. In contrast, staining for carcinoembryonic antigen favors a diagnosis of adenocarcinoma. In the mixed type of malignant mesothelioma, both sarcomatoid and epithelial patterns are observed. Malignant mesothelioma is an aggressive tumor that is only rarely survived longer than 2 years after diagnosis. The tumor tends to invade the lung directly and to metastasize first to hilar lymph nodes and then to the liver and other organs. The tumors often produce recurrent pleural effusions with chest pain and dyspnea. Malignant mesotheliomas can also arise in a variety of other sites, including the peritoneum, pericardium, and genital tract.

Pleuritis

Pleuritis, or inflammation of the pleura, is a cause of accumulation of exudative fluid within the pleural cavity. Pleuritis is conveniently classified by the character of the exudate produced. **Serofibrinous pleuritis** can be caused by inflammatory diseases within the lungs (pneumonia, tuberculosis, lung infarcts, bronchiectasis); systemic disorders (uremia, rheumatoid arthritis, lupus erythematosus, diffuse systemic infections); metastatic tumor; and radiation (radiotherapy of thoracic cancers). Early exudates tend to be serous or serofibrinous and are subsequently either resorbed (if small) or converted to fibrinous exudates, which can subsequently organize with formation of pleural adhesions.

Pleuritis may be serofibrinous, suppurative, or hemorrhagic.

Suppurative pleuritis (empyema) is almost always caused by bacterial or fungal infection that reaches the pleura either by contiguous spread from the lung (rarely, from the abdominal cavity through the diaphragm) or by lymphatic or hematogenous dissemination from a distant source. The fluid that accumulates in the pleural spaces is characteristically a yellow-green pus composed of masses of viable and necrotic neutrophils and other leukocytes. The infecting microorganisms can usually be cultured and can sometimes be visualized on smears of the exudate. Suppurative pleuritis often resolves with formation of tough, fibrous adhesions between the lung and chest wall.

In **hemorrhagic pleuritis,** inflammation produces a sanguinous exudate, which must be distinguished from the slight bleeding caused by a traumatic tap of the fluid. Sanguinous inflammatory exudates are uncommon, and are seen most frequently in neoplastic involvement of the pleural cavity, hemorrhagic diathesis, and rickettsial disease. Accumulations of large (1 liter or more) volumes of any pleural exudate can cause respiratory compromise by compression of the adjacent lung. Respiratory compromise can also be produced if the pleural exudate resolves with formation of heavy, fibrous adhesions, particularly if a thick connective tissue layer surrounding the lungs limits the ability of the lungs to expand.

Pneumothorax and Noninflammatory Pleural Effusions

The pleural space can become filled with substances other than inflammatory exudates. **Pneumothorax** occurs when air or gas is introduced into the pleural space by processes such as rupture of an emphysematous bullae or a puncture wound to the chest wall. Pneumothorax can cause sufficient compression and atelectasis of the adjacent lung to

The pleural space may be filled by air, serous fluid, blood, or lymph.

cause respiratory distress. If the process introducing the air is through a defect that acts as a valve by allowing air into the pleural cavity during inspiration, but does not allow its expulsion during expiration, the air pressure in the pleural space may increase, producing **tension pneumothorax.** Noninflammatory transudations of serous fluid (**hydrothorax**) may complicate cardiac failure, renal failure, hepatic cirrhosis, and other causes of generalized edema. Blood in the pleural cavity (**hemothorax**) can be caused by a ruptured aortic aneurysm. Lymphatic or other milky fluid accumulation (**chylothorax**) may be encountered in lymphatic obstruction by lymphomas and metastatic cancer; in many cases, the chylothorax is confined to the left thoracic cavity.

10
Nervous System

COMMON PATHOPHYSIOLOGIC COMPLICATIONS

Increased Intracranial Pressure

Intracranial pressure can rapidly increase in the fixed volume of the skull as a consequence of processes such as hemorrhage, cerebral abscess, edema, or hydrocephalus. Increased cranial pressure can produce brain herniations. **Subfalcine herniation** is the consequence of expansion of the cingulate gyrus of a cerebral hemisphere under the falx. **Uncinate or transtentorial herniation** is the consequence of expansion of a medial temporal lobe into the space between the tentorium and the cerebral peduncles. Uncinate herniation can compress the oculomotor (3rd) nerve, causing a fixed, dilated pupil. It can also compress the contralateral cerebral peduncle, causing an ipsilateral paralysis. **Coning** is the herniation of cerebellar tonsils into the foramen magnum with a consequent compression of the medulla. This medullary compression can cause death as the medullary respiratory center is compressed. **Upward herniation** of posterior fossa contents can occur when a mass occupies the posterior fossa. Other pathologic changes induced by increased intracranial pressure include flattening of cortical gyri; compression of surface arteries, which may in severe cases cause cortical infarction; and rupture of penetrating arteries (linear Duret hemorrhages) by downward displacement of the midbrain.

> Increased intracranial pressure can cause a variety of brain herniations.

Cerebral Edema

The brain is particularly vulnerable to damage by edema because of the confined space of the cranium and because the brain does not have a lymphatic system to drain excess fluid. **Vasogenic edema** is due to leakage of fluid from capillaries into the interstitial space. **Cytotoxic edema** is due to accumulation of intracellular fluid due primarily to either leakiness of the plasma membrane or impaired cellular metabo-

> Edema within the brain can be classified as vasogenic, cytotoxic, or interstitial.

175

lism that interferes with electrolyte or water homeostasis. **Interstitial edema** can be a consequence of noncommunicating hydrocephalus as cerebral spinal fluid crosses the ependymal lining of the ventricles.

Hydrocephalus

Hydrocephalus can be communicating or noncommunicating.

Marked increase in the volume of cerebral spinal fluid is called hydrocephalus. **Hydrocephalus** is usually the result of blockage of flow of cerebral spinal fluid through the ventricular system and subarachnoid space, although occasionally choroid plexus papillomas can cause hydrocephalus by producing excessive amounts of cerebral spinal fluid. Dilated ventricles are observed in all forms of hydrocephalus. **Noncommunicating hydrocephalus** is due to blockage of cerebral spinal fluid flow within the brain. **Communicating hydrocephalus** is usually due to obstruction of the subarachnoid space or malfunction of resorption of cerebral spinal fluid by the arachnoid villi. Both communicating and noncommunicating hydrocephalus have many causes. Hydrocephalus in infants and young children can cause enlargement of the head because the cranial sutures have not fused. In adults, the head is not enlarged. Hydrocephalus as a result of brain atrophy is called **hydrocephalus vacuo.**

MALFORMATIONS AND DEVELOPMENTAL DISEASES

The brain is vulnerable to many congenital malformations.

Many types of congenital brain malformations involve herniation of meninges or brain through defects in the skull or vertebrae.

The brain is vulnerable to a large variety of congenital malformations. The timing of damage to the brain during development tends to influence strongly the type of malformation, since different areas of the brain are most vulnerable at different gestational ages.

Anencephaly is a complete, or nearly complete, absence of the brain and spinal cord and is the most common congenital malformation of the brain. Defects in skull bones, most often in the occipital bone, can be associated with herniation of the meninges (**cranial meningocele**) or brain (**cranial encephalocele**) through the defect. Varying degrees of vertebral defects (**spina bifida**) can also occur. Spina bifida occulta is a small defect without herniation of the spinal cord or meninges. In a **meningocele,** dura and arachnoid herniate through the vertebral defect. In a meningomyelocele, both spinal cord and meninges herniate. In a **myelocele,** the defect includes skin, vertebrae, and meninges, and herniated spinal cord is exposed to the open air. The more serious of the forms of spina bifida can cause leg paralysis, sensory defects, and incontinence of bladder and stool. Additionally, trauma and infection may complicate the malformations and exacerbate the damage.

Arnold-Chiari malformations involve brain and spinal cord.

Arnold-Chiari malformations are complex abnormalities of the brain and spinal cord in which downward displacement of the vermis and tonsils of the cerebellum into the foramen magnum distorts the adjacent medulla. In **type I** Arnold-Chiari malformations, the cerebellar tonsils lie below the level of the foramen magnum; in **type II** (the most common form), the cerebellar vermis and fourth ventricle extend through the foramen magnum; in **type III,** part of the cerebellum and medulla lie within a cervico-occipital meningomyelocele. Hydrocephalus and a spinal dysraphism are also often present.

The entire brain may be abnormally small (**microcephaly**) or large (**megalencephaly**). The cerebral hemispheres may not form completely (**holoprosencephaly**), or the corpus callosum may be absent or hypoplastic. Neuronal precursors may fail to migrate correctly, producing ectopias and heterotopias. The cerebral gyri may fail to form (**agyria** or **lissencephaly**), form as a few broad gyri (**pachygyria**), or form as large numbers of narrow gyri (**polymicrogyria**). Clefts may form in the brain that are covered by cortex (**schizencephaly**), or that penetrate all layers of the brain so that the ventricles communicate with the subarachnoid space (**encephaloclastic porencephaly**). Hypoxia or ischemic insults that occur after formation of major brain structures can cause loss of most of the cerebral hemispheres (**hydroencephaly**), so that only the meninges and a glial layer remain; can selectively damage the cortex beneath the depths of the sulci (**ulegyria**); can cause white streaks and spots in the corpus striatum (**état marbre** or marbled state) due to focal loss of neurons with glial scarring and preservation of myelinated fibers; or can cause poorly defined areas of coagulative necrosis that characteristically are found in white matter near the angles of the ventricles (**periventricular leukomalacia**). The cerebellum may be absent, hypoplastic, or have an absent or severely hypoplastic vermis accompanied by a distended fourth ventricle (**Dandy-Walker malformation**). The spinal cord may have a tubular, fluid-filled cavity (**syringomyelia**) that may extend into the medulla (**syringobulbia**).

In addition to true malformations, the brain can be affected by slowly progressive, familial, neurocutaneous disorders called **phacomatoses**. The important phacomatoses include neurofibromatosis, von Hippel-Lindau syndrome, Sturge-Weber disease, and tuberous sclerosis. **Neurofibromatosis** is characterized by the presence of tumors (neurofibromas) in the skin and along peripheral nerves. **von Hippel-Lindau syndrome** is the association of angiomatosis of the retina, cerebellar angioma, and angiomas of visceral organs. **Sturge-Weber disease** is a form of neurocutaneous dysplasia characterized by port-wine nevus on the face or scalp, leptomeningeal angiomatosis, and sometimes cutaneous angiomatosis at other sites. **Tuberous sclerosis** is an autosomal disease characterized pathologically by firm, white nodules, up to 2 cm in diameter, that are composed of bizarre neurons and/or astrocytes, which are haphazardly oriented in a background of marked gliosis. The tuber tends to be found in the cortex and subependyma adjacent to (and sometimes projecting into) the ventricles. Clinically, patients have mental retardation and seizures that usually begin in infancy or childhood; other abnormalities can include skin lesions (adenoma sebaceum), pancreatic cysts, renal angiomyolipomas, and cardiac rhabdomyomas. Uncommonly, astrocytomas can arise in a tuber.

Many forms of cerebral cortex malformation also occur.

Phacomatoses are slowly progressive neurocutaneous disorders.

NUTRITIONAL, ENVIRONMENTAL, AND METABOLIC DISORDERS

Nutritional Disorders

Thiamine (see p. 15), nicotinamide (see p. 16), and vitamin B_{12} (cobalamin; see also p. 16) deficiencies can affect the nervous system. **Vitamin B_{12} deficiency** is the most common of these deficiencies; it causes degeneration of the posterior and lateral white columns of the

Deficiencies of thiamine, nicotinamide, and vitamin B₁₂ can affect the nervous system.

Toxic brain injury can be caused by ethyl alcohol, methyl alcohol, chemotherapy, and rapid correction of hyponatremia.

Defective mitochondria in Leigh's disease produce brain necrosis.

Deficiency of arylsulfatase A causes metachromatic leukodystrophy.

Deficiency of galactocerebroside B causes Krabbe's disease.

spinal cord. This degeneration produces spastic paraparesis, sensory ataxia, and lower extremity paresthesias, which may, in severe cases, progress to total paralysis with lower limb anesthesia. Vitamin B₁₂ therapy can correct early signs, but will only arrest disease progression if the axons have degenerated.

Environmental Disorders

Chronic use of **ethyl alcohol** (see p. 9), when coupled with thiamine deficiency, can cause cerebellar degeneration, a peripheral neuropathy, and the Wernicke-Korsakoff syndrome (see p. 9). **Methyl alcohol** (see p. 9) is toxic to the retina and the cerebral hemispheres. Therapeutic cranial **irradiation,** when coupled with some forms of **chemotherapy,** notably methotrexate, can cause foci of coagulative necrosis in periventricular and deep white matter. Demyelination in the central pons **(central pontine myelinolysis)** is observed when severe hyponatremia is corrected too rapidly. Disturbed cerebral function is observed in a variety of sick patients as a consequence of metabolic encephalopathy, which may be due to electrolyte disturbances, hepatic failure, uremia, hypoglycemia, hyperglycemia, hypoxia, or CO_2 narcosis.

Inborn Errors of Metabolism

Many genetic diseases produce central nervous system effects. Discussed here are those conditions not presented elsewhere in this book.

Disturbances of mitochondrial energy metabolism tend to produce combinations of muscle pathology and cerebral disease. **Leigh's disease** (subacute necrotizing encephalomyelopathy) is due, in at least some cases, to the autosomal recessive deficiency of cytochrome C oxidase activity in mitochondria of muscle and brain. Leigh's disease is characterized pathologically by areas of symmetric necrosis affecting the central areas of the central nervous system from the spinal cord to the thalamus. Clinically, patients have multiple symptoms including intellectual deterioration, weakness, ataxia, and seizures. Death usually occurs several years after symptoms appear.

Leukodystrophies are white matter diseases characterized by dysmyelination, probably as a consequence of a biochemical defect in myelin metabolism. **Metachromatic leukodystrophy** is due to the autosomal recessive deficiency of arylsulfatase A (cerebroside sulfatase), which causes accumulation of the sphingolipid galactosyl sulfatide as intra- and extracellular spherical masses that stain metachromatically with acid cresyl violet. These masses tend to be found free in tissue spaces, within perivascular macrophages, in the peripheral nervous system, or in Schwann cells. Widespread demyelination is observed in the cerebral hemispheres and the peripheral nervous system. Metachromic leukodystrophy causes mental deterioration and progressive motor impairment and presents in children aged 1 to 4 years.

Krabbe's disease (globoid cell leukodystrophy) is due to the autosomal recessive deficiency of galactocerebroside B galactosidase, which causes accumulation of galactocerebroside; produces demyelination; and is characterized histologically by the presence of large histiocytes (globoid cells) that contain cytoplasmic inclusions, often with longitudinal striations. Krabbe's disease presents with rigidity and decreased alertness and usually causes death with terminal blindness and deafness by 1 or 2 years of age.

Adrenoleukodystrophy/adrenomyeloneuropathy is an X-linked recessive disease in which long-chain fatty acid esters of cholesterol accumulate and are associated with adrenal insufficiency and nervous system manifestations. The juvenile form (adrenoleukodystrophy) usually affects preadolescent boys and leads to death within several years. It causes large plaques of demyelination, resembling those of multiple sclerosis, which usually involve the cerebral hemisphere. The adult form (adrenomyeloneuropathy) causes spastic paraparesis, peripheral neuropathy, cerebellar ataxia, intellectual deterioration, and hypogonadism. Both forms show characteristic inclusions composed of leaflets within an electron-lucent space that can be found in the adrenal cortex, Schwann cells, and cerebral macrophages.

Accumulation of long-chain fatty acid esters of cholesterol occurs in adrenoleukodystrophy.

MENINGITIS

Infection can reach the central nervous system by several routes, including a **blood-borne route,** either through the arterial system or retrograde through the venous sinuses that anastomose with face veins; or **direct implantation,** usually as a result of either trauma or medical procedures; or **local extension,** often from infected air sinuses; or via the **peripheral nervous system,** as occurs in infection by rabies and herpes viruses. Most central nervous system infections can be classified as either meningitis, in which the meninges are principally involved, or encephalitis, in which the brain parenchyma is principally involved.

Infection can reach the brain by many routes.

Meningitis is an inflammation of the leptomeninges and subarachnoid space. While most meningitis is the result of bacterial, viral, or fungal infection, meningitis can also be caused by drugs or toxins (chemical meningitis) or tumor (carcinomatous meningitis). **Acute pyogenic meningitis** is usually due to bacterial infection and is associated with neutrophil infiltration around leptomeningeal vessels and in the subarachnoid space. In severe cases, the cerebrospinal fluid may become frankly purulent. Common organisms isolated in acute pyogenic meningitis include *Escherichia coli* in neonates; *Haemophilus influenzae* in both infants and children; *Neisseria meningitis* in the second and third decades of life; and *Pneumococcus* in infants, the elderly, and after trauma. Irritating substances (methotrexate) injected into the brain may cause a chemical meningitis that histologically resembles acute pyogenic meningitis due to bacterial infection. **Acute lymphocytic meningitis** is usually the result of viral infection and is characterized by lymphocytic rather than neutrophilic infiltration. Many viruses have been implicated, including mumps, herpes, Epstein-Barr, echovirus, and coxsackievirus. **Chronic meningitis** is classically related to tuberculosis infection, but other indolent meningeal infections (syphilis, brucellosis, and chronic fungal infections) may produce a similar histologic picture characterized by the presence of a chronic inflammatory infiltrate with lymphocytes, plasma cells, macrophages, and fibroblasts. Granulomas and an obliterative endarteritis are also often encountered.

Meningitis may be the result of infections, drugs, or tumor.

Spread of infection from bones or sinuses of the skull sometimes produces a subdural collection of pus known as a **subdural empyema.** The underlying arachnoid mater, subarachnoid space, and brain parenchyma may be compressed, but are usually not otherwise affected. Spread of the infection to the cerebral vein may cause thrombophlebitis, sometimes with brain infarction.

ENCEPHALITIS

A parenchymal infection of the brain is termed encephalitis. Encephalitis can be classified as bacterial, brain abscess, viral, and slow viral.

Bacterial Encephalitides

Tuberculosis and syphilis are important bacterial encephalitides.

Bacterial encephalitides are primary bacterial infections of the brain that do not progress to formation of a brain abscess. The only relatively common bacterial encephalitides are those produced by tuberculosis and syphilis. **Tubercular** involvement of brain parenchyma produces granulomas similar to those seen in other organs (see p. 55). In children, the granulomas are often found in the posterior fossa; in adults, the granulomas are often supratentorial. Tuberculomas remain a common cause of intracranial masses in developing countries. Tuberculosis can also cause chronic meningitis. **Syphilis** (see p. 53) can affect the brain in its tertiary stage. Three clinicohistologic patterns are observed. Chronic meningitis due to syphilis is distinctive because of the prominent obliterative endarteritis with perivascular plasma cells. Paretic neurosyphilis is characterized by widespred parenchymal infection causing brain atrophy secondary to individual neuronal death. Tabes dorsalis is characterized by spirochete infection of the dorsal spinal roots with consequent loss of axons and myelin in the roots and atrophy of the dorsal columns of the spinal cord.

Brain Abscess

Brain abscesses resemble abscesses in other sites.

Brain abscesses resemble abscesses in other organs. The abscess cavity is surrounded by collagen-producing fibroblasts that are probably derived from blood vessels, since glial cells do not produce collagen. Newly formed blood vessels are a prominent component of this layer. Outside the fibrosis is a zone of glial proliferation (gliosis). The surrounding tissue is usually edematous, probably as a consequence of fluid leakage from the sites of neovascularization. Conditions associated with cerebral abscesses include acute bacterial endocarditis, congenital heart disease, and bronchiectasis. Common causative organisms include staphylococci, aerobic and anaerobic streptococci, and *Bacteroides fragilis*.

Viral Encephalitis

Viral brain infections tend to cause glial nodules, neuronophagia, and perivascular infiltrates containing lymphocytes, plasma cells, and macrophages.

Viral encephalitis is usually associated with a primary viral infection or colonization elsewhere in the body. Histologically, viral diseases of the brain tend to have perivascular and parenchymal infiltrates composed of lymphocytes, plasma cells, and macrophages; clusters of microglia (**glial nodules**); and foci of necrotic neurons (**neuronophagia**). With some viral infections, intranuclear inclusion bodies can be seen. Immunohistochemical techniques using antibodies to specific viruses can often be helpful in establishing a diagnosis.

Arboviruses cause epidemic encephalitis.

Arthropod-borne (arbovirus) **encephalitides** are a group of viral panencephalitides that cause outbreaks of epidemic encephalitis (see also p. 31). These encephalitides characteristically produce global neurologic deficits such as seizures or coma. All of these viruses have vertebrate hosts and mosquito or tick vectors. Types include eastern and western equine, Venezuelan, St. Louis, California, Japanese B, Murray Valley, and tickborne.

Herpesviruses that can cause encephalitis include herpes simplex type I, herpes simplex type II, and herpes zoster-varicella viruses (see also pp. 29). **Herpes simplex type II** usually causes herpetic viral meningitis, but can cause a severe, generalized encephalitis, usually in neonates born by vaginal delivery from mothers with primary genital herpes infection. **Herpes simplex type I** can cause a similar severe panencephalitis in neonates, but is more often encountered as a more localized encephalitis in children and young adults. In young adults, the localized form tends to cause necrosis and hemorrhage that most severely involves the temporal and frontal lobes. **Herpes zoster-varicella virus** usually affects adults by involving the peripheral nerves, causing a painful, vesicular skin eruption ("shingles") that characteristically follows a dermatome. Herpes zoster also uncommonly causes hemiparesis due to a predominantly unilateral vasculopathy that tends to follow shingles involving the distribution of the trigeminal (usually ophthalmic division) nerve. In acquired immunodeficiency syndrome (AIDS) patients, herpes zoster can cause a severe, multifocal encephalitis with sharply circumscribed areas of demyelination and necrosis. The antiviral agent **acyclovir** can often modify the severity of herpes central nervous system infections.

Poliomyelitis is now uncommon as a result of widespread immunization. Poliomyelitis infection usually begins with a nonspecific gastroenteritis that progresses in only a small percentage of cases to nervous system involvement. Acutely, poliomyelitis induces perivascular cuffing by lymphocytes, plasma cells, and macrophages, accompanied by death of isolated neurons (neuronophagia) localized to the anterior horn motor neurons of the spinal cord. Long-term survivors of symptomatic poliomyelitis clinically have a flaccid paralysis with muscle wasting. These patients have neuronal loss and gliosis in affected anterior horns and secondary atrophy of motor (anterior) spinal roots and muscles.

Rabies virus usually enters the body through a site from an infected animal, which is usually a dog but may also be a wild mammal. The virus is transmitted along peripheral nerves from the wound to the central nervous system; this period of progression is associated clinically with a several-month asymptomatic period. When symptomatic rabies develops, the patient characteristically has local paresthesias around the wound and nonspecific systemic symptoms including nausea, fever, and headache. Pathologically, inflammation and neuronal degeneration occur predominantly in the brainstem, sometimes with involvement of the spinal cord and dorsal root ganglia. Viral aggregates are visible in some neurons (notably the pyramidal neurons of the hippocampus and the Purkinje cells) as characteristic eosinophilic, round to bullet-shaped, cytoplasmic inclusions known as Negri bodies. As the disease progresses, the patient develops extreme sensitivity to sensory stimuli, and may go into convulsions after minimal stimuli. Death almost always occurs, often as a consequence of respiratory center failure.

Cytomegalovirus is an important cause of central nervous system infection in fetuses and in immunosuppressed patients (see also p. 30). In utero, infection can produce devastating brain destruction with microcephaly. The infection begins in the ependyma of the ventricles

Herpesviruses can produce panencephalitis.

Poliomyelitis causes neurophagia of anterior horn motor neurons.

Rabies usually involves the brainstem.

and then extends to the subependymal parenchyma, which may later calcify. In severely immunosuppressed patients, particularly those with AIDS, infection produces collections of microglia (microglial nodules). In both fetuses and immunosuppressed adults, cells infected with cytomegalovirus may contain both intranuclear and cytoplasmic inclusions.

AIDS virus (human immunodeficiency virus; see also p. 23) can affect the nervous system of infected patients in a variety of ways. An acute **aseptic meningitis** can occur early in the infection. **Subacute encephalitis** tends to occur later and has distinctive pathologic findings characterized by foci containing giant cells, mononuclear cells, and glia. The adjacent neuropil shows vacuolation and pallor. The giant cells may contain viral particles seen on electron microscopy. These foci may be found throughout the brain, with common sites including the cerebral and cerebellar white matter. Clinically, most patients have at least some degree of **AIDS-related dementia.** At autopsy, many AIDS patients are observed to have vacuolar myelopathy, characterized by vacuolization with accumulated macrophages that typically most severely involves the lateral columns of the spinal cord. **Peripheral neuropathy** is also observed in AIDS patients and may involve either demyelination or axonal loss. **Secondary infection** by neurotropic infectious agents (cytomegalovirus, herpesviruses, toxoplasmosis, *Cryptococcus*) and primary central nervous system lymphoma may also contribute to central nervous system pathology in AIDS patients.

Slow Virus Infections

A few viruses, called **"slow viruses,"** cause diseases characterized by very long latent periods followed by slowly evolving diseases.

Subacute sclerosing panencephalitis (Dawson's encephalitis) is caused by **measles virus** infection of the brain that apparently persists in some patients after an attack of measles in the distant past. The reason for the persistence of the virus in brain is not fully understood. The persistence appears to be related to the production by the brain of defective virus particles that lack an M-protein, which is usually a site of antibody binding. Subacute sclerosing panencephalitis is characterized clinically by personality changes followed by involuntary movements and a general neurologic deterioration. Pathologically, the brain shows foci of perivascular and parenchymal mononuclear cell infiltration with neuronal loss and a compensatory gliosis in severely affected areas. Oligodendroglia, neurons, and astrocytes may contain inclusion bodies that by electron microscopy can be shown to contain paramyxovirus nucleocapsid tubules typical of measles virus.

Progressive multifocal leukoencephalopathy is a slow virus encephalopathy caused by **papovaviruses** (types Jc and simian virus 40 [SV40]) that is usually observed in patients with AIDS or other severe immunodeficiencies. The viruses kill oligodendrocytes and consequently produce areas of demyelination that may be either microscopic or involve large areas of the brain. At the edges of the lesions, oligodendrocytes contain nuclear inclusion particles composed of viral particles. Also present are reactive astrocytes, foamy macrophages, and bizarre, sometimes multinucleate, giant astrocytes. The axons in the lesions are preserved. Patients with progressive multifocal leukoencephalopathy experience multiple focal neurologic signs that progress with time.

In addition to the slow viral encephalopathies described above in which the etiologic agent has been identified, several neurologic diseases are suspected of being due to transmissible agents that somewhat resemble slow viruses. Human diseases due to this type of transmissible agent include **kuru** and **Creutzfeldt-Jakob disease;** similar animal diseases include **scrapie** in sheep and **transmissible encephalopathy** in minks. All four of these diseases have long latent periods and may be caused by similar, or possibly the same, agent. The diseases cause spongiform change in gray matter that consists initially of a variable vacuolation of the neuropil, which may progress to severe neuronal loss with reactive astrocytosis. A distinctive feature of the lesions is the absence of inflammatory infiltrate. Amyloid deposits (kuru plaques) may involve the cerebellum.

Kuru and Creutzfeldt-Jakob disease are also suspected of being slow viral diseases.

Creutzfeldt-Jakob disease (subacute spongiform encephalopathy) is a rare cause of rapidly progressive dementia that is usually observed in sporadic form, although rare causes of iatrogenic transmission (corneal transplants, contaminated growth hormone, deeply implanted cortical electrodes) are clearly documented. A pronounced startle myoclonus may be a prominent clinical feature, and death usually occurs in less than 1 year.

Kuru is a progressive neurologic disease with prominent cerebellar ataxia leading to death that has been observed only in a single primitive New Guinea tribe that formerly practiced ritual cannibalism of the raw brains of their relatives. Kuru is historically important because it was the first of these diseases in which transmissibility of the disease was demonstrated.

Fungal and Miscellaneous Infections

Fungal infections of the central nervous system are most commonly encountered in immunosuppressed patients with cancer, lymphoma, or AIDS. Fungal infection of the brain is usually a complication of disseminated fungal infection by *Candida, Mucor* species, *Aspergillus,* or *Cryptococcus.* Many other agents are occasionally encountered, including *Histoplasma, Coccidioides,* and *Blastomyces.* Fungal infection of the brain can occur as chronic meningitis, vasculitis, or parenchymal invasion. Other agents that can infect brain include protozoa (malaria, toxoplasmosis, amebiasis, trypanosomiasis); *Rickettsia* (typhus, Rocky Mountain spotted fever); and parasitic worms (cysticercosis, echinococcosis). In the developing world, malaria, cysticercosis, and tuberculosis are common central nervous system infections. Toxoplasmosis in fetuses is an important cause of severe congenital brain disease; in immunosuppressed adults, it is a treatable cause of progressive encephalitis. In addition to true infections of the nervous system, central nervous system disease may follow systemic infections, possibly as a consequence of autoimmune mechanisms or toxins. Examples include postencephalitic parkinsonism, which appears to be related to prior viral influenza infection; Reye syndrome following influenza or chicken pox; and immune-mediated perivenous encephalitis.

Fungal and parasitic infections of the brain also occur.

CENTRAL NERVOUS SYSTEM TRAUMA

Brain trauma is a major cause, particularly in adolescents and young adults, of persistent neurologic symptoms. **Skull fractures** may cause

Epidural hematomas usually occur as a result of arterial bleeding, while subdural hematomas usually occur as a result of venous bleeding.

Brain parenchymal injuries include concussions, contusions, lacerations, hemorrhages, and diffuse axonal injury.

epidural hematoma or may directly injure the brain with bone fragments. **Epidural hematomas** occur as a result of arterial bleeding, often from the middle meningeal artery into the potential space between the skull and the dura mater. The typical clinical presentation is of a patient who recovers from an initial unconsciousness following trauma, only to become unconscious again minutes to hours later. Epidural hematomas are a surgical emergency that can cause rapid increase in intracranial pressure leading to brain herniation and death.

Subdural hematomas typically result from tear of penetrating veins that cross the skull to connect to the cranial venous sinuses. These sites bleed into the subdural space between the dura and arachnoid mater. The area over the convexities of the cerebral hemispheres is most commonly involved. **Acute subdural hematomas** usually occur after obvious trauma; tend to develop more slowly than epidural hematomas, since the bleeding is from veins; and usually produce slowly developing coma. **Chronic subdural hematomas** occur most often in older people and alcoholics, who may have some degree of brain atrophy that increases the risk that brain movement within the skull may rupture a bridging vein. The patients may not give a history of obvious cranial trauma. Chronic subdural hematomas develop slowly and may become quite large since the brain is able to accommodate the slowly developing mass effect. Symptoms tend to be vague (confusion, inattention) and may not be recognized.

Parenchymal injuries can also follow trauma. **Concussion** is a transient loss of consciousness, possibly due to torsion of the midbrain that disrupts the function of the reticular-activating system. **Contusions** are bruises of brain tissue that may occur at the site of impact (coup lesions); on the opposite side of the skull (contrecoup lesions); or adjacent to bony irregularities such as the orbital ridges or the lesser wing of the sphenoid. **Lacerations** are tears in brain tissue. Healing of both contusions and lacerations is by macrophage clearing of hemorrhagic gray matter to produce a crater that is lined by reactive glial tissue. **Traumatic intracerebral hemorrhages** appear to result from trauma to intraparenchymal vessels and are most commonly observed in the frontal lobes, temporal lobes, and deep structures of the brain. **Diffuse axonal injury** is characterized by widespread rupture of axons with formation of spheroids in a traumatized brain that does not show grossly visible damage. These patients usually become comatose at the time of injury and progress to a persistent vegetative state. Complications of brain trauma include brain edema, infection, hydrocephalus, epilepsy, and delayed intracerebral hemorrhage.

Spinal cord trauma can occur either from penetrating wounds or compression secondary to spine injury. Transient compression of the cord produces transient loss of function ("concussion") followed by complete recovery. Vertebral displacements or fractures may bruise, lacerate, or transect the spinal cord, often resulting in severe, permanent injury such as paralysis. Vascular damage with resulting local ischemia can also occur; edema or hemorrhage often contribute to the damage.

INTRACRANIAL HEMORRHAGE

Nontraumatic intracranial hemorrhage occurs most often in three clinicopathologic situations: intraparenchymal hemorrhage as a consequence of hypertension; subarachnoid hemorrhage as a consequence of rupture of a berry aneurysm; and mixed intraparenchymal and subarachnoid hemorrhage as a consequence of leakage or rupture of an arteriovenous malformation.

Intraparenchymal Hemorrhage

Spontaneous hemorrhage within the brain is usually related to **hypertension,** with less common causes including bleeding associated with tumors such as angiomas; clotting disorders; and amyloid angiopathy. Hypertension apparently causes brain hemorrhages by first inducing formation of tiny intraparenchymal aneurysms **(Charcot-Bouchard aneurysms)** at the branch points of arteries, which may subsequently rupture with continued hypertension. Roughly one-half of hypertensive hemorrhages involve the putamen, with most of the remainder occurring in the lobar white matter, thalamus, pons, and cerebellar cortex. **Mild intraparenchymal hemorrhages,** which are usually diagnosed by computed tomography or magnetic resonance imaging, can cause stroke symptoms. **Larger hemorrhages** are very often fatal as a consequence of hemispheric expansion by blood, which causes a mass effect, often with herniation of brain structures. The ventricles may also be filled with blood if rupture into them has occurred. With many intraparenchymal hemorrhages, most of the blood dissects between adjacent structures with relatively little gross tissue destruction. Microscopically, the parenchyma adjacent to the clot initially shows hemorrhage and later may contain hemosiderin-laden macrophages. Dissection of blood along vessels produces small ring-like hemorrhages **(Virchow-Robin hemorrhages).** With time, a zone of fibrillary astrocytosis forms between the digested clot and the adjacent parenchyma, leaving a slit-like space.

While the initial prognosis for severe intracranial hemorrhage is poor, patients who survive the initial insult have a relatively good prognosis because the dissection of the parenchyma by blood destroys only a relatively small number of neurons compared with those destroyed in an infarction. Recurrent intraparenchymal hemorrhage occurs infrequently. Almost all severe hemorrhages produce a mass effect with intracranial pressure leading to coma and brain herniation. Additionally, supratentorial hemorrhages often cause progressive hemiplegias, and posterior fossa hemorrhages often cause intractable vomiting secondary to brainstem compression, eye movement abnormalities secondary to cranial nerve compression, and cerebellar involvement and ataxia secondary to cerebellar involvement.

Subarachnoid Hemorrhage

Subarachnoid hemorrhage is usually the consequence of rupture of an **aneurysmal vessel.** The blood vessels at the base of the brain associated with the small circle of Willis are particularly vulnerable to aneurysm formation because they have only minimal mechanical support by adjacent tissues. Common aneurysm sites include the anterior cerebral artery; the junctions between a carotid and a posterior communicating artery; and the major bifurcation of the middle cerebral artery. Berry aneurysms develop after birth at congenitally located sites of smooth muscle discontinuity associated with arterial branch points. Sudden increases in blood pressure, due to activities such as weight lift-

Spontaneous intraparenchymal hemorrhage is usually related to hypertension.

Large hemorrhages may cause brain herniation.

Patients who survive the initial period following a severe intracranial hemorrhage have a relatively good prognosis.

Rupture of an aneurysm associated with the circle of Willis can cause subarachnoid hemorrhage.

ing, sex, or difficult defecation, can cause rupture of an aneurysm. Chronic hypertension does not appear to be a risk factor for berry aneurysm formation or rupture. Berry aneurysms are usually isolated findings, but can also be associated with polycystic kidney disease and cerebral arteriovenous malformation. Typically, the berry aneurysm has a thin-walled saccular fundus that may be filled with laminated blood clot and fibrin. When an aneurysm ruptures, the pathologic consequences vary with the direction of the rupture. When the rupture is directed away from the brain parenchyma, subarachnoid hemorrhage is produced. When the rupture is directed toward the brain parenchyma, both subarachnoid and intraparenchymal hemorrhage may be produced, since the high-pressure escaping blood can penetrate the parenchyma, sometimes reaching the ventricles. Rupture of a berry aneurysm typically presents with a sudden severe headache and may cause rapid death in up to one-quarter to one-half of patients on the first bleeding. Patients improve rapidly but commonly rebleed with recurrent risk of rapid death.

Mixed Parenchymal and Subarachnoid Hemorrhage

Vascular malformations tend to cause mixed parenchymal and subarachnoid hemorrhage.

Vascular malformations are the principal source of mixed hemorrhage. **Arteriovenous malformations** are composed of congenitally malformed vessels intermediate between arteries and veins that form complex tangles, usually in either the superficial or deep cerebral hemispheres. Arteriovenous malformations have moderate male predominance, bleed most commonly in adolescence and young adulthood, and usually present clinically with seizures or symptoms of subarachnoid hemorrhages. **Cavernous hemangiomas,** similar to those found elsewhere in the body, occasionally occur in the brain and may cause localized bleeding, which is often asymptomatic. **Capillary hemangiomas,** composed of nets of capillarylike vessels, occur in the brain, but are almost always asymptomatic. Berry aneurysms, as discussed in the preceding section, can also be a source of mixed parenchymal and subarachnoid hemorrhage.

VASCULAR DISEASES OF THE BRAIN

Cerebral anoxia can be produced by a variety of mechanisms.

Cerebrovascular disease accounts for approximately one-half of neurologic problems observed in general hospitals. Despite the brain's relatively small size, it is a major consumer of oxygen and is particularly vulnerable to interruption of aerobic metabolism by a variety of mechanisms. Inadequate oxygen content of inspired air produces **anoxic anoxia. Anemic anoxia** is the result of inadequate oxygen-carrying hemoglobin. Impaired oxygen use by tissues as a consequence of poisons or toxins such as cyanide causes **histotoxic anoxia. Stagnant** (ischemic) **anoxia** is the result of inadequate blood flow. Hypoglycemia, not anoxia, also interrupts aerobic metabolism and produces similar metabolic and pathologic damage. Stagnant (ischemic) anoxia tends to produce more severe damage than the other processes mentioned above, because toxic metabolites rapidly contribute to tissue damage. However, the distinction between types becomes blurred because severe anoxia of any form tends to impair cardiovascular function, leading to hypotension and sometimes cardiac arrest. Ischemic injury is clinically classified as either generalized ischemic (hypoxic) encephalopathy or focal cerebral infarction.

ISCHEMIC ENCEPHALOPATHY

Ischemic (hypoxic) **encephalopathy** occurs when ischemia or hypoxia causes widespread, bilateral damage to the brain. Systemic hypotension is a common cause of ischemic encephalopathy. Neurons are more vulnerable to ischemic damage than are glial cells, and permanent neuronal damage can occur within minutes. Some neurons, notably **Purkinje cells** of the cerebellum and **pyramidal cells** of the hippocampus, are particularly vulnerable to ischemia for reasons that are still unclear but may involve the toxicity of prolonged action by some neurotransmitters (possibly glutamate and aspartate).

Ischemic damage to the brain is usually pathologically observed at autopsy, and histologic damage is observed only if the patient survives over 12 hours. The earliest histologic changes, called ischemic cell change, are eosinophilia of the neuronal cytoplasm, which is accompanied by nuclear shrinkage, producing a small, pyknotic nucleus. Characteristically, the damage in less severe cases tends to be spotty and involve isolated or small clusters of neurons. In the cortex, the **pyramidal cell layers** tend to be most severely affected, and the loss of most of the pyramidal cell layer is called laminar necrosis. With severe ischemia, the junctional zones between major arterial territories may undergo coagulative necrosis producing **border zone** (watershed) **infarcts.** In the cerebral cortex, severe ischemic damage typically produces linear, parasagittal infarctions that form in the border zone between the anterior and medial cerebral arterial systems. Long-term survivors of severe ischemia may have cortical atrophy. Clinically, mild ischemia may produce only confusion with later complete recovery; severe ischemia can produce coma, which may progress to death or persistent vegetative state with loss of most cortical functions.

> Mild ischemic encephalopathy damages small clusters of neurons; more severe ischemia produces border zone infarcts.

Cerebral Infarction

Cerebral infarctions are caused by a failure of adequate quantities of blood to flow through a cerebral artery, usually as a consequence of thrombosis, embolus, or severe atherosclerosis coupled with hypotension. Less common causes include vessel compression during brain herniation and vessel occlusion secondary to tumor or infection. Clinically, infarctions of the brain can produce **strokes,** characterized by acute onset of focal neurologic signs. Strokes can also be caused by intracerebral hemorrhage. Pathologically, cerebral infarctions can be classified as anemic and hemorrhagic infarcts.

Anemic infarcts are first recognizable about 12 hours after the infarction occurs, when the affected brain becomes slightly softened and discolored, and histologically shows slight blurring of the architecture. Later, the tissue undergoes coagulative necrosis and grossly becomes softened and edematous, sometimes causing herniation of adjacent structures. Resolution of the infarction is similar to resolution of infarctions in other organs, with the exception that no fibrosis occurs since the repair is performed by astrocytes, which do not produce collagen, rather

> Cerebral infarctions can be of the anemic or hemorrhagic types.

than fibroblasts. Since no fibrosis occurs, healing of infarcted brain often causes cyst formation as the liquified tissue is removed by macrophages. In more superficial cysts, thickened leptomeninges often form the outer wall of the cyst.

Hemorrhagic infarcts are similar to anemic infarcts but additionally show extensive hemorrhage. Hemorrhagic infarction requires a route of blood to enter the necrotic tissue and is most often observed following venous occlusion or breakup of a cerebral embolus. Since the venous system of the brain has extensive collateralization, venous occlusion is relatively uncommon and tends to be seen either with occlusion of a large venous sinus or when there is widespread thrombosis of small veins. Often in these cases, there is a predisposition for thrombosis, which is caused most frequently by cancer.

Hypertensive Vascular Disease

Hypertension adversely affects the brain in a variety of ways. Hypertensive intracerebral hemorrhage has been discussed in a previous section. Hypertension is a risk factor for atherosclerosis with related atherosclerotic vascular disease and atheroembolic infarcts. **Lacunae** (little lakes) are small necrotic foci that are probably the result of occlusion of arterioles deep in the brain by emboli or hypertensive arteriosclerosis. Common sites for lacunae formation include the basal ganglia, thalamus, internal capsule, pons, and cerebral white matter. Lacunae are typically asymptomatic, but may cause symptoms (such as monoplegia) if they are located in a critical spot such as the internal capsule. **Subcortical leukoencephalopathy** (Binswanger's disease) is a diffuse loss of deep hemispheric white matter, possibly the result of severe arteriolar sclerosis, which produces progressive dementia in some hypertensive patients. Histologically, subcortical leukoencephalopathy is characterized by diffuse, irregular loss of axons and myelin that is accompanied by widespread gliosis. **Hypertensive encephalopathy** is observed in acute, severe hypertension such as can occur in eclampsia, acute nephritis, and malignant hypertension. The typical presentation is of generalized neurologic symptoms (headache, drowsiness, vomiting, convulsions) that may progress to coma. The etiology appears to involve high cerebral blood flow and breakdown of the blood–brain barrier. Pathologically, the brain shows cerebral edema and petechial hemorrhages. Walls of small arteries and arterioles may show fibrinoid necrosis.

Hypertension can cause lacunae formation, subcortical leukoencephalopathy and hypertensive encephalopathy.

Vascular Disease of the Spinal Cord

The spinal cord is supplied by one anterior and two posterior spinal arteries, which receive part of their blood supply from intercostal and lumbar arteries. **Dissecting aortic aneurysms** can interrupt this supply, causing damage that is usually most severe in the anterior horn gray matter of the thoracic cord. Less commonly, the **anterior spinal artery** may be occluded by emboli, thrombosis, or compression by a herniated disc. Trauma, vascular malformations, and tumors may cause spinal cord hemorrhage.

The blood supply of the spinal cord can be compromised by aortic aneurysm or occlusion of the anterior spinal artery.

DEMYELINATING DISEASES

The **demyelinating diseases** include a number of diseases whose etiologies are not yet understood, but that characteristically cause loss of axonal myelin sheaths, either as the result of direct damage to myelin or from damage to the oligodendrocytes that form the myelin. Multiple sclerosis and the perivenous encephalomyelitides are the most clinically important of these diseases.

Multiple Sclerosis

Multiple sclerosis is characterized by the formation of multiple, irregular areas of demyelination **(plaques)**. The plaques may occur anywhere in the central nervous system, with a particular predilection for the tissue at the angles of the cerebral ventricles. Each plaque has a natural history that begins with perivenous demyelination. The demyelination progresses to form microscopically visible plaques characterized by a central loss of oligodendroglia accompanied by a reactive astrocytosis with a peripheral border containing a predominantly lymphocytic infiltrate. In old plaques, oligodendroglia and myelin are nearly absent; some axons are usually lost; and a few fibrillary astrocytes may be present.

Multiple sclerosis is characterized by the formation of demyelinating plaques in the central nervous system.

Characteristically, multiple sclerosis is observed in young adults who develop a varied pattern of relapsing and remitting neurologic symptoms (paresthesias, retrobulbar neuritis, mild sensory or motor symptoms, incoordination). Some patients experience only brief episodes of neurologic symptoms, while others develop progressive symptoms that can eventually produce paralysis, incontinence, and mental dysfunction. Adrenocorticotropic hormone (ACTH) and other immunosuppressive agents can sometimes produce remissions, but no definitive therapy for multiple sclerosis has been found. The classic form of multiple sclerosis, described above, is also known as **Charcot type** multiple sclerosis. Variants include the acutely progressive **Marburg type; Devic's disease** (neuromyelitis optica) with demyelination of optic nerves and spinal cord lesions in addition to typical multiple sclerosis plaques; and one form of **Schilder's disease** (diffuse sclerosis) characterized by giant multiple sclerosis plaques. A second form of Schilder's disease is actually the quite different syndrome adrenoleukodystrophy (see p. 179).

Perivenous Encephalomyelitis

Perivenous and perivenular demyelination is observed in two rapidly progressive illnesses that can follow viral infections or vaccinations: acute disseminated encephalomyelitis and acute necrotizing hemorrhagic leukoencephalitis. Both of these conditions are thought to be the result of allergic reactions to the central nervous system.

Demyelination adjacent to veins and venules can be observed in acute and disseminated encephalomyelitis and acute necrotizing hemorrhagic leukoencephalitis.

In **acute disseminated encephalomyelitis** (postinfectious and postvaccinial encephalitis), demyelination, accompanied initially by neutrophilic and later by lymphocytic infiltration, is observed adjacent to veins and venules in many central nervous system foci. Clinically, headache and lethargy progressing to coma develop 1 to 2 weeks after virus infection, whooping cough, or vaccination. Up to one-fifth of patients may die, usually as a result of brain swelling, but survivors may have only mild residual disease.

In **acute necrotizing hemorrhagic leukoencephalitis,** the central nervous system develops multiple foci of perivenular demyelination with a prominent, initially neutrophilic and later lymphocytic and plasmacytic infiltration, acute necrosis of small blood vessels, and hemorrhage. Clinically, patients develop headache, fever, coma, and usually death following a nonspecific respiratory infection.

DEGENERATIVE DISEASES

The degenerative neurologic diseases are a group of central nervous system disorders characterized by a selective loss of neurons. The etiology of these disorders is typically unknown, and may be varied. Once an etiology is proved, a particular degenerative disease tends to be moved to an etiology-based category.

Spinocerebellar Degeneration

The spinocerebellar degenerations are characterized by neuronal atrophy in many sites.

The **spinocerebellar degenerations** are a group of diseases in which neurons atrophy and degenerate in varying degrees in many brain sites, including basal ganglion, brainstem, cerebellum, spinal cord, and peripheral nerves. Patients tend to have complex symptoms including parkinsonism symptoms, ataxia, spasticity, and peripheral motor and sensory deficits. These symptoms may change with time. A recessive or dominant genetic component is sometimes present. While the spinocerebellar degenerations have sometimes been extensively subclassified, many neurologists now simply classify then as dominant, recessive, or sporadic ataxia. Two types of spinocerebellar degenerations that are commonly still discussed as separate categories include Friedreich's ataxia and olivopontocerebellar atrophy.

Friedreich's ataxia and olivopontocerebellar atrophy are spinocerebellar degenerations with distinctive clinical patterns.

Friedreich's ataxia is usually an autosomal recessive condition that manifests initially as a gait ataxia in early adolescence and progresses to paralysis in about 20 years. Patients with Friedreich's ataxia often also have diabetes, cardiac arrhythmias, or congestive heart failure. **Olivopontocerebellar atrophy** ("heterogeneous system degeneration") has variable genetics; is associated with neuronal loss that usually most markedly affects the olive, pons, and cerebellum; and causes a variable pattern of symptoms that usually include ataxia, eye and body movement abnormalities, and rigidity.

Degenerative Diseases Primarily Affecting Cerebral Cortex

Alzheimer's disease is a form of cortical atrophy characterized histologically by neurofibrillary tangles, senile plaques, granulovacuolar degeneration, and amyloid angiopathy.

Alzheimer's disease causes a variable degree of cortical atrophy with widening of cerebral sulci and compensatory ventricular enlargement. Microscopic features characteristic of Alzheimer's disease, but that are present to a lesser degree in older people who are not demented, include bundles of cytoplasmic filaments that can displace the neuron nucleus (**neurofibrillary tangles**) and may persist after the death of the neuron; amyloid deposition within intracortical and small subarachnoid arteries (**amyloid angiopathy**); formation of cytoplasmic vacuoles containing granules that stain with silver stains (**granulovacuolar degeneration**) with neurons; glassy eosinophilic inclusions in proximal dendrites (**Hirano bodies**); and focal collections of silver-staining neuritic processes surrounded by microglial cells and reactive astrocytes (senile or neuritic plaques).

Neurofibrillary tangles and senile plaques can be found throughout the cerebral cortex and particularly in the hippocampus and amygdala. Granulovacular degeneration and Hirano bodies are usually most prominent in the pyramidal cells of the hippocampus. The basic etiology of Alzheimer's disease is unknown and is a subject of active research. Clinically, patients who are usually at least 50 years of age initially experience a subtle impairment of affect or higher intellectual functions. Over the subsequent 5 to 10 years, the neurologic symptoms can progress to the point that the patient is severely demented, mute, and immobile; death is often the result of infection, to which the patient may be predisposed by dehydration and malnutrition. While most cases of Alzheimer's disease are observed in older people without obvious predisposing conditions, some cases appear to be familial, and apparently identical pathologic changes are observed in patients with Down syndrome (trisomy 21) who survive more than 45 years.

Pick's disease clinically resembles the more common Alzheimer's disease, from which it cannot always be reliably distinguished before death. Pick's disease causes a pronounced brain atrophy (**"walnut brain"**) that usually most severely involves the frontal and temporal lobes with characteristic sparing of the posterior two-thirds of the superior temporal gyrus. Microscopically, severe neuronal loss tends to involve the outer three layers of the cortex, and some surviving neurons may show ballooning degeneration (**Pick's cells**) or contain silver-stain cytoplasmic filamentous inclusions (**Pick's bodies**) that are immunocytochemically similar to those observed in Alzheimer's patients.

Pick's disease differs from Alzheimer's disease by a preferential atrophy of the frontal and temporal lobes and the histologic presence of balloon degeneration of neurons.

Degenerative Diseases of Basal Ganglia and Brainstem

The basal ganglia and brainstem contain portions of the extrapyramidal motor system, and diseases involving these brain regions consequently frequently cause movement disorders.

Huntington's disease is an autosomal dominant disease (chromosome 4) characterized clinically by a progressive dementia accompanied by choreiform movements. The disease typically does not become clinically evident until midlife, after the gene may have been passed to the patient's children. The etiologic biochemical defect is still being investigated; the nervous system metabolism of many neurotransmitters appears to be altered in Huntington's disease. Pathologically, the brains of patients dying of the disease (about 15 years after symptoms develop) show marked atrophy of the caudate nucleus with somewhat less atrophy of the putamen, globus pallidus, and cerebral cortex. Microscopically, affected areas show a severe loss of neurons that is more pronounced among smaller neurons and is accompanied by a reactive fibrillary gliosis.

Autosomal dominant Huntington's disease causes marked atrophy of the caudate nucleus characterized histologically by neuronal loss and reactive fibrillary gliosis.

Parkinsonism (Parkinson's disease) is a heterogeneous group of diseases characterized pathologically by damage to the **nigrostriatal dopaminergic system** and clinically by the cluster of stooped posture, slow voluntary movements, expressionless facies, and rigidity. A characteristic "pill-rolling" tremor is often present, as is a distinctive festinating gait characterized by progressively shortened, accelerated steps.

Parkinsonism is a heterogeneous group of diseases in which damage to the nigrostriatal dopaminergic system causes tremor and slowed voluntary movements.

Idiopathic Parkinson's disease (paralysis agitans) is the prototype and is the most common of these diseases. Idiopathic Parkinson's disease is observed in older age groups and is characterized histologically by a loss of the pigmented neurons of the substantia nigra and locus coeruleus. Intracytoplasmic eosinophilic inclusions **(Lewy bodies),** often with a dense core surrounded by a paler rim, may be present in some remaining neurons in the cholinergic cells of the basal nucleus of Meynert, and occasionally, in large numbers in the cerebral cortex. In the early stages, idiopathic Parkinson's disease can be ameliorated by replacement therapy with levodopa, which is the immediate precursor of dopamine; as the disease progresses, drug therapy tends to become less effective. Parkinson's disease also occurs in a **postencephalitic** form that is presently rare but was common following encephalitis during the great "influenza" epidemic of 1914 to 1918.

Striatonigral degeneration clinically resembles idiopathic Parkinson's disease but does not respond to levodopa therapy. Pathologic changes include loss of predominantly small neurons with reactive gliosis that causes grossly visible atrophy of the caudate and putamen; loss of pigmented neurons also occurs in the zona compacta of the substantia nigra. **Shy-Drager syndrome** is characterized by parkinsonism plus autonomic nervous system failure, and pathologic changes similar to those of idiopathic Parkinson's disease are accompanied by loss of sympathetic neurons from the interomediolateral column of the spinal cord. **Progressive supranuclear palsy** is characterized by widespread neuronal loss that is most marked in the globus pallidus, subthalamic nucleus, periaqueductal gray matter, substantia nigra, and dentate nucleus. Symptoms related to eye movement difficulties are often the initial complaint. An acute parkinsonism syndrome has also been observed in young patients who were exposed to the contaminant MPTP in illicit meperidine analogs.

Degenerative Disease Affecting Motor Neurons

Lower motor neuron loss causes muscle atrophy, while upper motor neuron loss causes spasticity.

The pyramidal motor system includes upper motor neurons in the motor cortex; lower motor neurons in cranial nerve nuclei and the anterior horns of the spinal cord; and the axons of the upper motor neurons that traverse the internal capsule, brainstem, and corticospinal tract. Symptoms associated with loss of lower motor neurons include weakness, muscular atrophy, and muscle fasiculations. Symptoms associated with loss of upper motor neurons include hyper-reflexia, spasticity, and a Babinski reflex. Several variants of motor neuron disease can occur, all of which can cause paralysis.

Different diseases have different patterns of neuron degeneration.

In the most common of these diseases, **amyotrophic lateral sclerosis,** both upper and lower motor neurons degenerate. In **progressive bulbar palsy,** the cranial nerves and brainstem are selectively affected. In **progressive muscular atrophy,** lower motor neurons selectively degenerate. In **primary lateral sclerosis,** upper motor neurons are selectively affected. Degeneration of upper motor neurons leads to loss of their axons and a consequent atrophy and pallor of the corticospinal tracts. Degeneration of lower motor neurons leads to loss of their predominantly myelinated axons with gray discoloration and atrophy of the motor (anterior) roots of the spinal cord. The etiology of these degenerative diseases is still unknown. Clinically, patients usually present in late middle age with progressive weakness and then paralysis, which eventually causes death; patients with progressive bulbar palsy usually have a more rapid course because of early involvement of respiratory and pharyngeal muscles.

Werdnig-Hoffman disease (infantile progressive spinal muscular atrophy) is an autosomal recessive disease that causes severe lower motor neuron atrophy that begins in infancy. Affected infants are "floppy" from birth or shortly thereafter and develop progressive muscular weakness that leads to death, typically from either pneumonia or respiratory failure, within a few months.

> **Motor neuron disease in infancy presents as a "floppy" infant.**

CENTRAL NERVOUS SYSTEM TUMORS

Both primary intracranial tumors and metastatic tumors can involve the central nervous system. Tumors of glial origin include astrocytoma, glioblastoma multiforme, oligodendroglioma, ependymoma, and choroid plexus papilloma. Tumors of neuronal origin include neuroblastoma, ganglioneuroma, and ganglioglioma. Other tumors of the nervous system include medulloblastoma, meningioma, lymphoma, leukemia, and metastatic tumor.

Astrocytoma and Glioblastoma Multiforme

Astrocytoma and glioblastoma multiforme are the most common adult primary brain tumors. These tumors are graded by degree of anaplasia and prognosis; astrocytic tumors tend to become more anaplastic with time. **Astrocytomas** are the least anaplastic of this group and form poorly defined, infiltrative masses within the brain. They are composed of uniform populations of cells that may resemble protoplasmic, fibrillary, or gemistocytic astrocytes. The background between the cells is usually composed of packed fibrillary astrocytic processes. Pilocytic astrocytomas are a subtype composed of bipolar cells with long cell processes (pilocytic astrocytes). Pilocytic astrocytomas occur most often in the cerebellum of children and young adults and have a better prognosis than do other astrocytomas. **Anaplastic astrocytomas** grossly resemble other astrocytomas, but histologically show more pleomorphism, nuclear hyperchromatism, and mitoses. A characteristic feature that is often seen is hyperplasia of capillary endothelial cells.

Glioblastoma multiforme is the most aggressive of the tumors of the astrocyte line. Glioblastoma is characterized grossly by a variegated (multiforme) appearance with areas of necrosis, hemorrhage, and cyst formation. Glioblastoma is histologically similar to anaplastic astrocytomas, but contains areas of necrosis, which may be surrounded by pseudopalisading. Endothelial proliferation is often prominent. The clinical presentation of astrocytic tumors depends predominantly on their size and location. In adults, astrocytic tumors most often occur in the cerebral hemispheres and less often in the spinal cord. Astrocytomas often remain static or progress slowly for years, but then the patient

> **Astrocytoma and glioblastoma multiforme are both tumors in the astrocyte line.**

may rapidly deteriorate as the tumor becomes anaplastic. The prognosis for glioblastoma is dismal, even with aggressive palliative resection, radiotherapy, and steroids. **Brainstem gliomas** are a major cause of childhood primary brain tumors; roughly one-half of brainstem gliomas are glioblastomas.

Oligodendroglioma

Oligodendrogliomas tend to form well-circumscribed gelatinous masses.

Oligodendrogliomas are less common than astrocytomas, tend to occur in middle age in both sexes, and are usually found in the cerebral hemispheres. Oligodendrogliomas tend to form well-circumscribed, gelatinous masses that may contain calcification, cysts, or hemorrhage. Oligodendrogliomas are composed of clusters of tumor cells with round nuclei and cleared cytoplasm (**"fried egg" cells**) that are usually separated by anastomosing capillaries. Calcification, present in most cases, is a helpful diagnostic feature, both radiologically and histologically. The more anaplastic tumors may contain areas of astrocyte differentiation and may be difficult to identify as oligodendrogliomas. The prognosis for treated oligodendrogliomas is better than that for astrocytomas, with an average survival of 5 years.

Ependymoma

Ependymomas are typically found in the fourth ventricle in children and in the spinal cord in adults.

The ependyma lines the ventricles and central canal of the spinal cord; **ependymomas** are derived from these relatively few cells. Ependymomas are most frequently found in children in the fourth ventricle and in adults in the spinal cord. The cells in ependymomas usually have round to elongated nuclei, and their processes form a dense fibrillary background between the nuclei. The tumor cells may form structures resembling ependymal canals, and may also produce characteristic ependymal pseudorosettes, in which a blood vessel is surrounded by tumor cell nuclei that are slightly separated from the vessel by dense fibrillary processes. About one-half of ependymomas produce glial fibrillary acidic protein, which can be stained with immunohistochemical techniques. Staining by phosphotungstic acid–hematoxylin (PTAH) sometimes shows pathognomic ciliary basal bodies (**blepharoblasts).**

Ependymomas involving the fourth ventricle (**posterior fossa ependymomas)** tend to have a poor long-term prognosis because they cannot be adequately excised without endangering vital pontine and medullary nuclei. The prognosis of the spinal cord tumors is much better. A subtype of the **spinal cord ependymomas,** myxopapillary ependymoma, can involve the filum terminale and differs histologically from ependymomas in other locations by the inclusion of myxoid or papillary elements in addition to typical ependymomal cells. **Myxopapillary ependymomas** are usually histologically benign, but adequate excision may be difficult if the tumor involves the nerve roots of the cauda equina. Another subtype of ependymoma, **subependymomas,** typically produces slow growing, solid (sometimes calcified) nodules composed of clumps of nuclei in a dense fibrillary background. Subependymomas are typically found at autopsy but occasionally cause hydrocephalus.

Choroid Plexus Papilloma

Tissue that strongly resembles normal choroid plexus can form markedly papillary growths, known as **choroid plexus papillomas,** that are found most often in the lateral ventricles in children and in the fourth ventricle in adults. The vast majority of these tumors are benign but may cause hydrocephalus; very rare malignant choroid plexus tumors histologically resemble metastatic adenocarcinoma.

Choroid plexus papillomas are usually found in ventricles.

Tumors of Neuronal Origin

Tumors of neuronal origin rarely affect the central nervous system and usually appear in children or young adults. **Neuroblastomas** similar to peripheral neuroblastomas (see p. 126) are observed most frequently in the cerebral hemispheres in children. Histologically, they contain small, undifferentiated cells that often form rosettes. **Ganglioneuromas** (gangliocytomas) and **gangliogliomas** (see also p. 126) are tumors that contain cells resembling mature neurons admixed with an either benign (ganglioneuroma) or malignant (ganglioglioma) glial stroma. These tumors tend to grow slowly unless the glial component becomes anaplastic. They are found most frequently in the floor of the third ventricle, the hypothalamus, and the temporal lobe, where they usually form well-circumscribed masses.

Neuroblastomas and ganglioneuromas are both tumors of neuronal origin.

Tumors of Primitive or Undifferentiated Cells

Medulloblastoma is the important example of a tumor of undifferentiated cells. Medulloblastomas are an important cause of primary brain tumor in children, in whom the tumors tend to occur in the cerebellum, where they form gray-white masses. The tumors are more common in the cerebral hemispheres in adults. Medulloblastomas are composed of sheets of densely packed, small nuclei with little cytoplasm. These cells have the capacity for both glial and neuronal differentiation, as demonstrated by the occasional presence of spindle cells containing glial fibrillary acid protein and of Homer-Wright rosettes showing neuronal differentiation. Cerebral dysfunction and hydrocephalus are common presenting complaints. About one-half of patients treated with both surgery and radiation survive for 10 years.

Medulloblastoma is derived from primitive cells.

Tumors of Meninges

Primary tumors involving the meninges (**meningiomas**) usually arise from arachnoid cap cells and a common primary intracranial tumor. Meningiomas tend to form slowly growing masses that are well tolerated and may become quite large before they cause obvious symptoms. The masses are typically located in the meninges around the front half of the head. Uncommonly, meningiomas are found in other clinically important sites, including adjacent to the brainstem or spinal cord, and within the ventricular system. Multiple meningiomas are occasionally observed, particularly when associated with **von Recklinghausen's neurofibromatosis.** Meningiomas usually form bosselated, solid masses with a gritty texture that are attached to the dura and compress without invading the adjacent brain.

Several histologic patterns are observed in benign meningiomas. **Syncytial meningiomas** are composed of cells with indistinct cell borders that grow in whorls and nodules. **Fibroblastic meningiomas** have cells resembling fibroblasts that grow in bands. **Transitional**

Meningiomas often form well-circumscribed masses that compress the adjacent brain without infiltrating it.

meningiomas resemble both syncytial and fibroblastic meningiomas and may contain psammoma bodies. Uncommonly, meningiomas are **malignant,** with well-differentiated tumors resembling their benign counterparts except for a higher mitotic rate as well as poorly differentiated tumors resembling fibrosarcomas. **Malignant meningiomas** do not usually metastasize, but do tend to invade the adjacent brain. **Hemangiopericytomas,** while not technically meningiomas, can involve the meninges, where they produce masses that grossly resemble meningiomas but are more apt to recur and to become increasingly anaplastic with time than are meningiomas.

Lymphomas and Leukemias

Both primary and secondary lymphomas can involve the central nervous system.

Secondary (systemic) **lymphomas** can involve the meninges, or, less commonly, the brain parenchyma. **Primary lymphomas** can also arise in the brain, and are becoming increasingly frequent because as many as 5 percent of AIDS patients eventually develop a primary brain lymphoma. Histologically, the lymphomas resemble non-Hodgkin's lymphoma found throughout the body. These primary lymphomas tend to arise near the ventricles, sometimes multifocally, and may be either nodular or so diffusely infiltrative that it may be difficult to delineate the tumor borders. Microscopically, the lymphoma cells are often found in blood vessel walls and the parenchyma adjacent to the vessels. Central nervous system lymphomas tend to respond initially to steroid or radiation therapy but have a poor prognosis because of subsequent tumor recurrence. **Leukemias** can also involve the central nervous system, usually in the meninges, where a leukemia-associated bleeding diathesis may cause life-threatening intracerebral hemorrhages.

Other Intracranial Tumors

Metastatic tumors are relatively common in the brain.

Roughly one-quarter of intracranial tumors are due to metastasis. **Metastatic tumors** frequently encountered include lung carcinoma, breast carcinoma, melanoma, renal cell carcinoma, and gastrointestinal carcinomas. **Colloid cysts** are fibrous capsules up to about 4 cm in diameter that are filled with jelly-like material; they are most often encountered in the third ventricle of young adults, where they can obstruct cerebrospinal fluid circulation, causing a dangerous intermittent hydrocephalus.

PERIPHERAL NERVOUS SYSTEM

Degenerative Processes

Peripheral nerves can undergo wallerian degeneration, segmented demyelination, axon degeneration, and regeneration.

Peripheral nerves undergo a relatively small number of degenerative processes. Following transection, an axon undergoes **wallerian degeneration,** characterized by disintegration of both the axon and myelin sheath distal to the transection. If the transection is close to the cell body, the neuron will undergo chromatolysis; more distant transections cause a proximal degeneration back to the nearest node of Ranvier. **Segmental demyelination** is characterized by demyelination between nodes of Ranvier with preservation of the axon. If at least some

Schwann cells survive, myelin can be reconstituted by the remaining Schwann cells. The new myelin can be recognized microscopically because it has characteristically thinner sheaths and shorter internodal lengths. Repeated demyelination and remyelination can produce "onion bulbs" of concentrically arranged Schwann cell processes. **Axonal degeneration** occurs as the axon degenerates from its periphery as a consequence of damage to the neuron cell body (which may show chromatolysis); such damage limits the neuron's ability to maintain the axon.

Regeneration of axons can be observed in favorable cases following both wallerian degeneration and axonal degeneration. The regeneration occurs by the formation of several nerve sprouts, which can subsequently grow about 1 mm/day down the nerve trunk. If the nerve is interrupted by clot or fibrosis, the regenerating sprouts may form a painful **traumatic** (amputation) **neuroma.**

Peripheral Neuropathies

Peripheral neuropathies can be caused either by diffuse demyelination or diffuse axonal degeneration. The longest axons in the limbs tend to be most vulnerable and to cause symptoms first. Patients typically experience symmetrical limb weakness, paresthesias, and a distal ("glove and stocking") sensory loss. Impotence, constipation, or postural hypotension may be present if autonomic nerves are involved. In general, peripheral neuropathies due to axonal degeneration can be clinically distinguished from those due to demyelination by the presence in the former of muscle fasciculation and wasting.

Diseases that tend to produce an **acute demyelinating neuropathy** characterized by an acute, ascending motor paralysis, with or without sensory disturbance, include acute idiopathic polyneuritis (Landry-Guillain-Barré syndrome); infectious mononucleosis with polyneuritis; hepatitis with polyneuritis; diphtheria; and some toxic agents (triorthocresyl phosphate). Diseases that tend to cause a **symmetric, subacute sensimotor polyneuropathy** are usually due to axonal neuropathy caused by toxins (alcohol, arsenic, lead, vinca alkaloids) or vitamin deficiency (beriberi). **Asymmetric subacute sensorimotor polyneuropathy** tends to be caused by axonal neuropathy that may be focal or diffuse and is associated with some systemic diseases, including diabetes, polyarteritis nodosa, and sarcoidosis. **Acquired chronic sensimotor polyneuropathy** is usually also due to axonal neuropathy that may be focal or diffuse and can be caused by a variety of systemic conditions including cancer, uremia, diabetes, amyloidosis, leprosy, and connective tissue diseases.

Inherited forms of chronic sensimotor polyneuropathy are often associated with chronic demyelination and can be due to peroneal muscular atrophy (Charcot-Marie-Tooth disease), hypertrophic polyneuropathy (Dejerine-Sottas syndrome), or Refsum's disease. **Chronic relapsing polyneuropathy** can be idiopathic or caused by beriberi or by porphyria. **Mononeuropathy and multiple neuropathies** can be caused by trauma, serum neuritis, herpes zoster, tumor invasion, or leprosy. While this list of possible causes of neuropathies is very long, **diabetes** and **alcoholism** are the most commonly encountered neuropathies, both of which cause nonspecific, predominantly axonal neuropathies.

Peripheral neuropathies can be caused by either diffuse demyelination or diffuse axonal degeneration.

Diabetes and alcoholism are the most common of the very many causes of neuropathies.

Acute idiopathic polyneuritis appears to be an autoimmune disease that causes a progressive neuropathy characterized histologically by endoneural lymphocytic infiltration.

Acute idiopathic polyneuritis (Landry-Guillain-Barré syndrome) appears to be an autoimmune disease that can be either idiopathic or triggered by viral or other infections (cytomegalovirus, Epstein-Barr virus, mycoplasma), allergies, surgery, or other antecedent conditions. Acute idiopathic polyneuritis is characterized pathologically by lymphocytic infiltration of the endoneurium of peripheral nerves, particularly in the proximal nerve trunks; widespread focal demyelination that begins with splitting of myelin lamellae; and phagocytosis of damaged myelin by macrophages. Clinically, patients experience a rapidly progressive neuropathy that involves the motor system (causing weakness) more than the sensory system. Cerebrospinal fluid albumin levels are often significantly increased. Acute idiopathic polyneuritis can progress to a potentially fatal respiratory paralysis.

Peroneal muscular atrophy characteristically first involves the lower legs.

Peroneal muscular atrophy (hypertrophic type of Charcot-Marie-Tooth disease, type I hereditary sensory motor neuropathy) is an autosomal dominant neuropathy in which repeated episodes of demyelination followed by remyelination cause the formation of "onion bulb" hypertrophy of myelin around peripheral nerve axons. Peroneal muscular atrophy manifests with lower leg and foot wasting that causes the leg to resemble an "inverted champagne bottle." Other forms of hypertrophic neuropathy include Dejerine-Sottas syndrome, which affects young children, and Retsum's disease, which is due to impaired metabolism of phytanic acid.

PERIPHERAL NERVE TUMORS

Neurilemmomas are typically solitary tumors on proximal nerves or spinal nerve roots; neurofibromas are often multiple and tend to involve the nerve more intimately.

Neurilemmomas (schwannomas) and neurofibromas are both tumors derived from Schwann cells that may represent extremes of a common pathologic process, but that tend to have distinct clinical and histologic features. **Neurilemmomas** usually occur as solitary tumors that are found most commonly on proximal nerves or spinal nerve roots. The neurilemmomas tend to be well circumscribed and located eccentrically on the nerves. Neurilemmomas are composed of two distinct histologic patterns. **Antoni A areas** contain a high density of cells that may contain Verocay bodies composed of foci of palisading nuclei. **Antoni B areas** have much lower cellularity.

In contrast, **neurofibromas** are often multiple; may occur in large numbers as part of the familial disorder neurofibromatosis (von Recklinghausen's disease); and tend to be intimately interspersed with the nerve on which they arise rather than at the edge of the nerve. Histologically, tumor spindle cells form a loose pattern of interlacing bands in which are embedded scattered nerve fibers. Malignant transformation of neurofibromas, particularly in neurofibromatosis, is more common than in neurilemmomas. Both neurofibromas and neurolemmomas stain immunocytochemically for S100 protein. Surgical removal of neurolemmomas is easier than surgical removal of neurofibromas, in which the nerve cannot be separated from the tumor. Acoustic neurolemmomas can cause deafness and tinnitus. Large acoustic neuromas may also cause hydrocephalus or cmpress the brainstem or cranial nerves V and VII. Neurilemmomas involving peripheral nerve roots tend to compress the spinal cord or cause cauda equina syndrome. In contrast, neurofibromas usually involve more distal areas of peripheral nerves and cause subcutaneous "lumps and bumps."

11

Cardiovascular System

BLOOD VESSELS

CONGENITAL DISEASES OF ARTERIES

The complicated vascular system is vulnerable to many developmental aberrations including anomalous branching and duplications of vessels. These aberrations are discussed with the organs supplied. **Arteriovenous fistulas** are abnormal communications between arteries and veins that may have a diverse etiology, including anomalous development, penetrating injuries, and necrosis through adjacent arteries and veins. Large arteriovenous fistulas provide sufficient low-resistance blood flow to predispose for cardiac failure.

ARTERIOSCLEROSIS

Arteriosclerosis refers to a group of diseases that includes atherosclerosis, Mönckeberg's arteriosclerosis, and arterioloscerlosis. These disorders have differing etiologies but may coexist in a patient. Atherosclerosis, the most prevalent of these diseases, will be discussed separately in the next section.

Mönckeberg's Arteriosclerosis

Mönckeberg's arteriosclerosis (**medial calcific sclerosis**) is a disease of medium-sized to small muscular arteries characterized by ringlike calcifications of the vessel media. The calcifications are not accompanied by inflammation, but may form bone and even marrow. The disease occurs in older individuals. The arteries most commonly affected include those of the extremities (femoral, tibial, radial, and ulnar) and the male and female genital tracts. Mönckeberg's arteriosclerosis can be a cause of cal-

199

cifications visible by radiography, but is usually of no other clinical significance as the vessel lumina are not markedly narrowed.

Arteriolosclerosis

Arteriolosclerosis includes two lesions of small arteries and arterioles that are encountered in hypertensive patients. **Hyaline arteriolosclerosis** is a microangiopathy characterized by thickening and partial replacement of arteriole walls by homogenous, pink, hyaline material. The hyaline material is thought to be the result of the combination of leakage into the vessel wall of plasma components and increased deposition of extracellular matrix. Hyaline arteriolosclerosis is seen in elderly patients; the more severe and generalized lesions are seen in patients with hypertension, diabetes, or both conditions. The changes tend to be particularly pronounced in the kidneys, where the arteriolar narrowing causes benign nephrosclerosis, characterized by symmetric contraction of the kidneys as a consequence of diffuse renal ischemia.

Hyperplastic arteriolosclerosis is an arteriolar disease characterized by significant luminal narrowing as a result of concentric, laminated thickening ("onion skin") of arteriolar walls by proliferation of smooth muscle cells. The vessel walls may additionally show necrotizing arteriolitis, caused by acute necrosis with deposition of fibrin. Hyperplastic arteriolosclerosis is associated with severe (malignant) hypertension and can affect arterioles throughout the body, particularly in the kidneys, intestine, and gallbladder.

Atherosclerosis

In **atherosclerosis,** the lumina of large and medium-sized muscular arteries is narrowed by fibrofatty plaque (atheroma) within the intima. Atherosclerosis-related diseases, notably myocardial and cerebral infarctions, account for about 50 percent of deaths in the United States. Many risk factors have been identified or postulated for development of atherosclerosis, of which the most important are older age, male sex, familial tendency, cigarette smoking, diabetes, hyperlipidemia, and hypertension. Hyperlipidemia is discussed in greater detail in the next section (see p. 201).

The pathologic lesions in atherosclerosis take the form of fatty streaks and atheromatous plaques. While any large or medium-sized artery is potentially affected, the most important sites are the cerebral arteries in the circle of Willis (generalized chronic ischemia of the brain, cerebral infarction); the coronary arteries (chronic myocardial ischemia, myocardial infarction); the aorta (aneurysm, emboli to legs); the renal arteries (chronic renal ischemia); the visceral arteries (chronic bowel ischemia); and the lower limb arteries (claudication, gangrene).

Fatty streaks are elongated, yellow streaks, composed histologically of foamy macrophages and lipid-containing smooth muscle cells, found in the intima of aortas of virtually all people over the age of 1 year. Fatty streaks are important because their presence can affect blood flow and consequently predispose for plaque formation. It is still disputed whether some fatty streaks are the precursors of atheromatous plaques.

Atheromatous plaques are white to yellow lesions found in the intima of large and medium-sized arteries, particularly the aorta and the arteries arising from it. A well-developed atheromatous plaque is usually an asymmetric intimal lesion with several layers. A fibrous cap on the intimal surface covers an often necrotic center that may contain foam cells, cellular debris, cholesterol crystals, and calcium. The vessel media can be markedly thinned adjacent to the plaque. Plaques are considered **"complicated"** when they show calcification, luminal ulceration, superimposed thrombosis, intraplaque hemorrhage, or aneurysmal dilation of the vessel wall. The most important complication of atheromatous plaque formation is ischemia or infarction of the tissue supplied by the occluded artery.

Hyperlipidemia

Increased serum levels of cholesterol, particularly in the form of elevated low-density lipoprotein (LDL), and increased serum levels of triglycerides, in the form of elevated very low-density lipoprotein (VLDL), both predispose for coronary atherosclerosis. In contrast, increased levels of high-density lipoprotein (HDL) are associated with lower risk of developing severe atherosclerosis. Elevations of serum cholesterol and triglycerides can be the consequence of either excessive dietary intake or genetic disorders. Hyperlipoproteinemias have been classified based upon the types of excessive serum lipids. In **type 1** hyperlipoproteinemia, the deficiency of lipoprotein lipase causes elevated chylomicrons. Type 1 disease can be seen in familial lipoprotein lipase deficiency and secondary to systemic lupus erythematosus. In **type 2a** disease, the deficiency of an LDL receptor, seen in familial hypercholesterolemia and secondary to nephrotic syndrome and hyperthyroidism, causes elevated cholesterol in the form of increased LDL. In **type 2b** disease, an unknown mechanism causes elevation of both cholesterol and triglycerides, in the form of LDL and VLDL, in familial combined hyperlipidemia and secondary to nephrotic syndrome, stress, and diet. In **type 3** disease, abnormal lipoprotein E, seen in familial type 3 hyperlipoproteinemia and secondary to hypothyroidism, causes elevation of triglycerides and cholesterol in the form of chylomicron remnants and intermediate-density lipoprotein (IDL). In **type 4** disease, an unknown mechanism causes triglyceride elevation, in the form of VLDL, in familial hypertriglyceridemia and secondary to diabetes mellitus and alcoholism. In **type 5** disease, familial apoprotein CII deficiency (and other unknown mechanisms) cause elevation of triglycerides and cholesterol, in the form of VLDL and chylomicrons, in familial combined hyperlipidemia and secondary to alcoholism, diabetes, and oral contraceptive use.

Hyperlipidemias are subclassified based upon the type of serum lipid that is elevated.

ANEURYSMS

Aneurysms are abnormal, localized dilations of blood vessels. This section discusses mainly aortic aneurysms.

Atherosclerotic Aneurysms

The majority of aortic aneurysms are a complication of atherosclerosis. **Atherosclerotic aneurysm** is most commonly a disease of men over the age of 50, many of whom have histories of hypertension. Because of the increased hydrostatic pressures of the abdomen compared with the chest, the abdominal aorta or common iliac arteries are most commonly affected, although the thoracic aorta can also be involved. The aneurysms can have a fusiform, cylindroid, or saccular form.

Atherosclerosis is the most common cause of aortic aneurysm.

Atherosclerotic aneurysms form as a consequence of thinning of the aortic media by the atherosclerotic plaque. Atheromatous ulcers covered by mural thrombi (which may fill the aneurysmal dilation) are commonly found within the aneurysm. Rupture of an aneurysm can cause fatal hemorrhage. Pressure on adjacent structures can cause ureteral compression and vertebral erosion. Emboli can break off the mural thrombi, often lodging in lower extremities or other sites. Vessels arising from the aorta can become occluded by either direct pressure or mural thrombus formation. Treatment of large atherosclerotic aneurysms is by replacement with prosthetic grafts, preferably before rupture since repair after rupture has a much higher mortality rate.

Syphilitic Aneurysms

Syphilitic aneurysms characteristically involve the aortic arch.

Tertiary syphilis can cause aortic aneurysms that involve the ascending or transverse portions of the **aortic arch,** but can also extend distally to the level of the diaphragm. The aortic valve can also be involved with aneurysmal dilation, causing valvular insufficiency and then left ventricular volume overload hypertrophy, sometimes with massively enlarged heart **("cor bovinum").** An infiltration of lymphocytes and plasma cells begins in the adventitia of the aorta and produces obliterative endarteritis of the vasa vasorum. The resulting luminal narrowing of the vasa causes ischemic injury to the aortic media, characterized by loss of myocytes and elastic fibers followed by scarring. Revascularization of the damaged media may also be seen. **"Tree-barking,"** or wrinkling, of the aortic intima follows as the medial scars contract. The damaged intima additionally becomes a favored site for superimposed atherosclerosis, which may involve the aortic root.

Syphilitic aneurysms are now uncommon because of the decline of tertiary syphilis. When they do occur, they tend to cause more prominent symptoms than do abdominal aneurysms. Symptoms include respiratory and swallowing difficulties, chronic cough, pain secondary to erosion of ribs or vertebrae, and cardiac complaints. Therapy is with antibiotics for control of the syphilis, followed by surgical replacement of the affected aorta and aortic valve. Therapy is most successful when it is performed before significant secondary cardiac disease has occurred.

Cystic Medial Necrosis and Aortic Dissection

Aortic dissection usually involves an aorta previously weakened by cystic medial necrosis.

Aortic dissection (dissecting hematoma, dissecting aneurysm) refers to the formation of a blood-filled channel in the aortic wall. The blood is introduced through an intimal tear, then dissects along the media, and may or may not re-enter the aortic lumen through a second intimal tear. While the term "dissecting aneurysm" is often used, aneurysmal dilation of the aorta may or may not be present. The channel characteristically occurs between the middle and outer thirds of the media, in an area that has often been previously weakened by **cystic medial necrosis.** Cystic medial necrosis is a process of unknown etiology that damages the media by causing focal fragmentation of the elastic elements; deposition of mucoid material; focal fibrosis; and formation of small cystic (often cleft-like) spaces in areas of focal separation of elastic and fibromuscular elements. Aortic dissections that involve the ascending aorta, whether or not they extend into the descending aorta, are classified as **type A** or proximal dissections; those that do not involve the ascending aorta are classified as **type B.** Type A dissections, in which an intimal tear is often identified within 10 cm of the aortic valve, are much more common than type B dissections. If a second intimal tear is present distally (often at the level of the iliac vessels), a **double-barreled aorta** can be produced. A small percentage of dissections do not have an obvious endothelial tear, possibly as a result of healing, with re-epithelialization of the intima.

Blood may come through the tear in a double-barreled aorta.

Aortic dissection can cause sudden onset of excruciating pain referred to the chest and back if the dissection develops abruptly. Death can be caused by rupture of the aorta with extravasation of blood, often into the pericardial sac. Extension of the dissection into the major arteries arising from the arch can cause ischemia in the arms or head. Retrograde involvement of a major coronary artery can cause cardiac ischemia. Involvement of the aortic root can cause aortic regurgitation. Type A dissections require immediate emergency reparative surgery. Uncomplicated type B dissections, which are less dangerous, are treated with hypotensive therapy followed by reparative surgery after the patient's condition has stabilized. Treated in this manner, roughly two-thirds of patients survive aortic dissection for 2 or more years, while previously only 5 percent survived 1 year.

VASCULITIDES

The noninfectious systemic **necrotizing vasculitides** are inflammatory diseases characterized by inflammation and necrosis of blood vessels (vasculitis). Many of the vasculitides appear to have an immunologic basis, possibly related to deposition of antigen–antibody complexes in vessel walls. The vasculitides characteristically respond to corticosteroid therapy. The vascular lesions usually have a patchy, segmental distribution, and symptoms tend to be related to organ damage distal to a site of partial or complete obstruction of a blood vessel. The different vasculitides are distinguished by the vessels most severely affected, the presence or absence of granulomas, and related clinical associations.

Many vasculitides have an immunologic basis.

Polyarteritis Nodosa

Polyarteritis nodosa can be considered the prototype for the vasculitides. Classic polyarteritis nodosa characteristically affects small or medium-sized muscular arteries, often at branch points, in the renal and visceral circulations. Pulmonary vessels are usually selectively spared. The disease has a predisposition for young, male adults, although both sexes and all ages can be affected. The appearance of the individual, sharply localized, vascular lesions varies with the age of the lesion. **Acute** lesions are characterized by fibrinoid necrosis of much or all of the thickness of the arterial wall; such necrosis may cause an aneurysmal dilation that can be demonstrated by angiography. The fibrinoid necrosis is often accompanied by a leukocytic (neutrophils, eosinophils, and mononuclear cells) infiltration in and around the vessel. In **healing** lesions, the inflammatory cell infiltrate shifts to principally macrophages and plasma cells. Fibroblasts can be found in and adjacent to the vessel wall, sometimes producing sufficient fibrosis to produce a grossly palpable nodule. Any thrombus within the vessel adjacent to the site of injury

Polyarteritis nodosa typically causes small lesions at branch points of muscular arteries.

Acute, healing, and healed lesions often coexist.

becomes organized. In **healed** lesions, the leukocytic infiltration has cleared, and the remaining pathology consists of fragmentation of the internal elastic lamina and fibrous replacement of a part or all of the thickness of the vessel wall. The healed lesion can involve the vessel wall asymmetrically.

Lesions of all stages can be found concurrently. Since the lesions can affect muscular arteries throughout the body, the clinical signs and symptoms can be varied and difficult to interpret. Nonspecific systemic reactions that are usually present include fever, malaise, weakness, and leukocytosis. Other manifestations frequently relate to involvement of specific organs. Renal manifestations include hematuria, albuminuria, hypertension, and renal failure. Alimentary manifestations include abdominal pain and melena (often with anemia). Neuromuscular manifestations include diffuse muscular aches and peripheral neuritis. The prognosis was formerly poor but has markedly improved with corticosteroid and cyclophosphamide therapy.

Allergic Granulomatosis and Angiitis

Churg-Strauss syndrome is similar to polyarteritis nodosa, but is associated with asthma and eosinophilia.

Allergic granulomatosis and angiitis **(Churg-Strauss syndrome)** is a variant of polyarteritis nodosa that is strongly associated with bronchial asthma and eosinophilia. The disease is characterized by vascular lesions that may be histologically identical to those of polyarteritis nodosa; intra- and extravascular granulomas that may involve lungs, peripheral nerves, and skin; a heavy infiltration with eosinophils of vessels and perivascular tissues; and frequent involvement, unlike polyarteritis nodosa, of pulmonary and splenic vessels.

Hypersensitivity Angiitis

Hypersensitivity angiitis tends to affect small blood vessels.

Hypersensitivity angiitis (leukocytoclastic angiitis, microscopic polyarteritis) is characterized by vascular lesions of smaller vessels (arterioles, venules, and capillaries) than those affected by polyarteritis nodosa. When confined to the skin, the disease forms palpable purpura known as cutaneous vasculitis. Almost any other organ system can also be affected. The term hypersensitivity angiitis is used because specific antigens (penicillin, streptococci, tumor antigens, heterologous proteins) are often implicated as possible triggers. The term leukocytoclastic angiitis is based on the histologic appearance of the lesions: a vessel wall that may or may not show fibrinoid necrosis is infiltrated by neutrophils, some of which become fragmented **(leukocytoclasis).** Lesions less than 24 hours old can contain immunoglobulins and complement, which are subsequently cleared. Since the affected vessels are small, infarction of tissue distal to the lesion is less common than in polyarteritis nodosa. Patients usually improve if the antigenic trigger is removed, unless widespread brain or renal lesions are present. Hypersensitivity angiitis is also seen as a component of a variety of other syndromes, including malignancy, connective tissue disorders, essential mixed cryoglobulinemia, and Henoch-Schönlein purpura.

Wegener's Granulomatosis

Wegener's granulomatosis is a rare vasculitis of still unclear etiology that produces prominent pathology in the upper airways, lungs, and kidneys. **Focal necrotizing vasculitis,** which microscopically resembles the vasculitis of polyarteritis nodosa, with fibrinoid necrosis of the vessel wall, can be found in small arteries and veins throughout the body, with favored sites being the upper and lower respiratory tract, spleen, and kidneys. **Acute necrotizing granulomas,** which resemble the granulomas of tuberculosis, can be found both associated with vessels and as separate lesions. Involvement of the upper and lower respiratory tract is particularly prominent. **Renal disease** may be either mild, with acute focal proliferation and necrosis of some glomeruli (focal necrotizing glomerulonephritis), or severe, with diffuse proliferative glomerulonephritis accompanied by prominent crescent formation. Focal renal lesions can produce hematuria and proteinuria; crescenteric glomerulonephritis can progress rapidly to renal failure.

Wegener's granulomatosis affects upper airways, lungs, and kidneys.

Wegener's granulomatosis is principally a disease of middle-aged men. A wide variety of clinical signs and symptoms may be present depending upon the location of the vascular and granulomatous lesions; common features include pneumonitis with pulmonary infiltrates, chronic sinusitis with mucosal ulcerations of the nasopharynx, and renal disease. The formerly dismal prognosis of Wegener's granulomatosis has been modified by corticosteroid and cyclophosphamide therapy. Wegener's granulomatosis must be distinguished from the rare disease **lymphomatoid granulomatosis,** which is characterized by nodules of lymphoid and plasmacytoid cells in the lungs and other organs. These nodules may involve vessels but do not produce a true vasculitis with fibrinoid necrosis.

Temporal Arteritis

Temporal (giant cell) **arteritis** can occlude arteries of medium and small size (notably the temporal arteries) with focal, granulomatous inflammation. Temporal arteritis is a disease of unknown etiology that affects elderly individuals and may cause facial pain, headache, and ocular symptoms. Vigorous attempts at diagnosis and therapy with corticosteroids are important since involvement of the ophthalmic arteries can (rarely) cause blindness. Some cases are accompanied by generalized muscle pains and systemic malaise (polymyalgia rheumatica).

Temporal arteritis tends to involve the muscular arteries of the head.

Takayasu's Arteritis

Takayasu's arteritis is a granulomatous vasculitis that preferentially affects medium and larger arteries, particularly the aortic arch and the roots of vessels arising from it. The descending thoracic and abdominal aorta can also be affected. The disease is also called **pulseless disease** because irregular fibrous thickening of the aorta can markedly narrow the orifices of the vessels arising from the arch, rendering the peripheral pulses of the upper extremities difficult to palpate. Ocular defects (retinal hemorrhage, visual defects including blindness) and neurologic defects (dizziness, focal weakness, hemiparesis) can be produced by limitation of blood flow to the head. Hypertension can follow narrowing of the orifice of the renal arteries. The histologic changes observed are conveniently divided into early and later stages.

Takayasu's arteritis tends to involve the roots of arteries arising from the aortic arch.

Early in the disease, a perivascular mononuclear cell infiltrate cuffs small vessels of the vasa vasorum, which supplies blood to the aortic wall. The aortic media may show granulomatous changes with necrosis and Langhan's giant cells. **Later** in the disease, medial fibrosis and acellular deposition of collagen in the intima markedly thicken the aortic wall and involve the orifices of its major branches. Takayasu's arteritis may cause death within the first few years or may stabilize as fibrosis progresses, although patients that survive often have distressing neurologic and visual complaints.

Kawasaki Disease

Kawasaki disease is an acute febrile illness that may cause coronary artery aneurysms to form.

Kawasaki disease (mucocutaneous lymph node syndrome) is an acute illness of young children and infants that causes lymph node enlargement, skin rash, conjunctival and oral erythema, and fever. The disease is also characterized by a vasculitis resembling polyarteritis nodosa that has a particular affinity for cardiac involvement and can cause coronary artery aneurysms whose rupture or thrombosis can cause death. The etiology may involve retroviral infection. An immunologic process may contribute to the vascular injury, as these patients have T- and B-cell activation and circulating immune complexes.

Thromboangiitis Obliterans

Thromboangiitis obliterans is a vasculitis affecting heavy smokers.

Thromboangiitis obliterans (Buerger's disease) is a segmental inflammation of intermediate and small arteries and veins of the extremities of heavy smokers, principally younger men. The patients experience severe pain in the legs and sometimes arms, which usually remits with cessation of smoking. A genetic predisposition may also be a factor, as thromboangiitis obliterans has geographic variations (common in Israel, Japan, and India) and an increased prevalence of HLA-A9 and HLA-B5 antigens. The affected vessels show sharply segmental lesions characterized by neutrophilic infiltration of all layers of the vessel wall and mural thrombi characteristically containing small microabscesses surrounded by a granulomatous reaction that may contain giant cells. The disease is associated with migratory thrombophlebitis and may lead to gangrene of the extremities. Cigarette smoking cessation is considered mandatory.

Secondary Vasculitis

Vasculitis can also complicate a variety of systemic diseases.

Vasculitis is also seen in association with a variety of underlying disorders including malignancies, particularly lymphoproliferative disorders; immunologic and connective tissue diseases such as systemic lupus erythematosus and rheumatoid arthritis; and systemic diseases including mixed cryoglobulinemia and Henoch-Schönlein purpura. Arteritis can also be seen as a consequence of direct invasion of the vessel wall by bacteria and fungi. Such infection may spread to the vessels by direct extension from locally infected sites or by hematogenous spread from sites such as vegetative valves in endocarditis.

Raynaud's Disease and Raynaud's Phenomenon

Raynaud's phenomenon refers to a characteristic sequence of color changes of the fingers and hands (white to blue to red) seen as a consequence of vasospasm induced by cold or emotional stress. Raynaud's phenomenon must be distinguished from **Raynaud's disease:** Raynaud's phenomenon occurs secondary to an organic lesion in the vessel wall, while Raynaud's disease refers to a functional process, possibly due to hyper-reactivity of vessels to autonomic stimulation, producing vasospasm with similar skin changes, usually in young, apparently healthy women. Processes that can cause Raynaud's phenomenon include arteriosclerosis; scleroderma (in which Raynaud's phenomenon may precede visible skin changes) and other connective tissue diseases including systemic lupus erythematosus; thromboangiitis obliterans (Buerger's disease); diseases producing abnormal plasma proteins, including multiple myeloma and cryoglobulinemia; occult carcinoma; drugs (ergotamine) and poisonings (lead); and idiopathic pulmonary hypertension. Both Raynaud's phenomenon and Raynaud's disease can lead to tropic changes causing atrophy of skin, subcutaneous tissues, and muscle. Ulcerations and gangrene of the fingers and hands are seen less commonly.

Raynaud's phenomenon occurs secondary to a vascular lesion, while Raynaud's disease appears to be a functional process.

BLOOD VESSEL TUMORS

Vascular tumors range in aggressiveness from benign to locally invasive to frankly malignant. The benign tumors and tumorlike conditions include hemangiomas, glomus tumors, and vascular ectasias. Intermediate-grade tumors that are locally invasive include hemangioendothelioma and epithelioid hemangioendothelioma. Malignant tumors with high potentials for metastasis include angiosarcoma, hemangiopericytoma, and Kaposi sarcoma. Tumors can also form channels resembling lymphatics, including benign lymphangiomas and malignant lymphangiosarcomas.

Vascular tumors may be benign, locally invasive, or frankly malignant.

Hemangiomas

Hemangiomas are common, benign proliferations of blood vessels that are most prevalent in infancy and childhood. Histologic variants of hemangiomas include capillary hemangioma, cavernous hemangioma, and granuloma pyogenicum.

Capillary hemangiomas are composed of closely packed aggregations of narrow, thin-walled blood vessels that resemble capillaries and are separated by a scant connective tissue stroma. The tumors can be found in skin, mucous membranes, subcutaneous tissues, and visceral organs. The gross appearance is of a red to blue lesion ranging from a few millimeters to several centimeters in diameter. The lesion is usually well defined but is not encapsulated. **Juvenile hemangiomas** ("strawberry" hemangiomas) are a variant of capillary hemangioma observed in the skin of infants. These hemangiomas characteristically increase in size during the first few months of life, and then, in most cases, regress by the age of 5 years.

Capillary hemangiomas are composed of vessels that resemble capillaries.

Cavernous hemangiomas are composed of large, cavernous vascular spaces filled with blood and embedded in a matrix of scant connective tissue. The gross appearance is of a red-blue, spongy mass that is typically 1 to 2 cm in diameter and (rarely) much larger (giant cavernous hemangioma). Cavernous hemangiomas can be found throughout the body, including both skin and visceral organs. Cavernous hemangiomas of the skin, particularly in the head and neck, are usually identified in

Cavernous hemangiomas have large vascular spaces.

childhood. In the rare syndrome **von Hippel-Lindau disease,** the hemangiomas are found in multiple locations, including the cerebellum, brainstem, eye grounds, pancreas, and liver. Other visceral neoplasms can also be found in von Hippel-Lindau disease. Most cavernous hemangiomas have little clinical significance; cavernous hemangiomas of the brain can become clinically important when they bleed or cause increased intracranial pressure.

Granuloma pyogenicum (granulation tissue-type hemangioma) produces small red nodules on the skin and oral mucous membranes. The lesions often develop following trauma and may not represent true neoplastic growths, as they histologically strongly resemble exuberant granulation tissue with proliferating capillaries, edema, and an acute and chronic inflammatory infiltrate. When they occur in the gingiva of pregnant women, they are called **pregnancy tumor** or granuloma gravidarum.

A **glomus tumor** (glomangioma) is a small (often less than 3 mm), exquisitely painful, benign tumor found most commonly in the fingers and toes, particularly under the nails. The tumors arise in small vascular structures, known as glomus bodies, which regulate arteriolar flow in response to temperature changes. The glomus tumor has branching vascular channels separated by connective tissue stroma. Modified smooth muscle cells known as glomus cells are found as aggregates, nests, and masses of regular sized, round, or cuboidal cells within the connective tissue stroma. Resection is curative.

Telangiectasias

Telangiectasias (vascular ectasias) are benign lesions characterized by dilated or prominent vessels of the skin or mucous membranes that are probably not true neoplasms, but rather congenital anomalies or dilations of pre-existing vessels.

Nevus flammeus is a pink to purple, flat telangiectasia found most commonly on the head or neck of newborns. Nevus flammeus is composed histologically of dilated vessels in the dermis. Most of these lesions fade and regress as the child becomes older. One subtype, the **port-wine stain,** may become unsightly as it grows proportionately with the child. Port-wine stains are also clinically significant because those in the distribution of the trigeminal nerve can be associated with venous angiomatous masses involving the leptomeninges of the brain (Sturge-Weber syndrome or encephalotrigeminal angiomatosis). Sturge-Weber syndrome is an uncommon congenital disorder possibly caused by faulty embryologic development of mesoderm and ectoderm; it can cause a variety of neurologic problems including mental retardation, seizures, and hemiplegia.

Spider telangiectasias are radially arranged, tiny networks of dilated small arteries that can be seen to pulsate in the skin of patients with hyperestrinism, particularly in pregnant women and patients with hepatic cirrhosis.

Hereditary hemorrhagic telangiectasia (Osler-Weber-Rendu disease) is a rare, sometimes autosomal dominant disorder characterized by multiple, small, aneurysmal dilations of vessels found throughout the body. The most frequent sites are directly below skin and mucosal surfaces, including those of the respiratory, alimentary, and urinary tracts. Patients with hereditary hemorrhagic telangiectasias have an increasing tendency with age to bleed from these lesions. The patients have a nor-

Granuloma pyogenicum may be a reactive process rather than a true tumor.

Glomus tumors are tiny but painful tumors arising in glomus bodies.

Telangiectasias are composed of dilated vessels.

Nevus flammeus telangiectasia may either regress or grow proportionately with the child.

Hereditary hemorrhagic telangiectasia may require frequent blood transfusions.

mal life expectancy but may require frequent transfusions. Hepatomegaly is common, both as a result of transfusion-related hepatitis B infection and focal fibrovascular lesions in the liver.

Hemangioendothelioma and Epithelial Hemangioendothelioma

Hemangioendotheliomas are vascular neoplasms of intermediate-grade neoplastic potential, more invasive than well-differentiated hemangiomas, but with less metastatic potential than the frankly anaplastic angiosarcomas. The tumors are found most frequently in the skin, but may also be seen in the liver and spleen. Histologically, the tumors are composed of masses and sheets of spindle-shaped endothelial cells growing in and around vascular channels. Mitotic figures and some pleomorphism of the endothelial cells can be encountered. The tumors are important principally because they can resemble highly malignant angiosarcomas and lymphangiosarcomas (if bleeding in the lymphatic channels has occurred).

Hemangioendotheliomas have intermediate-grade malignant potential.

Epithelioid hemangioendotheliomas are a variant of hemangioendothelioma with somewhat greater malignant potential, since 40 percent recur after excision and 20 percent eventually metastasize. Epithelioid hemangioendotheliomas are composed of inconspicuous vascular channels within masses of cuboidal cells that resemble epithelial cells, but that can be demonstrated to be of endothelial origin by the presence of Weibel-Palade bodies and factor VIII-associated antigens.

The variant epitheloid hemangioendothelioma has a worse prognosis.

DISEASES OF VEINS AND LYMPHATICS

Ninety percent of clinically significant venous disease is caused by varicose veins and phlebothrombosis.

Varicose Veins

A prolonged increase in intraluminal pressure within a vein can cause abnormal dilation, producing a **varicose vein.** The superficial leg veins are most commonly affected, but other sites may also be involved, for example, the esophageal and hemorrhoidal varices seen in portal hypertension. Risk factors for varicosities in the superficial veins of the legs include increasing age (the incidence in age groups over 50 years approaches 50 percent); venous obstruction or compression by pregnancy, tumor masses, occupations that require long periods of standing or sitting, and intravascular thromboses; obesity; and familial tendency. Varicose veins characteristically show marked variation in wall thickness, with dilated, tortuous areas being thinned compared with less involved areas. Long-standing disease may produce a thickened, opaque vessel wall by compensatory hypertrophy of the medial muscle accompanied by intramural fibrosis. Major veins may also show degeneration of elastic tissue and focal medial calcifications **(phlebosclerosis).** Valvular deformities secondary to dilation of the vein and intramural thrombosis are often found. The marked venous stasis that accompanies varicose veins produces persistent leg edema with stasis dermatitis and skin ulcerations. Injuries to the involved extremity heal poorly.

Degeneration of elastic tissue and focal medial calcification are histologic characteristics of varicose veins.

Thrombophlebitis

Phlebothrombosis is thrombus formation in veins; **thrombophlebitis** is the inflammatory change observed in a vessel wall following thrombosis. The terms are in practice synonymous since venous thrombosis inevitably leads to inflammation. Commonly encountered factors predisposing for venous thrombosis include prolonged bed rest or immobilization, including the postoperative state; cardiac failure with slowed venous return; and hypercoagulable states including those produced by pregnancy and malignant tumors. Important sites of venous thrombosis include the deep leg veins, where the vast majority of clinically significant thrombophlebitis is observed; the periprostatic plexus in men and the pelvic veins in women; the dural sinuses and large veins of the skull, particularly if bacterial or fungal infection is present; and the portal vein and its tributaries, particularly if intra-abdominal infection is present.

The release of part or all of an intravascular thrombus from a systemic vein can produce **emboli,** which can pass through the heart to lodge in the pulmonary circulation. Emboli from deep leg veins are particularly significant because some of them are of a size to lodge at branch points in the pulmonary arterial circulation (saddle emboli), potentially causing pulmonary infarction or even sudden death. An embolic phenomenon may be the first clinical sign or symptom produced by thrombophlebitis. An **infected thrombus** may cause bacteremia and be a source of septic emboli. Infected thrombi are particularly important in the portal veins, where they may produce multiple liver abscesses, and in the dural sinuses, where they may cause meningitis and brain abscesses.

Thrombi can, but do not always, produce local clinical signs and symptoms. The most dependable clinical sign is the elicitation of pain when external pressure is applied to an affected vessel. In the case of thrombi in deep leg veins, this pain can sometimes be elicited by squeezing the calf muscles or dorsiflexing the foot. Other local manifestations that may or may not be present in the affected area include edema, dusky cyanosis, and dilation of superficial veins. In addition to the local signs and symptoms described above, venous thrombi can be demonstrated by invasive (venous angiography) and noninvasive (^{125}I-labeled fibrinogen, ultrasound, plethysmography) methods. Since the clinical consequences of thrombophlebitis, particularly embolic phenomena, are so severe, effort should be directed at preventing thrombus formation in vulnerable individuals.

Two variants of obscure etiology of primary phlebothrombosis are migratory phlebitis and phlegmasia alba dolens. **Migratory phlebitis** is the sequential occurrence and then disappearance of multiple venous thrombi, often as a paraneoplastic syndrome in patients with a visceral, pancreatic, pulmonary, or colonic cancer. **Phlegmasia alba dolens** (painful white leg or milk leg) is a disease of pregnant women, usually in the third trimester or early postpartum period, in which thrombosis at the iliofemoral venous system causes marked, painful swelling of the leg. The thrombosis is apparently due in part to the combination of the hypercoagulable state induced by pregnancy and pressure by the gravid uterus on the inferior vena cava and other pelvic vessels.

Lymphangitis and Lymphedema

Secondary involvement of lymphatics commonly occurs as a consequence of lymphatic drainage of sites containing infection or tumor, and can produce either lymphangitis or lymphedema. **Lymphangitis** is the acute inflammatory involvement of lymphatic channels secondary to infection by bacterial organisms, most often group A β-hemolytic streptococci, although almost any bacterial infection can cause lymphangitis. The lymphatic channels dilate and form painful, subcutaneous, red streaks with enlarged regional lymph nodes. Acute inflammatory cells (neutrophils, histiocytes) can be found in the lymphatic lumina, walls, and perilymphatic tissues. Involved lymph nodes also show acute inflammation. **Lymphedema** refers to the accumulation of interstitial fluid in areas drained by an obstructed lymphatic channel. Lymphatic channels can be obstructed by malignant tumors; surgical removal of lymph nodes (e.g., radical mastectomy); fibrosis (radiation therapy, inflammation); and filarial parasites. In addition to edema of deeper tissues, lymphedema characteristically causes skin changes including increased subcutaneous interstitial fibrosis, brawny induration, and skin ulcers; these skin changes are sometimes described as "peau d'orange" (orange peel). Rupture of obstructed, dilated lymphatics can cause chylous ascites, chylothorax, and chylopericardium. Lymphedema rarely occurs in idiopathic form.

Lymphedema praecox is a progressive, unremitting edema that usually manifests in women in their second or third decade; it begins with edema of one or both feet that may, with time, progress into the lower trunk and other sites. **Milroy's disease** is an inherited condition that possibly evolves as a result of development of structurally weak lymphatic channels; it presents at birth and causes predominantly lower extremity edema. **Simple congenital lymphedema** is similar to Milroy's disease, but only one family member is affected, and a possible genetic basis has not been identified.

Lymphangitis is often caused by group A β-hemolytic streptococci.

Lymphedema may induce skin changes.

HEART

CONGENITAL HEART DISEASE

The heart is vulnerable to many developmental defects. They are conveniently subclassified as defects causing right-to-left shunts; left-to-right shunts; obstructive noncyanotic congenital anomalies; and malpositions of the heart.

Right-to-Left Shunts

Early development of cyanosis is characteristic of right-to-left shunts.

Congenital cardiac lesions associated with flow of blood from the right to the left sides of the heart characteristically cause early development of cyanosis.

The cluster of defects observed in tetralogy of Fallot can produce either left-to-right or right-to-left shunts.

Tetralogy of Fallot is a cluster of defects including ventricular septal defects; dextraposed aorta overriding an interventricular septal defect; obstruction to the right ventricular outflow, commonly by a narrowed pulmonary artery or valve; and right ventricular hypertrophy. Mild tetralogy of Fallot with a large septal defect and mild pulmonic stenosis produces a left-to-right shunt without cyanosis. Severe tetralogy of Fallot, characterized by severe pulmonic stenosis, causes right-sided hypertension with reverse of flow through the septal defect (right-to-left shunting). Severe tetralogy of Fallot consequently produces cyanosis from birth or shortly thereafter. The timing of surgical repair, which may be complete or partial, is still controversial. Complications of untreated tetralogy of Fallot include polycythemia, infective endocarditis, paradoxic embolism, and cerebral abscess.

Transpositions of the great arteries occur in several forms, some of which are more dangerous than others.

Transpositions of the great arteries are a group of malformations in which the aorta arises from the morphologic right ventricle and the pulmonary artery arises from the morphologic left ventricle. In the most **common pattern,** the morphologic right ventricle is on the right side of the heart, and the morphologic left ventricle is on the left. This arrangement produces independent left and right circulations and is compatible with a postnatal life only if a large communication (interatrial, patent ductus, or ventricular septal defect) between the circulations is present. This form of transposition of the great arteries is a major cause of death in the first two months of life. Other variants include **"corrected" transposition,** in which the morphogenic right ventricle is on the left and the morphogenic left ventricle is on the right, and **Taussig-Bing malformation,** in which the aorta arises from the right ventricle and the pulmonary artery overrides a ventricular septal defect.

Truncus arteriosus is a serious defect that can sometimes be surgically corrected.

Truncus arteriosus is characterized by a single large vessel that overlies a ventricular septal defect and receives blood from both ventricles. The defect occurs as a failure of separation of the aorta from the pulmonary artery and has a poor prognosis because it is often associated with multiple concomitant defects of the heart and vasculature. Early surgical correction is sometimes successful.

Tricuspid atresia refers to the congenital complete absence of the tricuspid valve, which is usually associated with an underdeveloped right ventricle and an atrial septal defect with associated right-to-left shunt. Other congenital defects may also be present and the prognosis is poor unless palliative surgery is possible.

Patients with tricuspid atresia often have a poor prognosis.

Left-to-Right Shunts

Cardiac malformations that produce left-to-right shunts have a better prognosis and produce cyanosis later than do those that produce right-to-left shunts.

Ventricular septal defect is the most common congenital cardiac malformation and is frequently associated with other defects including patent ductus arteriosus, tetralogy of Fallot, atrial septal defects, coarctation of the aorta, and transposition of the great arteries. Most ventricular septal defects are found within or adjacent to the membranous septum. The clinical significance of a ventricular septal defect varies with its size. Defects less than 0.5 cm (Roger's disease) may close spontaneously or may be well tolerated for years, producing only a loud pansystolic murmur. Larger defects permit significant left-to-right flow, and cause a secondary right ventricular hypertrophy with pulmonary hypertension. As the right ventricle hypertrophy becomes increasingly severe, the flow of blood may shift to right-to-left, producing cyanosis leading to finger clubbing and polycythemia. Very large defects may cause fulminant cardiac failure at birth. Infective endocarditis is sometimes encountered in patients with small to moderate-sized defects.

Ventricular septal defect is the most common congenital cardiac malformation.

Atrial septal defect is a common congenital anomaly that is often first recognized in adulthood. The defects may take three forms. **Ostium primum defects** in the atrial septum occur low and may be associated with Down syndrome and defects of the atrioventricular valves. **Ostium secundum defects** including patent foramen ovale are the most common atrial septal defects and occur in the upper half of the atrial septum, because of juxtaposed defects in the primary and secondary septa. Many other defects may be associated, including patent ductus arteriosus, ventricular septal defect, transposition of the great arteries, and tetralogy of Fallot. Sinus venosus defects are found near the top of the atrial septum. The defects are near the entrance of the superior vena cava. Associated defects can include an anomalous connection of the right pulmonary veins to the superior vena cava or right atrium. Small atrial defects are well tolerated. Larger defects can produce significant left-to-right flow, which eventually causes right ventricular hypertrophy with cor pulmonale and a late reversal of the shunt, producing cyanosis. Surgical correction early in life prevents the development of right ventricular hypertrophy.

Atrial septal defect is also common.

Patent ductus arteriosus refers to a postnatal failure to close of the ductus arteriosus, which in intrauterine life permits the flow of blood from the pulmonary to the aortic systems. Functional closure of the ductus usually occurs within the first day or two of life. Patent ductus arteriosus most often occurs as an isolated anomaly but can be seen in infants with respiratory distress syndrome (the low oxygen tension mimics that in the uterus), septal defects, coarctation, pulmonary stenosis, or aortic stenosis. When the patent ductus arteriosus is seen with other cardiac anomalies, it is often functionally necessary to compensate for the other defects by providing flow of blood from the systemic to pulmonary circulations. Early correction of isolated patent ductus arteriosus is recommended to prevent pulmonary hypertension.

Patent ductus arteriosus can be functionally appropriate compensation for other circulatory problems.

Obstructive Noncyanotic Congenital Anomalies

Preductal aortic coarctation often involves large aortic segments, while postductal coarctation is typically a ridgelike aortic constriction.

Congenital defects that can produce circulatory obstruction without cyanosis affect the aorta, the pulmonary trunk, or valves. **Coarctation of the aorta** is a narrowing or constriction of the aorta. Coarctation proximal to the ductus arteriosus (**preductal** or "infantile form") tends to involve large segments of the aortic root and is almost always associated with a patent ductus arteriosus. It frequently causes death in infancy due to right ventricular hypertrophy with congestive heart failure. The more common **postductal coarctation** ("adult form") is usually a localized, ridgelike constriction of the aorta that is often found just distal to the ductus arteriosus. The ductus may or may not be patent. Postductal coarctation, unless unusually severe, may be asymptomatic for years due to the development of collateral circulation including dilation of the internal mammary arteries. Symptoms, when present, are those of arterial insufficiency of the lower extremities. Coarctation of the aorta characteristically produces hypertension in arteries of the upper extremities and hypotension in arteries of the lower extremities. Surgical treatment of significant adult coarctation is recommended since death can occur after about age 40 due to congestive heart failure, infective aortitis, sequelae of hypertension including intracranial hemorrhage, and rupture of the precoarctation aorta.

Pulmonary valvular stenosis or atresia, when accompanied by an intact interventricular septum, can cause obstruction without cyanosis. Atresia of the pulmonic valve is commonly accompanied by a hypoplastic right ventricle and an atrial septal defect. In atresia, blood reaches the pulmonary circulation by bypassing the right ventricle through an atrial septal defect and then entering the pulmonary vasculature via a patent ductus arteriosus. When the pulmonary valve or artery is only stenosed, right ventricular hypertrophy, which may lead to right heart failure, develops. Mild pulmonary stenosis may be asymptomatic; more severe stenosis usually requires surgical correction.

Aortic valvular stenosis or atresia can occur as a consequence of a variety of congenital anomalies including bicuspid aortic valve and subvalvular or valvular congenital aortic stenosis. Congenital aortic atresia occurs rarely and causes death in infancy. Mild to moderate stenoses are well tolerated, but may require antibiotic prophylaxis against infective endocarditis. Surgical correction of both mild and severe disease is recommended.

Malpositions of the Heart

Dextrocardia may be an isolated finding or part of situs inversus totalis.

Occasionally, the heart is found in an unusual position or orientation. **Dextrocardia** is an inversion of the heart, which is often otherwise normal, such that the morphologic left side heart is on the right and is in the right hemithorax. Dextrocardia is usually an anatomic curiosity and may be accompanied by inversion of all of the viscera (**situs inversus totalis**), which creates "mirror image" chest and abdominal cavities. **Kartagener syndrome** is the cluster of situs inversus, sinusitis, and bronchiectasis. When the dextrocardia is isolated, the heart is almost always abnormal, with associated defects including transposition of the atria and transposition of the great arteries. Asplenia and polysplenia are also associated with malpositions of the heart. Rarely, the heart is found outside the body (**ectopia cordis**) or in the abdomen if a diaphragmatic hernia is present.

ISCHEMIC AND HYPERTENSIVE HEART DISEASE

Chronic Ischemic Heart Disease

Some, usually elderly, patients will experience **insidiously developing congestive heart failure** following repeated injury to the myocardium by ischemia. While many of these patients have experienced angina or obvious prior episodes of myocardial infarction, a few individuals may have been asymptomatic, or had only an arrhythmia, before developing congestive failure. The hearts of these patients show diffuse **myocardial atrophy** with a diffuse, predominantly perivascular, **interstitial fibrosis**. Necrosis of individual or small groups of myocytes can also be seen; healed scars from previous acute infarctions may or may not be present. Grossly, the heart may be small, of normal size, or hypertrophied. Stenosing atherosclerosis of the coronary arteries is almost always observed. These elderly patients may die either of the congestive failure or of unrelated medical causes.

> Chronic ischemic heart disease is observed in patients who have not experienced frank myocardial infarction.

Sudden Cardiac Death

Sudden cardiac death is an unexpected death due to cardiac causes that occurs shortly (1 to 24 hours, depending upon the exact definition chosen) after onset of acute symptoms. Ischemic heart disease (e.g., massive myocardial infarction) is the overwhelmingly most common cause of sudden cardiac death. Less frequent causes include marked aortic valve stenosis, abnormal cardiac conduction systems, and electrolyte derangements. Rare causes include myocarditis, mitral valve prolapse, and hypertrophic cardiomyopathies. The immediate cause of death is almost always a lethal arrhythmia such as asystole or ventricular fibrillation.

> Sudden cardiac death is usually due to a lethal arrhythmia that may have many causes.

Angina Pectoris

Myocardial ischemia can cause paroxysmal attacks of substernal or precordial chest discomfort known as **angina pectoris.** Descriptions of the discomfort vary; the terms constricting, squeezing, choking, and knife-like are commonly used. The significance of angina pectoris is that it suggests that severe myocardial ischemia, which may be just short of that necessary to cause myocardial infarction, is occurring. **Stable (typical) angina** is the most common clinical pattern and occurs following exertion that would usually be tolerated. Other causes of increased cardiac work load (e.g., emotional excitement) can also induce stable angina. Atheromatous stenosis of coronary arteries is almost always present. **Prinzmetal's variant angina** is angina that occurs at rest as a consequence of coronary artery spasm by unknown mechanisms. Coronary atherosclerosis may be present but does not appear to be part of the etiology. **Unstable or crescendo angina** is a pattern of worsening angina triggered by progressively less effort; it may occur at rest. It tends to have a longer duration than stable angina. The presence of unstable angina suggests impending myocardial infarction. The etiology is usually atherosclerosis, which may be complicated by thrombosis or platelet aggregation on a fractured or ulcerated atheromatous plaque. Vasospasm may also play a role.

> Stable angina occurs after exertion; Prinzmetal's variant angina occurs at rest; and unstable angina is triggered by progressively less effort.

Myocardial Infarction

Acute myocardial infarctions occur when the perfusion of a portion of the heart falls below the level needed to sustain a viable myocardium. Acute myocardial infarction is a very common disease; approximately 20 percent of American men experience a myocardial infarction or die from an acute ischemic event before age 65. Coronary **atherosclerosis** is a major contributor to myocardial infarction, and the risk factors for myocardial infarction are similar to those for atherosclerosis. Factors strongly predisposing for atherosclerosis include hypertension, cigarette smoking, diabetes mellitus, and increased levels of serum cholesterol and lipids. Men experience more myocardial infarctions than do women; this predisposition diminishes with age after female menopause. The older, higher estrogen formulations of oral contraceptives predisposed for myocardial infarction. Newer formulations significantly predispose for myocardial infarction only in women who smoke. Regular exercise, possibly by increasing development of collateral blood supply to the myocardium, appears to lessen both the risk of myocardial infarction and the risk of developing fatal arrhythmias if myocardial infarction does occur.

Myocardial infarctions commonly occur in two morphologic patterns. **Transmural infarctions** involve the full or nearly full thickness of the myocardium and are usually associated with thrombosis superimposed on severe coronary atherosclerosis. Common sites of occlusion (in order of frequency) include the anterior descending branch of the left coronary artery (apex and anterior septal infarct), the right coronary artery (posterior wall), and the circumflex branch of the left coronary artery (lateral wall of left ventricle). **Subendocardial infarcts** are limited to the inner one-third to one-half of the myocardium. While coronary atherosclerosis is commonly present, the usual event initiating this type of infarction is a process, such as shock, that causes a generalized decrease in perfusion. The subendocardial myocardium is most vulnerable to ischemia because its collateral circulation is less well developed than that in the subpericardial portions of the myocardial wall. The distinction between subendocardial and transmural infarcts can be less clear than implied above, since the cellular necrosis in transmural infarcts usually begins in the subendocardium, and, if the infarction is interrupted by therapy, the necrosis may not extend to the pericardium.

Similar gross and microscopic findings are observed in both transmural and subendocardial infarctions. A nonspecific waviness of myocardial fibers at the border of the infarct may be visible after 1 hour. Coagulative necrosis is first detectable after 4 to 8 hours. Over the next few days, muscle fibers begin to disintegrate, and a predominantly neutrophilic infiltrate enters the infarct from the margins. By about 10 days, the infarcted tissue is being replaced by granulation tissue that over a period of months forms fibrotic scar tissue.

Early complications of myocardial infarctions include arrhythmias, cardiogenic shock, mural thrombosis with risk of systemic emboli, and pulmonary embolism from leg vein thrombosis. Acute pericarditis and rupture of affected myocardium (wall, papillary muscles, or septum) are most apt to occur several days to weeks after infarction. During the weeks to months after infarction, chronic congestive heart failure or cardiac aneurysm may develop. Recurrence or extension of the infarction can occur at any time. Many of the complications mentioned above are potentially fatal.

Hypertensive Heart Disease

Long-standing hypertension can be associated with a **left ventricular hypertrophy** that is usually concentric. Furthermore, since hypertension strongly predisposes for atherosclerosis, many of these patients have significant accompanying coronary **atherosclerosis.** The mechanism by which hypertension produces left ventricular hypertrophy is still not fully elucidated, but appears to be a compensatory response to pressure overload, possibly with an additional direct contribution by adrenergic stimulation. The gross appearance and functioning of the heart vary with the stage of the left ventricular hypertrophy. In **early compensated hypertensive heart disease,** the left ventricular wall is thickened and chamber size is roughly normal. In **late compensated hypertensive heart disease,** the thickened left ventricular wall is sufficiently stiffer than normal to limit diastolic filling and consequently stroke volume. With the onset of cardiac decompensation, the failure of the myocardium to contract adequately leads to a dilated left ventricle with corresponding thinning of the ventricular wall and enlargement of the cardiac profile. Microscopic changes observed include an early increase in myocyte size; a later disorganization of myocyte arrangement secondary to variations in myocyte transverse diameter; and a late increase in interstitial fibrosis secondary to random myocyte atrophy and death.

Untreated hypertrophic heart disease may be asymptomatic or may cause atrial fibrillation or lead to cardiac decompensation with cardiac dilation. There is an increased risk of sudden cardiac death. The patient may be vulnerable to hypertensive symptoms including headache, dizziness, or nosebleeds. The patient's atherosclerosis, for which hypertension is a risk factor, may lead to ischemic heart disease, stroke, or progressive renal failure. Effective pharmacologic control of the hypertension causes regression of the hypertrophy in some patients.

Hypertension can produce a concentric left ventricular hypertrophy.

COR PULMONALE

Right ventricular enlargement secondary to lung disease is called **cor pulmonale** (pulmonary heart disease). Cor pulmonale can be considered to be analogous to the left ventricular hypertrophy observed in systemic hypertension, since the pressure overload produced by increased pulmonary blood pressure causes right ventricular enlargement. **Acute cor pulmonale** is the abruptly developing right ventricular dilation caused by the interruption of pulmonary blood flow by a massive pulmonary embolus. The more common **chronic cor pulmonale** is right ventricular hypertrophy associated with chronic hypertension. Many diseases predispose for chronic cor pulmonale including disorders affecting the lung parenchyma (chronic obstructive pulmonary disease, pulmonary interstitial fibrosis, cystic fibrosis); pulmonary vessels (pulmonary emboli, vasculitides); chest wall movement (poliomyelitis and other neuromuscular disease, marked obesity, scoliosis); and the constriction of pulmonary arterioles (hypoxemia, metabolic acidosis). Cor pulmonale is a common disorder because it is associated with common diseases such as chronic obstructive pulmonary disease. In addition to right ventricular hypertrophy, the lungs will show the vascular changes associated with pulmonary hypertension known as pulmonary vascular sclerosis.

Chronic lung disease can cause right ventricular enlargement.

CONGESTIVE HEART FAILURE

Congestive heart failure is a common end point of most forms of serious heart disease. In severe congestive heart failure, both the left and the right ventricles are usually performing inadequately. However, with most disease processes, one or the other chamber will usually become compromised first, and it is consequently convenient to discuss congestive heart failure in terms of right- or left-sided failure.

Left-Sided Heart Failure

The function of the left atrium and ventricle is to supply an adequate volume and pressure of blood to the systemic circulation. The ability to do this is most commonly compromised by hypertension and ischemic heart disease, acting either together or independently; aortic and mitral valvular diseases, notably rheumatic heart disease and calcific aortic stenosis; and cardiomyopathies, which compromise myocardial function. The appearance of the heart in **left-sided congestive failure** varies with the disease causing the pathology. Most commonly, the left ventricle is dilated, sometimes massively. However, if the underlying disease restricts ventricular expansion (restrictive cardiomyopathies) or blood flow into the ventricle (mitral stenosis), the left ventricle may be small and the left atrium dilated.

Left-sided congestive heart failure has prominent distant effects. In the **systemic circulation,** decreased cardiac output can compromise the function of many organ systems. Of particular importance are the effects on the **brain** and **kidney.** In severe congestive heart failure, cerebral hypoxia may cause a variety of symptoms such as irritability and loss of attention span, and may even progress to stupor and coma. The kidneys are usually affected by even relatively mild left-sided failure, since a reduction in renal perfusion activates the renin-angiotensin-aldosterone system, causing retention of salt and water. In more severe failure and in kidneys already damaged by shock or hypertensive arteriolar narrowing, ischemic acute tubular necrosis and/or prerenal azotemia may occur. In the **pulmonic circulation,** the failure of blood to be pumped at an adequate rate and pressure through the systemic circulation tends to cause blood to "back up" into the pulmonic circulation. This process first increases the pressure and volume in the pulmonary veins, which, if the congestive failure worsens, then involves the alveolar capillaries, producing pulmonary congestion and edema. Transudate accumulation in the pleural spaces can also occur, sometimes producing significant pleural effusions. Clinically, the patient may experience dyspnea, orthopnea, paroxysmal nocturnal dyspnea, and cough, which is sometimes productive of frothy, blood-tinged sputum.

Right-Sided Heart Failure

Right-sided heart failure develops most frequently as a consequence of left-sided failure, which increases the burden on the right side of the heart by increasing pressures in the pulmonic circulation. Failure of the right side of the heart occurs in the pure form most commonly in cor pulmonale when right ventricular hypertrophy develops secondary to pulmonary diseases that induce pulmonary hypertension. Other causes of pure right-sided failure include tricuspid or pulmonic valvular lesions and some cardiomyopathies. Constrictive pericarditis may also simulate right-sided failure by restricting right ventricular filling and consequently damming blood into the systemic venous system. With the exception of diseases that restrict right ventricular filling (e.g., tricuspid stenosis or restrictive cardiomyopathies), the right ventricle and sometimes the right atrium dilate in right-sided congestive failure.

The disruption of function of the right heart causes systemic venous congestion with significant effects on many organs. The **liver** and portal system of drainage become congested. On cut section, the liver displays a "nutmeg" pattern caused by congestive accentuation of the centers of the lobules around the branches of the hepatic veins, surrounded by the paler periphery of the lobules.

Histologically, the centrilobular sinusoids are congested, and, depending on the duration and severity of the congestion, the hepatocytes near the centers of the lobules may be atrophic or necrosed. When the hepatic congestion is severe, flow through the portal system of drainage also becomes impaired, which can cause ascites, an enlarged (up to 500 g or more) congested spleen, and congestion of the gut with intestinal disturbances. The **kidneys** can develop marked congestion and hypoxia with right-sided failure, which, like left-sided failure, stimulates fluid retention, leading to peripheral edema. Prerenal azotemia can also be produced. The **subcutaneous tissues** can develop edema, which may range from intermittent peripheral edema of the dependent regions (usually legs) of the body to the massive, generalized edema (anasarca) seen in severe, prolonged congestion. Other sites that can be affected by right-sided failure include the **central nervous system,** which can develop symptoms similar to those seen in left-sided failure, and the **pleural spaces,** which may develop effusions.

Right heart failure is associated with hepatic congestion, ascites, and peripheral edema.

MYOCARDITIS

Myocarditis is a broad category of heart disease characterized by an inflammatory infiltrate with myocyte necrosis in the myocardium. Causes of myocarditis are diverse. Most well-documented cases of myocarditis are caused by **viruses,** including coxsackie A and B, polio, influenza A and B, human immunodeficiency (HIV), and echoviruses. The primary infection usually involves the respiratory tract, with the exception of poliovirus; the initial infection is neuromuscular. Viral myocarditis usually causes isolated myofiber necrosis accompanied by interstitial edema and an inflammatory infiltrate composed of lymphocytes, macrophages, and plasma cells. Uncommonly, **other infectious agents** can cause myocarditis, including *Corynebacterium, Salmonella, Mycobacterium,* streptococci, *Neisseria, Leptospira, Borrelia, Rickettsia typhi,* and *Rickettsia tsutsugamushi.* Fungal agents include *Aspergillus, Blastomyces, Cryptococcus, Candida,* and *Coccidioides immitis.* The protozoa *Trypanosoma* (Chagas disease) is an important cause of myocarditis in South America, causing death in 10 percent of acute attacks or a late (10 to 20 years later) cardiac insufficiency in many patients who survive the acute disease. The metazoa *Trichinella* and *Echinococcus* can also cause myocarditis. The histologic pattern associated with nonviral infectious myocarditis varies with the etiologic agent.

Myocarditis can be caused by viruses, other infectious agents, and immune-mediated reactions.

A variety of **immune-mediated reactions** can cause noninfectious inflammation of the myocardium, including immune-mediated systemic diseases such as rheumatic fever, systemic lupus erythematosus, and systemic sclerosis; allergic reactions to drugs including methyldopa, sulfonamides, penicillin, streptomycin, and para-aminosalicylic acid; and rejection of a cardiac transplant. These immune-related reactions tend to produce a myocarditis with an inflammatory infiltrate that can contain lymphocytes, plasma cells, macrophages, and eosinophils. The inflammatory infiltrate is frequently perivascular, and a true acute vasculitis with vessel necrosis is occasionally seen. **Miscellaneous causes** of myocarditis include radiation, heat stroke, sarcoidosis, giant cell myocarditis, Fiedler's myocarditis, and Kawasaki disease.

CARDIOMYOPATHY

Cardiomyopathies are noninflammatory processes that affect cardiac muscle.

The term **cardiomyopathy** is used for a group of noninflammatory processes that affect the heart muscle. Explicitly excluded are myocardial diseases related to hypertension, congenital pathology, and valvular or epicardial pathology. Cardiomyopathies of idiopathic origin are called primary cardiomyopathies. Secondary cardiomyopathies can be due to causes such as cobalt toxicity, lithium toxicity, muscular dystrophy, or hemochromatosis. The cardiomyopathies have been traditionally subdivided into dilated (congestive), hypertrophic, and restrictive (obliterative).

Dilated Cardiomyopathy

Dilated cardiopathy can be related to alcohol abuse, pregnancy, or other causes.

In **dilated** (congestive) **cardiomyopathy,** the heart is large, (up to 900 g), flabby, and shows at most only vague, nonspecific changes, such as hypertrophy or atrophy of occasional myocytes and slight increase in interstitial fibrous tissue. Functionally, patients with dilated cardiomyopathy have hypocontracting hearts and develop slowly progressive congestive heart failure. Only one-quarter of patients survive for 5 years. Death may be the result of cardiac failure, arrhythmias, or intracardiac thrombi with resulting systemic or pulmonary emboli. Dilated cardiomyopathy can present at any age, including childhood. While the etiology is unknown, several pathogenic pathways are suspected as contributing to some cases.

Alcohol abuse appears to be a contributing factor in some cases, with possible pathologic mechanisms including direct alcohol toxicity, nutritional deficits, or cobalt (a former additive to beer) toxicity. Dilated cardiomyopathy is sometimes identified in the **peripartum** period between 1 month before and 1 month after delivery, most often in impoverished patients who have had multiple pregnancies. Some patients recover from peripartum cardiomyopathy, but others do not and may die during a subsequent pregnancy. Suspected causes include nutritional deficiency, hypertension, and volume overload. **Genetic influences** are suspected when dilated cardiomyopathy is found in multiple family members, but no consistent inheritance pattern or biochemical defect has been identified. **Postviral myocarditis,** possibly with an autoimmune component, has also been postulated as a cause for some cases of dilated cardiomyopathy.

Hypertrophic Cardiomyopathy

Hypertrophic cardiomyopathy (idiopathic hypertrophic subaortic stenosis, asymmetric septal hypertrophy, hypertrophic obstructive cardiomyopathy) is an idiopathic condition characterized by cardiac enlargement with myocardial hypertrophy. This hypertrophy produces a hypercontracting heart in contrast to the hypocontracting heart of dilated cardiomyopathy. Often, but not always, there is a disproportionate hypertrophy of the interventricular septum compared with the left ventricular free wall.

In some cases, thickening of the septum at the level of the mitral valve can alter the cardiac hemodynamics sufficiently to produce **obstructive hypertrophic cardiomyopathy.** Microscopically, many of the myocytes are hypertrophied, show disarray of myofilaments, and are arranged in a haphazard pattern. A delicate interstitial fibrosis is usually present. These changes may be absent in some affected hearts. Hypertrophic cardiomyopathy is usually seen in young adults, but may also present in the elderly. In many patients, a genetic predisposition (autosomal dominant) appears to be present. The cardiomyopathy is often asymptomatic. Clinical manifestations can include dyspnea, angina, dizziness, and congestive heart failure. Since the cardiac output is characterized by rapid emptying of a small stroke volume, the patient's symptoms may paradoxically improve as mild congestive failure develops. **Sudden death** can occur in affected patients who exercise strenuously. Death can also occur as a consequence of either infective endocarditis involving the mitral valve or of atrial fibrillation with mural thrombus formation and subsequent embolization.

> The myocardial hypertrophy in hypertrophic cardiopathy may alter cardiac hemodynamics.

Restrictive Cardiomyopathy

Restrictive (infiltrative, obliterative) **cardiomyopathy** refers to a group of rare conditions characterized by restriction of cardiac filling. **Cardiac amyloidosis** may affect only the heart, or it may be a manifestation of systemic amyloidosis. Mild, asymptomatic cardiac amyloid deposition is frequently seen in the hearts of elderly individuals (**senile isolated cardiac amyloidosis**). More severe cardiac amyloidosis can restrict the heart's ability to dilate and induce arrhythmias.

Endomyocardial fibrosis is an idiopathic disease observed in African children and young adults and is characterized by a predominantly subendocardial fibrosis that may extend into the myocardium. An inflammatory infiltrate, which may contain eosinophils, is often present at the junction between the scarring and the preserved myocardium. Contraction of the scars produces a restrictive cardiomyopathy.

Löffler's endocarditis also produces an endomyocardial fibrosis. The fibrosis is similar to that observed in the African form of endomyocardial fibrosis, and it is thought that the two diseases may by variants of a single pathologic process. Löffler's endocarditis is observed principally in the temperate zones. The disease is characterized by focal myocardial necrosis with a prominent eosinophilic infiltrate that progresses to scarring of the necrotic areas. The endocardium becomes layered with thrombus, which subsequently organizes to produce endomyocardial fibrosis. Löffler's endocarditis is frequently accompanied by eosinophilic leukocytosis accompanied by eosinophilic infiltration of visceral organs. The clinical course tends to progress rapidly to death.

> Restrictive cardiomyopathy may be due to amyloidosis, endomyocardial fibrosis, Löffler's endocarditis, or endocardial fibroelastosis.

Endocardial fibroelastosis is an uncommon idiopathic disease characterized by a diffuse or patchy thickening of the endocardium. The thickening is due to a marked increase of collagenous and elastic fibers that sometimes extend into the left ventricle; other cardiac chambers may also be involved. Additional findings may include mural thrombi, flattened trabeculae cornae, aortic or mitral stenosis, and cardiac enlargement secondary to left ventricular hypertrophy or dilation. The etiology of endocardial fibroelastosis is unclear, and may be a common final pathway that can be triggered by a variety of diseases. Endocardial fibroelastosis is most common in the first 2 years of life. About one-third of cases are accompanied by congenital heart defects. In infants with diffuse fibroelastosis, cardiac failure can progress rapidly to death. The disease progresses more slowly in older children and adults, and patients with only focal fibroelastosis may be asymptomatic and have normal longevity.

Secondary Cardiomyopathy

Secondary cardiomyopathy has many causes.

Secondary cardiomyopathy can be caused by many pathologic processes. **Toxic agents** that have been associated with cardiomyopathies include alcohol, chemotherapeutic agents (cyclophosphamides, doxorubicin, daunorubicin), other drugs (catecholamines, lithium), and poisons (cobalt, carbon monoxide, hydrocarbons, arsenic). **Metabolic diseases** associated with cardiomyopathy include hyperthyroidism, hypothyroidism, hyperkalemia, hypokalemia, hemochromatosis, and nutritional deficiencies. **Neuromuscular diseases** (Friedreich's ataxia, muscular dystrophy, congenital anomalies) and **storage disorders** (Hunter-Hurler syndrome, glycogen storage disease, Fabry's disease, Sandhoff's disease) can also cause cardiomyopathies. Miscellaneous causes include leukemia, carcinomatosis, and sarcoidosis. Of these causes, the pattern of injury seen after toxic injury to the myocardium is best defined; it typically consists of mitochondrial changes followed by myofiber swelling with fatty change and myocyte necrosis. In patients who survive, the healing may be complete, or a mild interstitial fibrosis may develop.

CARDIAC TUMORS

Benign primary cardiac tumors include myxomas, lipomas, papillary fibroelastomas, and rhabdomyomas.

Metastatic disease affects the heart far more commonly than do primary tumors. Pericardial involvement can produce arrhythmias, congestive heart failure, and obstruction of blood flow through the heart. Tumors that commonly metastasize to the to the heart include lung cancer, breast cancer, melanoma, lymphoma, and leukemia. Primary tumors of the heart are rare. **Myxomas** are the most common primary tumor of the heart. These benign tumors are composed of abundant mucopolysaccharide ground substance and a variety of cells derived from primitive mesenchymal cells, including stellate or globular myxoma cells, mature or immature smooth muscle cells, endothelial cells, and macrophages. The tumors can form sometimes large (up to 10 cm) sessile or pedunculated, subendocardial masses. The sessile lesions may grossly resemble an organizing thrombus. The pedunculated lesions often have a soft, translucent, myxoid appearance. Myxomas can occur at any age and have a female predominance. The lesions, particularly the pedunculated myxomas, are significant primarily because they can create ball-valve obstructions that can damage cardiac valves and block blood flow, causing syncopal attacks and even sudden death in apparently healthy children and adults. Surgical removal is the treatment of choice, although local recurrence can occur.

Lipomas are benign, poorly encapsulated proliferations of fat cells that can be found in the myocardium from subendocardial to subpericardial sites. The tumors can be up to 10 cm in diameter and can cause ball-valve obstructions and arrhythmias. **Papillary fibroelastomas** are usually incidental lesions found most often on the cardiac valves. Papillary fibroelastomas have a distinctive, fuzzy, gross appearance produced by clustering of hairlike projections. The projections are covered with endothelium and contain myxoid connective tissue, smooth muscle cells, and fibroblasts. **Rhabdomyomas** are uncommon, benign tumors composed of a mixed population of cells that can be demonstrated to be of myocyte lineage by the presence of myofibrils. One distinctive cell type seen is the "spider cell," which is a large, polygonal cell containing a central nucleus and glycogen-laden vacuoles separated by cytoplasmic strands (resembling spider legs). Other cells can be spindle-shaped or resemble histiocytes. The tumors form gray-white myocardial masses that can obstruct valves or cardiac chambers. Tuberous sclerosis can coexist with cardiac rhabdomyomas, which suggests that the tumors may actually be hamartomas. **Malignant angiosarcomas and rhabdomyosarcomas,** resembling those seen elsewhere in the body, affect the heart less commonly than do benign tumors.

Malignant tumors uncommonly affect the heart.

RHEUMATOID HEART DISEASE

Rheumatoid arthritis is a systemic disease that can involve the heart in 20 to 40 percent of severe cases. Cardiac findings that can be observed include fibrinous pericarditis, which sometimes heals as dense fibrous pericardial adhesions; rheumatoid nodules of the myocardium, endocardium, valves, or root of the aorta; and rheumatoid valvulitis that resembles chronic rheumatic valvular disease.

Rheumatoid arthritis, like rheumatic fever, can affect all layers of the heart.

ENDOCARDIAL AND VALVULAR DISEASE

Calcific Aortic Valve Stenosis

Age-related degenerative calcifications can affect the aortic valve, producing **calcific aortic valve stenosis.** These calcifications most frequently become clinically significant in the eighth and ninth decades of life in patients with previously normal valves, and one or two decades earlier in patients with congenital bicuspid valves. The valves in calcific aortic stenosis become fibrotically thickened and contain calcified masses that distort the cusp architecture and limit left ventricular outflow. Compensation occurs by development of concentric left ventricular hypertrophy. As the stenosis progresses, the patient may experience

Calcific aortic valve stenosis is observed in elderly individuals.

angina, syncope, sudden death, or cardiac decompensation. Treatment is by surgical replacement of the valve, or, in selected cases, balloon aortic valvuloplasty.

Mitral Valve Prolapse

Mitral valve prolapse is characterized by ballooning of one or both valve leaflets back into the left atrium during cardiac systole. The ballooning occurs because the valve leaflet is structurally weakened by changes including degeneration and thinning of the zona fibrosa and compensatory thickening of the weaker zona spongiosa. Replacement of muscle by loose connective tissue causes lengthening and sometimes rupture of adjacent chordae tendinea. The basis for the histologic changes is unknown. Mitral valve prolapse is a very common disorder with a modest female predominance. Patients are usually identified when a distinctive **midsystolic click** is heard on auscultation. Most individuals with mitral valve prolapse are asymptomatic throughout their lives. A small percentage experience complications including infective endocarditis, insufficiency, arrhythmias, and (rarely) sudden death.

Rheumatic Fever and Rheumatic Heart Disease

Pharyngeal infection with **group A streptococci** can be followed by the acute inflammatory disease **rheumatic fever,** which can affect many organ systems. Rheumatic fever is probably a result of either cross-reactivity of tissue antigens with streptococcal antigens, or triggering of an autoimmune response by an unknown mechanism. Acute rheumatic fever is most frequently observed in children and adolescents 1 to 5 weeks after streptococcal pharyngitis.

Acute rheumatic fever can cause a variety of problems. **Acute carditis** affects over one-half of children, and somewhat fewer adults, during the first attack of acute rheumatic fever. The pathognomonic lesions in the acute carditis, **Aschoff bodies,** are foci of fibrinoid necrosis within an inflammatory infiltrate that initially contains predominantly lymphocytes and macrophages and may later contain multinucleate giant cells. The infiltrate later also contains plump cells (**Anitschkow or Aschoff cells)** with abundant cytoplasm and distinctive nuclei containing a ("caterpillar"-like) wavy ribbon of chromatin. The carditis of acute rheumatic fever may involve all tissue layers of the heart, producing fibrinous or serofibrinous pericarditis, myocarditis, and endocarditis. Maplike subendocardial thickenings, particularly in the left atrium, are called **MacCallum's plaques. Veruccae,** which are small foci of fibrinoid necrosis covered with small, wartlike, friable vegetations, are found most often on the cardiac valves, particularly along the lines of cusp closure where the leaflets touch. Acute involvement of the mitral and aortic valves can produce regurgitation, which can be heard on auscultation as murmurs.

A **migratory polyarthritis** that affects the large joints, (e.g., knees), usually accompanied by **fever,** is often the presenting complaint. The arthritis is characterized histologically by edema, focal fibrinoid deposits, and a nonspecific mononuclear inflammatory infiltrate. Damage to synovial membranes or articular cartilage does not usually occur. The **skin** in acute rheumatic fever may show either subcutaneous nodules, com-

Mitral valve prolapse is characterized by degeneration of the zona fibrosa.

Rheumatic fever may be related to cross-reactivity of tissue antigens with streptococcal antigens.

The carditis of acute rheumatic fever may involve all tissue layers of the heart.

Other features of acute rheumatic fever can include arthritis, rash, arteritis, pneumonitis, and Sydenham's chorea.

posed of a central area of fibrin and necrosis surrounded by cells similar to those seen in Aschoff bodies, or erythema marginatum, which is a distinctive rash with a cleared center and darkly erythematous edges. The coronary, renal, mesenteric, and cerebral arteries may show **rheumatoid arteritis,** which strongly resembles hypersensitivity angitis. The lungs rarely develop pleuritis or a **pneumonitis** that resembles viral pneumonia. **Sydenham's chorea** is a neurologic disorder observed in acute rheumatic fever and characterized by rapid, purposeless, involuntary movements.

A few patients die from fulminant rheumatic fever, usually of cardiac complications. The remaining patients are vulnerable to recurrence of acute rheumatic fever with subsequent pharyngeal infections. Patients who do not experience carditis on the first attack usually do not experience it on subsequent attacks, and may have no long-term sequelae. Patients with carditis tend to have progressive cardiac involvement, and, in particular, valvular disease, with each recurrence. In time, the heart may develop **chronic rheumatic heart disease** characterized by thickened, blunted cardiac valve leaflets, often with calcifications and fibrous bridging between leaflets, which creates **stenotic valves** described as "fish mouth" or "buttonhole." The mitral valve is most frequently involved without accompanying aortic valve involvement; tricuspid valve involvement occurs rarely. The mitral stenosis causes left atrial dilation, and, eventually, pulmonary congestion with right ventricular hypertrophy. Histologically, Aschoff bodies are no longer recognizable, and the rheumatic heart disease is most easily identified by the characteristic appearance of involved valves. Rheumatic heart disease was formerly a major cause of cardiac death. This pattern has been markedly modified by the use of antibiotics for prophylaxis against streptococcal pharyngitis with risk of recurrent acute rheumatic fever. Additionally, early diagnosis of rheumatic valvular disease can permit surgical replacement of the valves before irreparable damage to the myocardium has occurred.

Chronic rheumatic heart disease is predominantly a valvular disease.

Infective Endocarditis

In **infective endocarditis,** friable vegetations develop on heart valves or mural endocardium as a consequence of colonization or invasion by bacteria or (rarely) fungi. The morphology of the vegetative lesions is similar, with different pathogens. The vegetations are friable, bulky masses, up to several centimeters in diameter, that are found at the free margins of the valve leaflets. Histologically, they are composed of fibrinous deposits that often contain large numbers of bacteria. Infective endocarditis is classified based on the clinical setting in which it is observed. In **acute endocarditis,** virulent organisms (*Staphylococcus aureus*) usually infect a previously normal heart, causing valvular disease with bulky vegetations and a predisposition for complications related to necrotizing infection, such as valve perforation or myocardial abscess. Acute endocarditis tends to present fulminantly with fever, chills, and weakness; complications generally occur within several weeks of onset of the disease. In **subacute endocarditis,** less virulent organisms (streptococcal species) usually colonize a heart previously damaged by diseases such as rheumatic fever or congenital heart disease. The vegetations are usually smaller and the necrotizing complications less common than in acute endocarditis, but they are more apt to involve the mural endocardium adjacent to the valve. In hearts with nonvalvular

Friable vegetations develop on valves in endocarditis.

Acute endocarditis has a more fulminant course than subacute endocarditis.

congenital defects such as a ventricular septal defect, the vegetations are usually located near the defect in areas "downstream" in the aberrant blood flow. Subacute endocarditis may cause only fatigue and weight loss.

Intravenous drug abusers, as a consequence of introduction of organisms (*Staphylococcus aureus, Candida, Aspergillus*) by injection, are prone to develop an endocarditis that characteristically affects the right side of the heart. **Prosthetic valve recipients** can have colonization of the prosthesis by organisms (*Staphylococcus aureus*) that are sometimes sufficiently resistant to antibiotic therapy to require replacement of the prosthesis. The vegetations are usually located at the interface between the prosthesis and the host heart, where they can cause a ring abscess that may progress to paravalvular perforation, sometimes with dislocation of the prosthesis. Other predisposing factors for endocarditis include neutropenia, immunodeficiency, and indwelling catheter use. With any form of endocarditis, a positive blood culture is considered necessary to prove the presence of infective endocarditis. A wide variety of bacteria, and some fungi, have been isolated from patients with infective endocarditis. Commonly encountered bacteria in addition to those mentioned above include *Streptococcus pneumoniae* and gram-negative bacilli such as *Escherichia coli* and *Neisseria gonorrhoeae*.

Endocarditis can produce a variety of complications. Cardiac complications include valvular insufficiency, myocardial abscess, suppurative pericarditis, and artificial valve dehiscence. Embolic complications and metastatic infections can arise as bacteria or vegetations are released into the blood stream. Right-sided vegetations seed to the lungs, while left-sided lesions seed to the body; brain, spleen, and kidneys are favored sites. Renal complications, in addition to embolic infarction and metastatic abscess formation, include focal or diffuse glomerulonephritis, which may cause nephrotic syndrome or renal failure. The prognosis of endocarditis was formerly poor, but has been markedly modified by aggressive antibiotic therapy coupled with, when appropriate, surgical replacement of damaged valves before intractable cardiac failure develops.

Nonbacterial Thrombotic Endocarditis

Nonbacterial thrombotic endocarditis (marantic endocarditis) is characterized by small, sterile vegetations that form as fibrin and other blood elements precipitate, most commonly along the line of closure of valve leaflets. A single, loosely attached, vegetation is seen more commonly than multiple vegetations. Nonbacterial thrombotic endocarditis is usually observed at autopsy in patients who have died after protracted illness (e.g., cancer, renal failure, or sepsis) and who may have had a hypercoaguable state or possible endocardial trauma secondary to Swan-Ganz catheterization. The vegetations are usually of little clinical significance but can produce embolic infarction in sites such as the brain, kidneys, or lungs.

Endocarditis of Systemic Lupus Erythematosus

Systemic lupus erythematosus can produce sterile vegetations (**Libman-Sacks disease**) that can resemble either those of ineffective

---

Intravenous drug abusers and prosthetic valve recipients may develop endocarditis.

Endocarditis has many complications.

Nonbacterial thrombotic endocarditis may be related to a hypercoagulable state or endocardial trauma.

endocarditis or nonbacterial thrombotic endocarditis. The subjacent valves can develop fibrinoid necrosis with mucoid pooling, which can progress to collagenous fibrosis. Surgical repair or replacement of the affected valves is sometimes required.

Calcification of the Mitral Anulus

Calcium can be deposited as irregular beads in the **anulus of the mitral valve.** This condition is seen most often in elderly individuals with ischemic heart disease. The deposits may become sufficiently severe to interfere with systolic contraction of the mitral valve ring, leading to mitral regurgitation. Other complications occasionally encountered include arrhythmias and infective endocarditis in the overlying endothelium.

The mitral anulus of elderly individuals may calcify.

Carcinoid Heart Disease

The **carcinoid syndrome** is a cluster of distinctive **physiologic symptoms** characterized by flushing of skin; vomiting and diarrhea; and asthmalike bronchoconstrictive episodes. The carcinoid syndrome is observed in some patients with carcinoid tumors (argentaffinomas), particularly those with liver metastases, and is thought to be secondary to release of a wide variety of bioactive products, including serotonin and bradykinin. In addition to the physiologic symptoms, **cardiac lesions** are present in about one-half of patients with carcinoid syndrome. The carcinoid lesions usually take the form of plaquelike thickenings resembling atheromas and involve the endocardium of the cardiac chambers and valvular cusps. The outflow tract of the right ventricle is most commonly affected. The pathogenesis of the lesions is still unclear, but may be related to one or more of the bioactive products released by the tumors.

Bioactive products produced by carcinoid tumors may produce endocardial lesions.

Complications of Artificial Valves

While **prosthetic replacement** of damaged cardiac valves can be life-saving, it can also predispose for a variety of complications including ineffective endocarditis, paravalvular leaks, thromboemboli, and structural deterioration.

PERICARDIAL DISEASE

Pericardial Effusions and Hemopericardium

The pericardial sac can accumulate fluid. **Pericardial effusions** are accumulations of noninflammatory fluid that may take several forms. The most common are **serous effusions,** which are sterile, watery, clear to straw-colored fluid accumulations caused by hydrostatic processes favoring flow of fluid into the extravascular space, including congestive heart failure and hypoproteinemia secondary to renal, hepatic, or nutritional disease. Much less common are serosanguineous effusions

Both effusions and blood may fill the pericardial sac, sometimes compromising cardiac function.

secondary to blunt trauma including cardiopulmonary resuscitation; chylous effusions secondary to lymphatic obstruction; and effusions containing cholesterol crystals of idiopathic etiology or secondary to myxedema. Small effusions do not usually produce symptoms; large effusions, most commonly serous effusions, may require withdrawal, as they can compromise cardiac filling. **Hemopericardium** is the accumulation of pure blood in the pericardial sac. Common causes of hemopericardium include rupture of a dissecting aortic aneurysm within the pericardial sac, and rupture of the cardiac wall secondary to trauma or myocardial infarction. Less common causes include cardiopulmonary resuscitation, tumor, and bleeding diatheses. Like pericardial effusions, large volumes of blood in the pericardial sac, which may accumulate rapidly, can compromise cardiac filling, potentially leading to death.

Pericarditis

Pericarditis is subclassified based upon the type of exudate produced.

Pericarditis is inflammation of the pericardium. **Serous pericarditis** is characterized by the presence of a serous effusion in the pericardial sac and a scant inflammatory infiltrate (neutrophils, histiocytes, lymphocytes) in the epicardial and pericardial surfaces. Many pathologic processes can cause pericarditis, including systemic diseases such as rheumatic fever, systemic lupus erythematosus, and progressive systemic sclerosis; uremia; tumors; an adjacent bacterial pleuritis; and viruses including coxsackie A or B virus, Echovirus type 8, adenovirus, influenza virus, and mumps virus. Serous pericarditis can also be idiopathic. Serous pericarditis usually develops slowly and does not cause cardiac compromise. When the underlying disease remits, the serous effusion is often resorbed without development of fibrous adhesions.

Unlike the serous form, fibrinous pericarditis and purulent pericarditis tend to produce fibrous adhesions.

Fibrinous pericarditis and serofibrinous pericarditis are characterized by accumulation of a fibrinous exudate containing more or less admixed serous fluid. With time, the fibrinous exudate may either be digested or may organize, producing delicate, fibrous adhesions (adhesive pericarditis), which do not usually restrict cardiac motion. Causes of fibrinous and serofibrinous pericarditis include myocardial infarction; uremia; radiotherapy; rheumatic fever and systemic lupus erythematosus; bacterial or viral infection; and trauma including cardiac surgery. Fibrinous pericarditis characteristically produces a loud pericardial friction rub that may be accompanied, depending on the etiology, by pain, fever, or signs of cardiac failure.

Purulent or suppurative pericarditis causes the accumulation of a thin to creamy, puslike exudate that has a strong tendency to heal with formation of dense fibrous adhesions, causing **constrictive pericarditis.** Purulent pericarditis is usually caused by infections from bacteria, fungi, or parasites; less common causes include severe viral infections of the heart and sterile inflammation such as myocardial infarction or uremia. **Mediastinopericarditis** is produced if the inflammatory process extends outside the pericardial sac. The clinical findings in purulent pericarditis are similar to those in fibrinous pericarditis, although the friction rub is usually less prominent.

Hemorrhagic and caseous pericarditis can both be observed in tuberculosis.

Hemorrhagic pericarditis produces an exudate containing both blood and a fibrinous or suppurative effusion. Tubercular or tumorous involvement of the pericardial space are the most common causes, but hemorrhagic pericarditis can also be caused by bleeding diatheses, cardiac surgery, and bacterial infections. **Caseous pericarditis** refers to the presence of caseating granulomas in the pericardium. The cause is usually tuberculosis, but may rarely be mycotic infections. Caseous pericarditis tends to progress to constrictive pericarditis that may contain calcifications.

Pericarditis can resolve completely or can heal with varying degrees of fibrous adhesions. Clinically important forms of healed pericarditis include adhesive mediastinopericarditis and constrictive pericarditis. In **adhesive mediastinopericarditis,** the pericardial sac is obliterated by adherence of the parietal to the visceral pericardium. This produces a great strain on the heart, leading to massive cardiac hypertrophy and dilation, since each contraction must move both the cardiac wall and all of the adjacent thoracic structures. Adhesive mediastinopericarditis can be seen following suppurative or caseous pericarditis; cardiac surgery; or radiotherapy to the mediastinum. In **constrictive pericarditis,** the pericardium is replaced by a dense, fibrous, or fibrocalcific scar that restricts cardiac output by limiting the degree to which the heart can expand during diastole. While in some cases a history of suppurative or caseous pericarditis can be elicited, no pertinent history is identified in many cases, suggesting that the original damage may have been relatively mild and occurred many years previously. In extreme cases, the calcifications and fibrosis become so severe that the heart appears to be encased in plaster **(concretiocordis).** In contrast to adhesive mediastinopericarditis, the heart is usually small in constrictive pericarditis.

Adhesive mediastinopericarditis and constrictive pericarditis are both characterized by extensive fibrosis.

12

Digestive System
ESOPHAGUS

NONTUMOROUS CONDITIONS

Congenital Anomalies

The esophagus is vulnerable to congenital defects. The defects can be accompanied by other congenital malformations, particularly of the trachea, bronchi, heart, and other parts of the gastrointestinal tract. Severe congenital defects of the esophagus are typically identified shortly after birth when feeding is attempted and the infant experiences symptoms such as excessive salivation, vomiting, coughing, or paroxysmal suffocation secondary to aspiration. True **agenesis** (or absence) of the esophagus is very rare and may be either partial or complete. **Atresia,** which is more common than agenesis, is congenital narrowing of the esophagus, typically at the level of the tracheal bifurcation, to form a lumenless cord. Tracheoesophageal and bronchoesophageal **fistulae** may coexist with atresia or may occur independently. Many variants exist; in the most common, the proximal esophagus ends in a blind pouch and the distal esophagus communicates superiorly with the trachea or a bronchus. **Stenosis** of the esophagus can be either congenital or acquired secondary to tumor, scleroderma, or scarring.

> Congenital anomalies of the esophagus often coexist with other congenital anomalies.

Acquired Anatomic Defects

A variety of acquired anatomic defects, in addition to the stenosis described above, can be seen in the esophagus. **Esophageal webs** are smooth mucosal ledges present most typically in the upper esophagus of women over 40. Webs were traditionally associated with iron deficiency anemia and atrophic glossitis (Plummer-Vinson syndrome), but this association may be coincidental. **Esophageal rings** (Schatzki's rings) are observed in the lower esophagus and consist of a rim of fibrovascular tissue that is typically covered superiorly by stratified squamous epithelium and inferiorly by columnar epithelium. Some patients have an accompanying hiatal hernia. **Sliding hiatal hernias** occur when the esophagus ends above the diaphragm secondary to either a congenitally

> Acquired anatomic defects include webs, rings, hernias, diverticula, and lacerations.

short esophagus or acquired fibrous scarring applying upward traction to the esophagus. The thoracic portion of the stomach forms a symmetric dilation. **Paraesophageal hiatal hernias** occur when the cardiac stomach dissects through a paraesophageal defect in the diaphragmatic hiatus. Paraesophageal hernias are much less common than sliding hernias and produce an asymmetrical outpouching vulnerable to strangulation and infarction.

Esophageal **diverticula** occur in two forms. **Pulsion** (Zenker's) diverticula are the result of chronic intrapharyngeal pressure and typically occur in the upper third of the esophagus at the insertion of the cricopharyngeal muscle. **Traction** diverticula are the result of extraesophageal traction by scar tissue and typically occur in the lower two-thirds of the esophagus. **Lacerations** of the esophagus typically occur at the gastroesophageal junction following prolonged vomiting (Mallory-Weiss syndrome), possibly as a result of failure of appropriately timed relaxation by the fatigued gastroesophageal junction. The lacerations are typically irregular, superficial or deep, longitudinal tears millimeters to centimeters in length. The lacerations are seen most commonly in chronic alcoholics and may cause massive hematemesis. **Scleroderma** can cause fibrosis throughout the gastrointestinal tract that is most severe in the lower two-thirds of the esophagus and is associated with mucosal thinning and ulceration, as well as "rubber-hose" inflexibility due to excessive collagenization of the lamina propria and submucosa.

Varices

Portal hypertension can cause esophageal varices.

Portal hypertension of any cause, notably alcoholic cirrhosis, induces formation of dilated shunts between the portal and systemic circulations. These shunts can occur between the coronary veins of the stomach and the plexus of esophageal submucosal veins, causing dilated tortuous vessels known as **esophageal varices.** Varices typically produce no symptoms until they rupture, when they can cause massive hematemesis, which may cause death. Approximately one-half of patients with massive hematemesis subsequently rebleed. Sclerotherapy, in which varices are thrombosed, delays rupture but is usually eventually unsuccessful due to formation of new varices.

Achalasia

Achalasia is a motor dysfunction that causes dysphagia.

Dysphagia, or difficult swallowing, can be seen with any of the tumors, congenital defects, or acquired anatomic defects described in this chapter. Alternatively, it can be the result of a motor dysfunction known as **achalasia.** Achalasia appears to involve a defect or derangement of innervation of the esophagus that leads to abnormalities identified by manometric studies. These abnormalities can include failure of peristalsis; partial or complete failure of relaxation of the lower esophageal sphincter; or increased basal tone of the lower esophageal sphincter. The etiology is unknown, with the exception of achalasia from infection with the parasite *Trypanosoma cruzi* (Chagas disease), which causes destruction of the myenteric plexus throughout the gut. Achalasia is associated with the retention of food in the esophagus, which increases the risk of aspiration and of development of squamous carcinoma.

Esophagitis

Inflammation of the esophagus may be asymptomatic or may cause dysphagia, retrosternal pain, hematemesis, or melena. **Esophagitis** is associated with many causes including gastric reflux; intubation; alcohol or smoking; ingestion of hot fluids (tea); bacterial, viral, or fungal infections (notably in immunosuppressed patients); suicide attempts by ingestion of acids or bases; uremia; and radiation or chemotherapy. Despite this diversity of causes, most esophagitis is associated with reflux of gastric contents. Reflux esophagitis alters the squamous epithelium of the esophagus, causing basal zone hyperplasia, extension of subepithelial papillae into the superficial third of the epithelium, and intraepithelial infiltration by eosinophils and sometimes neutrophils. Persistent gastroesophageal reflux can cause mucosal metaplasia with gastric or intestinal-type mucosa **(Barrett's mucosa).** Barrett's mucosa is associated with increased risk of dysplasia, ulceration, stricture, and adenocarcinoma.

Reflux of gastric contents is the most common cause of esophagitis.

TUMORS

Both benign and malignant tumors can affect the esophagus. **Benign tumors** are rarely large enough to cause symptoms and are typically located within the esophageal wall. Leiomyomas are most common, but many other benign tumors have been identified.

Squamous Cell Carcinoma

Squamous cell carcinoma is the most common malignant tumor of the esophagus. The tumors can arise throughout the esophagus, most commonly in the middle third. They are found in adults over 50 and are associated with many risk factors including diet (fungal contamination of food, nitrites and nitrosamines, vitamin and trace metal deficiencies); esophageal disorders that delay food transit (achalasia, diverticula); alcohol and tobacco use; and genetic predisposition (celiac disease, ectodermal dysplasia, epidermolysis bullosa). Early squamous cell carcinomas form small, plaquelike thickenings of the esophageal mucosa that may preferentially extend along the longitudinal axis of the esophagus. Larger lesions are usually moderately to well-differentiated squamous carcinomas that may take three morphologic forms, listed below in order of prevalence.

Squamous cell carcinoma often arises in the middle third of the esophagus.

    Polypoid fungating lesions protrude into the esophageal lumen causing dysphagia and obstruction earlier than other forms. **Deeply ulcerating lesions** invade the esophageal wall and can erode into the adjacent trachea or bronchi (causing aspiration with pneumonia or sepsis), aorta (causing hemorrhage), or mediastinum and pericardium. **Diffuse infiltrative lesions** cause thickening and rigidity of the esophageal wall and sometimes show superficial ulceration of the mucosa. Staging of esophageal carcinoma is based on length along the axis and extension into adjacent structures. Cervical lymph nodes drain the upper third of esophagus; mediastinal, paratracheal, and tracheobronchial nodes drain the middle third; and gastric and celiac nodes drain the lower third. The prognosis of squamous cell carcinoma of the esophagus is poor because resectable lesions are rarely identified, and radiation therapy is rarely curative.

Adenocarcinoma

Adenocarcinoma of the esophagus often arises in areas of mucosal metaplasia.

Adenocarcinoma of the esophagus usually arises in areas of gastric or intestinal mucosal metaplasia **(Barrett's mucosa)** in the lower or middle third of the esophagus. Adenocarcinomas typically occur after age 40 with a strong male predominance and are rare among blacks. The tumors may be multicentric. Histologic variants, usually composed of moderately to poorly differentiated cells, include the intestinal type, with well-formed glands lined by neoplastic cells; the adenosquamous type, composed of both adenocarcinoma and squamous carcinoma; and the diffuse type with infiltration of the esophageal wall by mucin-producing neoplastic cells that do not form well-defined glands. The clinical course, prognosis, and staging of adenocarcinoma of the esophagus are similar to squamous cell carcinoma.

STOMACH

CONGENITAL ANOMALIES AND MISCELLANEOUS LESIONS

Congenital anomalies that affect the stomach include diaphragmatic hernias and pyloric stenosis. **Diaphragmatic hernias** occur when congenital weakness or absence of a portion of the diaphragm (usually the left) allows herniation of the stomach and sometimes small intestine into the chest. Large diaphragmatic hernias compress the lungs and are incompatible with life after birth. **Congenital hypertrophic pyloric stenosis** is a hypertrophy of the muscularis propria of the pyloris that appears to have a multifactorial genetic basis. The stenosis causes regurgitation and vomiting in the second or third week of life and can be cured by incision of the pyloris **(pyloromyotomy).** Acquired forms of pyloric stenosis are seen in adulthood as complications of chronic lesions close to the pyloris (gastritis, peptic ulcers, carcinomas, lymphomas).

Miscellaneous lesions that can affect the stomach include gastric dilation and gastric rupture. **Massive gastric dilation** (up to 10 to 15 liters) can follow chronic organic or functional pyloric obstruction. The gastric wall is consequently markedly thinned and vulnerable to the medical emergency **gastric rupture,** which can cause massive internal hemorrhage. Gastric rupture can also occur following trauma, massive dietary consumption (beer-drinking competitions), pregnancy labor, and incorrectly performed cardiac resuscitation in which the stomach is inflated with air.

Gastric congenital anomalies include diaphragmatic hernias and congenital hypertrophic pyloric stenosis.

Miscellaneous lesions include massive gastric dilatation and gastric rupture.

GASTRITIS

The stomach is vulnerable to acute and chronic **gastritis.** Specific forms of chronic gastritis that are considered under separate headings are *Helicobacter*-associated, hypertrophic, granulomatous, and eosinophilic.

Acute Gastritis

Acute gastritis is an acute inflammatory process that is typically limited to the gastric mucosa. Mild forms of acute gastritis may show only edema, slight hyperemia, and scattered neutrophils in the lamina propria. In the most severe form, **acute hemorrhagic erosive gastritis,** the surface epithelium sloughs to denude large areas of gastric mucosa. The underlying lamina propria shows hemorrhage and an acute inflammatory infiltrate. Even in severe acute gastritis, the underlying gastric wall is usually spared. The clinical course varies with the severity of the gastritis from asymptomatic to massive hematemesis and acute abdominal pain. Many agents have been implicated in the etiology of acute gas-

Acute gastritis may be mild or may denude large areas of gastric mucosa.

tritis, including drugs (aspirin, cancer chemotherapy); infections and toxins (salmonellosis, staphylococcal food poisoning, uremia); smoking and alcohol use; severe stress (burns, trauma, surgery, shock); and physical damage (gastric irradiation or freezing). Mechanisms of injury typically involve breakdown of the mucosal barrier to acid, hypoperfusion or ischemia, or direct damage to epithelial cells.

Chronic Gastritis

Chronic gastritis can be subclassified based on the severity of the inflammation.

Chronic gastritis is a continuum of lesions that are semiarbitrarily divided into stages. In **chronic superficial gastritis,** the lamina propria and upper third of the gastric mucosa contain an inflammatory infiltrate composed of lymphocytes and plasma cells. Some flattening of the mucosa may be present, but this is not prominent. In **chronic atrophic gastritis,** the chronic inflammatory infiltrate extends to deeper areas of glands. The mucosa becomes thinned and flattened, with glandular atrophy, loss of parietal cells, and increased numbers of either gastric mucous cells or metaplastic intestinal cells with microvilli. In **chronic gastric atrophy,** nearly complete glandular atrophy produces a shiny, glazed mucosa with flattened or absent rugal folds. The epithelial cells are nearly all mucus-secreting goblet cells or metaplastic intestinal cells. A few scattered, cystically dilated glands and abortive, villus-like projections may be present.

Chronic gastritis can alternatively be subclassified based on the sites of worst pathology.

In addition to the stages of chronic gastritis described above, chronic gastritis has been categorized by the sites of worst pathology. **Type A (fundal) gastritis,** also known as autoimmune gastritis, preferentially involves the body-fundic mucosa, with less severe antral involvement. Patients with type A gastritis often have circulating antibodies to intrinsic factor; these antibodies induce an immune response that destroys intrinsic factor-producing gastric parietal cells, secondarily causing decreased acid secretion and a reactive increase in serum gastrin levels. The high gastric pH predisposes for gastric atrophy and intestinal metaplasia. Frank pernicious anemia develops in about one-tenth of cases, and vitamin B_{12} cannot be absorbed by the mucosa. Type A gastritis is associated with other autoimmune diseases, notably Hashimoto's thyroiditis and Addison's disease.

Type B (antral) gastritis principally involves the gastric antrum and is more common than type A gastritis. Type B gastritis is divided into two subtypes: hypersecretory gastritis and environmental (type AB) gastritis. **Hypersecretory gastritis** is characterized by excess acid production, which decreases stomach pH and predisposes for duodenal ulcer (and less commonly gastric ulcer) formation. Gastrin levels are typically normal, and no antibodies or associations with autoimmune diseases are observed. **Type AB (environmental) gastritis** is the most common subgroup of chronic gastritis, has worldwide distribution, and affects all age groups, particularly the elderly. Environmental gastritis is multifactorial, with causes varying throughout the world; it has a strong association with gastric atrophy, intestinal metaplasia, gastric polyps, and gastric cancer. Environmental gastritis is sometimes called chronic atrophic gastritis because of these strong associations. All of the different stages of chronic gastritis discussed previously can coexist in the same stomach. Some parietal cell loss related to the chronic gastric atrophy is often observed, associated with decreased gastric production, but true achlorhydria and pernicious anemia are not observed. There is no association with autoimmune diseases, and antibodies to intrinsic factor are not seen.

Helicobacter Gastritis

Helicobacter (formerly *Campylobacter*) *pyloris* is a curved, spiral or S-shaped bacteria that can colonize the mucous layer overlying the gastric epithelium and surface of the gastric pits. The organism disrupts the mucosal barrier but does not penetrate into the underlying tissue. Neutrophils may be found in the adjacent epithelial lining and superficial lamina propria. *Helicobacter pyloris* has worldwide distribution and has been associated with a variety of gastric conditions including chronic gastritis, gastric and duodenal ulcer disease, and gastric cancer.

The bacteria *Helicobacter pyloris* has been associated with several gastric conditions.

Hypertrophic Gastritis

Several conditions can produce enlarged rugal folds by causing severe hyperplasia of the gastric epithelial cells. These changes are traditionally called **hypertrophic gastritis,** although neither hypertrophy nor inflammatory gastritis are present. Hypertrophic gastritis is important because it must be distinguished from infiltrative cancer or lymphoma of the stomach. The following conditions can cause hypertrophic gastritis. **Menetrier's disease** is an idiopathic hyperplasia of surface mucous cells seen most commonly in older adults; it is associated with excessive mucus secretion. Decreased gastric acid secretion is also seen, secondary to replacement of parietal cells by mucous cells. Menetrier's disease may be asymptomatic or may cause epigastric symptoms; bleeding from rugal erosions; and a protein-losing gastroenteropathy secondary to extensive protein losses in mucus. The mucosa may also become metaplastic, predisposing for gastric carcinoma. **Hypersecretory gastropathy** can be associated with parietal and chief cell hyperplasia and the associated extensive acid and pepsin production. **Gastrinomas** (Zollinger-Ellison syndrome) can cause excessive gastrin secretion leading to gastric gland hyperplasia with excessive acid secretion and sometimes multiple peptic ulcers.

Causes of hypertrophic gastritis include Menetrier's disease, hypersecretory gastropathy, and gastrinomas.

Other Forms of Gastritis

Two other forms of gastritis are less well understood but deserve specific mention. **Granulomatous gastritis** may be seen in younger adults secondary to sarcoidosis or regional enteritis. Alternatively, it may occur as an isolated disorder in middle-aged or older adults. **Eosinophilic gastritis** is characterized by prominent eosinophilic infiltration that may be confined to the mucosa or may penetrate into the gastric wall. Granuloma formation (allergic granulomatosis) or acute vasculitis may also be present.

Granulomatous and eosinophilic gastritis are uncommon forms.

ACUTE GASTRIC EROSIONS AND ULCERATIONS

Severe stress, in many different forms, is associated with the acute development of **focal gastric mucosal defects.** These lesions are acute lesions that are not related to peptic ulcer disease. The lesions form a continuum, with the more superficial lesions being termed acute gastric erosions and the deeper lesions being termed acute ("stress") ulcers. While the mechanisms of injury have not been fully defined, a variety of etiologic factors have been identified. **Intracranial lesions** that can

Severe stress, in many different forms, is associated with the development of acute gastric erosions.

increase intracranial pressure (trauma, tumors, surgery) directly stimulate vagal nuclei to induce acid hypersecretion, with the resultant formation of acute erosions and ulcers. Ulcers associated with increased intracranial pressure are called **Cushing's ulcers** and are contrasted with other acute ulcers by the low gastric pH. Processes causing **mucosal hypoxia,** possibly due to catecholamine-induced or neurogenic vasoconstriction, are associated with direct injury to mucosal cells and with indirect damage secondary to back-diffusion of hydrogen ions through a damaged mucosal barrier. These problems can be exacerbated if systemic acidosis, which is common in shock states, is also present. **Exogenous agents** have also been associated with acute ulcers. These agents include smoking, alcohol, and caffeine. Drugs associated with acute ulcer formation include aspirin, corticosteroids, indomethacin, and phenylbutazone.

Acute stress ulcers are usually small (less than 1 cm), often multiple, circular lesions found throughout the stomach. The ulcer base is often dark-brown due to digestion of blood; the margins are usually poorly defined. Scarring of the adjacent base and wall are absent, although a mild to moderate inflammatory infiltrate may be present. The ulcers are usually asymptomatic and can heal completely in days to weeks with removal of the causative factors. Rarely, the ulcers are associated with massive gastrointestinal bleeding.

GASTRIC AND DUODENAL PEPTIC ULCERS

Gastric peptic ulcers are often related to disruption of the mucosal barrier, while duodenal ulcers are often related to excess acid.

Peptic ulcers are chronic, usually solitary lesions that can be observed at any level in the gastrointestinal tract exposed to acid and pepsin. Almost all peptic ulcers occur in the duodenum and stomach (with a 4:1 duodenal ulcer predominance). Gastric peptic ulcer disease is often related to disruption of the mucosal barrier; duodenal peptic ulcer disease is often related to excessive acid secretion. The remainder are found in sites such as gastric mucosa containing Meckel's diverticula, Barrett's esophagus, and gastroenterostomy stoma.

Independently of site, peptic ulcers have a similar appearance. A peptic ulcer is typically a "hole" in the mucosa and underlying tissue with round-to-oval shape, perpendicular walls, and a smooth base due to pepsin-acid digestion of necrotic tissue. The size is usually small, although a few peptic ulcers are larger than 4 cm. Scarring of the adjacent tissues can cause puckering of the surrounding mucosa. The margins may be slightly elevated, but only rarely appear "heaped-up," as they can in the ulcers associated with gastric cancer. A thrombosed or bleeding vessel may be present in the base. The classic histologic appearance of the base of a peptic ulcer, from superficial to deep, shows a thin (microscopic) layer of necrotic fibrinoid debris; an active neutrophilic infiltrate; active granulation tissue infiltrated with mononuclear leukocytes; and a fibrous scar with blood vessels with thickened walls. The lamina propria of the mucosa adjacent to the ulcer may contain plasma cells, lymphocytes, and neutrophils. Peptic ulcers can be complicated by perforation, leading to peritonitis or massive hemorrhage.

BENIGN GASTRIC TUMORS

Benign tumors of the stomach are less common than malignant ones. Benign polyps are mucosal proliferations that commonly take two forms. **Hyperplastic** (inflammatory) **polyps** are an exaggerated regenerative response to mucosal injury; they tend to occur as multiple, soft, small (less than 1 cm) mucosal elevations composed of hyperplastic glands with cells resembling those in gastric pits. Hyperplastic polyps have no malignant potential, but they do suggest chronic irritation, and a search for carcinoma may be warranted. **Neoplastic polyps** (tubular adenomas or villous adenomas) are less common and resemble neoplastic polyps seen in the colon. The lesions contain atypical or dysplastic cells and may undergo malignant change. Multiple gastric polyps are sometimes observed in familial multiple polyposis and Peutz-Jeghers syndrome. **Benign stromal** (spindle) **cell tumors** are well-demarcated, firm nodules arising within the muscularis and composed of spindle-shaped cells. Stromal cell tumors include a variety of tumors (leiomyomas, neurofibromas, fibromas, etc.) and are clinically important primarily because they must be distinguished from their malignant counterparts. Larger lesions can produce bleeding (sometimes massive) and symptoms resembling those of peptic ulcer.

> **Benign tumors of the stomach include hyperplastic polyps, neoplastic polyps, and benign stromal cell tumors.**

MALIGNANT GASTRIC TUMORS

Malignant tumors found in the stomach include carcinomas, sarcomas, lymphomas, endocrine cell tumors, and metastatic tumors.

Gastric Carcinoma

Gastric carcinoma is the most common malignant gastric tumor, is almost always **adenocarcinoma,** and may contain cells resembling either gastric mucous cells or metaplastic intestinal cells (or both types). The metaplastic intestinal (goblet) cells can contain large mucin droplets that may stain for acidic intestinal mucin or neutral gastric mucin. In some cells, the mucin droplets may be so large as to flatten the nucleus against the plasma membrane (signet-ring cells). The **"intestinal-type"** tumors tend to be associated with chronic gastritis (and intestinal metaplasia) and also tend to have a better prognosis than the **"gastric-infiltrative"** tumors. The intestinal-type lesions are associated with many risk factors including high salt, nitrate, grain, or tuber intake; chronic gastritis; pernicious anemia; achlorhydria; bacterial overgrowth; and neoplastic polyps. The intestinal-type tumors appear to account for the marked variation in gastric carcinoma incidence worldwide, while the gastric-infiltrative tumors have a similar incidence throughout the world.

Gastric carcinomas occur throughout the stomach with a predilection for the lesser curvature of the antropyloric region. As a group, the ulcers formed by gastric carcinomas differ from peptic ulcers by location and usually by having raised edges. However, there is enough overlap in the radiologic and endoscopic appearance of the two types of lesions that biopsy is considered necessary to establish either diagnosis definitively.

Gastric carcinoma can also be classified by morphologic form. Advanced gastric carcinoma was formerly categorized as ulcerative,

> **Gastric carcinoma is the most common malignant gastric tumor.**

Gastric carcinomas can be subclassified into expanding, infiltrative, and undifferentiated types.

ulcerated-infiltrative, polypoid, and diffusely infiltrative. However, the simpler classification of expanding carcinomas and infiltrative carcinomas appears adequate. **Expanding carcinomas** have cohesive masses of tumor cells and are more apt to be surgically resectable because the tumor margin is well defined. In **infiltrative carcinomas,** poorly differentiated individual and small groups of tumor cells penetrate between adjacent muscle and fibrous tissue. If the infiltrative pattern is accompanied by an exuberant desmoplastic (fibrous) reaction, the stomach may resemble a leather bottle (linitis plastica). The **undifferentiated carcinomas** constitute an additional variant of gastric carcinoma composed of sheets of small cells with hyperchromatic nuclei. These tumors are probably neuroendocrine tumors, as the cells contain secretory granules and can secrete a variety of amine and polypeptide hormones.

The prognosis for gastric carcinoma is poor, as gastric carcinomas tend to metastasize widely to involve regional lymph nodes, liver, lungs, ovaries (Krukenberg tumors), and other organs. The supraclavicular and scalene lymph nodes may enlarge early. Early lesions are often asymptomatic; advanced lesions tend to produce weight loss and gastrointestinal symptoms. In Japan, where gastric carcinoma is common, routine screening by endoscopy identifies a larger percentage of early, treatable cancers.

Primary Gastrointestinal Lymphomas

Primary gastrointestinal lymphomas may be sporadic or associated with malabsorption.

Primary gastrointestinal lymphomas can arise in lymphoid tissue throughout the gut. These lymphomas comprise a small percentage of gastric malignancies. **Sporadic** (Western) **lymphoma** is of unknown etiology, with no identified risk factors, and is seen most commonly in the Western hemisphere in adults of both sexes. Sporadic lymphomas arise most commonly in the stomach and small intestine (although they can arise throughout the gut). Sporadic lymphomas are typically B-cell lesions derived from follicular center cells and consist of a mixture of cleaved cells, noncleaved cells, and immunoblasts. **Sprue-associated lymphoma** arises in the small intestine (notably the duodenal–jejunal segment) in patients of both sexes with 10- to 20-year histories of malabsorption syndromes, which are not always due to sprue. The relationship to malabsorption syndromes appears to be through a malabsorption-associated proliferation of plasma cells. **Mediterranean lymphomas** are more common in patients with Mediterranean ancestry, occur in children and young adults of both sexes, and, like sprue-associated lymphomas, may be associated with long-standing malabsorption and an accompanying proliferation of plasma cells. Mediterranean lymphomas are usually B-cell lesions and may show plasma cell differentiation. Lymphomas throughout the gastrointestinal tract have a poor prognosis; the worst prognosis occurs with the small and large intestine lymphomas.

Other Malignant Tumors

Malignant stromal (spindle) **cell tumors** (leiomyosarcomas, fibrosarcomas, endothelial sarcomas, etc.) account for a small percentage of malignant gastric tumors. They have a poor prognosis; occur in all ages and both sexes; and tend to be bulky masses with soft, "fish-flesh" appearance when cut. Intramural tumors will often fungate and ulcerate into the gastric lumen; subserosal tumors form masses that project into the peritoneal cavity. They are composed of malignant spindle cells of which a few may show differentiation, permitting more definitive tumor typing. Treatment is usually surgical removal, but only about one-half of patients survive for 5 years. **Endocrine cell tumors** (carcinoids) account for an additional small percentage of gastric malignancies and have a histologic appearance and aggressive behavior similar to endocrine cell tumors of the intestine. **Metastatic tumors** rarely involve the stomach. The most common sources are leukemias, lymphomas, breast carcinomas, and malignant melanomas.

Other tumors that can involve the stomach include malignant stromal cell tumors, endocrine cell tumors, and metastatic tumors.

SMALL INTESTINE

CONGENITAL ANOMALIES

Congenital anomalies can involve the small intestine.

Congenital anomalies can affect the small intestine. **Atresia** refers to developmental absence of a segment of bowel. The segment can be either completely absent or may be represented by a noncanalized cord connecting adjacent bowel segments. **Stenosis** refers to narrowing of an already canalized bowel segment, as by fibrosis or tumor. **Diverticula** are focal defects in the muscular wall of the small intestine, usually at points where mesenteric nerves and vessels enter the intestinal wall; such defects permit herniation of the musoca and submucosa into the mesentery. Small intestinal diverticula are similar to colonic diverticula but occur much less commonly. **Meckel's diverticulum** is a persistence of the vestige of the omphalomesenteric duct that is typically found within 12 inches of the ileocecal valve. A Meckel's diverticulum is not a true diverticulum because the wall is fully formed and is not a herniation. A Meckel's diverticulum can contain heterotropic rests of gastric mucosa or pancreatic tissue. Small rests of essentially normal **pancreatic tissue** can occur under the mucosa anywhere in the small bowel. **Malrotations and duplications** are rarely encountered in the small bowel.

ISCHEMIC BOWEL DISEASE

Hypoxic injury can affect the small intestine, colon, or both. In the colon, the watershed area of the splenic flexure is particularly vulnerable to ischemic injury. In the small intestine, injury can occur in either a patchy distribution or in a single, often long, intestinal segment.

Transmural Infarction

Transmural infarctions are more common in the small intestine than colon.

Transmural infarction, or infarction of the entire intestinal wall including the serosa, is less common in the colon than in the small intestine, possibly because much of the colonic mucosa has an accessory blood supply derived from the posterior abdominal wall. Transmural infarction can be caused by arterial thromboses (atherosclerosis); embolic arterial occlusion (endocarditis, intracardiac mural thromboses); and venous thrombosis (cardiac failure, polycythemia, portal stasis, hypercoagulable states). Additional causes of transmural infarction include mechanical occlusion of arterial or venous vessels (strangulated hernias, torsions, or intestinal adhesions); and vasospasm or hypotension, particularly when superimposed on pre-existing narrowed vessels (atherosclerosis, fibromuscular dysplasia, dissecting aortic aneurysm, arteritis).

Transmural infarction of the bowel has a poor prognosis and may be difficult to diagnose because the abdominal symptoms mimic those of more common abdominal disorders. In the early stages of transmural infarction, the bowel has a dusky to purple-red, congested appearance. Large serosal ecchymoses may be present. The histologic appearance is of extensive hemorrhage and ischemic necrosis. Death may occur before an inflammatory response develops. Later, the lumen typically contains blood or blood-stained mucus, and the bowel wall is edematous and hemorrhagic. Areas of transmural infarction following arterial occlusion are typically sharply demarcated from healthy bowel, while transmural infarction following venous occlusion gradually fades into adjacent bowel. Later lesions show inflammatory infiltrations and ulcerations. Secondary bacterial contamination may cause perforation with peritonitis.

Mucosal and Mural Infarction

Less severe ischemic injury throughout the gastrointestinal tract can cause **mucosal and mural infarctions,** which are also known as hemorrhagic gastroenteropathy since hemorrhage into the gut lumen is a prominent feature. This type of injury is usually associated with hypoperfusion rather than frank occlusion of vessels. The inner layers of the gut are most vulnerable, and there is relative sparing of the deeper levels of the muscularis and the serosa. The lesions are typically in a patchy or continuous distribution through the gastrointestinal tract. The mucosa is hemorrhagic, edematous, and sometimes ulcerated. Histologically, hemorrhagic necrosis involves the mucosa (mucosal infarction) and may extend to the submucosa and superficial muscularis (mural infarction). Bacterial superinfection may induce pseudomembranous inflammation. Depending principally upon the patient's general health and whether the hypoperfusion persists, mucosal and mural infarctions may resolve completely, cause scarring of the involved gut, or contribute to the death of the patient.

> **Mucosal and mural infarctions are usually associated with hypoperfusion.**

INFECTIVE GASTROENTEROCOLITIS

Many infective agents can cause inflammatory gastric and diarrheal disease by several mechanisms. **Preformed bacterial toxins,** caused by bacteria such as *Clostridium botulinum* and *Staphylococcus aureus,* can cause mild to severe (even fatal) gastroenterocolitis. **Bacterial toxigenic enterocolitis,** in which bacterial toxins are derived from organisms growing within the gut lumen, can be caused by *Vibrio cholerae* and some serotypes of *Escherichia coli.* **Bacterial invasive enterocolitis,** in which bacterial pathogens are found within the surface glycocalyx or mucosal epithelium, can be caused by *Helicobacter jejuni,* some serotypes of *Escherichia coli, Salmonella, Shigella, Yersinia enterocolitica,* and *Aeromonas hydrophila* (see also p. 43). **Tuberculosis** may involve the bowel following either primary infection (usually by contaminated milk products) or secondary infection after swallowing organisms in sputum. **Viral causes** of gastroenterocolitis include parvoviruslike agents (adults), reoviruslike agents (infants), and rotavirus (infants and children). **Fungi** that can invade the small and large intestine, usually in immunocompromised hosts, include *Candida* and Mucormycetes. **Parasitic agents** causing enterocolitis include *Entamoeba histolytica, Giardia lamblia, Schistosoma mansoni,* and cryptosporidia. In general, the changes produced by the above agents are nonspecific and may include focal areas of hyperemia, lymphoid tissue

> **Bacterial gastroenterocolitis may be caused by preformed toxins, toxins produced by intestinal organisms, and bacterial invasion of the gut mucosa or wall.**

> **Viruses, fungi, and parasites can also cause gastroenterocolitis.**

proliferation, ulceration, or pseudomembrane formation. The lesions may be focal or involve long segments of bowel. The adjacent serosa may be normal or covered by exudate.

MALABSORPTION SYNDROMES

Malabsorption may induce protein and vitamin deficiencies.

Malabsorption syndromes of many etiologies are characterized by a failure to absorb adequate nutrients from the gut. They tend to produce anorexia, weight loss, and muscle wasting. Abdominal distention, with passage of abnormally bulky stool, also occurs. When severe, malabsorption syndromes can also produce symptoms related to failure to absorb key nutrients. Inadequate **protein** absorption can cause edema and ascites. Inadequate fat absorption can cause deficiencies of **vitamins A** (skin and vision changes), **K** (bleeding tendency), and **D** (skeletal changes and hypocalcemia). Inadequate absorption of folate and vitamin B_{12} can produce megaloblastic anemia. Inadequate resorption of fluids and electrolytes can produce a profuse diarrhea that may be life-threatening.

Malabsorption may be due to inadequate solubilization of luminal contents, mucus cell abnormalities, lymphatic obstruction, or a variety of other causes.

The many etiologies of malabsorption syndromes can be grouped into broad classes. **Inadequate hydrolysis or solubilization** of intraluminal contents is caused most commonly by inadequate lumenal concentrations of pancreatic enzymes or bile salts. These inadequate concentrations may be the result of primary or secondary pancreatic insufficiency; bacterial overgrowth causing bile salt deconjugation (blind intestinal loops, intestinal strictures or diverticula, postgastrectomy syndromes, scleroderma); or deficient secretion of conjugated bile salts (liver and biliary tract disease, intestinal resection leading to decreased resorption of conjugated bile salts). **Abnormalities of mucosal cells** can limit nutrient absorption either by a specific failure of transport of nutrients (disaccharidase deficiency, abetalipoproteinemia, vitamin B_{12} malabsorption, cystinuria, Hartnup's disease) or by a generalized loss in mucosal cell surface area (celiac disease, Whipple's disease, eosinophilic gastroenteritis, Crohn's disease). **Lymphatic obstruction,** by lymphoma, tuberculosis, or lymphangiectasia, can cause malabsorption by blocking transport of nutrients from the gut to the systemic circulation.

Other causes of malabsorption include loss of significant portions of the gastrointestinal tract (subtotal gastrectomy, distal ileal resection, radiation enteritis); infection (acute infectious enteritis, tropical sprue, parasitic diseases); and drugs (cholestyramine, colchicine, some laxatives, neomycin). Unexplained causes of malabsorption include diabetes mellitus, carcinoid syndrome, hypogammaglobulinemia, and many endocrine disorders. Among these many disorders, only a few will be discussed in detail in this section.

Bacterial Overgrowth Syndrome

Bacterial overgrowth is an important cause of malabsorption.

Bacterial overgrowth syndrome occurs whenever lumenal stasis is present (blind loops, motility disorders). Bacterial overgrowth causes many absorptive defects as a consequence of competition by bacteria for nutrients (proteins, fats, carbohydrates); deconjugation of bile salts and inactivation of lipase (fat, vitamins); and direct and indirect mucosal damage (water, electrolytes). Small bowel biopsy specimens in bacterial overgrowth syndrome tend to show nonspecific changes such as increased inflammatory infiltrates in the lamina propria.

Celiac Sprue

Celiac sprue (gluten-sensitive enteropathy, nontropical sprue, adult and childhood celiac disease) is a malabsorption syndrome characterized by a striking loss of small intestinal villi, with consequent marked loss of absorptive surface. The disease is usually diagnosed in childhood. It can be cured or markedly ameliorated by removal from the diet of gluten and its derivative gliadin, which are found in wheat, barley, and rye. The specific mechanism by which gluten causes loss of intestinal villi is still not fully elucidated, but appears to involve an IgA-mediated hypersensitivity reaction to gliadin.

Microscopic features include marked villus atrophy with flattening of the columnar epithelial cells and increased numbers of lymphocytes in the epithelium; hyperplasia and increased mitotic activity of the deeper epithelium to form elongated and tortuous crypts; and increased inflammatory infiltrate (plasma cells, lymphocytes, macrophages, eosinophils, and mast cells) in the lamina propria. Electron microscopy additionally shows markedly distorted and shortened microvilli and abnormal mitochondria. The proximal small bowel is usually more severely affected than the distal bowel because the gluten exposure to the proximal bowel is greater.

Celiac sprue is a malabsorption syndrome that appears to involve an IgA-mediated hypersensitivity reaction to gliadin.

Tropical Sprue

Tropical sprue resembles celiac sprue but is unrelated to gluten ingestion. The etiology is still undetermined, but may be related to enterotoxigenic *Escherichia coli* species. The intestinal pathology ranges from mild, nonspecific changes to severe disease closely resembling celiac sprue. Unlike celiac sprue, the worst pathology tends to occur in the distal small bowel, and the jejunum may be uninvolved. The histologic appearance also tends to differ from celiac sprue by the presence of larger numbers of lymphocytes and eosinophils in the lamina propria. The epithelial nuclei are frequently enlarged (analogous to megaloblastic anemia) as a consequence of diminished folate or vitamin B_{12} absorption in the distal small bowel.

Tropical sprue clinically resembles celiac sprue, but tends to involve the distal small bowel.

Whipple's Disease

Whipple's disease is a multisystem disease with prominent malabsorption symptoms caused by bacilli that have long been observed by electron microscopy but have only recently been successfully cultured. These bacilli are found near and within macrophages throughout the body, particularly the small bowel. In the small intestine, the most striking histologic feature of Whipple's disease is clusters within the lamina propria of distended, periodic acid-Schiff (PAS)-positive (glycoprotein-laden) macrophages that contain occasional bacillary bodies. These macrophages distend the villi to produce a "bear-skin rug" gross appearance to the intestinal mucosa. The mucosal lymphatics are often dilated and may contain lipid droplets; rupture of the lymphatics can

Whipple's disease is a malabsorption syndrome caused by bacilli.

induce occasional small granulomas. The mesenteric lymph nodes may also have dilated channels and contain small granulomas. Macrophages containing bacillary bodies resembling those in the small intestine can also be found in many other sites, including synovial membranes, the central nervous system, the heart, and throughout the gastrointestinal system.

Whipple's disease is seen most frequently in white males in the fourth and fifth decades of life. While malabsorption symptoms are the most common presentation, the disease can also be found in patients with polyarthritis or obscure central nervous system complaints. The condition was formerly fatal but now responds promptly to antibiotic therapy.

Disaccharidase Deficiency

Lactase deficiency produces diarrhea secondary to a failure to absorb lactose.

Disaccharidase deficiency refers to congenital (hereditary) or acquired deficiency of one of the disacharidases located on the lumenal membrane of the intestinal epithelial cells. The most common and important form of disacharidase deficiency is an **acquired deficiency of lactase** seen frequently among North American blacks. The normal action of lactase is to hydrolyze lactose (principally from milk products) into glucose and galactose, for which intestinal molecular transport systems exist. In the absence or deficiency of lactase, nonabsorbable dietary lactose is not cleared from the gut lumen and acts as an osmotic laxative, producing malabsorption and a watery diarrhea. The intestinal mucosa appears histologically normal. Bacterial digestion of the lactose produces hydrogen and the disease can be suspected by a positive hydrogen breath test. The symptoms vanish with removal of lactose from the diet.

Abetalipoproteinemia

Abetalipoproteinemia leads to fat accumulation in epithelial cells and a failure to synthesize chylomicrons.

Abetalipoproteinemia is an autosomal recessive failure to synthesize the apoprotein component needed for formation of chylomicrons by intestinal mucosal cells. The result is that while dietary fat can be digested and free fatty acids can be absorbed by epithelial cells, chylomicrons cannot be synthesized and the dietary fat cannot enter the circulatory system. Fat accumulation within epithelial cells causes lipid vacuolation, which is easily visualized by fat stains. Other changes observed in the disease include markedly decreased serum levels of chylomicrons, very low density lipoproteins, and low density lipoproteins. Red cells develop a "burr cell" appearance as a consequence of insufficient absorption of essential fatty acids. The disease is identified in infancy when it produces diarrhea, steatorrhea, and failure to thrive.

OBSTRUCTIVE LESIONS OF THE SMALL BOWEL

Obstructive lesions of the small bowel include hernias, intestinal adhesions, intussusception, and volvulus.

Obstructive lesions can affect the small bowel. A **hernia** is an outpouching of bowel, usually small intestine, into a weakened or defective area of the peritoneal cavity such as the inguinal and femoral canals, umbilicus, or a surgical scar. The most serious complications of hernias are intestinal obstruction and infarction. **Intestinal adhesions** are fibrous bands between the bowel and adjacent structures. Predisposing factors include peritonitis and abdominal surgery. Complications of adhesions include intestinal obstruction and strangulation. **Intussusception** is telescoping of a segment of bowel by a wave of peristalsis into the immediately distal segment of bowel. Intussusception is observed most commonly in infants and children, but can also be encountered in adults in which an intraluminal mass (e.g., tumor) is dragged into an adjacent bowel segment. The vascular supply of the entrapped bowel can be compromised, leading to infarction. **Volvulus** refers to twisting of a bowel loop about its mesentery and is a cause of intestinal obstruction and infarction.

CROHN'S DISEASE

Crohn's disease is a primarily enteric disorder with sometimes prominent systemic effects that can affect any segment of the gastrointestinal tract, but most commonly affects the terminal ileum, colon and rectum, or both. The etiology of Crohn's disease is unclear, but may involve still poorly defined immunologic mechanisms that may or may not be triggered by a still unidentified pathogen. The disease typically manifests in the second decade of life. Transmural inflammatory lesions, composed of chronic inflammatory infiltrates and fibrosis, occur in a segmental distribution ("skip" lesions), with sharp demarcations between severely affected and more nearly normal small or large intestine. **Noncaseating granulomas,** resembling those of sarcoidosis, are a helpful feature in identifying Crohn's disease, but they may be small, uncommon, or even completely absent. **Lymphoid aggregates,** which may contain germinal centers, are prominent and dilated, or sclerosed lymphatic channels may be present.

> Crohn's disease is an enteric disorder with sometimes prominent systemic effects.

> Granulomas, while helpful in identifying Crohn's disease, may be small or even absent.

In early Crohn's disease, the small intestinal wall may be thickened and edematous. The mucosa may be disrupted only by small ulcers. Later, chronic inflammation and fibrosis produces "lead pipe" or **"rubber hose" rigidity** with narrowed lumen of affected segments. The mucosa at this stage may be edematous, ulcerated, or sloughed. Deep penetration of ulcers may cause fistula formation with connections to adjacent bowel loops, the abdominal cavity, or other abdominal or pelvic organs. Involvement of the serosa and adjacent mesentery may "bury" the affected segment in mesenteric fat.

In some cases, Crohn's disease can be difficult to distinguish from ulcerative colitis (see p. 251). It is now thought that these two diseases may represent two extremes of a spectrum of pathologic change known as **"inflammatory bowel disease."** Features that tend to substantiate a diagnosis of Crohn's disease include more severe involvement of the ileum and right colon, skip lesions, granulomas, fistulas, and transmural inflammation. Some cases are best classified as "inflammatory bowel disease, type unspecified" since they exhibit overlap characteristics or do not exhibit the full range of characteristics of either Crohn's disease or ulcerative colitis.

> Crohn's disease and ulcerative colitis may represent extremes of a spectrum of inflammatory bowel disease.

The clinical course of Crohn's disease may range from occasional diarrhea to severe disease with complications including anemia, weight loss, intestinal obstruction, and fistula formation. Systemic manifestations, some of which may be immunologically mediated, include migratory polyarthritis, sacroileitis, ankylosing spondylitis, erythema nodosum, uveitis, hepatic inflammations, gallstones, ureteral obstruction by fibrosis, amyloidosis, and finger clubbing. A few patients with long-standing, progressive Crohn's disease develop gastrointestinal cancer in either involved or uninvolved intestinal segments.

> Crohn's disease may have many complications.

TUMORS OF THE SMALL INTESTINE

Despite the length of the small intestine and the rapid turnover of its mucosa, both benign and malignant tumors of the small intestine are rare. **Benign stromal tumors, adenomatous polyps,** and **angiomas** are uncommonly encountered in the small intestine. All of these tumors resemble their counterparts in other parts of the gastrointestinal tract. Small benign tumors are asymptomatic; larger tumors can cause partial obstruction, bleeding, intussusception, and volvulus. Malignant tumors include carcinomas, carcinoids, and lymphomas (see p. 240).

Carcinomas

Adenocarcinomas uncommonly affect the small intestine (notably the duodenum), where they can either encircle the intestine or form polypoid fungating masses. Symptoms (cramping pain, vomiting, weight loss) tend to occur late, unless obstruction of the adjacent biliary tree causes jaundice. A 70 percent 5-year survival is seen if extensive resection is performed.

Gastrointestinal Carcinoid Tumors

Carcinoid (neuroendocrine) **tumors** can arise throughout the gut and can also arise in other sites such as the lungs, biliary tract, and ovaries. In the gastrointestinal tract, the lesions are found most frequently in the terminal ileum and in the appendix. Carcinoid tumors arise from **neuroendocrine cells** or their precursors and are best considered as potentially malignant tumors. Carcinoids in the appendix and rectum rarely metastasize, but do show extensive local spread. In contrast, carcinoids of similar histologic appearance in the ileum, stomach, or colon have often metastasized at the time of diagnosis. Size larger than 1 to 2 cm and deep local invasion are also associated with substantially increased risk of metastasis before detection. The gross appearance of carcinoids is of a small submucosal elevation that appears yellowish-gray to bright yellow on transection and often deeply infiltrates the adjacent gut wall. The tumor cells tend to be monotonously similar, with pale-pink, granular cytoplasm and round to ovoid nuclei with stippled chromatin. Characteristically, the usual cytologic stigmata of an aggressive tumor, such as prominent mitotic activity, nuclear pleomorphism, or cytologic atypia, are absent. The tumor cells can grow in a variety of patterns, including trabecular, insular, glandular, mixed, and undifferentiated.

Gastrointestinal carcinoids are conveniently subclassified by site of origin. **Foregut carcinoids** are the least common gastrointestinal carcinoids and tend to grow in a trabecular or mixed pattern. Gastric carcinoids, the most common of the foregut carcinoids, tend to arise in patients with pre-existing endocrine cell hyperplasia and are often multicentric in origin. **Midgut carcinoids,** particularly in the terminal ileum and appendix, are the most commonly encountered carcinoids and tend to grow in an insular pattern. Appendiceal carcinoids are characteristically located at the tip of the appendix. **Hindgut carcinoids,** particularly from the rectum, usually show a trabecular or mixed growth pattern. Many carcinoids are hormonally nonfunctional. Others can secrete any of a large number of hormones including adrenocorticotropic hormone (ACTH), serotonin, gastrin, somatostatin, glucagon, insulin, calcitonin, substance P, and pancreatic polypeptide. Secretory granules containing specific hormones can be identified in these tumors by immunoreactive methods.

COLON

DISEASES OF THE APPENDIX

The appendix is commonly affected by only a small number of conditions, of which the most important is appendicitis. **Simple acute appendicitis** produces colicky abdominal pain that later localizes (usually to the lower right quadrant) as the adjacent peritoneum becomes inflamed. The appendix is swollen, and the vessels in the mesoappendix are congested. Microscopically, large numbers of neutrophils are found in the appendiceal wall and lumen, often adjacent to a focus of mucosal ulceration. Fibrin may be present on the peritoneal surface. **Suppurative appendicitis,** with abscess formation, may either complicate simple acute appendicitis, or may be associated with an impacted fecalith in the appendix. Suppurative appendicitis may be complicated by necrosis and appendiceal perforation with risk of peritonitis. **Gangrenous appendicitis** occurs either following vascular damage (typically thrombosis) or severe obstruction by stricture or a fecalith. Complications of acute appendicitis include peritonitis, appendiceal abscess, adhesions, and liver abscess. **Chronic appendicitis** is usually related to appendiceal fibrosis, which interferes with peristalsis within the appendix, predisposing for recurrent inflammation, mucocele formation, and gangrene. In addition to appendicitis, the appendix is vulnerable to tumors (notably carcinoid), tuberculosis, and *Actinomyces* infections (which may spread to the liver).

> **Appendicitis is the most important condition that affects the appendix.**

CONGENITAL ANOMALIES OF THE COLON

The colon is vulnerable to a variety of uncommon congenital anomalies including malrotations, reduplications, imperforate anus, and fistulous communications between the gastrointestinal and genitourinary tracts.

    Megacolon, or marked dilation of the colon, is observed in both congenital and acquired forms. When acquired, the dilation may be proximal to a site of obstruction due to fibrosis or neoplasia, or it may be related to motility dysfunction. With the exception of the megacolon observed in parasitic infection by *Trypanosoma cruzi* (Chagas disease), the intrinsic innervation of the bowel appears normal.

    In contrast to acquired megacolon, congenital megacolon (Hirschsprung's disease) is characterized by the absence of ganglion cells in both Meissner's (submucosal) plexus and Auerbach's (intramuscular) plexus. There is an accompanying erratic proliferation of nonmyelinated nerve fibers. Commonly, the rectum or sigmoid colon contains the proximal border of the aganglionic segment. The aberrant innervation causes a defect in peristalsis leading to functional colonic obstruction with dila-

> **Megacolon may be either congenital or acquired.**

tion of the colon. The diagnosis can often be excluded by the demonstration of ganglion cells in **Meissner's plexus** in submucosal biopsies. Definitive diagnosis of **Hirschsprung's disease** can be made at time of surgery to resect the affected bowel by the demonstration of absence of Auerbach's plexus in transmural biopsies of adjacent, nondilated colon. Hirschsprung's disease is usually identified in neonates who experience either obstructive constipation or, if only a small segment of rectum is involved, intermittent constipation and diarrhea. Treatment is surgical resection of the affected bowel; untreated cases are associated with enterocolitis and (rarely) colonic perforation with accompanying peritonitis.

MISCELLANEOUS LESIONS

Miscellaneous lesions to which the colon is prone include melanosis coli, hemorrhoids, and angiodysplasia.

Melanosis coli is an asymptomatic colonic discoloration.

Melanosis coli is an idiopathic, asymptomatic, brown-black discoloration of most or all of the colonic mucosa due to pigment granules within macrophages in the lamina propria. This pigment deposition has been associated in some cases with coronic abuse of some organic laxatives, and may represent phagocytized material from damaged mucosal cells.

Hemorrhoids tend to develop when venous pressures are chronically elevated.

Hemorrhoids are mucosa-covered dilations of the anal and perianal venous plexuses. Hemorrhoids affect 5 percent of the general population and are uncommon at ages less than 30, except in pregnant women. When the varicosities develop below the anorectal line in the inferior hemorrhoidal plexus, they are called "external hemorrhoids." Dilations that develop in the superior hemorrhoidal plexus are called "internal hemorrhoids." Hemorrhoids develop in a setting of persistently elevated venous pressure, due most commonly to constipation with straining at stool, venous stasis of pregnancy, or portal hypertension. Histologically, varices are thin-walled, dilated veins located in the submucosa of the anus or rectum. They tend to protrude into the anal canal, where they are easily traumatized and may become thrombosed, ulcerated, or infarcted.

Angiodysplasia may be the cause of significant gastrointestinal bleeding in the elderly.

Angiodysplasias are abnormal, tortuous, thin-walled, dilations of the submucosal veins of the cecum and ascending colon. These lesions appear to be acquired vascular ectasias that are rare before the seventh decade of life and can cause significant gastrointestinal bleeding and anemia. The lesions are best diagnosed by colonoscopy or selective mesenteric angiography. They may be difficult to identify in surgical or postmortem pathologic specimens because of collapse of the vessels during dissection.

DIVERTICULAR DISEASE

Diverticular disease may be asymptomatic or may require surgery for obstructive or inflammatory complications.

Colonic **diverticula** are acquired saccular outpouchings of the colon that tend to develop with advancing age and are rare at ages less than 30 years. The presence of diverticula, or **diverticulosis,** has traditionally been distinguished from the inflammation of diverticula, or **diverticulitis;** but this distinction now appears less clinically useful than before, and the unspecified term **diverticular disease** is often now used to refer to the presence of either or both conditions. Most diverticula are located in the rectosigmoid colon, although the entire colon can be affected by a few to hundreds of diverticula. Diverticula tend to form at the edge of the taenia coli where the arterial vasa recta penetrate the muscularis.

Microscopically, a diverticulum has a thin wall with flattened, atrophic mucosa. The submucosa is usually compressed and the muscularis may be attenuated or totally absent. Acute or chronic inflammatory changes (including fibrotic thickening of the colonic wall) are often present in the inflamed diverticulum and may extend into the pericolic fat. Most patients with diverticular disease are asymptomatic or have relatively mild symptoms of cramping or abdominal discomfort, constipation, or the sensation of a chronically full rectum. These symptoms can often be ameliorated with increased dietary fiber. Patients with more severe disease occasionally require surgery for obstructive or inflammatory complications, including rupture of an infected diverticulum, which produces peritonitis in a syndrome resembling acute appendicitis.

INFLAMMATIONS OF THE COLON

The colon is vulnerable to a variety of inflammations, many of which have been discussed together with those of the small intestine. This section discusses ulcerative colitis, pseudomembranous colitis, necrotizing enterocolitis, and collagenous colitis.

Ulcerative Colitis

Idiopathic ulcerative colitis is an inflammatory bowel disease characterized by recurrent acute and chronic ulceration and inflammation of the large bowel, particularly the rectum and left colon. Patients are typically young adults who experience recurrent, sometimes bloody, diarrhea. Fulminant disease may be complicated by colonic distention and perforation. In addition to the colonic disease, ulcerative colitis is associated with systemic complaints similar to those of Crohn's disease, including skin lesions, migratory polyarthritis, ankylosing spondylitis, sacroileitis, hepatic inflammations, and uveitis (see p. 247). Ulcerative colitis begins in the rectum and extends proximally. The terminal ileum can be involved in severe cases. Ulcerative colitis differs from Crohn's disease in that the lesions are superficial; the ulcerated mucosa often shows inflammatory polyposis and does not show skip lesions; and fibrous strictures or fistulae are rare. Malignant change is more common than in Crohn's disease.

> **Ulcerative colitis is an inflammatory bowel disease that may have systemic effects.**

Pseudomembranous Colitis

Pseudomembranous colitis is a distinctive severe form of colitis that is most frequently caused by the toxin of *Clostridium difficile*. The characteristic pathologic feature is a "pseudomembrane," composed of a coagulum of fibrin, inflammatory cells, and cellular debris, which coalesces on the surface of an inflamed and sometimes ulcerated mucosa. The disease is most commonly seen following treatment with broad-spectrum antibiotics, notably clindamycin and lincomycin, and appears to be the result of bacterial overgrowth with toxin formation by the antibiotic-

> **The pseudomembrane of pseudomembranous colitis is composed of fibrin, inflammatory cells, and cellular debris.**

resistant *Clostridium.* The toxin can be identified in stool to establish the diagnosis. While pseudomembranous colitis is usually associated with *Clostridium difficile,* other conditions (ischemic injury and infections with staphylococci, *Shigella,* or *Candida*) can also induce pseudomembrane formation.

Necrotizing Enterocolitis

Necrotizing enterocolitis causes a common gastrointestinal emergency in premature and low-birthweight neonates. The disease produces an acute necrotizing inflammation of the small and large bowel that may cause abdominal distress, gastrointestinal bleeding, gangrene, intestinal perforation, and sepsis. Many factors can contribute to the development of necrotizing enterocolitis including intestinal ischemia, microbial agents, and the poor gastrointestinal immune response of neonates. The disease is most commonly seen in bottle-fed infants in the first week of life when the infants are started on oral foods. The histologic appearance of necrotizing enterocolitis varies with the stage of the disease from edema, hemorrhage, and necrosis of the mucosa; to necrotic mucosa covered by pseudomembrane composed of coagulated fibrin, neutrophils, and cellular debris; to transmural necrosis and inflammation, which may be accompanied by perforation and peritonitis. Treatment involves stabilization of shock and electrolyte disorders; surgical intervention may be required if gangrene or peritonitis develops. Survivors of severe necrotizing enterocolitis may have malabsorption and stricture formation.

Collagenous Colitis

Collagenous colitis is a recently described form of colitis characterized histologically by a distinctive, thick, hypocellular collagenous band located between the surface epithelial cells and the lamina propria. The surface epithelial cells may be abnormal (shortened, with decreased mucin and increased vacuolization) and a mixed inflammatory infiltrate (lymphocytes, neutrophils, eosinophils) may be prominent in both the surface epithelium and lamina propria. The crypt epithelium is usually well preserved, although a few crypt abscesses may be seen.

Collagenous colitis produces a chronic or episodic watery diarrhea by an unknown mechanism. The disease may have an autoimmune foundation, since it has been associated with a variety of diseases, many of which are known to have an immune basis. These associated diseases include rheumatoid arthritis, thyroiditis, temporal arteritis, myasthenia gravis, diabetes mellitus, atrophic gastritis, chronic hepatitis, duodenal ulcer, and obstructive pulmonary disease. Many patients with collagenous colitis are positive for rheumatoid factor and antinuclear antibody.

COLONIC POLYPS

Benign Polyps

A variety of **colonic polyps** and polypoid lesions can affect the colon. Benign polyps may be of the hyperplastic, hamartomatous, inflammatory, or lymphoid type.

Hyperplastic polyps are completely benign epithelial polyps found principally in the rectosigmoid colon; they can also be seen in other colonic locations. The polyps are small (less than 1 cm), round lesions that characteristically sit on mucosal folds and are composed of mature glands and crypts. The epithelial lining may contain either goblet cells or absorptive cells; crowding of these cells produces a characteristic "sawtooth pattern."

Hamartomatous polyps are developmental malformations, rather than true polyps, that consist of abnormal arrangements of essentially normal glands and lamina propria. Several forms of hamartomatous polyps have been described. **Juvenile polyps** are rounded lesions up to 2 cm in diameter that may or may not have a stalk and that are vulnerable to ulceration, inflammation, bleeding, torsion, and infarction. The polyps consist of mucus-filled tubules that are lined by normal or inflamed mucosa with abundant intervening lamina propria. The polyps can occur as an isolated finding or as part of the **juvenile polyposis syndrome,** in which multiple polyps are found throughout the gastrointestinal tract, particularly in the colon and stomach. **Peutz-Jeghers polyps** are large and pedunculated; they are composed of an arborizing framework of connective tissue containing smooth muscle. The intestinal epithelium is characteristically rich in goblet cells but otherwise normal. Peutz-Jeghers polyps can be either an isolated finding or can occur as part of Peutz-Jegher syndrome. In this autosomal dominant syndrome, multiple polyps (observed throughout the gastrointestinal tract) can be accompanied by melanotic pigmentation of the mouth, face, genitalia, and palmar sufaces of the hands. While Peutz-Jegher's polyps have no neoplastic potential, the syndrome is associated, for unknown reasons, with increased risk of carcinomas of the pancreas, breast, ovary, uterus, and lung.

Inflammatory polyps (pseudopolyps) are mucosal tags that develop following re-epithelialization of ulcers with overhanging margins. Inflammatory polyps are often multiple and are seen most commonly following severe mucosal damage by ulcerative colitis. These polyps have no malignant potential; the carcinomas associated with inflammatory bowel disease arise from other, dysplastic epithelium.

Lymphoid polyps are benign mucosal elevations above sites of enlarged lymphoid follicles, often with prominent germinal centers.

Neoplastic Polyps

Neoplastic polyps have a malignant potential. They are characterized by a proliferation of dysplastic epithelium around a fibrovascular core that may form either a sessile or a pedunculated polyp. These polyps are subclassified based upon whether the predominant growth pattern of the dysplastic epithelium is in a tubular or a villous growth pattern. A polyp is considered a **tubular adenoma** when at least three-fourths of the epithelium is growing in tubular patterns. **Tubulovillous adenomas** have dysplastic epithelium with one-fourth to one-half growing in a villous pattern. **Villous adenomas** have dysplastic epithelium with more than one-half growing in a villous pattern. More severe atypia is associated with disordered alignment of cells in the epithelium and greater numbers of mitotic figures and hyperchromatic nuclei. Both carcinoma in situ, with or without invasion of the fibrovascular core of the

Hyperplastic polyps have a crowded epithelial lining that forms a "sawtooth pattern."

Hamartomatous polyps are actually developmental malformations.

Inflammatory polyps are mucosal tags.

Neoplastic polyps include tubular adenomas, tubulovillous adenomas, and villous adenomas.

polyp, and frank invasive carcinoma can arise in the dysplastic epithelium. In general, the larger the adenoma, the greater the percentage of villous growth pattern, and the greater the villous component, the greater the malignant potential. Polypoid carcinomas, which often arise in adenomas, represent the extreme end of this spectrum of lesions: the dysplastic epithelium has become frankly carcinomatous.

A few patients have very large numbers of neoplastic polyps as part of a familial (usually autosomal dominant) polyposis syndrome. In **familial polyposis coli,** the colon is virtually carpeted (average 1,000) with adenomas, most of which are tubular adenomas. Smaller numbers of polyps can also be found in the stomach, duodenum, and small intestine. The disease is closely monitored, and early resection of the entire involved colon is usually performed, as these patients will almost all eventually develop colon cancer if left untreated. In **Gardner syndrome,** what appears to be nearly the same genetic defect as seen in familial polyposis coli causes colonic polyposis with extracolonic manifestations including multiple osteomas, epidermal cysts, fibromatosis, abnormal teeth, duodenal cancer, and thyroid cancer. Treatment of the colonic adenomas is by early surgical resection of the entire involved colon to reduce the risk of colon cancer. In the rare **Turcot syndrome,** colonic polyposis is seen in association with central nervous system tumors.

COLON CANCER

The colon, rectum, and anal regions are vulnerable to many malignant tumors, including spindle cell tumors (sarcomas), lymphomas, carcinoids, squamous cell carcinomas, transitional cell carcinomas, and melanomas. However, the overwhelmingly most common malignancy affecting the colon is **adenocarcinoma,** and the unqualified phrase "colon cancer" consequently almost always refers to adenocarcinoma of the colon.

Colorectal cancer is the second leading cause (behind lung cancer) of cancer deaths in the United States. Diets low in vegetable fiber and high in fats and refined carbohydrates appear to predispose for colon cancer, possibly by decreasing stool transit time and thereby modifying the intestinal bacterial flora population and potentially increasing the number and time of contact of dietary carcinogens. Other risk factors include familial polyposis syndromes and inflammatory bowel disease, with ulcerative colitis having a greater risk than Crohn's disease.

It is convenient to subdivide colon cancer into tumors arising in the right and left sides of the large bowel. Colon cancers arising in the **cecum and ascending colon** tend to produce polypoid fungating masses that project into the gut lumen. Obstruction is uncommon, and the cancers of the right colon can remain asymptomatic for long periods of time. Cancers of the right colon are seen commonly in countries with a low incidence of colon cancer; interestingly, for unknown reasons, the proportion of right-sided colon cancers has also been increasing in the United States and other developed countries. Colon cancers arising in the **left side of the colon** tend to encircle the bowel to form "napkin-ring" constrictions that cause early obstructive symptoms. These tumors tend to ulcerate and bleed, but do not usually project into the bowel lumen.

Familial forms of colonic polyposis include famlial polyposis coli, Gardner syndrome, and Turcot syndrome.

While many tumors can be found in the colon, adenocarcinoma is the overwhelmingly most common malignancy.

Adenocarcinomas arising in the right side of the colon tend to form intraluminal masses, while those arising in the left side tend to encircle the bowel.

While the gross pathology of colon cancers arising in the right and left sides of the colon tends to differ, the microscopic appearance is similar. Ninety-five percent of the colon carcinomas are adenocarcinomas, many of which contain mucin-producing tumor cells. Significant mucin production is associated with a worse prognosis because the pockets of mucin can mechanically dissect the bowel wall, facilitating the extension of the malignancy.

Several variants of adenocarcinoma of the colon are worth noting. If the adenocarcinoma has foci of squamous cell differentiation, it is termed **"adenosquamous" carcinoma.** Infrequently, the colon cancer is composed of small, undifferentiated cells, which presumably arise from neuroendocrine cells and are capable of secreting hormonal products. These tumors can be considered undifferentiated carcinoid tumors, but are usually called **small cell undifferentiated carcinomas.** In another variety, seen most commonly in patients with ulcerative colitis, long tapered strictures are produced by infiltration of **poorly differentiated carcinomas.**

The prognosis and clinical course of colon cancer depends on the stage and location of the tumor. Tumors from the left side of the colon tend to be symptomatic (melena, diarrhea, constipation) earlier, but are often deeply infiltrative (particularly in the rectum and sigmoid) and may be difficult to resect adequately. In contrast, cecal and right colonic cancers tend to be asymptomatic until late in their course, but do not bleed easily. The detection of occult gastrointestinal bleeding or anemia can lead to their early discovery. Staging of colorectal cancer is based on the depth of tumor penetration, presence of fistula or extension to adjacent structures, nodal involvement, and presence of distant metastases. Metastases can occur through both the lymphatics and blood vessels; common distant sites of metastasis include the liver, lungs, and bone.

Variants of colon cancer include adenosquamous, small cell, and undifferentiated carcinomas.

Tumors from the left side of the colon tend to be symptomatic earlier than are tumors from the right side.

LIVER

BASIC CLINICAL PATTERNS OF LIVER DISEASE

The liver and extrahepatic biliary system are vulnerable to a variety of diseases. However, severe hepatobiliary disease, independently of etiology, tends to produce several clinical patterns that are related to disruption of normal hepatic function, including jaundice, liver failure, cirrhosis, and portal hypertension.

Jaundice

Jaundice is produced by many hematologic and hepatobiliary diseases.

Jaundice, or icterus, is a yellow-green pigmentation of the skin or sclera that becomes noticeable when the serum bilirubin level exceeds 2 mg/dl. Jaundice is produced by many hematologic and hepatobiliary diseases. Predominantly unconjugated hyperbilirubinemia can be produced by overproduction of unconjugated bilirubin (hemolysis, internal bleeding, ineffective erythropoiesis); decreased hepatocellular uptake of bilirubin (drugs, near starvation, sepsis); or decreased hepatocellular conjugation (Gilbert syndrome, Crigler-Najjar syndrome, neonatal jaundice, chloramphenicol, diffuse hepatocellular disease). Predominantly conjugated hyperbilirubinemia (cholestasis) is produced by impaired hepatocellular secretion (Dubin-Johnson syndrome, Rotor syndrome, hepatitis); drugs (sex steroid); damage to intrahepatic ducts (early biliary cirrhosis, cystic fibrosis, congenital atresia of intrahepatic ducts); and extrahepatic obstruction (gallstones, tumor, stricture, inflammation).

Liver Failure

Liver failure disrupts many normal metabolic functions.

Liver failure occurs when the liver is so badly damaged that it can no longer perform its metabolic functions. End-stage liver failure of many causes has similar clinical consequences, related to disruption of normal hepatic function. **Diminished hepatic protein synthesis** causes decreased albumin synthesis with consequent ascites and generalized edema; decreased synthesis of clotting factors with consequent coagulopathy; impaired toxin degradation; impaired urea cycle function with consequent hyperammonemia; impaired estrogen metabolism leading to gynecomastia and gonadal atrophy; and impaired bilirubin metabolism with consequent jaundice. Damage to the **hepatocyte plasma membrane,** as seen in many forms of acutely developing hepatic failure, may cause increased serum levels of many hepatic cytosolic enzymes, notably lactic dehydrogenase, alanine transaminase, and aspartate transaminase.

Hepatorenal syndrome refers to the appearance of renal failure that cannot be attributed to other causes in patients with coexisting severe liver disease. The specific etiology is still disputed, but is probably the result of toxic injury to the kidney. Clinically, diminished urine output is associated with a rising blood urea nitrogen and serum creatinine. The urine is hyperosmolar, with low concentrations of sodium, and contains no proteins or abnormal sediment. **Hepatic encephalopathy** refers to a reversible pattern of central nervous system and neuromuscular dysfunction seen in patients with severe hepatic disease, probably related to elevated serum levels of toxic metabolites. The syndrome is characterized by asterixis, fluctuating neurologic signs, and progressive confusion, which may progress to coma and death. High protein intake, either through diet or digestion of blood following massive gastrointestinal bleeding, tends to precipitate or exacerbate the hepatic encephalopathy.

Severe liver failure also induces renal and central nervous system dysfunction.

Cirrhosis

Cirrhosis is a severe fibrosis of the liver characterized by a disorganization of the architecture of the entire liver caused by hepatocyte injury and loss followed by replacement with interconnecting fibrous scars. Cirrhosis is the end stage of many liver diseases. Fibrosis extends from one lobule into another and may take the form of either delicate bands or broad scars. Reorganization of the vascular architecture may cause abnormal anastomoses between the arterial and venous systems, bypassing areas disrupted by scars. Regenerative nodules form in the hepatic parenchyma as less severely affected hepatocytes regenerate. The term **micronodular cirrhosis** is used when the nodules have a diameter less than 3 mm; **macronodular cirrhosis** refers to cirrhosis with larger nodules. Mixed micronodular and macronodular cirrhosis can also be encountered.

Cirrhosis is the end stage of many liver diseases.

Alcoholic, postnecrotic, biliary, and cryptogenic cirrhoses are common as is cirrhosis following hemochromatosis and α_1-antitrypsin deficiency. The complications seen in severe cirrhosis are hepatic failure, portal hypertension, and, uncommonly, hepatocellular carcinoma.

Portal Hypertension

Portal hypertension, or increased pressure in the portal system, can occur as a consequence of prehepatic, intrahepatic, or posthepatic obstruction. **Prehepatic** causes include partial or complete occlusion of the portal vein (thrombosis, tumor, enlarged portohepatic nodes), and increased inflow into the portal system (massive splenomegaly). **Intrahepatic** causes include cirrhosis, schistosomiasis, veno-occlusive disease, massive fatty change, granulomatous disease, focal nodular hyperplasia, and idiopathic portal hypertension. **Posthepatic** causes include severe right-sided failure, Budd-Chiari syndrome, and constrictive pericarditis. Despite this variety, hepatic cirrhosis is the overwhelming cause of portal hypertension and is usually assumed to be present unless convincing evidence is presented that it is not.

Portal hypertension has many causes, of which the most common is cirrhosis.

Portal hypertension is associated with portosystemic shunts (gastroesophageal varices, hemorrhoids, caput medusa), and splenomegaly. Hepatic encephalopathy is seen most commonly in advanced cirrhosis complicated by diffuse parenchymal damage and portosystemic shunting.

HEPATITIS

Hepatotropic Viruses

A variety of viruses can infect the liver. **Hepatitis A** is an RNA virus transmitted principally by an anal-oral route. Hepatitis A infection produces acute hepatitis, which is usually a mild febrile illness (or asymptomatic in children) but rarely is fulminant and can cause death. Chronic infection and progression to cirrhosis are not seen. **Hepatitis B** is a DNA virus transmitted principally by parenteral routes. Since hepatitis B can produce chronic infection, all of the viral hepatitis syndromes discussed in this chapter can be seen. **Hepatitis D** is a defective RNA virus that replicates only if hepatitis B is present. Compared with patients who have hepatitis B alone, coinfection or superinfection with hepatitis D tends to produce more severe hepatitis and to predispose for chronic disease leading to cirrhosis. **Hepatitis C** (an RNA virus) and the other hepatitis **non-A, non-B viruses** can also infect the liver; they are important causes of post-transfusion acute and chronic hepatitis. In the United States, other viral causes of hepatitis are seen primarily in severely immunosuppressed patients. Important viruses include cytomegalovirus, Epstein-Barr virus, herpes simplex virus, and herpes varicella-zoster virus. The yellow fever virus causes hepatitis in tropical countries.

Acute Viral Hepatitis

Acute viral hepatitis can be considered to be the prototype for acute hepatitis. The general disease pattern is similar for each viral cause although the time course may differ. An asymptomatic **incubation period** follows viral exposure. For all hepatotropic viruses, the peak infectivity occurs toward the end of the incubation period and in the early symptomatic period. During the **symptomatic preicteric phase,** a patient usually experiences nonspecific symptoms including malaise, fatigue, anorexia, and nausea. Some patients additionally experience low-grade fever, headache, or muscle pain. Elevation of the serum levels of alanine transaminase and aspartate transaminase is seen as hepatocyte injury occurs. A **symptomatic icteric phase,** if seen, is characterized clinically by jaundice, conjugated hyperbilirubinemia, and itching due to retained bile salts. Patients who are apt to experience jaundice include almost all adults (but not children) with hepatitis A and many patients with hepatitis B, C, and non-A, non-B. The combined symptomatic preicteric and icteric phases typically last a few weeks to several months and tend to be somewhat longer in patients with hepatitis B (with or without D) than in other forms. A **convalescent phase,** lasting weeks to months, is seen following the symptomatic phase. Liver function tests remain somewhat elevated, and the patient may experience residual constitutional symptoms.

The classic form of acute viral hepatitis is seen in almost all cases of hepatitis A infection and most cases of hepatitis non-A, non-B infection. Histologic features include acidophilic and ballooning degeneration of hepatocytes, focal necrosis of hepatocytes producing lobular disarray, predominantly mononuclear inflammation involving the portal triads, binucleation and mitoses as the remaining liver regenerates, and Kuppfer cell enlargement. Grossly, the liver in milder forms of acute viral hepatitis may show only mild abnormalities including bile staining, congestion, and swelling.

One form of acute viral hepatitis, icteric hepatitis, can mimic extrahepatic mechanical obstruction. The histology resembles that of the classic form of acute viral hepatitis, but bile stasis is more prominent. Proliferation of bile ductules and neutrophilic infiltration may be present.

Fulminant Hepatitis

Fulminant hepatitis is severe acute hepatitis with submassive to massive necrosis. While complete massive necrosis is uniformly fatal, about one-fourth of affected people, particularly young, healthy individuals, can recover from nearly complete necrosis. Recovery, if it occurs, is usually complete, and progression to chronic disease or cirrhosis is unusual. **Submassive necrosis** is present when large areas of hepatocytes are necrotic. Patchy involvement of the central and midzonal regions is typical. Features seen in addition to those present in classic acute viral hepatitis include collapse of portions of the reticular network, inflammation of central veins, and bridging necrosis between lobules. The collapse of the reticular framework and development of fibrosis can progress eventually to cirrhosis.

Fulminant hepatitis can produce submassive to massive necrosis.

Chronic Hepatic Viral Infection

Hepatitis B virus, with or without coexistent hepatitis D virus, is capable of inducing **chronic hepatic infection,** which may produce a wide range of disease states from asymptomatic carrier to cirrhosis or hepatocellular carcinoma. Hepatitis C and other hepatitis non-A, non-B viruses can also produce chronic infective states. Chronic infection with hepatitis A virus apparently does not occur. While carrier states for a few other viruses (cytomegalovirus, herpesvirus, Epstein-Barr virus) exist, these viruses become clinically significant only in severely immunocompromised patients such as organ transplant recipients.

Chronic hepatic viral infections include carrier states, chronic persistent viral hepatitis, and chronic active viral hepatitis.

A person who does not exhibit symptoms but harbors a virus is a **"carrier"** and may transmit virus to other individuals. All hepatotropic viruses except hepatitis A can produce a carrier state. Carriers may experience no adverse affects or may have low level chronic disease.

Failure to develop immunity, usually to hepatitis B virus, can cause **chronic persistent viral hepatitis,** which clinically and histologically resembles classic viral hepatitis. This form of hepatitis may be viewed as a prolonged recovery period (up to years) following acute hepatitis that is not associated with progressive liver damage. The patient typically feels well but has elevated serum transaminase levels. Morphologic changes that are suggestive but not pathognomic of chronic persistent viral hepatitis include a chronic inflammatory infiltrate limited to the portal tracts, and absence of significant hepatocyte necrosis.

Chronic persistent viral hepatitis has a benign course, while chronic active viral hepatitis tends to progress to cirrhosis and liver failure.

Development of **chronic active viral hepatitis,** particularly that caused by hepatitis B, appears to be related to an autoimmune mechanism, as similar reactions may be triggered by drugs such as isoniazide, methyldopa, and aspirin. Chronic active viral hepatitis may be asymptomatic or may cause nonspecific symptoms similar to those seen in acute hepatitis. Immune complex diseases, such as polyarteritis nodosa and glomerulonephritis, rarely coexist with chronic active hepatitis. Elevated serum transaminase levels and prolonged prothrombin time are consistently present; increased serum bilirubin and serum globulin levels are sometimes seen. Up to one-half of patients with chronic active hepatitis die within 5 years; major causes of death include liver failure, cirrhosis with massive gastrointestinal bleeding, and hepatocellular carcinoma. A small number with milder disease experience spontaneous remission.

Chronic active hepatitis is usually identified by liver biopsy, which may show a predominantly lymphocytic and plasmocytic inflammatory infiltrate located mainly in portal tracts, but which characteristically "spills" into the adjacent liver parenchyma. Also present is marked hepatocyte necrosis, which may be either "piecemeal" at the limiting plates adjacent to the portal tracts or "bridging," with formation of tracts of collapsed reticulum network between lobules as a result of necrosis of intervening hepatocytes. Fibrosis can extend from the portal tracts into the adjacent hepatocyte parenchyma, and may progress to cirrhosis. Hepatitis B and D viruses can often be identified by immunocytochemical or in situ hybridization techniques.

While chronic persistent hepatitis and chronic active hepatitis are considered distinct clinicopathologic forms, some cases of chronic persistent hepatitis progress to chronic active hepatitis, and treatment of chronic active hepatitis will sometimes convert it to chronic persistent hepatitis.

Chronic hepatitis B infection, with or without coexistent hepatitis D infection, is associated with both post-necrotic cirrhosis (see p. 263) and hepatocellular carcinoma (see p. 269).

Nonviral Causes of Hepatitis

Many agents can produce syndromes resembling viral hepatitis.

Syndromes resembling fulminant viral hepatitis can be produced by a variety of etiologies. **Drugs and chemicals** that cause acute pathology include isoniazide, antidepressants, acetaminophen, nonsteroidal anti-inflammatory agents, methyldopa, halothane, chlorinated hydrocarbons, phosphorus, and mycotoxins derived from mushrooms. **Impaired perfusion** due to ischemia, Budd-Chiari syndrome, or veno-occlusive disease can cause significant hepatocyte necrosis. Causes of severe **microvesicular steatosis** can also produce fulminant liver failure, such as acute fatty liver of pregnancy, Reye syndrome, and drug-induced microvesicular steatosis. **Autoimmune** chronic active hepatitis can progress to fulminant hepatitis.

Miscellaneous causes include massive malignant infiltration of the liver, Wilson's disease, hyperthermia, liver transplantation, and partial hepatectomy. Many of these causes of fulminant hepatitis will also produce milder forms of disease resembling acute viral hepatitis. Nonviral causes are seen more commonly with chronic active hepatitis than chronic persistent hepatitis. Chronic active hepatitis may be seen with drugs, metabolic disorders, autoimmune diseases, or idiopathically. Note that chronic autoimmune ("lupoid") hepatitis is a syndrome with a variety of nonspecific autoantibodies (antinuclear, anti-smooth muscle, and antimitochondrial antibodies) and organ-specific autoantibodies (to liver-specific protein, liver membrane antigen, and liver microsomes) seen principally in young and perimenopausal women who may have other forms of autoimmune disease such as thyroiditis, arthritis, vasculitis, and Sjögren syndrome. Alcohol use is an additional important cause of acute and chronic hepatitis, and is discussed later (see p. 262).

Other Hepatic Inflammations

Other inflammations that can affect the liver include pericholangitis, ascending cholangitis, primary sclerosing cholangitis, and liver abscess. Also included in this section, although not technically inflammations, are parasitic infestations.

Pericholangitis is inflammation of the portal tracts without involvement of bile duct lumina or the adjacent hepatic parenchyma. The inflammation usually consists mainly of lymphocytes and macrophages, and is typically of little or no clinical significance. Clinical findings that are occasionally present are almost always mild and may include fever, pruritis, jaundice, and elevated alkaline phosphatase. Pericholangitis is associated with inflammatory bowel disease, sepsis, and pancreatitis. The inflammation is not relieved by antibiotics and is possibly related to drainage of bacterial products into the liver.

Inflammation (usually due to infection) within bile ducts is termed **cholangitis.** It most frequently develops following bile stasis due to extrahepatic biliary obstruction, leading to the use of the term **ascending cholangitis.** Causes of extrahepatic duct obstruction include gallstones, tumors, pancreatitis, and benign strictures. A wide variety of bacterial agents have been implicated, including *E. coli, Klebsiella,* and *Enterobacter.* Less common pathogens include staphylococci, streptococci, and anaerobes. Cholangitis has also been seen following toxic shock syndrome, possibly related to circulating toxins. The patient with cholangitis is usually quite ill and experiences leukocytosis, high fever, and jaundice. Therapy consists of surgical drainage of the extrahepatic biliary system.

Primary sclerosing cholangitis is an uncommon condition in which fibrosis narrows or may even obliterate the lumina of bile ducts. The process is of unknown etiology and can affect either or both extrahepatic and intrahepatic bile ducts. The diagnosis is usually made by cholangiography, where the ducts may appear "beaded" due to the segmental, uneven pattern of duct involvement. Microscopically, a principally mononuclear cell inflammatory infiltrate is associated with fibrosis of the ducts. The clinical presentation is similar to other causes of obstructive jaundice. The disease occurs most commonly in young to middle-aged men and is associated with ulcerative colitis and a variety of autoimmune diseases. Primary sclerosing cholangitis usually progresses to biliary cirrhosis and liver failure within 4 or 5 years.

In the United States, **liver abscesses** most commonly develop by arterial-borne spread of infection in immunocompromised patients or following ascending cholangitis. Common organisms seen in these settings include enteric organisms, fungi, and streptococci. Antibiotic-resistant species (including staphylococci, *Pseudomonas,* and *Enterobacter*) are often important in patients who have been hospitalized before developing hepatic abscess. In developing countries, parasitic infections by echinococci, amoeba, other protozoa, or helminths are additional common causes of hepatic abscesses. Regardless of etiology, liver abscess clinically resembles ascending cholangitis, with fever, hepatomegaly, right upper quadrant pain, and (rarely) jaundice. Even with appropriate therapy including surgical drainage, the mortality of liver abscesses is 20 to 30 percent.

Pericholangitis is often of little or no clinical significance.

Ascending cholangitis typically occurs when bile stasis predisposes for bacterial infection.

Primary sclerosing cholangitis has a segmental pattern of duct involvement.

Liver abscesses can be caused by bacteria, protozoa, fungi, and metazoal parasites.

Many parasites may infest the liver.

The liver can be infested with **parasites.** Protozoa species include plasmodia species (malaria), *Entamoeba histolytica* (amebic hepatitis, amebic liver abscess), *Leishmania donovani* (kala-azar), and *Trypanosoma cruzi* (Chagas disease). Trematodes include *Schistosoma* species (schistosomiasis, bilharziasis), *Clonorchis sinensis, Fasciola hepatica, Opisthorchis felineus,* and *Dicrocoelium dendriticum.* Cestodes include *Taenia solium* (cysticercosis), and *Echinococcus* species (hydatid cyst, echinococcosis). Nematodes include agents causing visceral larva migrans (*Toxocara* species, *Ancyclostoma* species, *Strongyloides stercoralis*), and *Capillaria hepatica.* The reader is referred to the chapter on parasitology for more information about these infestations and the diseases they cause (see pp. 63).

ALCOHOLIC LIVER DISEASE

Three patterns of liver disease, which sometimes overlap, can be seen in chronic alcohol users: fatty liver, alcoholic hepatitis, and cirrhosis.

Fatty Liver

Fatty liver is the earliest change observed in alcoholic liver disease.

Fatty liver (alcoholic steatosis) is the earliest change. Early fatty liver is present in normal volunteers following several days of alcohol consumption. Grossly, the fatty liver is enlarged (up to 4 or more kg), soft, yellow, and has a greasy cut surface. Histologically, the cytoplasmic coalescence of small lipid droplets (**microvesicular steatosis**) into larger droplets (**macrovesicular steatosis**) can displace hepatocyte nuclei to the cell periphery. Rupture of lipid-filled hepatocytes uncommonly induces lipogranulomas, which are focal aggregations of lymphocytes, macrophages, and sometimes multinucleated giant cells. The biochemical basis of fatty change is still disputed, but appears to involve direct hepatotoxicity of either ethanol or its metabolites, possibly aggravated by malnutrition. In its milder forms, fatty liver is a benign, reversible condition. Severe fatty liver change will sometimes produce signs and symptoms associated with hepatic dysfunction including malaise, nausea, tender hepatomegaly, jaundice and elevated serum transaminase levels. Rarely, fatty liver may progress directly to cirrhosis, possibly as a result of fibrosis beginning in the perivenular and perisinusoidal areas.

Alcoholic Hepatitis

Alcoholic hepatitis, characterized by scattered hepatocyte necrosis, can follow "binge" drinking.

Alcoholic hepatitis is characterized by acutely developing hepatocyte necrosis, and typically begins after an episode of heavy ("binge") drinking in a patient with pre-existing fatty liver or cirrhosis. Histologically, alcoholic hepatitis is characterized by single cell or scattered foci of hepatocyte necrosis; an inflammatory cell infiltrate, mainly neutrophils, which is found near the degenerating liver cells; scattered, damaged hepatocytes with eosinophilic cytoplasmic inclusions known as Mallory bodies or "alcoholic hyaline" (although similar structures can sometimes be seen in other liver diseases); and perisinusoidal and perivenular fibrosis. The mechanism causing hepatocyte necrosis and Mallory body formation is still unknown, but may involve toxic damage to the hepatocyte cytoskeleton by alcohol or its metabolites. The fibrosis seen after alcoholic hepatitis appears to be a forerunner of cirrhosis, which can eventually develop after repeated episodes of alcoholic hepatitis.

Depending upon severity and remaining functional liver reserve, alcoholic hepatitis may be asymptomatic or may produce a range of signs and symptoms (malaise, anorexia, tender hepatomegaly, jaundice, elevated transaminase levels) that may culminate in fulminant hepatic failure. A significant risk of death (10 to 20 percent per bout) is associated with symptomatic alcoholic hepatitis. Of the individuals who survive repeated bouts of alcoholic hepatitis, approximately one-third subsequently develop hepatic cirrhosis. The presence of fever and a neutrophilic leukocytosis may help to distinguish moderately severe alcoholic hepatitis from symptomatic fatty liver.

Alcoholic Cirrhosis

It is convenient to consider alcoholic cirrhosis in early and late stages. **Early alcoholic cirrhosis** is characterized by a large (more than 2 kg) fatty liver with a micronodular pattern of cirrhosis. It may be histologically recognizable as probably due to alcohol consumption if the changes associated with alcoholic fatty liver or alcoholic hepatitis are seen. The fibrous septa in early alcoholic cirrhosis are typically delicate and extend between portal tracts and from central veins to portal tracts. **Late alcoholic cirrhosis** is characterized by a much smaller liver, produced as portions of the liver exhibiting fatty change are replaced by fibrous scar. The liver may eventually develop macronodular cirrhosis as regeneration of the few remaining viable nodules produces large nodules separated by broad bands of fibrosis. Bile stasis may be prominent, and cytoplasmic hemosiderin deposition may occur. The distinctive features of alcoholic fatty change and alcoholic hepatitis tend to be absent, and consequently the end-stage alcoholic cirrhotic liver may be indistinguishable from the end-stage postnecrotic cirrhotic liver.

Early alcoholic cirrhosis usually has a micronodular pattern, while late alcoholic cirrhosis may have a macronodular pattern.

Alcoholic cirrhosis is the most common cause of cirrhosis in the Western world. Surprisingly, only about 10 to 15 percent of heavy alcohol users develop alcoholic cirrhosis, and it has proved difficult to define which alcohol users are most at risk. The clinical course of severe alcoholic cirrhosis is similar to that of other severe cirrhoses. The prognosis for patients who stop drinking before jaundice and ascites develop is much better (90 percent 5-year survival rate) than it is for those who continue to drink or who start drinking again (50 to 60 percent 5-year survival).

POSTNECROTIC CIRRHOSIS

Postnecrotic cirrhosis is a macronodular cirrhosis characterized by irregular nodules separated by broad bands of fibrosis. At the end stage, the liver is typically small and has nodules up to several centimeters in diameter. Microscopic characteristics include broad bands of fibrosis surrounding large nodules of regenerating hepatocytes. The distorted portal triads may lie close together as a result of destruction of intervening hepatic lobules. Bile ductule proliferation and a principally lymphocytic and histiocytic infiltrate may be present within the fibrotic bands. The cirrhosis usually results from necrosis of hepatocytes followed by heal-

Postnecrotic cirrhosis has many causes.

ing, with scar formation. Causes of postnecrotic cirrhosis include viruses (hepatitis B, C, D, and non-A, non-B virus) and hepatotoxins (phosphorus, carbon tetrachloride, mushroom poisoning, acetaminophen, oxyphenisatin, methyldopa). Often, damage has occurred over years. Chronic active hepatitis B infection can be demonstrated in about 20 to 25 percent of cases of postnecrotic cirrhosis. Other etiologies are less common, and in a substantial fraction of cases, the etiology remains undetermined. Since end-stage alcoholic cirrhosis develops a similar gross and microscopic appearance, some cases of postnecrotic cirrhosis may actually be alcoholic cirrhosis in which alcohol use was denied. Submassive hepatic necrosis tends to produce cirrhosis more often than does massive hepatic necrosis, since massive hepatic necrosis usually causes either death or recovery as nearly complete regeneration occurs.

The clinical course varies with the etiology.

The clinical course of postnecrotic cirrhosis varies with etiology and the presence of continued liver damage. Postnecrotic cirrhosis, particularly when associated with chronic hepatitis B virus infection acquired early in life, is the most common form of cirrhosis to progress to hepatocellular carcinoma.

OTHER FORMS OF CIRRHOSIS

Hemochromatosis

The excessive iron deposition observed in hemochromatosis can also cause cirrhosis.

When the total body iron is substantially increased over the normal range of 2 to 6 g, iron deposition can occur in tissues, notably the liver and pancreas. This process is called **hemochromatosis** and may occur either in an idiopathic or a secondary form. Idiopathic hemochromatosis tends to be more severe than secondary hemochromatosis. The biochemical defect(s) that produces idiopathic hemochromatosis is still unproved, but it may be due to either excessive iron absorption by the intestine or a failure to excrete excess iron promptly following intestinal absorption. The total body iron stores may be increased to as much as 50 to 60 g in idiopathic hemochromatosis. This excess iron is preferentially deposited in the cytoplasm of parenchymal cells in organs such as the liver, pancreas, endocrine glands, or heart, rather than being preferentially deposited in cells in the reticular endothelial system, as occurs in secondary systemic hemosiderosis following iron liberation from red cells by processes such as hemolytic anemias or multiple transfusions.

The involved liver may be large, dense, and chocolate brown. Micronodular cirrhosis, which may be complicated by primary liver cancer, may eventually develop. Diffuse pancreatic fibrosis may be associated with deranged glucose metabolism or frank diabetes mellitus. Hemosiderin deposition in myocardial fibers can produce cardiomyopathy and arrhythmias. Skin discoloration may range from golden-brown to slate-gray. Hemosiderin deposition in joint synovial lining can be accompanied by deposition of calcium pyrophosphate, producing pseudogout, a disabling arthritis. Many endocrine glands, particularly the adrenals, may also show hemosiderin deposition, and the hypogonadism seen in many patients of both sexes may be a consequence of disruption of the hypothalmic-pituitary axis. In general, patients with primary hemochromatosis tend to experience more complications than do patients with secondary hemochromatosis. Progression of the disease can be slowed by lowering body iron stores with repeated phlebotomy or the use of iron chelates such as desferrioxamine.

Wilson's Disease

Wilson's disease is an autosomal recessive biochemical failure to synthesize adequate levels of the serum protein ceruloplasmin, which normally binds plasma copper. Any excess copper bound to ceruloplasmin is normally processed by liver and excreted into bile. In the absence of adequate serum ceruloplasmin, excess copper accumulates in many tissues, notably liver, brain, and eye. In the **liver,** a variety of clinicopathologic syndromes can be seen, including fatty change, acute hepatitis, chronic active hepatitis, cirrhosis, and (rarely) massive liver necrosis. In the **brain,** toxic injury, sometimes leading to grossly visible cavitations, involves neurons of the basal ganglia, particularly the putamen. These changes are associated with movement disorder and psychiatric disturbances. In the **eye,** green-brown copper deposits in Descemet's membrane of the cornea are known as Kayser-Fleischer rings. The formerly dismal prognosis of Wilson's disease has been modified by the use of copper chelators, such as penicillamine, early in the disease.

> Copper accumulation in Wilson's disease can cause cirrhosis and brain injury.

α₁-Antitrypsin Deficiency

α_1**-Antitrypsin** is a major serum protease inhibitor that is synthesized in liver. The gene that codes for α_1-antitrypsin has many genetic variations, which are given alphabetical designations. MM homozygotes are the normal phenotype and have normal serum α_1-antitrypsin. SS homozygotes have approximately 10 percent activity. Clinically significant disease is usually seen only in ZZ homozygotes, in whom it can cause emphysema and liver disease. Abnormal α_1-antitrypsin accumulates as round to oval, PAS-positive, cytoplasmic granules in **liver** cells due to a failure to secrete the abnormal protein. A wide range of hepatic syndromes can be produced, including neonatal hepatitis, childhood cirrhosis, and adult cirrhosis. Factors contributing to the expression of the liver disease remain unelucidated. In the **lung,** lack of sufficient serum α_1-antitrypsin causes exaggerated activity of proteases leading to alveolar destruction with the development of panlobular emphysema (see p. 164).

> α_1-Antitrypsin deficiency can cause both emphysema and liver disease.

Primary Biliary Cirrhosis

Primary biliary cirrhosis is a severe, progressive cholestatic condition that appears to begin as a destructive sclerosing cholangitis and cholangiolitis. While the etiology remains undetermined, primary biliary cirrhosis appears to have an autoimmune basis, and patients with primary biliary cirrhosis often have other immunologic diseases. The disease is seen most frequently in perimenopausal and postmenopausal women, although any adult age group can be affected. The clinical course of primary biliary cirrhosis is primarily of progressive cholestasis leading eventually to cirrhosis.

The pathology involves intrahepatic duct and ductule inflammation that can eventually progress to cirrhosis; it may be considered to occur in four stages. In stage I, **florid inflammation** is confined to the portal triads and is accompanied by focal destruction of septal and interlobular bile ducts. Granulomas can sometimes be seen in the inflammatory infiltrate. In stage II, **proliferation of ducts** is accompanied by a more severe inflammatory infiltrate that extends beyond the portal triads to involve the limiting plates of the surrounding parenchyma in a manner

> Primary biliary cirrhosis appears to have an autoimmune basis.

> The pathology begins with portal tract inflammation and bile duct proliferation, and later progresses to fibrosis and cirrhosis.

similar to that seen in chronic active hepatitis. Mallory bodies are sometimes seen in damaged liver cells. Cholestasis is more prominent than in stage I, and granulomas are seen less frequently. In stage III, **fibrosis** is accompanied by less prominent inflammatory infiltrate with marked reduction of granulomas, distinct reduction in the number of bile ducts, replacement of portal tracts by fibrous septa that may sometimes extend into the parenchyma to interconnect adjacent lobules, and increasingly prominent cholestasis. In stage IV, **cirrhosis,** caused by extension of the changes seen in stage III, eventually creates an overt micronodular cirrhosis characterized by nearly complete disappearance of larger bile ducts. Copper retention due to impaired excretion through damaged ducts can occur.

Secondary Biliary Cirrhosis

Bile and outflow obstruction can cause secondary biliary cirrhosis.

Secondary biliary cirrhosis results from obstruction of the major extrahepatic ducts and can follow any cause of bile outflow obstruction. Ductal damage caused by bile stasis induces a secondary inflammatory reaction that culminates in a micronodular cirrhosis. Ascending cholangitis and cholangiolitis, often with enteric organisms such as coliforms and enterococci, can also cause secondary biliary cirrhosis, with or without bile stasis.

Miscellaneous Forms of Cirrhosis

A variety of other processes can also cause cirrhosis.

Cirrhosis can be seen in other diseases than those described above. Galactosemia, tyrosinosis, and other **inborn metabolic disorders** may cause cirrhosis in children who survive infancy. **Cardiac sclerosis** may uncommonly become sufficiently severe to produce true cirrhosis. **Carcinomatous cirrhosis** is caused by a severe desmoplastic reaction to a diffusely infiltrative primary or secondary cancer involving the liver. **Syphilis,** in both the congenital and tertiary adult forms, may mimic cirrhosis by causing severe scarring of the liver. **Liver fluke infestations** can obstruct larger bile ducts, mimicking secondary biliary cirrhosis. **Cystic fibrosis** rarely leads to biliary cirrhosis as a consequence of plugging of bile canaliculi by mucinous material. **Cryptogenic cirrhosis,** in which no cause is identified, remains relatively common.

HEPATIC VASCULAR DISEASE

Passive Congestion

Passive congestion occurs when cardiac decompensation increases the pressure in central veins.

Cardiac decompensation, particularly right heart failure, can cause passive congestion of the liver by increasing the pressure in the central veins. **Acute passive congestion** follows acutely developing cardiac decompensation. Grossly, the liver typically shows dusky red cyanosis, slight enlargement with rounded edges, and prominent central veins in cut section. Microscopically, centrilobular sinusoidal congestion is seen. Acute passive congestion is a frequent autopsy finding since preterminal circulatory failure is common. Obstruction of the inferior vena cava or hepatic veins is an uncommon cause of acute passive congestion.

Chronic passive congestion occurs when persistent right-sided heart failure causes progression of acute passive congestion to chronic passive congestion. Grossly, the liver has a fine, mottled appearance known as nutmeg liver, in which the central congested region of each lobule is dark red-blue and the peripheral portions of the lobule are pale. Microscopically, centrilobular congestion is present, but chronic passive congestion differs from acute passive congestion by the presence of atrophy of central hepatocytes secondary to severe chronic hypoxia and fatty change of peripheral hepatocytes secondary to mild chronic hypoxia.

Central hemorrhagic necrosis is a severe acute passive congestion of the liver, such as can occur following severe acute cardiac failure; it causes necrosis of the central lobular hepatocytes and extravasation of blood from sinusoids into the space of Disse. This central hemorrhagic necrosis may be due to severe hypoxia. **Cardiac sclerosis** is a severe chronic passive congestion that can eventually lead to a modest increase in fibrous tissue around the central veins. Typically, delicate strands of fibrous tissue, best seen with special stains to highlight collagen, extend into the hepatic parenchyma. These changes are known as cardiac sclerosis and only rarely become so severe as to cause portal hypertension.

Central hemorrhagic necrosis and cardiac sclerosis are severe forms of acute and chronic passive congestion, respectively.

Hepatic Infarction

True hepatic infarction is rare, since the liver has a dual blood supply from the portal vein and hepatic artery. Occlusion of an intrahepatic branch of the **portal vein** causes sinusoidal congestion and hepatocellular atrophy. This lesion, known inappropriately as an **infarct of Zahn,** appears grossly as a well-demarcated, red-blue discoloration. Infrequently, occlusion of an intrahepatic branch of the **hepatic artery** can cause a **small, true infarct** characterized by hepatocellular necrosis. Causes of such infarcts include polyarteritis nodosa, embolism, and neoplasia. **Larger infarctions** of the liver are usually seen only when the liver blood supply is compromised by several processes, as when septic shock develops in a patient with pre-existing cirrhosis.

Occlusion of a branch of the hepatic artery may cause a true infarction, while occlusion of a branch of the portal vein usually does not.

Hepatic Vein Thrombosis

Thrombosis of the hepatic veins or adjacent inferior vena cava **(Budd-Chiari syndrome)** can produce hepatomegaly, ascites, and abdominal pain that can lead to death. Acute passive congestion and sometimes central hemorrhagic necrosis are seen following sudden thrombosis. Chronic passive congestion and cardiac sclerosis are seen if the thrombosis develops more slowly. Predisposing conditions are associated with thrombotic tendencies and include polycythemia vera, high estrogen states (e.g., oral contraceptive use), intra-abdominal carcinomas (e.g., hepatocellular carcinoma), and paroxysmal nocturnal hemoglobinuria. Outside the United States, membranous webs in the major hepatic veins or inferior vena cava are a common cause of Budd-Chiari syndrome. The chronic form of the syndrome has about a 50 percent 5-year survival rate, while the acute form has a very high mortality rate. Prompt surgical intervention to remove the thrombosis or to establish alternative blood flow can decrease mortality.

Thrombosis of the hepatic veins can cause death.

Hepatic Veno-Occlusive Disease

Rarely, intrahepatic central veins may become obliterated following subendothelial thickening and sclerosis. The basis for such **hepatic veno-occlusive disease** appears to be toxic, as these changes can be seen following exposure to some plant alkaloids, irradiation, and antineoplastic drugs. Graft-versus-host disease following bone marrow transplantation is also a risk factor.

Portal Vein Obstruction

Intrahepatic portal vein obstruction is typically caused by cirrhosis, with tumor invasion or compression of the vessels being the only other common cause. **Extrahepatic** causes of portal vein obstruction include abdominal cancers, infection of the portal vein (pyelophlebitis) following peritonitis, pancreatitis, and postsurgical thromboses. Portal vein obstruction is better tolerated than hepatic vein obstruction. Portal vein obstruction produces abdominal pain, massive ascites, and portal hypertension. Bowel infarction secondary to impaired portal drainage and liver abscesses secondary to pyelophlebitis can also be seen. Therapy involves surgical resection of the infarcted bowel and shunting procedures to ameliorate the venous obstruction.

HEPATIC CYSTS AND TUMORS

Benign Cysts

Simple cysts of the liver are lined with flattened, atrophic biliary epithelium and may occur singly or in clusters. **Caroli's disease** involves congenital intrahepatic dilations of the biliary tree. Individual cysts are lined by biliary epithelium and, because of their connection to the remainder of the biliary tree, may contain bile or inflammatory exudate. This pattern of cysts may be seen in association with polycystic kidney disease. **Choledochal cysts** are large (up to 6 cm) dilations of the common bile duct. These cysts are more common in children, predispose to biliary tract obstruction and gallstones, and may contain carcinoma. **Polycystic liver disease** is an inherited disorder, often associated with polycystic kidney disease, in which the liver can contain large numbers of cysts (up to several centimeters in diameter). Like polycystic kidney disease, the inheritance pattern of disease first recognizable in childhood appears to be autosomal recessive, while the adult variant is autosomal dominant.

Benign Tumors

Focal nodular hyperplasia is a benign proliferation of the liver parenchyma. It is more common in women than men and is possibly associated with oral contraceptive use. The characteristic gross appearance is of a poorly encapsulated yellow, brown, or bile-stained nodule that may range up to many centimeters in diameter. The nodule contains a central stellate scar that sends fibrous projections to the periphery of the nodule. These fibrous septae typically contain large numbers of lymphocytes and bile ducts. The intervening parenchyma consists of normal appearing plates of hepatocytes that may contain increased glycogen or lipid. **Bile duct adenomas** are benign hamartomatous proliferations of bile ducts that can produce small nodules of no clinical significance. The nodules are composed of epithelium-lined channels separated by connective tissue stroma. The lesions are almost never bile stained and characteristically are firm, pale nodules of diameter less than 1 cm.

Liver cell adenomas are benign proliferations of hepatocytes that are most often seen in young women with a history of oral contraceptive use. They are vulnerable to rupture, particularly during pregnancy, with resulting severe intraperitoneal hemorrhage. Liver cell adenomas are typically large (up to 30 cm), yellow-tan, or bile-stained nodules with irregular borders that may not grossly appear to be encapsulated. The microscopic appearance is of sheets or cords of hepatocytes with abnormally arranged, dilated sinusoids. The hepatocytes may appear normal or may vary in nuclear and cell size and shape. A characteristic feature is the absence of bile ducts. A connective tissue capsule, which may be incomplete, separates the adenoma from the surrounding hepatic parenchyma. **Cavernous hemangiomas** are benign, usually small (less than 2 cm), red-blue, soft nodules composed of dilated vascular channels that are similar to cavernous hemangiomas found elsewhere in the body.

Hepatocellular Carcinoma

Ninety percent of all primary liver tumors are **hepatocellular carcinomas.** These tumors are strongly associated with carcinogenic agents, notably hepatitis B viral infection and the mycotoxin aflatoxin B_1, which is produced by *Aspergillus flavus.* In the United States and Western Europe, hepatocellular carcinoma typically arises in cirrhotic livers in men (male/female ratio of 6:1) and is rare before age 60. In less developed countries, where hepatitis B virus infection often occurs in infancy or childhood, hepatocellular carcinoma tends to occur in young to middle adulthood, with less male predominance, and cirrhosis may not be present.

Hepatocellular carcinomas are the most common primary liver tumor.

Hepatocellular carcinomas are malignant proliferations of hepatocytes that do not usually contain bile ducts. Both the gross and microscopic appearance can vary markedly. Grossly, hepatocellular carcinomas may be unifocal, multifocal, or diffusely infiltrative. When hepatocellular carcinoma occurs in a cirrhotic liver, the tumor may be difficult to distinguish from adjacent cirrhotic nodules. Unlike cholangiocarcinomas, which are rarely bile stained, hepatocellular carcinomas may be tan, yellow-white, or have a green hue. Focal hemorrhage and necrosis may be present.

Hepatocellular carcinoma has many gross and microscopic appearances.

Microscopically, the tumor has many variations including a trabecular pattern; a pseudoglandular pattern; a "clear cell" variant of the pseudoglandular pattern with cells having a high cytoplasmic glycogen content; fibrolamellar carcinoma with acidophilic cells in nests or cords separated by fibrous stroma; and poorly differentiated carcinomas that can contain giant cells, spindle cells, and small undifferentiated cells.

Histologic features that may be helpful, when present, in establishing that a hepatic tumor is hepatocellular carcinoma include **bile pigment, bile canaliculi,** inclusions resembling Mallory's alcoholic hyaline, and vascular invasion. Immunohistochemical stains for α_1-antitrypsin, α-fetoprotein, and carcinoembryonic antigen may be positive, although not all hepatocellular carcinomas may express these markers. Hepatitis B virus may also be stained immunohistochemically in some cancers.

The presence of bile or bile canaliculi may help to establish the diagnosis.

Hepatocellular carcinoma is an aggressive tumor whose early symptoms are often masked by coexisting cirrhosis or chronic hepatitis. Patients with hepatocellular carcinoma have ill-defined upper abdominal pain. Enlargement of the liver, with typically an irregular nodular anterior edge, can be palpated in most cases. Mass lesions of the liver can be detected with ultrasonography, hepatic angiography, and computed tomography. Elevated serum α-fetoprotein or carcinoembryonic antigen may suggest, but does not prove, hepatocellular carcinoma, as many other tumors express these markers, and small hepatocellular carcinomas may not elevate serum levels. A precursor of prothrombin, **des-γ-carboxy prothrombin,** has been suggested as a potentially useful new serum marker. Biopsy of a mass lesion is usually necessary to establish the tumor diagnosis.

With the exception of the **fibrolamellar variant,** the prognosis of hepatocellular carcinoma is very poor, with death typically occurring within 6 months owing to liver failure, gastrointestinal bleeding, or cachexia. Hepatocellular carcinomas tend to metastasize late in the course of the disease, with the most common site of hematogenous spread being the lung. The fibrolamellar variant typically arises in the absence of cirrhosis in children, adolescents, and young adults. It may be amenable to surgical resection, with resulting increased survival.

The prognosis of the fibrolamellar variant is better than that of other forms of hepatocellular carcinoma.

Cholangiocarcinoma

Cholangiocarcinomas are rarely bile-stained.

Roughly 10 percent of primary carcinomas of the liver are **cholangiocarcinomas.** These tumors are composed of cells resembling bile-duct epithelium. The gross appearance of cholangiocarcinomas resembles that of hepatocellular carcinomas with the exception that the tumors are rarely bile stained, since bile is not synthesized by differentiated bile duct epithelium. The histologic appearance of cholangiocarcinoma is typically of a well-differentiated adenocarcinoma with prominent dense collagenous stroma. Well-defined glandular and tubular structures are lined by cuboidal to columnar epithelial cells that may appear anaplastic or contain mucus. Vascular invasion can occur, but is less common than in hepatocellular carcinoma.

Cholangiocarcinomas have been associated with invasion of the biliary tract by **liver flukes** (*Opisthorchis sinensis*) and also with the use of the contrast agent **thorotrast,** which was formerly used to delineate the biliary tract. Unlike hepatocellular carcinoma, hepatitis B viral infection and aflatoxin exposure do not appear to increase the risk of cholangiocarcinoma. These tumors have a poor prognosis. Metastases to lymph nodes, lungs, bones, adrenals and brain are more common than in hepatocellular carcinomas. Rarely, mixed tumors are observed that contain areas resembling both cholangiocarcinoma and hepatocellular carcinoma.

Other Primary Tumors

Other malignant hepatic tumors include hepatoblastoma and angiosarcoma.

Almost all primary tumors of the liver are either hepatocellular carcinomas or cholangiocarcinomas. However, two additional forms of primary liver cancer are rarely seen. **Hepatoblastomas** occur in infants in two anatomic variants, the epithelial type, composed of cells resembling small fetal hepatocytes; and the mixed type, composed of cells resembling fetal hepatocytes mixed with more mature-appearing hepatocytes and mesenchymal tissue, which may show striated muscle, cartilage, or osteoid differentiation. Hepatoblastomas are fatal if untreated but can sometimes be resected before metastasis has occurred. **Angiosarcomas,** or sarcomatous proliferations of blood vessels, are highly aggressive neoplasms that can involve the liver and have been associated with exposures to vinyl chloride, arsenic, and thorotrast.

Metastatic Tumors

A variety of tumors can metastasize to the liver; the most common primary tumors include **breast, lung,** and **colon cancer.** These metastatic tumors are much more common than is primary neoplasia. In the absence of coexisting primary hepatic disease, the liver can often tolerate a surprisingly large number of metastatic tumor nodules before abnormal liver function tests are seen as major bile ducts become obstructed. Metastatic tumor nodules identified by computed tomography or magnetic resonance can be biopsied, although it may not prove possible to identify definitively the primary tumor in the metastatic lesion.

Metastatic involvement of the liver is common.

HEREDITARY HYPERBILIRUBINEMIAS

The hereditary hyperbilirubinemias are biochemical disorders associated with jaundice and increased serum bilirubin levels. With the exception of Crigler-Najjar syndrome type I, which produces death in neonates, all of these diseases are relatively benign, and are clinically significant primarily because they must be distinguished from more serious causes of jaundice.

Hereditary hyperbilirubinemias, with the exception of Crigler-Najjar syndrome type I, are relatively benign biochemical disorders.

Crigler-Najjar syndrome type I is a rare autosomal recessive absence of the enzyme that catalyzes the conjugation of bilirubin, glucuronyl transferase. The resulting very high serum levels of unconjugated bilirubin (20 mg/dl) cause bilirubin accumulation in the central nervous system (kernicterus) leading to death in the neonatal period. The liver may be morphologically normal or may show canalicular cholestasis. A few patients appear to have a somewhat less severe form of the disease that produces death in adolescence.

Crigler-Najjar and Gilbert syndromes produce unconjugated hyperbilirubinemias.

Crigler-Najjar syndrome type II is a mild unconjugated hyperbilirubinemia due to an autosomal dominant partial absence of glucuronyl transferase. It is associated with jaundice, often with morphologically normal liver, without illness or shortening of the lifespan. In children, the jaundice will often respond to barbiturate therapy, which stimulates synthesis of glucuronyl transferase.

Gilbert's syndrome is a benign form of unconjugated hyperbilirubinemia of unknown etiology. The disease is characterized by both reduced uptake by hepatocytes of unconjugated bilirubin and reduced glucuronyl transferase activity. The syndrome is typically recognized as an incidental finding in late adolescence or early adulthood, frequently when jaundice appears following hemolysis due to some unrelated cause. The only morphologic abnormality in the liver is some increase in lipofuscin pigment.

Dubin-Johnson syndrome is a chronic or intermittent conjugated hyperbilirubinemia characterized by autosomal recessive inheritance and dark gray discoloration of the liver. The genetic defect may be impaired canalicular transport of organic anions, including conjugated

Dubin-Johnson and Rotor syndromes produce conjugated hyperbilirubinemia.

bilirubin, which leads to the accumulation of coarse pigment granules within the liver cells. The patient typically experiences fluctuating jaundice, but feels well. These patients are also unable to excrete the dyes used in oral cholecystography, and their biliary systems can consequently not be visualized with this technique.

Rotor syndrome is a rare asymptomatic conjugated hyperbilirubinemia of unclear etiology that differs from Dubin-Johnson syndrome in that the liver is not pigmented.

REYE SYNDROME

Reye syndrome is characterized by mitochondrial damage in liver and brain.

Reye syndrome is an acute postviral illness that mainly affects children, although adult cases have been described. In the typical presentation, pernicious vomiting develops 3 to 5 days following one of a variety of viral illnesses (notably varicella and influenza A and B) in a previously healthy child who may have been treated with aspirin or other salicylates. As the disease progresses, lethargy occurs that may progress to coma. Serum levels of bilirubin, transaminases, and ammonia are elevated. While many cases are mild, fatality can occur as a consequence of nervous system depression or liver failure. The etiology of the syndrome, and in particular the relationship to salicylate therapy, remains unclear. However, the disease is characterized by mitochondrial damage, with the most severe injury occurring in the liver (microvesicular steatosis). Less severe mitochondrial damage involves the brain, skeletal muscle, heart, and kidneys. In the United States, the incidence of Reye syndrome has diminished with decreased use of aspirin in children.

NEONATAL CHOLESTASIS

Neonatal cholestasis has many causes.

Neonates can experience prolonged conjugated hyperbilirubinemia for a variety of reasons. **Extrahepatic biliary atresia** is uncommonly encountered in normal weight female infants, and, if untreated, may cause secondary biliary cirrhosis. **Infectious neonatal hepatitis** can be caused by a large variety of congenital and neonatal infections, including viruses (hepatitis A and B, echoviruses 11, 14, and 19, coxsackie B, cytomegalovirus, herpes simplex), syphilis, gram-negative sepsis, toxoplasmosis, and endotoxemia. **Genetic and metabolic** causes of neonatal hepatitis and cholestasis include α-antitrypsin deficiency, cystic fibrosis, tyrosinemia, galactosemia, Niemann-Pick disease, and total parenteral nutrition. **Idiopathic neonatal hepatitis** accounts for over one-half of cases. The prognosis of prolonged neonatal hepatitis varies with etiology. The development of cirrhosis is an ominous sign. Many cases of idiopathic neonatal hepatitis will spontaneously remit with supportive therapy.

ADDITIONAL DISEASES THAT CAN AFFECT THE LIVER

In addition to the hereditary hyperbilirubinemias, a variety of metabolic diseases can affect the liver. **Galactosemia** is a form of hepatitis related to enzymatic deficiency in galactose metabolism (galactosyl-1-phosphate uridylyl transferase). The liver develops fatty change, both canalicular and ductal bile stasis, cellular necrosis, and, ultimately, scarring. Removal of lactose from the diet is therapeutic. Many varieties of **glycogenoses** that affect the liver are now described. Types I (von Gierke's), III, IV, and VI most often affect the liver. Normal or abnormal glycogen is stored, causing hepatomegaly and hepatic functional impairment. Types III and VI tend to produce mild disease; type I produces severe disease; and type IV is fatal early in life. **Lipid-storage diseases** (Niemann-Pick disease, Gaucher's disease, Fabry's disease, and gangliosidoses) can cause hepatomegaly, jaundice, and sometimes cirrhosis as abnormal substances are stored in hepatocytes. **Mucopolysaccharidoses** do not significantly functionally impair the liver, although liver cell storage of abnormal mucopolysaccharides may be present. **Tyrosinosis** can cause fatty change and fibrosis of the liver.

Hemochromatosis, Wilson's disease, and α_1-antitrypsin deficiency are hereditary causes of cirrhosis discussed previously (see p. 264). Cystic fibrosis is discussed in the chapter on the pancreas (see p. 278). **Amyloidosis** is an acquired systemic disease (see p. 26) that can affect the liver. Amyloid deposition between the sinusoidal membrane and the hepatocyte plates can cause hepatocyte atrophy. These changes are usually of little functional significance unless the liver becomes massively involved. The massively involved liver enlarges and may become pale and friable. **Granulomatous diseases** that can cause liver disease include tuberculosis, histoplasmosis, brucellosis, tularemia, sarcoidosis, lymphogranuloma venerum, and syphilis.

Many metabolic diseases affect the liver.

DRUG-RELATED INJURY

Drugs can cause hepatic injury. Focal nodular hyperplasia, adenomas, and **hepatocellular carcinoma** are associated with estrogen use, including oral contraceptives. Anabolic steroids have also been questionably implicated in hepatocellular carcinogenesis. **Steatosis** can be caused by tetracycline, salicylates, methotrexate, and ethanol. Cholestasis can be caused by chlorpromazine and sex steroids, including oral contraceptives. Acute and chronic **hepatitis** can be caused by isoniazide, phenytoin, and cinchopen. Centrilobular or massive necrosis can be seen with acetaminophen, halothane, and methyldopa. Fibrosis or **cirrhosis** can be caused by methotrexate, cinchopen, and amiodarone. Granuloma formation can be caused by sulfonamides, methyldopa, quinidine, phenylbutazone, hydralazine, and allopurinol. Veno-occlusive disease can be caused by cytotoxic drugs. Hepatic or portal vein thrombosis can be caused by estrogens, including oral contraceptives.

Drugs can damage liver in a variety of ways.

EXTRAHEPATIC BILIARY SYSTEM AND EXOCRINE PANCREAS

CHOLECYSTITIS

Cholecystitis is acute or chronic inflammation of the gallbladder. If gallstones are present, the cholecystitis is termed calculous; if not, it is termed acalculous.

Acute Calculous Cholecystitis

Acute cholecystitis is typically caused by lodging of a gallstone.

Acute inflammation of the gallbladder is most commonly caused by the lodging of a gallstone within either the neck of the gallbladder or the cystic duct. Such **acute calculous cholecystitis** is a major complication of cholelithiasis and is consequently seen most commonly in older, obese, female patients. Since the stone may impact in the biliary tree abruptly, the clinical presentation of acute calculous cholecystitis may be of an acute abdomen with right upper quadrant tenderness requiring surgery because of the risk of rupture of the gallbladder. Bacterial infection with colonic organisms (gram-negative rods, enterococci, anaerobic organisms) is seen in many, but not all, inflamed gallbladders. The gross presentation of acute calculous cholecystitis is an enlarged and tense gallbladder containing bile and one or more gallstones. The bile may be cloudy or turbid and contain pus (empyema), fibrin, or hemorrhage. The gallbladder wall may be thickened, edematous, hyperemic, or even gangrenous. The serosal covering may be covered by fibrin or a suppurative exudate. Microscopically, the wall usually shows acute inflammation, sometimes with frank abscess formation or gangrenous necrosis. Infection can spread across the wall of the acutely inflamed gallbladder to cause generalized peritonitis or local abscesses.

Whether acute calculous cholecystitis should be treated medically or surgically remains controversial since emergency surgery for acute cholecystitis may have a 3 to 5 percent perioperative mortality, while 25 percent of medically treated patients develop significant complications. Acutely inflamed gallbladders may resolve or progress to chronic cholecystitis. In some cases, "porcelain gallbladder" develops following deposition of calcium in the gallbladder wall.

Acute Acalculous Cholecystitis

No stone is present in some cases of acute cholecystitis.

In approximately 10 percent of cases of acute cholecystitis, no stone is present. Such **acute acalculous cholecystitis** tends to occur in children and older men. Acute acalculous cholecystitis is associated with a large variety of conditions that tend to favor cystic duct obstruction or hematogenous seeding of bacteria into the gallbladder secondary to bacteremia. Acalculous cholecystitis has a gross and microscopic appearance similar to that of calculous cholecystitis, except for the absence of stones. The complications and prognosis of acalculous cholecystitis are also similar to the calculus variant.

Chronic Cholecystitis

Chronic cholecystitis may follow acute cholecystitis or may develop in the apparent absence of previous acute inflammation. Gallstones are usually present, and the patients are most often older, obese women. Enteric organisms are present in the bile in about one-third of patients. The chronically inflamed gallbladder typically contains stones and has a thickened, fibrotic wall. The mucosal folds may have a normal appearance or may be flattened. Microscopically, the wall shows variable numbers of chronic inflammatory cells and may show increased fibrous tissue. The mucosal epithelium may penetrate into the wall to produce epithelial crypts known as cholecystitis glandularis. Acute inflammation is also sometimes observed, producing acute exacerbation of chronic cholecystitis. A **"porcelain gallbladder,"** similar to that which can follow acute cholecystitis, can be seen if dystrophic calcification is deposited in the gallbladder wall. Chronic cholecystitis is clinically significant because the accompanying gallstones may be a source of complications such as biliary obstruction.

Chronically inflamed gallbladders often contain stones.

CHOLELITHIASIS

Gallstone formation **(cholelithiasis)** can occur when bile becomes supersaturated with relatively insoluble cholesterol or bile pigments. Gallstones frequently form over a period of years as the initial nucleation or initiation of stone formation is followed by growth by accretion. The resulting stones may have pure cholesterol, mixed but principally cholesterol, or principally bile pigment composition. Passage of small gallstones through the extrahepatic biliary tree can produce excruciating biliary colic. Obstructions by stones of the extrahepatic biliary tree can produce obstructive cholestasis or infection of the gallbladder (cholecystitis). If infection does not occur, mucus filling of the gallbladder can produce **hydrops** (mucocele). Partial obstruction of the biliary tree predisposes for ascending suppurative cholangitis. Rarely, a large stone may erode through the gallbladder wall and into the adjacent intestine, causing **"gallstone ileus"** by obstruction of the intestinal lumen. While the evidence is still controversial, it also appears that gallstones may be a risk factor for carcinoma of the gallbladder.

Gallstones may cause a variety of complications.

Cholesterol and Mixed Stones

The majority of gallstones vary from a pure to mixed cholesterol composition. **Pure cholesterol stones** are radiolucent, up to several centimeters in diameter, round or ovoid, pale yellow stones that often have a glistening crystalline structure when transected. **Mixed stones** are radiolucent or radio-opaque, round or faceted, gray-white to black stones with a lamellated appearance on transection. Mixed stones are often

Most gallstones have a pure to mixed cholesterol composition.

found in one or several distinct sizes, suggesting that nucleation of the stones occurred at several distinct times. Risk factors for cholesterol and mixed stones include increasing age, female sex and multiple pregnancies, obesity and high calorie diet, gastrointestinal disorders such as Crohn's disease that impair resorption of bile salts, drugs, notably clofibrate and estrogens, biliary tract infection, and genetic predisposition, notably American Indian women. Cholesterol stones are much more common than pigment stones in the Americas and Northern Europe.

Pigment Stones

Pigment stones contain calcium bilirubinate.

Pigment stones are composed of relatively pure calcium bilirubinate. These stones are small, typically occur in large numbers, and may be either ovoid or irregular in shape. Less is known about the formation and treatment of pigment stones than about the formation and treatment of cholesterol stones. Risk factors include hepatic cirrhosis (mechanism unknown), disorders causing red cell hemolysis, and infestation by the liver fluke *Opisthorchis sinensis* (Oriental countries; see p. 74).

TUMORS OF THE GALLBLADDER AND EXTRAHEPATIC BILIARY SYSTEM

The gallbladder and extrahepatic biliary system can be affected by both benign and malignant tumors.

Benign Tumors

Papillomas and adenomas can involve the gallbladder.

Benign tumors of the gallbladder include papillomas, adenomas, and adenomyomas. **Papillomas** form from localized overgrowths of the gallbladder lining epithelium. Papillomas are small (less than 1 cm in diameter), branching, pedunculated masses with a fibrovascular core covered by a single layer of columnar epithelium. Papillomas project into the gallbladder lumen and can occur singly or multiply. Fragments of a papilloma sometimes provide a nidus for crystallization of a gallstone. **Adenomas** of the gallbladder are broad-based, rather than pedunculated, benign epithelial proliferations that strongly resemble papillomas, but may also show stromal glands. **Adenomyomas** are an uncommon variation of adenomas in which the stroma is composed in part of proliferating smooth muscle cells. Adenomyomas may be associated with carcinoma of the gallbladder.

Carcinoma of the Gallbladder

Carcinoma of the gallbladder has a poor prognosis because it tends to extend to the liver.

Carcinoma of the gallbladder is an uncommon tumor with a very poor (1 percent 5-year survival) prognosis because it is only rarely identified before it has invaded the adjacent liver and is no longer resectable. Gallstones and chronic cholecystitis are associated with carcinoma of the gallbladder, and some derivatives of cholic acid are known to be experimental carcinogens. Carcinoma of the gallbladder is a disease of older adults (peak in the seventh decade), with women having twice the incidence of men. Most carcinomas of the gallbladder are adenocarcinomas, although approximately 5 percent are squamous or adenosquamous carcinomas that arise in metaplastic epithelium. Grossly, the tumors can be either infiltrating with diffuse thickening and induration of the gallbladder wall or fungating with papillary projections into the lumen. With both growth patterns, the carcinomas may remain asymptomatic until after either metastasis or direct extension into adjacent structures has occurred. Common sites affected by direct extension include the liver, cystic and bile ducts, and adjacent viscera. Common metastatic sites include portahepatic lymph nodes, liver, peritoneum, lungs, and gastrointestinal tract.

Carcinoma of Bile Ducts and Ampulla of Vater

Carcinomas can arise throughout the extrahepatic biliary system; common sites (in descending order of frequency) are the gallbladder, ampulla of Vater, common duct, hepatic ducts, and junction between the hepatic and common ducts (Klatskin tumor). Predisposing factors for **carcinomas of the extrahepatic biliary ducts** include chronic inflammation of the ducts, ulcerative colitis, and, in the Orient, infections by *Ascaris* and *Opisthorchis sinensis*. Gallstones do not appear to be as significant a contributor to carcinoma of the extrahepatic biliary ducts as does carcinoma of the gallbladder. Most of these carcinomas are **adenocarcinomas,** although a few **squamous cell** or **adenosquamous carcinomas** arise in metaplastic epithelium. The adenocarcinomas may or may not be mucin secreting and commonly have an abundant fibrous stroma. Gross patterns of proliferation can be papillary fungating, intraductal nodules, or diffusely infiltrating into the duct wall. These cancers can produce the signs and symptoms of obstructive jaundice by occluding the extrahepatic biliary system. Unfortunately, by the time they are recognized, approximately three-fourths of them have metastasized or directly invaded adjacent structures such as the liver. Common sites of metastasis are the liver, lungs, and regional lymph nodes. Therapy is by extensive surgical resection (Whipple procedure) with an 85 percent 5-year survival for localized lesions but only 10 to 25 percent 5-year survival for more extensive lesions.

Carcinomas can arise throughout the extrahepatic biliary system.

MISCELLANEOUS DISORDERS OF THE GALLBLADDER

Anatomic Variants

The gallbladder and extrahepatic biliary tree may uncommonly show a variety of developmental anomalies. **Agenesis** or atretic narrowing of any portion of the extrahepatic bile ducts may cause obstructive cholestasis and require surgical correction. The gallbladder may be found in **aberrant locations** or may be congenitally absent, duplicated, or bilobed. The most common anomaly of the gallbladder is a **folded fundus,** which can create a terminal saccule or phrygian cap, which may not empty properly and can consequently provide a site for gallstone formation.

Anatomic variants of the gallbladder and extrahepatic biliary tree occur uncommonly.

Cholesterolosis

Cholesterolosis of the gallbladder is a common condition of unknown etiology and no clinical significance in which lipid-laden macrophages accumulate below the columnar epithelium in the tips of mucosal folds. This accumulation causes the mucosal surface to be studded with tiny, yellow lesions, producing the so-called strawberry gallbladder.

Polyps

Sessile mucosal inflammatory polyps can protrude into the gallbladder lumen and are clinically significant because they must be distinguished from malignant tumors when the gallbladder is visualized with ultrasound or radiographic techniques. The polyps consist of a chronically inflamed fibrous stroma covered by columnar epithelial cells. The stroma may contain lipid-laden macrophages similar to those seen in cholesterolosis; granulomas are sometimes also seen and appear to form following the rupture of these macrophages.

CONGENITAL DISORDERS OF THE PANCREAS

Congenital anomalies of the pancreas include complete agenesis, hypoplasia, persistent separate dorsal and ventral pancreas (pancreas divisum), and anular pancreas in which the duodenum is encircled by the head of the pancreas. **Ectopic pancreatic tissue,** ranging up to 3 to 4 cm in diameter, can sometimes be found in the stomach, duodenum, jejunum, Meckel's diverticulum, or ileum. **Congenital cysts** of the pancreas are associated with polycystic disease of the liver and kidney. These cysts are usually multiple, have atrophic lining epithelium, and appear to result from anomalous development of pancreatic ducts. Congenital cysts of the pancreas, together with cysts of liver and kidney, can also be seen in association with angiomas of the retina, cerebellum, or brain stem (von Hippel-Lindau disease).

Cystic Fibrosis

Cystic fibrosis is a systemic, autosomal recessive disease that is seen most frequently in whites. The protein product of an abnormal gene located on chromosome 7 alters anion transport in both mucus-secreting glands and eccrine sweat glands, affecting a variety of organs. Increased NaCl concentration in sweat forms the basis of a screening test for cystic fibrosis, but does not cause microscopically visible changes in sweat ducts, probably because even highly saline sweat will still flow freely through sweat ducts. Decreased passive transport of sodium and water in the pancreas and lung produces abnormally viscid mucus. **Pancreatic changes** seen include mucus-filled, dilated ducts whose lining epithelium may show squamous metaplasia, atrophic pancreatic acini that may be completely replaced by fibrous tissue, and a relative sparing of pancreatic islets. **Pulmonary changes** (see also p. 166) seen include hypertrophy of mucus-secreting glands, mucus plugging of bronchioles leading to dilation termed bronchiectasis, and lung abscesses following pulmonary infection by bacteria such as *Staphylococcus aureus,*

Pseudomonas aeruginosa, or *Pseudomonas cepacia.* Organs less severely affected include the **liver,** in which mucinous material can plug bile canaliculi and in a few cases lead to biliary cirrhosis; the **testes,** in which obstruction of the epididymis and vas deferens by mucus produces infertility; and the **salivary glands,** in which the changes resemble those in the pancreas.

The clinical course of cystic fibrosis is highly variable. Meconium ileus, caused by viscid plugs of mucus in the small intestine, is seen in severely affected infants. Malabsorption syndromes develop in moderately affected infants in the first year of life. Children with mild disease often survive to adolescence or young adulthood, when they may die of respiratory complications, particularly infarction. Better nutritional support, aggressive therapy of infection, and physical therapy to remove pulmonary secretions have contributed to marked improvements in survival of children with cystic fibrosis, most of whom formerly died in infancy.

PANCREATITIS

Inflammation of the pancreas can be seen in both acute and chronic forms.

Acute Hemorrhagic Pancreatitis

The classic form of acute pancreatitis, **acute hemorrhagic pancreatitis,** is an abdominal emergency that can lead to the multiple complications of severe hypotension, including shock, adult respiratory distress syndrome, acute renal failure, and death. Risk factors for acute pancreatitis include biliary tract disease (female predominance) and alcoholism (male predominance). Patients with acute hemorrhagic pancreatitis often report having excessive alcohol or food consumption before developing symptoms. A large variety of other risk factors that may damage pancreatic tissue have also been demonstrated, including trauma, bacterial and viral infections, ischemia, vasculitis, hereditary factors, drugs, hyperlipidemias, and hypercalcemia.

The pathologic damage seen in acute hemorrhagic pancreatitis is principally the result of activated pancreatic enzymes acting on pancreatic tissues. The affected pancreas shows necrosis accompanied by hemorrhage and a leukocytic infiltrate involving both pancreatic acinar tissue and fat. The necrotic fat may contain chalky-white calcium deposits. Systemic effects of acute hemorrhagic pancreatitis can include severe pain referred to the upper back; hypocalcemia due to precipitation of calcium in necrotic fat; glucose intolerance due to islet damage; severe hypotension due to a combination of release of vasodilatory agents by damaged tissues, blood loss, and electrolyte disturbances; and jaundice due to bile duct obstruction by edema. Therapy of acute hemorrhagic pancreatitis is supportive. Despite aggressive therapy, 5 percent of patients with acute hemorrhagic pancreatitis die during the first week of shock or its complications. Patients that survive may develop pancreatic abscess, pseudocyst, or duodenal obstruction secondary to stricture formation.

Acute hemorrhagic pancreatitis may complicate biliary tract disease and alcoholism.

Milder Forms of Acute Pancreatitis

While acute hemorrhagic pancreatitis is the classic form of acute pancreatitis, it is clear that milder forms of acute pancreatitis also exist. The mild pancreatitis experienced by many alcoholics is an example of these milder forms and probably usually represents acute exacerbations of chronic pancreatitis.

Chronic Pancreatitis

Chronic pancreatitis may be calcifying or obstructive.

Repeated mild damage to the pancreas can progress to two forms of chronic pancreatitis. **Chronic calcifying pancreatitis** is the most common morphologic form. Chronic calcifying pancreatitis is most often associated with alcoholism and may be the result of alcohol-induced pancreatic protein secretion leading to plug formation with subsequent lobular damage. Histologic features include protein plugs within ducts; damage to duct epithelium, which may manifest as atrophy, hypertrophy, or squamous metaplasia; atrophied acini; a chronic inflammatory infiltrate; and a marked increase in interlobular fibrous tissue. The damage is characteristically lobular. Pancreatic pseudocysts and calculi may be present. The islets are characteristically preserved, and can sometimes be seen surrounded by fibrosis or atrophic acinar tissue. The gross appearance of the pancreas is of sclerosis with focal calcification.

Chronic obstructive pancreatitis is the second common form of chronic pancreatitis. This form is associated with cholelithiasis and other causes (e.g., tumor) of stenosis of the distal pancreatic duct system. Since the obstruction is in the distal duct system, the damage is characteristically diffuse rather than lobular. Chronic obstructive pancreatitis also differs from chronic calcifying pancreatitis in that duct epithelial damage and calculi are less common.

The most common risk factors for chronic pancreatitis are **alcoholism** and **biliary tract disease.** Other risk factors include hypercalcemia, hyperlipidemia, and anomalous development of the pancreatic duct (pancreas divisum). Familial hereditary pancreatitis and nonalcoholic tropical pancreatitis are rare forms of chronic pancreatitis. Many patients do not have recognizable risk factors. Characteristically, acute hemorrhagic pancreatitis progresses directly to pseudocyst formation rather than chronic pancreatitis. Chronic pancreatitis is characterized by episodic attacks of upper abdominal pain that may be accompanied by mild fever, slight jaundice, and moderate elevations of serum amylase and alkaline phosphatase. A precipitating factor, such as overeating, alcohol use, or drug use, may be identified. Patients are usually initially asymptomatic between attacks, but as the pancreas becomes increasingly damaged and the attacks occur more frequently, long-term sequelae may be seen. Exocrine pancreatic insufficiency may cause profound steatorrhea, weight loss, and hypoalbuminemic edema. While the islets are initially relatively preserved, diabetes mellitus may eventually develop.

Pancreatic Pseudocysts

A **pancreatic pseudocyst** is an acquired loculation of fluid bound by a fibrous capsule (often inflamed) without an epithelial lining.

Pancreatitis and trauma are common predisposing factors. Pseudocysts are typically single and may be as large as 5 to 10 cm in diameter. Rupture can cause abdominal pain, intraperitoneal hemorrhage, and peritonitis.

Pancreatitis and trauma predispose for pancreatic pseudocysts.

TUMORS OF THE EXOCRINE PANCREAS

Benign Tumors

Benign tumors of the pancreas are much less common than pancreatic carcinoma. While many variants exist, only serous cystadenoma and solid-cystic tumors deserve specific mention. These tumors produce cystic structures that must be differentiated from other benign cysts and from cystic pancreatic cancers. **Serous cystadenoma** is a disease of elderly women in which large, multiloculated cysts are lined by a glycogen-rich, flattened cuboidal epithelium. Serous cystadenoma is usually an incidental finding at autopsy or during evaluation of abdominal disease. **Solid-cystic** (papillary-cystic) **tumor** is a disease of adolescent girls and young women that may cause abdominal pain. Small, uniform tumor cells with eosinophilic cytoplasm grow in sheets and in papillary projections into cystic zones. The resulting tumor is a large, well-circumscribed mass containing both solid and cystic zones.

The most important benign tumors of the pancreas are serous cystadenoma and solid-cystic tumor.

Carcinoma of the Pancreas

Carcinoma of the exocrine pancreas is seen in several forms, usually containing adenocarcinoma arising from the pancreatic duct epithelium. **Pure adenocarcinomas** often contain small bizarre glands lined by anaplastic epithelial cells that may or may not secrete mucin. **Adenosquamous carcinomas** contain both squamous and glandular differentiation. Highly **anaplastic tumors** may show giant cell formation. **Cystadenocarcinomas** are uncommon tumors arising in pancreatic cysts. **Acinar cell carcinomas** are uncommon tumors arising in pancreatic acini.

Pancreatic carcinomas may be diffuse (20 percent) or may arise in the head (60 percent), body (15 percent), or tail (5 percent) of the pancreas. On gross examination, small lesions may be inapparent; larger tumor infiltrates may be homogenous scirrhous masses with poorly defined margins. Pancreatic cancer can spread by direct extension, lymphatics, and vascular invasion, notably of the splenic vein, leading to massive liver metastases. Obstruction of the extrahepatic biliary system by tumor can cause hepatobiliary dysfunction leading to death. The prognosis for carcinomas of the pancreas is very poor, since most tumors are extensive or have metastasized before they become symptomatic.

Carcinoma of the pancreas has several histologic forms and often a poor prognosis.

13

Urinary Tract

KIDNEYS

CONGENITAL ANOMALIES

Urinary tract malformations are common. **Agenesis** of a single kidney is compatible with life and usually produces compensatory hypertrophy of the remaining kidney. Total bilateral agenesis is encountered in stillborn infants, who often have other congenital disorders. **Renal hypoplasia,** usually unilateral, occurs uncommonly, and most cases reported are probably the result of intrauterine damage to the kidney by vascular infections or other parenchymal diseases rather than the result of true hypoplasia. Bilateral renal hypoplasia can cause renal failure in early childhood. **Ectopic kidneys** are most commonly found slightly above or within the pelvis and are vulnerable to urinary obstruction secondary to kinking of the ureters. **Horseshoe kidney** is a single, large, midline kidney caused by fusion of the lower, or less commonly, upper poles of the kidneys. **Miscellaneous anomalies** include doubled pelvis, doubled ureters, and doubled renal vessels.

CYSTIC DISEASES OF THE KIDNEYS

Renal cysts can be either acquired or congenital. This section discusses the more important forms of renal cystic disease. Cystic renal dysplasia and polycystic kidney disease primarily affect the renal cortex. Medullary sponge kidney and the nephronophthisis uremic medullary cystic disease complex affect primarily the medulla. Simple cysts and dialysis-related cystic disease are the major forms of acquired cystic disease.

Cystic Renal Dysplasia

Renal dysplasia is a sporadic disorder characterized by the presence of abnormal tissues (cartilage, undifferentiated mesenchyma, immature collecting ductules) and abnormal lobar organization with large numbers of cysts of varying sizes lined by flattened epithelium. Cystic renal dysplasia appears to be an abnormality in metanephric differentiation that

283

is frequently associated with abnormalities of the ureter and lower urinary tract, which possibly cause intrauterine urinary obstruction. Unilateral disease is often discovered during evaluation of a flank mass and carries a good prognosis after nephrectomy of the affected kidney. Bilateral disease can cause renal failure.

Adult Polycystic Kidney Disease

Adult polycystic disease is autosomal dominant.

Adult polycystic kidney disease is an autosomal dominant, relatively common condition in which the kidneys become bilaterally massively enlarged and contain masses of cysts with small amounts of intervening renal tissue containing functioning nephrons. The cysts may be lined with either proximal or distal tubular epithelium. The cyst fluid can be clear, turbid, or hemorrhagic. Occasional papillary epithelial formations may project into the lumen. Clinically, patients are usually initially asymptomatic, but later develop hematuria, proteinuria, polyuria, and hypertension. A variety of other congenital anomalies can also be seen, including cysts in other organs, commonly the liver but also the spleen, pancreas, and lungs; intracranial berry aneurysms, which can cause subarachnoid hemorrhage leading to death; and mitral valve prolapse. Patients live into adulthood but eventually die of renal failure, hypertension (cardiac disease or rupture of berry aneurysm), or unrelated causes.

Childhood Polycystic Kidney Disease

Childhood polycystic kidney disease is autosomal recessive.

Childhood polycystic kidney disease is a rare, autosomal recessive disease that can present at neonatal, infantile, or juvenile ages. The kidneys contain saccular or cylindrical dilations of the collecting tubules that are lined by cuboidal cells. The dilations are perpendicular to the cortical surface, and the kidney cortex and medulla have a spongelike appearance. Multiple epithelium-lined cysts are also usually present in the liver. Patients who survive infancy can develop hepatic fibrosis (congenital hepatic fibrosis) with portal hypertension and splenomegaly.

Cystic Diseases of the Renal Medulla

Cystic diseases of the medulla include medullary sponge kidney and nephronophthisis uremic medullary cystic disease complex.

Medullary sponge kidney is a relatively common and usually innocuous condition found in adults (often as an incidental finding) in which the collecting ducts in the medulla have multiple cystic dilations lined by cuboidal or occasionally transitional epithelium. Renal function is typically normal; secondary complications include infection, calculi, and calcification of the ducts. **Nephronophthisis uremic medullary cystic disease complex** is a group of renal disorders characterized by medullary cysts, cortical tubular atrophy, and interstitial fibrosis that eventually cause renal insufficiency. Variants include autosomal recessive familial juvenile nephronophthisis; a sporadic, nonfamilial form; a recessive form associated with retinitis pigmentosa known as renal-retinal dysplasia; and a dominantly inherited adult onset form. This disease complex causes 20 percent of childhood and adolescent chronic renal failure. Affected children have a tubular defect in the distal tubules and collecting ducts that causes polyuria, polydipsia, sodium wasting, and tubular acidosis. Terminal renal failure typically occurs 5 to 10 years after the patient becomes symptomatic.

Dialysis-Associated Cystic Disease

Dialysis patients with end-stage renal disease sometimes develop numerous cortical and medullary cysts. The cysts appear to develop as a consequence of tubular obstruction; are lined by hyperplastic or flattened epithelium; and often contain calcium oxalate crystals. Renal adenomas and occasionally adenocarcinomas may be present in the cyst walls. Hematuria secondary to cyst bleeding is also sometimes observed.

Dialysis patients can develop renal cysts.

Simple Cysts

Single or multiple cystic spaces up to 5 (and rarely 10) cm are common postmortem findings in the cortex and rarely the medulla. Most simple cysts are without clinical significance. The cysts may occasionally become hemorrhagic, with subsequent calcification of the hemorrhage, which can produce bizarre radiographic shadows.

Simple cysts are a common postmortem finding.

HYPERTENSION AND RENAL FAILURE

Hypertension and renal disease are intimately inter-related, since some forms of renal disease can cause hypertension, and hypertension can cause renal pathology. The kidneys can affect blood pressure through the action of several mechanisms that can act synergistically, including activation of the renin-angiotensin system, sodium hemostasis, and renal vasodepressor substances.

Hypertension and renal disease are intimately related.

Renin-Angiotensin System

The **renin-angiotensin system** can raise blood pressure both by directly stimulating vasoconstriction of vascular smooth muscle and by stimulating aldosterone secretion, leading to an increase in blood volume. Diseases associated with increased renin secretion include unilateral renal artery stenosis, malignant hypertension, and other diseases. **Unilateral renal artery stenosis** can occur as a result of atheromatous plaque or fibromuscular thickening (fibromuscular dysplasia) of the renal artery wall. The stenosis causes hypoperfusion of the kidney, leading to increased renin secretion and diffuse ischemic atrophy characterized by crowded glomeruli, interstitial fibrosis, atrophic tubules, and a focal inflammatory infiltrate. The contralateral kidney is damaged by the hypertension induced by the high renin levels, and typically shows hyaline arteriolosclerosis. In **malignant hypertension,** very high levels of renin and aldosterone can be present, usually for unclear reasons. A variety of other diseases can activate the renin-angiotensin system, including vasculitides; renin-secreting tumors such as juxtaglomerular cell tumors, renal cell carcinoma, and Wilms tumors; and some cases of chronic pyelonephritis, reflux nephropathy, and chronic renal failure of varied causes.

Unilateral renal artery stenosis increases renin secretion.

Very high renin and aldosterone levels can be present in malignant hypertension.

Sodium Homeostasis

The kidney regulates body sodium.

The kidney regulates body **sodium** and, consequently, extracellular (and blood) volume. Activation of the **renin-angiotensin system** increases **aldosterone** release and thereby increases distal tubular reabsorption of sodium. A decreased glomerular filtration rate occurs as a consequence of decreased blood volume and leads to increased reabsorption of sodium by proximal tubules. Naturietic factors secreted by the heart atria inhibit sodium reabsorption in the distal nephron. Renal parenchymal diseases, including chronic renal failure, cause hypertension by a failure of the above homeostatic mechanisms, leading to marked retention of sodium and fluid. The hypertension is often markedly improved following removal of the excess fluid by diuresis or dialysis.

Renal Vasopressor Substances and Other Secondary Forms of Hypertension

Secondary hypertension has renal and hormonal causes.

A variety of **vasopressor** (antihypertensive) substances are produced by the kidney, including prostaglandins, a urinary kallikrein-kinin system, and platelet-activating factor. In theory, renal hypertension could result from decreased levels of these factors, but this mechanism has not been convincingly demonstrated to be a significant cause of hypertension. In addition to the renal causes of hypertension, secondary hypertension can also be caused by primary aldosteronism, via increased sodium retention; pheochromocytomas, via epinephrine and norepinephrine-induced vasoconstriction and increased cardiac output; oral contraceptives, possibly via activation of the renin-angiotensin system; and polyarteritis nodosa, associated with increased renin levels.

Benign Nephrosclerosis

Benign nephrosclerosis is characterized histologically by hyaline arteriolosclerosis, patchy ischemic atrophy, and fibroelastic hyperplasia.

Benign hypertension can cause benign nephrosclerosis. **Hyaline arteriolosclerosis,** almost invariably present, causes narrowing of the lumina of arterioles and small arteries as a consequence of thickening and hyalinization of the vessel walls. The hyaline material contains basement membrane components, lipid, and blood proteins. Some degree of hyaline arteriolosclerosis is often present with aging, but tends to be more severe if the patient is hypertensive, diabetic, or both. **Patchy ischemic atrophy** affects those portions of the kidney in which blood supply is compromised by hyaline arteriolosclerosis. The ischemic atrophy causes focal tubular atrophy and interstitial fibrosis, as well as glomerular alterations including basement membrane changes and degrees of fibrosis ranging from deposition of collagen within Bowman's space to total glomerular sclerosis.

Fibroelastic hyperplasia, characterized by reduplication of the elastic lamina and fibrosis of the media of larger interlobular and arcuate arteries, can accompany the hyaline arteriosclerosis and is more severe in hypertensive patients. The kidneys in benign nephrosclerosis are of normal to slightly reduced size (due to cortical narrowing) and have a finely granular surface caused by focal loss of cortex secondary to the patchy ischemic atrophy. Patients with uncomplicated benign nephrosclerosis do not usually develop renal insufficiency or uremia, but are more apt to develop azotemia if stressed by volume depletion, surgery, or gastrointestinal hemorrhage, possibly as a result of reduced renal reserve. Most patients who develop renal failure do so as a consequence of supervening malignant hypertension.

Malignant Nephrosclerosis

The malignant or accelerated phase of hypertension can cause severe renal disease known as **malignant nephrosclerosis.** The arterioles show fibrinoid necrosis, in which eosinophilic granular material, which stains for fibrin by histochemical techniques, is deposited in the vessel wall. An inflammatory infiltrate within or adjacent to the wall is also often present. Interlobular arteries and arterioles may alternatively show an intimal thickening known as **hyperplastic arteriolitis** ("onion-skinning"), characterized by collagen deposition and by the proliferation of smooth muscle and other concentrically arranged cells. The compromised blood flow, primarily as a result of hyperplastic arteriolitis, can cause ischemic atrophy and **infarction of renal tissue** supplied by the vessels. Additionally, some glomeruli may become necrotic, with neutrophilic infiltration and thrombosed capillaries, known as **necrotizing glomerulitis.**

Malignant hypertension is usually associated with very high serum concentrations of renin, angiotensin, and aldosterone. It occurs either in previously normal individuals (uncommonly) or in patients with pre-existing essential hypertension or renal disease (particularly glomerulonephritis and reflux nephropathy). In addition to renal failure, the diastolic pressures greater than 130 mmHg are associated with papilledema, encephalopathy, and cardiovascular abnormalities. Headaches, visual impairments (scotomas), nausea and vomiting, loss of consciousness, and seizures are related to increased intracranial pressure. The increased blood pressure to the kidneys causes early proteinuria and hematuria with progression to renal failure. The formerly dismal long-term prognosis for malignant hypertension has been modified by aggressive therapy with newer antihypertensive agents, but patients with malignant hypertension still have only a 50 percent 5-year survival. Most deaths are caused by uremia, cerebral hemorrhage, or cardiac failure.

MICROANGIOPATHIC HEMOLYTIC ANEMIA AND RENAL DISEASE

Several diseases associated with endothelial injury and intravascular coagulation produce morphologic changes in the kidney similar to those seen in malignant hypertension. Thickening of vessel walls is accompanied by thrombosis (and secondary necrosis) of interlobular arteries, afferent arterioles, and glomeruli. Microangiopathic hemolytic anemia (see also p. 78) occurs as a result of red cell destruction in narrowed vessels. Platelet consumption causes thrombocytopenia. Also seen are renal failure and manifestations of intravascular coagulations.

These manifestations can be seen in several vascular diseases. The common pathology in these diseases appears to be disseminated intravascular coagulation initiated at sites of endothelial injury by a variety of agents. **Childhood hemolytic uremic syndrome** is an

> **Malignant hypertension produces severe renal disease.**

> **Histologic changes observed include hyperplastic arteriolitis, infarction, and necrotizing glomerulitis.**

> **Microangiopathic hemolytic anemia occurs when red cells are destroyed in narrowed renal vessels.**

The childhood and adult forms of hemolytic uremic syndrome are life-threatening diseases.

Thrombotic thrombocytopenic purpura has a high mortality.

Atherosclerosis and emboli can involve the renal arteries.

Sickled cells can occlude the vasa recta.

Massive ischemic injury causes diffuse cortical necrosis.

uncommon disease that is a major cause of renal failure in children. The disease usually begins suddenly following a flulike or gastrointestinal prodome and is associated with infection by enterotoxin-producing *Escherichia coli*. Clinical manifestations include microangiopathic anemia, hematemesis, melena, oliguria, hematuria, and sometimes prominent neurologic manifestations. The kidneys show endothelial and subendothelial swelling of glomerular vessel walls with fibrin deposits in the capillary lumen, subendothelium, and mesangium. Interlobular arteries and afferent arterioles show intimal hyperplasia, fibrinoid necrosis, and thrombi. Renal cortical necrosis may be patchy or widespread. Even with aggressive therapy using dialysis, mortality is 10 to 15 percent. Most of the remaining patients recover completely, but a few develop chronic renal insufficiency and hypertension.

Adult hemolytic uremic syndrome is similar to that seen in childhood and can be encountered in pregnancies complicated by placental hemorrhage or retained placental fragments; in postpartum women; in women using oral contraceptives; and in some systemic infections (*E. coli* sepsis, typhoid fever, shigellosis, viral infections). **Thrombotic thrombocytopenic purpura** (see also p. 86) is seen most often in women less than 40 years of age. The dominant feature is central nervous system involvement. Symptoms include fever, neurologic symptoms, thrombocytopenic purpura, and hemolytic anemia. One-half of patients also have manifestations related to eosinophilic granular thrombi in interlobular arteries, afferent arterioles, and glomerular capillaries. Exchange transfusions and corticosteroid therapy have modified the formerly dismal prognosis, although mortality is still near fifty percent. Systemic sclerosis can also produce renal disease with microangiopathic anemia and is discussed further elsewhere (see p. 25).

OTHER RENAL VASCULAR DISEASES

Atheroembolic Renal Disease

Atheromatous plaques in the aorta and renal arteries can fragment, often after surgery on atherosclerotic aneurysms, producing **emboli** that usually lodge in arcuate and interlobular arteries. These emboli can have no clinical significance; can cause acute renal failure in elderly patients with marginal renal functions; or can heal, producing vascular fibrosis and narrowing with subsequent chronic ischemic injury to the kidney.

Sickle Cell Nephropathy

Blood passing through the vasa recta of the renal medulla is exposed to a hypertonic, hypoxic milieu that favors erythrocyte sickling in both homozygous and heterozygous forms of **sickle cell disease.** The sickled cells can cause focal occlusions of the vasa recta, which can produce a patchy papillary necrosis, proteinuria, and sometimes cortical scarring.

Diffuse Cortical Necrosis

Diffuse cortical necrosis appears to be the result of **massive ischemic injury** to the kidneys as a consequence of disseminated intravascular coagulation, vasoconstriction, or both. Diffuse cortical necrosis is uncommonly encountered in a variety of situations including abruptio placentae, septic shock, and extensive surgery. Survival of the patient is possible when the cortical necrosis is patchy.

Renal Infarction

Renal infarctions are usually the result of emboli from sites such as cardiac mural thrombi (typically secondary to myocardial infarction), vegetative endocarditis, and aortic atherosclerosis. The infarcts initially form patchy areas of acute ischemic necrosis ringed by hyperemic zones that usually have a wedge-shaped configuration with a base at the cortical surface and an apex that points toward the medulla. With time, the infarction undergoes progressive, fibrous scarring. Renal infarcts can be clinically silent; cause localized pain and tenderness at the costovertebral angle associated with intermittent hematuria; or cause hypertension when the infarct is large.

True renal infarctions also occur.

GLOMERULAR DISEASES

Nephrotic Syndrome

Urinary protein losses exceeding 3.5 g (less in children) are associated with a cluster of clinical findings known as the **nephrotic syndrome.** The urinary protein losses occur as a result of leakage of serum proteins across the glomerular capillary walls. Hypoalbuminemia is due to preferential loss into urine of serum albumen because of its relatively low molecular weight. Generalized edema follows loss of serum colloid oncotic pressure (principally due to hypoalbuminemia) coupled with sodium and water retention. Hyperlipidemia, possibly as a result of a stimulation of synthesis of lipoproteins by liver, is also seen in nephrotic syndrome, and the leak of lipoproteins across the glomerular capillary wall may cause lipiduria. Patients with nephrotic syndrome are also vulnerable to infections and thrombotic complications. Renal vein thrombosis can complicate the hypercoagulable state.

Massive leakage of proteins across glomerular capillary walls causes the nephrotic syndrome.

Diseases that typically produce nephrotic syndrome include membranous glomerulonephropathy (most common cause in adults), lipoid nephrosis (most common cause in children), and focal segmental glomerulosclerosis. Other causes of nephrotic syndrome, which typically can also produce other clinical renal syndromes, include membranoproliferative glomerulonephritis and other forms of proliferative glomerulonephritis. Systemic diseases that may cause nephrotic syndrome include diabetes mellitus, amyloidosis, systemic lupus erythematosus, malignancies (carcinoma, melanoma), infections (acquired immunodeficiency syndrome [AIDS], hepatitis B, malaria, syphilis), and drugs (gold, penicillamine, heroin).

Membranous Glomerulonephritis

Membranous glomerulonephritis (membranous nephropathy) is characterized by a uniform, diffuse thickening of the glomerular capillary wall caused by irregular deposits (seen by electron microscopy) between the basement membrane and overlying epithelial cells. The deposits contain immunoglobulins and complement and are interrupted

Membranous glomeru-lonephritis is characterized by electron-dense deposits between the basement membrane and overlying epithelial cells.

by irregular spikes of basement membrane material. As the lesions progress, these projections of glomerular basement membrane eventually cover the immune deposits with a thickened, irregular membrane. Other changes seen with progressive disease include narrowing of the capillary lumina by the thickened basement membrane, sclerosis of the mesangium, and, eventually, glomerular hyalinization. Protein reabsorption by the proximal tubules can be visualized in the form of epithelial hyaline droplets; with progressive disease, tubular atrophy and interstitial fibrosis are seen. Grossly, the kidney, with time, resembles that seen in other forms of chronic glomerulonephritis, with a small size and finely granular, scarred texture.

Membranous glomerulonephritis is a common cause of **nephrotic syndrome** in adults. It can occur idiopathically or secondary to a variety of disorders or etiologic agents, including tumors (melanoma, lung cancer, colon cancer), systemic diseases (hepatitis B, syphilis, schistosomiasis, malaria), and drugs or toxins (gold salts, mercury salts, penicillamine, captopril). In most cases, no predisposing etiology is identified. Depending upon the specific etiology, the **subepithelial deposits** are thought to be caused by both circulating immune complexes and in situ immune reactions. The leakiness of the glomerular capillary walls, which causes the proteinuria, is thought to be related to damage by activated complement factors (C5b-9). The clinical course of membranous glomerulonephritis is variable. Patients present with proteinuria, which is usually sufficiently severe to cause nephrotic syndrome. Hematuria and mild hypertension may also be present. In most patients, the proteinuria persists, and renal insufficiency eventually (2 to 20 years) develops in one-half of cases. A small percentage of patients experience partial or complete remissions. The hypercoagulable state associated with the nephrotic syndrome can cause renal vein thrombosis.

Lipoid Nephrosis

Lipoid nephrosis is characterized by diffuse effacement of podocyte foot processes.

Lipoid nephrosis (minimal change disease) is the major cause of nephrotic syndrome in children. Lipoid nephrosis is associated with a characteristic diffuse effacement ("fusion") of the foot processes of the visceral epithelial cells (podocytes) of the glomeruli. The glomerular basement membrane appears normal and without deposits by electron microscopy, but biochemical studies suggest that the increased permeability is associated with loss of glomerular polyanion. The proximal tubules contain hyaline droplets associated with reabsorption of filtered protein. Unlike many other glomerulonephropathies, complement and immunoglobulin deposition do not appear to be part of the pathology. Most cases of lipoid nephrosis occur in children, in whom the disease produces massive proteinuria but does not usually cause hematuria, hypertension, or renal failure. Most cases resolve with steroid therapy, although a few patients require continued steroid therapy ("steroid dependency"), as cessation of the drugs is associated with recurrence of the proteinuria.

Focal Segmental Glomerulosclerosis

Focal segmental glomerulosclerosis refers to the sclerosis of portions of the glomerular tuft (segmental lesions) found in some glomeruli (focal distribution). Focal segmental glomerulosclerosis is a frequent cause of heavy proteinuria and the nephrotic syndrome. The sclerotic portions of the glomeruli show increased mesangial matrix with deposition of hyaline masses (hyalinosis); collapse of basement membranes; and amorphous material that stains with immunochemical techniques for IgM and C3. Additional changes seen include hyaline thickening of afferent arterioles, as well as diffuse effacement of foot processes in nonsclerotic areas, analogous to that seen in lipoid nephrosis, which is probably associated with heavy proteinuria. With progression of disease, completely sclerosed glomeruli (global sclerosis) are seen, and are associated with tubular atrophy and interstitial fibrosis.

Focal segmental glomerulosclerosis involves portions of some glomeruli.

Focal segmental glomerulosclerosis can be subclassified. **Idiopathic focal segmental glomerulosclerosis** accounts for roughly one-tenth of cause of nephrotic syndrome. It is seen in both children and adults. It clinically resembles lipoid nephrosis, with heavy proteinuria and nephrotic syndrome, but is more apt to fail to respond to steroid therapy. Other clinical differences from lipoid nephrosis include a higher incidence of hematuria, reduced glomerular filtration rate, hypertension, and progression to chronic glomerulonephritis and end-stage renal disease. **Secondary focal segmental glomerulosclerosis** can be seen either in association with other primary glomerular lesions, notably IgA nephropathy, or in association with other disorders including AIDS, heroin abuse, reflux nephropathy, analgesic abuse nephropathy, and unilateral renal agenesis.

Focal segmental glomerulosclerosis may be idiopathic or secondary.

Both primary and secondary forms of focal segmental glomerulosclerosis tend to progress to renal failure. The intractable massive proteinuria does not usually respond to steroid therapy. About one-half of renal allograft recipients with pre-existing focal segmental glomerulonephritis will have a recurrence in the transplant.

Acute Poststreptococcal Glomerulonephritis

Acute poststreptococcal glomerulonephritis is a relatively common cause of acute nephritis that is most commonly seen in children following a streptococcal infection of the throat or occasionally skin. Certain strains of **group A β-hemolytic streptococci** (types 12, 4, and 1) apparently increase synthesis of antibodies that are associated with the glomerular disease, possibly either by cross-reaction with glomerular basement membrane or by deposition of circulating immune complexes. The process of antibody synthesis can be monitored by following the serum titers of antistreptolysin-O.

Glomerulonephritis may follow streptococcal throat infection.

The glomeruli affected by the disease are characteristically enlarged, hypercellular, and relatively bloodless as a consequence of endothelial and mesangial cell proliferation; neutrophil and monocyte infiltration; and a resulting obliteration of capillary lumen. Granular IgG and complement deposits can be found in the mesangium and adjacent to the basement membrane. Electron microscopy shows that these deposits form characteristic "humps" on the epithelial side of the basement membrane, which are presumably caused by trapping of antigen-antibody complexes. These changes usually subside by 2 months after the onset of clinical renal disease. Persistent hypercellularity of the mesangium may be associated with progression to chronic glomerulonephritis.

In children, the glomerulonephritis presents 1 to 2 weeks after a sore throat, when the child develops nausea, oliguria, hematuria with red cell casts, and a usually mild proteinuria. Periorbital edema and a mild to moderate hypertension may also be present. Adults may present with hypertension, edema, or elevated blood urea nitrogen. While the majority of patients recover with supportive therapy, a few children and more adults develop rapidly progressive or chronic glomerulonephritis. Poststreptococcal glomerulonephritis is sometimes encountered in epidemic forms, in which the overall prognosis tends to be better than in sporadic cases. Acute glomerulonephritis resembling poststreptococcal disease can also be caused by other bacteria (meningococcemia, pneumococcal pneumonia, staphylococcal endocarditis); viruses (hepatitis, mumps, varicella, infectious mononucleosis); and parasites (malaria, toxoplasmosis).

Rapidly Progressive Glomerulonephritis

Rapidly progressive glomerulonephritis may cause renal failure only weeks after becoming clinically evident.

Rapidly progressive (crescentic) **glomerulonephritis** is characterized by the partial or complete obliteration of Bowman's space by the accumulation of cells and fibrin deposits **(crescent formation).** The crescents include proliferating parietal epithelial cells, macrophages, neutrophils, and occasional lymphocytes. Electron microscopic studies characteristically show focal disruptions of the glomerular basement membranes.

Rapidly progressive glomerulonephritis has many causes.

Clinically, rapidly progressive glomerulonephritis can progress in a matter of weeks to renal failure requiring dialysis or renal transplantation. Rapidly progressive glomerulonephritis occurs in a small percentage of **postinfectious** (usually poststreptococcal) patients who develop glomerulonephritis. **Multisystem diseases** that can cause rapidly progressive glomerulonephritis notably include Goodpasture syndrome, but also systemic lupus erythematosus, vasculitis such as polyarteritis nodosa, Wegener's granulomatosis, Henoch-Schönlein purpura, and essential cryoglobulinemia. In Goodpasture syndrome, antibodies are directed against the basement membranes of both the pulmonary alveoli and the renal glomeruli, producing, respectively, pulmonary hemorrhage and crescenteric glomerulonephritis. Remission of both pulmonary and renal symptoms may follow plasma exchange combined with steroid and cytotoxic therapy, but many patients eventually require chronic dialysis or renal transplantation. Approximately one-half of cases of rapidly progressive glomerulonephritis are **idiopathic,** possibly due to a variety of initial renal insults.

GLOMERULAR LESIONS ASSOCIATED WITH SYSTEMIC DISEASE

Many systemic disorders can cause glomerular disease.

Systemic Lupus Erythematosus

Virtually all cases of **systemic lupus erythematosus** will show renal abnormalities by fluorescence and electron microscopy; in two-thirds of the cases, lesions are also visible by ordinary light microscopy. The renal lesions are thought to be associated with deposition of DNA–anti-DNA complexes within the glomeruli. The reasons for the different clinical and pathologic patterns are still not clear, but may reflect the physical and chemical characteristics of the complexes as well as the pre-existing state of the glomerular capillary wall.

The renal involvement can take a variety of forms. The mildest is **mesangial lupus glomerulonephritis,** which is characterized by granular mesangial deposits of immunoglobin and complement (probably filtered immune complexes) accompanied by a slight to moderate increase in the intercapillary mesangial matrix and number of mesangial cells. Mesangial lupus glomerulonephritis is usually observed in patients with mild hematuria or proteinuria and may also be a component of other forms of renal disease. **Focal proliferative glomerulonephritis** is characterized by swelling and proliferation of endothelial and mesangial cells in one or two glomerular tufts in some glomeruli. Other features include neutrophilic proliferation, fibrinoid deposits, intracapillary thrombi, hematoxylin bodies, and fragmented nuclei (nuclear dust). Focal proliferative glomerulonephritis is usually associated with recurrent hematuria and moderate proteinuria; mild renal insufficiency is also occasionally seen. **Diffuse proliferative glomerulonephritis** characteristically shows marked proliferation of endothelial, mesangial, and sometimes epithelial cells. The lesions involve the entire glomerulus, and may affect most or all glomeruli in both kidneys. Diffuse proliferative glomerulonephritis is associated with serious clinical disease, including microscopic or gross hematuria, proteinuria, which may be in the nephrotic range, hypertension, and often decreased glomerular filtration rate. Diffuse proliferative glomerulonephritis is the most common pattern seen in systemic lupus erythematosus; focal proliferative glomerulonephritis is also common. **Membranous glomerulonephritis** is characterized by widespread thickening of capillary walls, resembles idiopathic membranous glomerulonephritis, and is usually observed in patients with severe proteinuria or overt nephrotic syndrome.

Electron microscopy is often used to evaluate lupus renal disease. The **electron-dense deposits** observed are often thought to represent DNA–anti-DNA immune complexes. Mesangial deposits are found in all histologic types. Deposits between the basement membrane and visceral epithelial cell (subepithelial) are usually observed in membranous glomerulonephritis. Deposits between the endothelium and basement membrane (subendothelial) can also be seen in many types of systemic lupus erythematosus renal disease, and are particularly distinctive for systemic erythematosus, since they are usually not observed in glomerulonephritis due to other causes. Extensive subepithelial deposition can cause thickening of the capillary walls ("wire loop" lesions), most typical of the diffuse proliferative type of glomerulonephritis, but also observed in focal and membranous glomerulonephritis. Such "wire loops" usually indicate a poor prognosis because they reflect active disease. Individual patients may either have persistence of a single type of lesion throughout the course of their disease, or may initially have mesangial or focal glomerulonephritis that later progresses to diffuse proliferative glomerulonephritis, with worsening of the clinical course.

In addition to the glomerular lesions, vasculitis affecting the cortical arterioles can also sometimes be seen; it resembles the vasculitis

Systemic lupus erythematosus produces many renal abnormalities.

Relatively mild forms of involvement include mesangial lupus glomerulonephritis and focal proliferative glomerulonephritis.

More serious forms of lupus glomerulonephritis include diffuse proliferative and membranous glomerulonephritis.

Electron-dense deposits in many sites are often thought to represent DNA–anti-DNA immune complexes.

observed in other affected tissues and organs. While the glomerular disease is the most distinctive and pronounced change observed in the kidneys of patients with lupus nephritis, interstitium and tubules may also show disease, particularly in cases of diffuse proliferative glomerulonephritis. Uncommonly, the tubulointerstitial lesions, characterized by granular deposits of immunoglobulin and complement in the tubular basement membranes, may be the dominant abnormality.

Lupus also produces vasculitis.

Henoch-Schönlein Purpura

Henoch-Schönlein purpura is a systemic syndrome of unknown etiology observed in both adults and children (most commonly seen at ages 3 to 8 years). The syndrome consists of many features, not all of which may be present in an individual patient. Skin lesions due to necrotizing vasculitis and accompanying subepidermal hemorrhage may be present on the extremities and buttocks. Prominent gastrointestinal manifestations, possibly related to vasculitis, include pain, vomiting, and intestinal bleeding. Nonmigratory arthralgias may be present. Renal manifestations may include gross or microscopic hematuria; proteinuria that may be severe enough to cause nephrotic syndrome; and, in a few patients, rapidly progressive glomerulonephritis. Depending upon the severity of the disease, the renal lesions may include mild to diffuse mesangial proliferation or crescenteric glomerulonephritis. Since IgA deposits can always be identified, Henoch-Schönlein purpura may be part of the spectrum of IgA nephropathy.

Henoch-Schönlein purpura is a vasculitis with sometimes prominent renal manifestations.

Bacterial Endocarditis

Subacute **bacterial endocarditis** can cause a focal immune complex nephritis characterized clinically by hematuria, proteinuria, acute nephritis, or even rapidly progressive glomerulonephritis. The histology of the renal lesions varies with the severity of the presentation, from focal and segmental necrotizing glomerulonephritis to diffuse proliferative glomerulonephritis to rapidly progressive glomerulonephritis with crescent formation.

Endocarditis may cause immune complex nephritis.

Diabetic Glomerulosclerosis

Renal manifestations are prominent in diabetes. The glomerular pathology can take three forms. **Glomerular capillary basement membrane thickening,** often with mesangial widening, can be detected by electron microscopy in virtually all diabetics. **Diffuse glomerulosclerosis** increases mesangial volume by proliferation of mesangial cells together with a diffuse increase in periodic acid-Schiff (PAS)-positive mesangial deposits. The changes begin adjacent to the arterioles in the vascular stalk (which almost always show hyaline thickening) and may progress to the point that the entire glomerulus is involved (obliterative diabetic glomerulosclerosis). **Nodular glomerulosclerosis** (intercapillary glomerulosclerosis, Kimmelstiel-Wilson syndrome) produces ovoid, hyaline, PAS-positive masses usually found within the mesangial core at the periphery of the glomerulus. The nodular lesions usually coexist with diffuse glomerulosclerosis. With disease progression, enlarging nodules may obliterate the glomerular tuft. Other changes seen in the kidneys of

Diabetes is an important cause of renal disease.

diabetics include hyaline thickening of arterioles; tubular atrophy and interstitial fibrosis secondary to ischemia; eosinophilic fibrin caps found as a subendothelial deposit in the periphery of a lobule; and PAS-positive capsular drops in the parietal layer of Bowman's capsule. Diabetics are also vulnerable to pyelonephritis and papillary necrosis.

Clinically, diabetics can experience proteinuria, sometimes accompanied by nephrotic syndrome, which tends to occur 1 or 2 decades after onset of the diabetes and precedes progression to chronic renal failure within the subsequent 4 or 5 years. Juvenile onset diabetics experience more frequent and more severe renal disease than do adult onset diabetics.

Amyloidosis

Amyloid can be deposited in the mesangium and subendothelium of glomeruli, renal blood vessel walls, and renal interstitium. Patients with renal, particularly glomerular, amyloid deposits may experience proteinuria in the nephrotic range and later develop chronic renal failure secondary to glomerular destruction.

Amyloid deposition may eventually produce chronic renal failure.

Other Systemic Disorders

Other systemic disorders can cause glomerular lesions. **Goodpasture syndrome, polyarteritis nodosa, and Wegener's granulomatosis** can all produce a variety of glomerulonephropathies from focal and segmental glomerulonephritis to rapidly progressive glomerulonephritis with crescent formation. **Essential mixed cryoglobulinemia** is a rare disease in which IgG-IgM complexes induce focal or diffuse proliferative glomerulonephritis. Cutaneous vasculitis and synovitis are other features of this rare systemic condition. **Plasma cell dyscrasias,** including both multiple myeloma and light-chain nephropathy in the absence of overt multiple myeloma, can produce glomerular lesions characterized by amyloidosis, deposition of cryoglobulins, and nodular lesions resembling those seen in diabetics.

Other systemic disorders can damage glomeruli.

OTHER FORMS OF GLOMERULONEPHRITIS

Alport Syndrome

Alport syndrome is the best studied of a group of hereditary-familial renal diseases associated with glomerular injury that are known as hereditary nephritis. Alport syndrome consists of the cluster of nerve deafness, eye disorders (corneal dystrophy, cataracts, lens dislocation), and nephritis with hematuria, proteinuria, and eventual progression to overt renal failure. Glomerular changes begin with segmental proliferation or sclerosis and progress to increasing glomerulosclerosis with tubular atrophy and interstitial fibrosis. Some kidneys also show accumulation of fat and mucopolysaccharides in glomerular or tubular epithelial cells (foam cells). A characteristic irregular alternating thickening and attenuation of the glomerular, and sometimes tubular, basement membranes may be observed by electron microscopy.

Alport syndrome is a form of hereditary nephritis.

Membranoproliferative Glomerulonephritis

Membranoproliferative glomerulonephritis can be subdivided based on electron microscopic observations.

Membranoproliferative glomerulonephritis is a type of glomerulonephritis characterized by mesangial cell proliferation with accentuation of lobular architecture. The glomerular basement membrane is thickened, particularly in the peripheral capillary loops, which often gives the glomerular capillary wall a characteristic "train-track" appearance as a result of inclusion within the basement membrane of mesangial cell processes (mesangial interposition).

Membranoproliferative glomerulonephritis can be subdivided based on electron microscopic observations. **Type I** has prominent subendothelial electron-dense deposits (and a smaller number of deposits in other sites) and stains by immunofluorescence in a granular pattern for C3, IgG, and often the early complement components C1q and C4. **Type II** has deposition of dense material of unknown composition within the glomerular basement membrane, which causes the basement membrane to have a thickened, ribbonlike structure. While C3 can be identified along the basement membrane, IgG and the early complement components are usually not present. **Type III** is a rare variant characterized by both subendothelial and subepithelial deposits and disruption and reduplication of the glomerular basement membrane.

Membranoproliferative glomerulonephritis usually produces slowly progressive renal disease that can often be slowed by steroid therapy. The clinical presentation can be of nephrotic syndrome, nephritic syndrome, or both. A few patients will show crescent formation and rapidly progressive glomerulonephritis. The disease tends to recur in renal transplant patients. Glomerular changes similar to membranoproliferative glomerulonephritis can also be seen in a variety of diseases, including infections (infected ventriculoatrial shunts, schistosomiasis, hepatitis B), systemic lupus erythematosus, chronic liver diseases and α_1-antitrypsin deficiency, as well as malignancies.

IgA Nephropathy

Mesangial deposition of IgA is observed in Berger's disease.

IgA nephropathy (**Berger's disease**) is a common type of glomerulonephritis that usually causes gross or microscopic hematuria. IgA nephropathy is characterized by mesangial deposition of IgA. C3, properdin, IgG, and IgM can also often be identified, but the early complement components are usually absent. In some cases, particularly those that later progress to chronic renal failure, the arterioles show prominent hyaline thickening. The disease is thought to be due to trapping in the glomeruli of large IgA aggregates that activate the alternate complement pathway. IgA nephropathy often begins in children and young adults shortly after onset of respiratory, gastrointestinal, or urinary tract infections. Patients experience several days of hematuria, which then remits but may recur every few months. The disease often slowly (over decades) progresses, with eventual development of renal failure in about one-half of cases. Other pre-existing renal disease is associated with more rapid progression. If renal allograft transplantation is performed, IgA deposits may recur in the transplant, but usually do not cause significant disease.

Focal Proliferative Glomerulonephritis

Focal proliferative glomerulonephritis is characterized by proliferation of glomerular cells limited to only certain glomeruli and, often, only certain glomerular segments. Focal glomerular necrosis with fibrin deposition and neutrophilic infiltration is also often seen. Focal proliferative glomerulonephritis is seen in two circumstances. **Primary** focal glomerulonephritis can be subclinical or can cause recurrent hematuria or proteinuria that is usually nonnephrotic. **Secondary** focal glomerulonephritis occurs as an early or mild form of renal disease in many systemic diseases with prominent immunologic manifestations (IgA nephropathy, Goodpasture syndrome, Wegener's granulomatosis, Henoch-Schönlein purpura, systemic lupus erythematosus, polyarteritis nodosa, subacute bacterial endocarditis).

Focal proliferative glomerulonephritis occurs in both primary and secondary forms.

Chronic Glomerulonephritis

The end stage of most glomerular disease is **chronic glomerulonephritis,** in which the kidneys become small (often about 100 g) and have diffusely granular cortical surfaces. Hyaline obliteration of glomeruli occurs by trapping of plasma proteins and deposition of increased mesangial matrix, collagen, and material resembling basement membrane. The result is acellular, eosinophilic masses at sites of former glomeruli. Hypertension commonly accompanies chronic glomerulonephritis and produces conspicuous arterial and arteriolar sclerosis. The destruction of the glomeruli causes changes in the rest of the nephrons, manifested by marked tubular atrophy, interstitial fibrosis, and lymphocytic infiltration. Patients with chronic glomerulonephritis treated by dialysis also show tubular and interstitial deposition of calcium oxylate crystals; focal calcification; arterial changes including intimal thickening; and acquired cystic changes. Renal adenomas and borderline adenocarcinomas may also be seen. Patients dying of chronic renal disease also show secondary pathology in other organ systems, which may include pericarditis, hyperparathyroidism with renal osteodystrophy, gastroenteritis, and diffuse alveolar damage in the lungs. The initial cause of the chronic glomerulonephritis is known in many cases. In others, the chronic renal failure develops insidiously, perhaps as an exacerbation of what was initially subclinical disease, and the underlying etiology is never identified.

Chronic glomerulonephritis is the end stage of most glomerular disease.

TUBULOINTERSTITIAL NEPHRITIS

Hypersensitivity Interstitial Nephritis

Drugs can cause acute **tubulointerstitial nephritis** by an **IgE-mediated hypersensitivity reaction.** Drugs that have been implicated include antibiotics (sulfonamides, synthetic penicillins, rifampin), diuretics (furosemide, thiazides), nonsteroidal anti-inflammatory agents

Drugs can cause acute tubulointerstitial nephritis.

(phenylbutazone), and miscellaneous drugs (phenindione, cimetidine). The interstitial nephritis characteristically affects only a few individuals exposed to the drugs. The interstitial nephritis develops in the first 6 weeks (typically 2 weeks) after exposure to the drug and is characterized clinically by fever, (transient) eosinophilia, skin rash, and renal findings including sterile pyuria, mild proteinuria, hematuria, and, in about one-half of patients, oliguria accompanied by a rising serum creatinine level that may progress to acute renal failure. An interstitial edema is present containing a principally lymphocytic and histiocytic infiltrate that may also contain eosinophils, neutrophils, plasma cells, and basophils. Tubular necrosis or regeneration (or both) may also be seen. In cases initiated by a few drugs, notably methicillin and the thiazides, small granulomas containing giant cells may also be present in the interstitium. Hypersensitivity interstitial nephritis usually resolves with removal of the inciting agent, although return to normal renal function may take months. Older patients sometimes experience irreversible damage.

Analgesic Abuse Nephropathy

Chronic analgesic abuse may produce chronic tubulointerstitial nephritis.

Chronic tubulointerstitial nephritis with renal papillary necrosis can be observed in some patients who have had excessive intake of **analgesic mixtures** that may have contained phenacetin, aspirin, caffeine, acetaminophen, and codeine. The chronic renal disease is usually only observed after the phenacetin intake exceeds 2 to 3 kg ingested over 3 years; analgesic mixtures appear to be more toxic than pure aspirin, phenacetin, or acetaminophen. The renal papilla show changes that characteristically vary in stage from papilla to papilla and spare the cortical columns of Bertini. These changes include varying degrees of necrosis, fragmentation or **sloughing of the papilla,** and focal calcification of necrotic tissue. The cortex shows changes related to tubular obstruction (secondary to the papillary necrosis) that include loss and atrophy of tubules accompanied by interstitial fibrosis and inflammation. Papillary vessels, as well as those in the urinary tract submucosa, can show PAS-positive basement thickening considered characteristic of analgesic abuse (analgesic microangiopathy). A **secondary pyelonephritis** may be superimposed on the papillary and cortical changes. The pathology is associated with a variety of clinical problems. Papillary damage impairs urinary concentration. Distal renal tubular acidosis may be accompanied by development of renal stones. Pyuria, which may be either sterile or infected, is almost always present. Necrotic papillae may break off, potentially causing gross hematuria, renal colic, or ureteral obstruction. **Chronic renal failure** eventually develops. Urothelial carcinoma of the renal pelvis is observed as a late finding in some patients. Analgesic nephropathy is often accompanied by headache, anemia, hypertension, and gastrointestinal symptoms. Renal function can be stabilized, and will sometimes improve, with withdrawal of analgesics and treatment of urinary tract infections.

Renal papilla may slough into the urine.

ACUTE RENAL FAILURE

Acute renal failure has prerenal, renal, and postrenal causes.

Renal function can be acutely suppressed, usually causing oliguria and rarely causing anuria, by a variety of processes. **Prerenal causes** of acute renal failure include shock and bilateral occlusion of renal arteries by external compression or thromboemboli. **Intrarenal vascular caus-**

es include processes with diffuse involvement of vessels such as polyarteritis nodosa, malignant hypertension, hemolytic uremic syndrome, and disseminated intravascular coagulation. **Glomerular causes** include any of the diseases that produce rapidly progressive glomerulonephritis. **Tubular causes** include any of the causes of acute tubular necrosis or acute tubulointerstitial nephritis (particularly drug hypersensitivity). **Pyelonephritis** can cause papillary necrosis and acute renal failure. **Postrenal causes** include urinary obstruction by tumor, prostatic hypertrophy, or blood clots.

Acute Tubular Necrosis

In **acute tubular necrosis,** acute renal failure is associated with destruction of the renal tubular epithelium. It is convenient to subdivide acute tubular necrosis into ischemic and nephrotoxic forms.

Ischemic tubulorrhectic acute tubular necrosis is observed after processes causing renal hypoperfusion and ischemia, including cardiovascular shock, burns, and bacterial sepsis. **Pigment-induced acute tubular necrosis** is a special form seen after massive hemolysis or severe skeletal muscle injury have caused massive hemoglobinuria or myoglobinuria, respectively. Histologically, ischemic acute tubular necrosis is characterized by focal areas of tubular necrosis with intervening skip areas having lesser degrees of damage; rupture of tubular basement membranes (tubulorrhexis); and occlusion of tubular lumina by eosinophilic hyaline casts. The casts contain Tamm-Horsfall protein (derived from cells of the ascending thick limb and distal tubules), hemoglobin, myoglobin, and plasma proteins. Other findings may include interstitial edema and leukocytes within the vasa recta. In patients who survive, tubular epithelial regeneration occurs.

Ischemic acute tubular necrosis often causes skip areas of tubular damage.

Nephrotoxic acute tubular necrosis can be caused by poisons (mushrooms, insecticides, herbicides, mercury, lead, arsenic, carbon tetrachloride, methyl alcohol, ethylene glycol), antibiotics and chemotherapeutic agents (gentamicin, cephalosporin, cyclosporine), anesthetics (methoxyflurane), and contrast media. Nephrotoxic acute tubular necrosis, in contrast to ischemic acute tubular necrosis, tends to have more severe damage to the proximal convoluted tubules. Also, the tubular necrosis often involves extensive regions of the nephron, rather than showing the patchy distribution characteristic of ischemic acute tubular necrosis. Most often, the etiology of the acute tubular necrosis cannot be determined from the histologic presentation. However, a few agents produce distinctive or suggestive features. In mercuric chloride poisoning, large acidophilic inclusions may be present in injured tubular cells. Necrotic cells may form calcified intraluminal masses. In carbon tetrachloride poisoning, neutral fats accumulate in injured cells. In ethylene glycol poisoning, the proximal convoluted tubular epithelium shows ballooning, with hydropic or vacuolar degeneration. The tubular lumina often contain calcium oxalate crystals.

Nephrotoxic acute tubular necrosis preferentially damages proximal convoluted tubules.

The distinction between toxic and ischemic acute tubular necrosis is sometimes blurred because agents causing toxic acute tubular necrosis often also cause shock and consequently ischemic damage. The clinical course of both forms of acute tubular necrosis can be broadly classified into the following phases. The **initiating phase** is the time after injury during which the acute renal failure can be reversed by correcting the inciting ischemic or toxic cause. The **maintenance phase** is typically characterized by oliguria (40 to 400 ml urine/day) and its consequences,

Oliguria is followed by diuresis in patients who recover from acute tubular necrosis.

including uremia, salt and water overload, hyperkalemia, and metabolic acidosis. This phase is managed by appropriate supportive therapy, often including dialysis. The **recovery phase** usually begins with a diuresis that may reach 3 liters/day. Since tubular reabsorption is still impaired, sodium and potassium losses may be large. Patients in this phase are also particularly vulnerable to infection for unknown reasons. As recovery continues, the kidneys' ability to concentrate urine returns and the uremia resolves. While the above phases typically occur, up to one-half of patients may not have oliguria (nonoliguric acute tubular necrosis); these patients tend to have a more benign clinical course. The prognosis in acute tubular necrosis is dependent primarily upon the degree of coexisting damage to other major organ systems. In nephrotoxic acute tubular necrosis without damage to other organs, approximately 95 percent of patients recover.

TUMORS OF THE KIDNEY

The kidney is vulnerable to both benign and malignant tumors. The benign tumors are usually of little clinical significance, and include, among others, cortical adenomas and renomedullary interstitial cell tumor. Malignant tumors such as renal cell carcinoma, Wilms tumor, and urothelial carcinomas are clinically important.

Cortical Adenoma

Small, benign renal adenomas are common.

Small (usually under 2 cm), benign **adenomas** are found in roughly one-tenth to one-fifth of autopsy cases. The adenomas arise in the renal tubules and are composed of cuboidal to polygonal cells with regular, small, centrally located nuclei and lipid-laden cytoplasm. The cells are free of atypia and can grow in a variety of patterns including papillary fronds, tubules, glands, cords, and masses. Cortical adenomas have the same histologic structure as renal cell adenocarcinoma. Tumors less than 2 to 3 cm are unlikely to metastasize and are classified as benign. Some authors consider tumors of borderline size (2 to 3 cm) to be early cancers.

Renomedullary Interstitial Cell Tumor

Renomedullary interstitial cell tumor is a small, benign lesion.

Renomedullary interstitial cell tumors (renal fibroma or hamartoma) are small, benign, gray-white foci of tissue composed of collagenous tissue that contain cells resembling fibroblasts with ultrastructural features of renal interstitial cells. The renomedullary interstitial cell tumors are usually found in the renal pyramids. Rarely, small, gray hamartomatous nodules of fibrous tissue, tubular cells, and blood vessels can be found in the renal cortex.

Miscellaneous Benign Tumors

Other benign tumors also occur in the kidney.

Benign mesenchymal tumors of many types, notably **hemangiomas** and **angiomyolipomas,** occur in the kidney. Angiomyolipomas are harmatomatous malformations that contain vessels, smooth muscle, and fat. Angiomyolipomas are clinically significant because they may coexist with the cerebral cortical disease tuberous sclerosis. **Renin-producing jux-**

taglomerular cell tumors are rare tumors resembling hemangiopericytomas that can cause hypertension by activating the renin-angiotensin system. **Oncocytomas** are benign, sometimes large (up to 12 cm) tumors composed of markedly eosinophilic cells that ultrastructurally contain prominent mitochondria.

Renal Cell Carcinoma

About nine-tenths of all adult kidney cancers are **renal cell carcinomas** (hypernephroma, adenocarcinoma of the kidney). The tumors are found most frequently in men in their sixth and seventh decades. Tobacco use appears to be a risk factor, and many chemical and viral agents cause renal cell carcinomas in laboratory animals. Genetic predisposition may also play a role, since renal cell carcinoma is frequently seen in patients with von Hippel-Lindau syndrome (who may develop multiple renal cell carcinomas) and is sometimes found in familial form.

Most kidney cancers are renal cell carcinoma.

On gross examination, the tumors form bright yellow to gray-white spherical masses up to 15 cm in diameter that often contain areas of hemorrhage and necrosis. Satellite nodules are often found in the adjacent tissue, and the tumor may invade the renal vein (sometimes extending into the vena cava and then right atrium) or ureter. Renal cell carcinomas can grow in a variety of histologic patterns including papillary, solid, trabecular, and tubular; multiple patterns may be present in a single tumor. The cell type is most commonly a clear cell with abundant clear cytoplasm and a rounded or polygonal shape but can also be a granular cell with moderately eosinophilic cytoplasm or can be spindle-shaped. Significant nuclear atypia, if present, suggests a worse prognosis. The tumors also contain scanty, but highly vascularized, stroma.

Renal cell carcinomas may invade the vena cava.

Renal cell carcinomas have a highly variable clinical course. The tumors may be silent until after they have attained a large size or metastasized, or both. Costovertebral pain, palpable mass, and hematuria are considered classic diagnostic features but unfortunately are often (usually) not all present. Renal cell carcinomas may produce paraneoplastic syndromes as a consequence of hormone production, including hypertension (renin), polycythemia (erythropoietin), feminization or masculinization (sex steroids), Cushing syndrome (glucocorticoids), hypercalcemia, eosinophilia, leukemoid reactions, and amyloidosis. Tumor growth may be slow or explosively fast. Favored sites for metastases are lungs, bones, regional lymph nodes, liver, adrenals, brain, and the opposite kidney. Renal vein invasion and extension of the tumor into the perinephric fat are associated with poorer prognosis.

Some renal cell carcinomas produce paraneoplastic syndromes.

Wilms Tumor

Wilms tumor (nephroblastoma) is an aggressive childhood (peak incidence ages 2 to 4 years) cancer that can form large spherical masses composed of variegated tissues. Wilms tumor originates in the kidney, but can nearly fill one-half to all of the abdomen. In roughly one-tenth of cases, the tumors are bilateral. The tumor is derived from the primitive blastoma and characteristically produces a variety of tissues, including nests and sheets of primitive renal epithelial elements; intervening mesenchymal stroma that can resemble sarcoma; abortive tubules and glomeruli; and heterologous tissues such as striated or smooth muscle, cartilage, fat, fibrous connective tissue, and bone. High degrees of

Wilms tumor is an aggressive childhood cancer.

anaplasia of the stroma are associated with poorer prognosis. Children with Wilms tumor typically present with an (often large) abdominal mass. Alternative presentations include hematuria, abdominal pain, hypertension, and intestinal obstruction. Metastases, often in the lungs, are frequently present at the time of initial diagnosis. The formerly poor prognosis has been markedly modified by aggressive combined modality therapy with chemotherapy, radiotherapy, and surgery.

Urothelial Carcinomas of the Renal Pelvis

The **renal pelvis** is the site of origin of about one-tenth of primary renal tumors. Tumors of the renal pelvis resemble those of the urinary bladder and range from benign papillomas to frank papillary carcinomas. Distinguishing benign papillomas from low-grade papillary carcinomas can be difficult. Despite a tendency to produce early hematuria or obstruction of urine flow, only about one-half of patients survive for 5 or more years, in part because the tumors frequently invade the renal vein. A coexisting urothelial tumor involves the bladder in about one-half of cases.

URINARY TRACT OBSTRUCTION

Urinary tract obstruction can occur as a result of a variety of predisposing factors, including congenital anomalies, urinary calculi, tumors, benign prostatic hypertrophy, inflammation, pregnancy, blood clots, sloughed renal papillae (renal papillary necrosis), and bladder paralysis. Dilation of ureters, renal calyces, and renal pelvis (hydronephrosis) tends to be most severe after a subtotal intermittent obstruction, since complete urinary obstruction will completely suppress glomerular filtration, while a partial obstruction does not. In extreme cases, the kidney may be transformed into a large (up to 20 cm), dilated "sac" with total obliteration of pyramids and striking parenchymal atrophy. Urinary tract obstruction strongly predisposes for acute and chronic pyelonephritis, as discussed in a previous section. Complete or nearly complete bilateral obstruction is a cause of acute renal failure. A postobstructive diuresis can follow relief of the obstruction. Bilateral partial obstruction can produce polyuria, nocturia, distal tubular acidosis, renal salt wasting, secondary renal calculi, tubulointerstitial nephritis, and hypertension.

UROLITHIASIS

While stones can form throughout the urinary tract, the kidney is the most common site of origin. **Calcium oxalate,** with or without calcium phosphate, is the most common composition. Approximately half of patients with calcium oxalate stones have "idiopathic hypercalciuria," which is not accompanied by hypercalcemia and which may be related to factors such as increased intestinal absorption or impaired renal tubular reabsorption of calcium. About one-tenth of patients have both hypercalcemia and hypercalciuria and may have predisposing diseases such as hyperparathyroidism, bone disease, or sarcoidosis. Hyperuricosuria and hyperoxaluria also predispose for calcium oxalate stone formation. In about one-fourth of patients, both hypercalcemia and hypercalciuria are absent, and the stone formation is considered idiopathic.

"Triple stones," formed of magnesium ammonium phosphate are associated with renal infections by urea-splitting bacteria (*Proteus* and some staphylococci), which produces an alkaline urine secondary to conversion of urea to ammonia. Magnesium ammonium phosphate stones may be huge and tend to follow the outlines of the calyceal system (staghorn calculi). Uric acid stones are observed both idiopathically and in patients with hyperuricemia (gout) or rapid cell turnover (leukemias). Cystine stones are observed in patients who have a genetically impaired renal transport of cystine. Since many patients with hypercalciuria, hyperoxaluria, or hyperuricosuria do not develop stones, it has been postulated that normal urine contains inhibitors of stone formation (possibly mucoproteins). Stone formation would then be postulated to occur when these inhibitors were deficient. Urinary calculi are often asymptomatic as long as they remain in the renal calcyceal system. Entry of a stone into a ureter can cause renal colic, obstruction, or ulceration with bleeding. Stones also predispose for infection because of both the obstruction and the trauma they can cause.

PYELONEPHRITIS AND URINARY TRACT INFECTIONS

Urinary tract infections can involve either the bladder, producing cystitis, or the kidneys, producing pyelonephritis. The bacteria causing urinary tract infections are usually normal inhabitants of the gastrointestinal tract that usually seed the lower urinary tract via fecal contamination of the urethral orifice; renal infection, when it occurs, is by an ascending route. Hematogenous spread is an alternative, less common, route. Commonly isolated enteric organisms include *Escherichia coli, Proteus, Klebsiella, Enterobacter,* and *Streptococcus faecalis.* Staphylococci, along with almost every other bacteria and fungus, can also infect the urinary tract. Individuals at particular risk for developing ascending urinary tract infections include women (particularly between ages 15 and 40 years), patients with long-term urinary catheterization, and patients with urethral obstruction due to processes such as prostatic hypertrophy. Individuals at particular risk of hematogenous infection include patients with ureteral obstruction, debilitated or immunosuppressed patients, and those with septicemia or infective endocarditis.

Infections of the lower urinary tract may remain asymptomatic, may cause symptomatic disease (fever, dysuria) but remain localized to the bladder, or may spread via the ureters to one or both kidneys. Factors favoring spread to the kidneys are primarily those favoring reflux of urine back into the kidneys during voiding. Incompetence of the vesicoureteral junction can be due in children to congenital absence or shortening of the intravesicular portion of the ureter, and in adults to bladder diverticula and neurogenic factors. Infection of the kidneys is termed pyelonephritis and is conveniently divided into acute and chronic forms.

Bacteria causing urinary tract infection are often normal gastrointestinal inhabitants.

Acute Pyelonephritis

Acute suppurative inflammation of the kidneys can occur either by hematogenous spread or via an ascending urinary tract infection. **Acute pyelonephritis** causes patchy interstitial suppurative inflammation (abscesses); masses of neutrophils within tubules secondary to rupture of abscesses into engulfed tubules; and relative preservation of glomeruli unless the pyelonephritis is severe or due to fungal (*Candida*) infection. **Papillary necrosis** (necrotizing papillitis) refers to a coagulative infarctive necrosis with preservation of tubular outline in one or more pyramids in either or both kidneys. Papillary necrosis is seen most often in diabetics and patients with urinary tract obstruction. **Pyonephrosis** is the collection of large quantities of suppurative exudate (pus) in the renal pelvis, calyces, and ureter. Pyonephrosis occurs when obstruction, usually high in the urinary tract, prevents drainage of pus through the urinary tract. **Perinephric abscess** occurs when the suppurative inflammation (pus) extends through the renal capsules to involve the perinephric tissue.

Acute pyelonephritis may be subclinical or may present with fever, malaise, and pain at the costovertebral angle. Lower urinary tract symptoms (dysuria, increased frequency of urination) are often present due to coexisting cystitis. Urinary leukocyte casts, which are formed in renal tubules, indicate renal involvement; quantitative urinary cultures can determine the infecting organism. Uncomplicated acute pyelonephritis usually responds promptly to appropriate antibiotic therapy. Healing is by fibrosis (scar formation) of inflamed areas of the kidney. Complicated cases (diabetes mellitus, unrelieved urinary obstruction, immunocompromised or debilitated patients) may cause repeated septicemic episodes. Acute renal failure can occur in patients who develop papillary necrosis.

Chronic Pyelonephritis and Reflux Nephropathy

While chronic bacterial infection is a component of **chronic pyelonephritis,** it is clear that chronic urinary obstruction or chronic urinary reflux (or both) are as important as the bacteria in maintaining chronic pyelonephritis. Chronic pyelonephritis is characterized by complex histologic changes including chronic tubulointerstitial inflammation, renal scarring, a variety of tubular changes including colloid casts (renal "thyroidization"), obliterative endarteritis and hypertensive hyaline arteriolosclerosis, and lymphoid follicles. The renal pelvis and calyces may also be involved. Focal segmental glomerulosclerosis is present in some patients in advanced stages with proteinuria. The gross appearance of kidneys affected by chronic pyelonephritis is characteristic, and includes coarse, irregular, asymmetric scarring of the cortex and medulla that overlies a dilated, blunted, or otherwise deformed calyx.

It is convenient to subclassify chronic pyelonephritis into obstructive and chronic-reflux associated forms. **Chronic obstructive pyelonephritis** is characterized by renal damage by both recurrent infection, with inflammation and scarring, and obstruction, which causes parenchymal atrophy. **Reflux nephropathy** (chronic-reflux associated pyelonephritis) is the more common form of pyelonephritis and occurs in childhood when urinary infection is superimposed on congenital vesicular urinary reflux. Both forms of pyelonephritis can affect either or both kidneys. An uncommon form of pyelonephritis, **xanthogranulomatous pyelonephritis,** is associated with *Proteus* infections and obstruction and is characterized by the formation of large, yellow-orange nodules composed of foamy macrophages, plasma cells, lymphocytes, neutrophils, and occasional giant cells.

The typical clinical courses of reflux nephropathy and chronic obstructive pyelonephritis are somewhat different. Chronic obstructive pyelonephritis may be either initially subclinical or may present with recurrent episodes of acute pyelonephritis. Reflux nephropathy almost always has a silent insidious onset that begins in childhood and comes to medical attention when the children develop hypertension and renal insufficiency with polyuria and nocturia. Both forms of pyelonephritis may either stabilize or progress to chronic end-stage renal failure.

LOWER URINARY TRACT

DISEASES OF THE URETERS

The ureters are vulnerable to congenital anomalies, inflammation, tumors, and obstruction.

Congenital Anomalies

Ureters can be doubled through the entire or only portions (**bifid ureters**) of their course. **Ureteropelvic junction obstruction** occurs mainly in male infants and is characterized by hydronephrosis secondary to ureteral obstruction at the ureteropelvic junction by extrinsic compression of aberrant renal vessels; disorganized smooth muscle; or excessive collagen deposition in the smooth muscle. The ureters may have **congenital diverticula** or may be dilated (**hydroureter,** which when massive is termed megaloureter). Ureteral abnormalities are sometimes associated with congenital defects of the kidney.

Some forms of ureteral anomalies are associated with hydronephrosis.

Ureteritis

Ureters may become acutely inflamed as a part of upper or lower urinary tract infections. **Chronic ureteritis** can cause focal subepithelial aggregations of lymphocytes that give the mucosal surface a fine granular texture (ureteritis follicularis); or multiple cysts of 1 to 5 mm in diameter (ureteritis cystica) usually lined with transitional epithelium.

Acute inflammation of the ureters may accompany either upper or lower urinary tract infections.

Tumors

Metastatic tumor involvement of the ureters is more common than primary tumor involvement. **Benign tumors** are usually small; do not usually cause obstruction; and may be derived from fibrous tissue, blood vessels, lymphatics, or smooth muscle. The **malignant tumors** that rarely arise in ureters are of the same types that can arise in the urothelium of the bladder or renal calyces.

Metastatic tumors involve the ureters more often than do primary tumors.

Obstructive Lesions

Intrinsic lesions that can obstruct the ureters include calculi, strictures, tumors, and blood clots. **Extrinsic lesions** that can obstruct the ureter by compressing it include pregnancy, endometriosis, tumor, inflammation, and an obscure disease characterized by formation of ill-defined fibrous masses known as retroperitoneal fibromatosis (sclerosing retroperitonitis).

Many processes may cause ureteral obstruction.

URETHRAL PATHOLOGY

The principal diseases affecting the urethra include inflammations and tumor.

Inflammations

Urethritis is characterized by local pain, itchiness, and increased frequency of urination. Gonococcal urethritis can be one of the earliest manifestations of gonorrhea. The more common nongonococcal urethritis may be caused by a large number of bacteria including *Escherichia coli,* other enteric organisms, *Chlamydia,* and mycoplasma. In women, urethritis is associated with cystitis; in men, it is associated with prostatitis. **Reiter syndrome** is the cluster of arthritis, conjunctivitis, and urethritis.

Urethritis may be caused by many organisms.

Tumors

Benign tumors of the urethra include papillomas and venereal condylomas. **Carcinomas** may rarely affect the urethra and are usually squamous cell carcinomas but may also be transitional cell carcinomas or adenocarcinomas. Urethral **caruncles** are benign inflammatory lesions that resemble tumors and are composed of vascularized fibroblastic connective tissue usually containing large numbers of leukocytes.

Both benign and malignant tumors can involve the urethra.

CONGENITAL ANOMALIES OF THE BLADDER

Bladder Diverticula

Pouchlike evaginations of the bladder wall are known as bladder diverticula. **Congenital diverticula** are characterized by the presence of some muscle within a thinned portion of the bladder wall and may occur as a focal failure of musculature development, secondary to fetal urinary tract obstruction, or as a budlike outgrowth of the bladder. **Acquired diverticula** are almost always secondary to bladder outflow obstruction by processes such as prostatic hypertrophy. In contrast to congenital diverticula, advanced acquired diverticula may have a wall that contains a mucosa and tunica propria but no muscle. Diverticula may predispose for vesicoureteral reflux, infection, and bladder calculi.

Diverticula may be congenital or acquired.

Exstrophy

A failure in the development of the anterior wall of the abdomen and the bladder produces **exstrophy,** in which the bladder is open to the body surface. With the resulting recurrent infections, the exposed bladder mucosa becomes replaced by granulation tissue covered by stratified squamous epithelium. Exstrophy of the bladder predisposes for development of cancer, usually adenocarcinoma.

In exstrophy, the bladder is open to the body surface.

Miscellaneous Anomalies

Vesicoureteral reflux can occur as a result of a shortened course of a ureter through the bladder wall and is important because it predisposes

The bladder is also vulnerable to other anatomic defects.

Cystitis may take a variety of pathologic forms.

for chronic pyelonephritis. Uncommonly, the bladder may be absent, hypoplastic, contain an incomplete transverse septum (**"hourglass" deformity**), or have abnormal **fistulous connections** to nearby structures such as the vagina, rectum, or uterus. The **urachus** may persist focally, causing urachal cysts, or through its length, forming a fistulous urinary tract connecting the bladder to the umbilicus.

CYSTITIS

Inflammations of the bladder are termed **cystitis** and may occur in acute and chronic forms. Etiologic agents include coliform bacteria (*Escherichia coli, Proteus, Klebsiella, Enterobacter*); tuberculosis, usually following renal tuberculosis; fungi (*Candida albicans,* cryptococci) in immunosuppressed patients; schistosomiasis (in the Middle East); viruses, *Chlamydia,* and mycoplasma; and radiation or chemotherapy (cyclophosphamide, busulfan). A variety of special terms are used to describe different types of cystitis.

Hemorrhagic cystitis is a form of acute cystitis characterized by mucosal hyperemia, submucosal hemorrhage, and often epithelial atypia associated with radiation injury, antitumor chemotherapy, and adenovirus infection. **Suppurative cystitis** is accompanied by production of large amounts of pus. **Ulcerative cystitis** is characterized by ulceration of large areas of bladder mucosa. **Polypoid cystitis** has mucosal polyps and is associated with chronic use of indwelling catheters. **Chronic cystitis,** seen with persistent or repeated infections, is characterized by inelasticity of the bladder wall secondary to fibrous thickening of the tunica propria and a red, granular, often ulcerated mucosa. **Cystic follicularis** is a variant of chronic cystitis characterized by lymphoid aggregates within the bladder mucosa and wall.

Ulcerative interstitial cystitis (Hunner's ulcer) is a persistent chronic cystitis with bladder wall fibrosis and inflammation often accompanied by a localized ulcer. **Emphysematous cystitis** is seen most often in diabetics and consists of gas bubbles, often surrounded by giant cells, in the submucosal connective tissue that are presumed to be caused by gas-forming bacteria. **Cystitis cystica** are small cystic inclusions lined by transitional epithelium that are found in the submucosa in some longstanding chronic inflammations. **Eosinophilic cystitis** is a rare form of chronic cystitis of unknown etiology in which the subepithelial connective tissue contains many eosinophils, fibrosis, and rare giant cells. **Malakoplakia** is characterized by soft yellow, mucosal plaques up to 4 cm in diameter composed of closely packed foamy macrophages with occasional giant cells and some lymphocytes. The macrophages contain PAS-positive cytoplasmic granules possibly caused by phagocytosis of bacterial debris. The lesion is thought to be due to an acquired failure of normal phagocytosis and is more common in immunosuppressed transplant recipients.

BLADDER TUMORS

The vast majority of **bladder tumors** are epithelial neoplasms, which include transitional cell papilloma, transitional cell carcinoma, squamous cell carcinoma, adenocarcinoma, mixed carcinoma, and undifferentiated carcinoma. Nonepithelial neoplasms of the bladder are mainly mesenchymal tumors similar to those that arise throughout the body.

Transitional Cell Papilloma

Transitional cell papillomas are usually single, but sometimes multiple, branching structures that attach to the bladder mucosa by a slender stalk. The branches are composed of fibrovascular cores covered with normal appearing transitional epithelium. Transitional cell papillomas are considered benign lesions, but they may be difficult to distinguish from early papillary carcinomas. A helpful criterion is that the papilloma transitional epithelium is consistently seven or fewer layers in thickness. Treatment is usually by transurethral resection.

Transitional cell papillomas may be difficult to distinguish from early papillary carcinomas.

Carcinoma of the Bladder

Carcinoma of the bladder has a male predominance, and some cases appear to be associated with environmental risk factors including occupational exposures (β-naphthylamine, biphenyl compounds), *Schistosoma haematobium* infection of the bladder (or possibly its therapy), tryptophan metabolites, cyclophosphamide chemotherapy, smoking, and analgesic abuse. Nine-tenths of bladder carcinomas are transitional carcinomas; the remainder are squamous cell, mixed, or adenocarcinomas. Squamous cell carcinomas are most common in the Middle East, where *Schistosoma haematobium* infections are found.

Most bladder carcinomas are transitional cell carcinomas.

Vesicular cancers are categorized grossly as papillary or flat, and noninvasive or invasive. Staging for bladder cancer is the same for all types and is based on the depth of invasion into the bladder wall, involvement of the perivesical region, and presence of regional or distant metastases. Grading of transitional cell carcinomas is based on epithelial thickness and cellular atypia. Transitional cell carcinomas may show areas of squamous metaplasia. Pure squamous cell carcinomas may have widely varying levels of cytologic differentiation and may be in situ or grow invasively in fungating, infiltrative patterns. Adenocarcinomas of the bladder only rarely occur; variants include the highly malignant signet-ring cell carcinoma and the more clinically benign mesonephric or nephrogenic adenoma.

Squamous cell carcinoma of the bladder may be associated with *Schistosoma hematobium*.

Bladder tumors classically present with painless hematuria, but may also cause frequency, dysuria, pyelonephritis, or hydronephrosis. Transitional cell carcinomas tend to arise in dysplastic epithelium, and often recur (possibly due to a new, second primary tumor) after resection.

Other Bladder Tumors

Benign mesodermal tumors, most commonly leiomyomas, and sarcomas, notably adult or embryonal rhabdomyosarcomas, rarely arise in the bladder. Secondary malignant involvement of the bladder is usually by direct extension from adjacent organs rather than by metastatic spread.

Other bladder tumors also occur.

14

Male Genital System

PENIS

Congenital Anomalies

The penis can be affected by many congenital anomalies including rare congenital absence, hypoplasia, hyperplasia, or duplication. **Hypospadias** is a malformation of the urethral groove and urethral canal in which the urethra opens on the ventral surface of the penis. **Epispadias** is a similar malformation in which the urethra opens on the penile dorsal surface. Hypospadias and epispadias are significant because they may cause partial urinary obstruction with risk of urinary tract infection, as well as sterility by blocking normal ejaculation and insemination. **Phimosis** refers to a small prepuce that cannot be normally retracted and consequently can cause **paraphimosis,** in which a forcibly retracted prepuce constricts the glans penis causing extreme pain, urethral constriction, and acute urinary retention.

Relatively common congenital anomalies of the penis include hypospadias, epispadias, and phimosis.

Inflammations

Most specific inflammations of the penis are sexually transmitted and are discussed elsewhere (see p. 40, 52). **Balanoposthitis** is a nonspecific inflammation that can cause ulceration or scarring of the glans and prepuce. It is usually encountered in patients with penile structural abnormalities including phimosis and large, redundant prepuces. Infecting organisms can include staphylococci, streptococci, enteric organisms, and (less commonly) gonorrhea.

Balanoposthitis is a nonspecific inflammation of the glans and prepuce.

Penile Tumors

Tumors uncommonly affect the penis. The lesions range from clearly benign (condyloma acuminatum) to intermediate malignant potential

311

Condyloma acuminatum and giant condyloma are caused by papillomavirus.

Carcinoma in situ of the penis has several morphologic forms.

Penile carcinoma is almost always squamous cell and may be associated with papillomavirus infection.

(giant condyloma, carcinoma in situ) to clearly malignant (squamous cell carcinoma).

Condyloma acuminatum is a benign tumor caused by human papillomavirus (types 6 and 11). Condyloma acuminatum is similar to the common wart (verruca vulgaris), but is found on moist mucocutaneous surfaces of male or female external genitalia. The lesions tend to be red, papillary excrescences up to several millimeters diameter that are often located on the prepuce. Histologically, hyperplastic squamous epithelium, containing vacuolated cells (koilocytosis) characteristic of human papillomavirus infection, overlies a branching, papillary connective tissue stroma. Almost all of these lesions remain benign. Their occurrence in children suggests the possibility of sexual abuse.

Giant condyloma (Buschke-Loewenstein tumor, verrucous carcinoma) is also related to infection with human papillomavirus types 6 and 11, but tends to be much larger, locally invasive, and likely to recur if resected. Metastasis rarely, if ever, occurs. Histologically, giant condyloma is distinguished from condyloma acuminatum by the presence of both upward and downward growth patterns of the hyperplastic epithelium. It is distinguished from frank squamous cell carcinoma by the absence of cellular atypia.

Carcinoma in situ refers to the presence of cytologic changes associated with malignancy that are confined to the epithelium. **Bowen's disease** is characterized by gray-white, opaque plaques, usually on the penile shaft or scrotum, composed histologically of a dysplastic squamous cell epithelium with a sharply delineated dermal-epidermal border. Bowen's disease is thought to have a 10 percent chance of progressing to squamous cell carcinoma. It additionally has been linked, in some controversial studies, to visceral cancers. **Erythroplasia of Queyrat** presents as a red, soft plaque on the glans or prepuce composed histologically of dysplastic epithelium in which the dysplasia may range from a mild cellular disorientation to change indistinguishable from Bowen's disease. Like Bowen's disease, erythroplasia of Queyrat sometimes progresses to invasive carcinoma. **Bowenoid papulosis** is associated with human papillomavirus type 16. Multiple, reddish brown, papular lesions, which may be mistaken for condyloma acuminatum, are observed on the external genitalia of sexually active adults. Histologically, the lesions resemble those of Bowen's disease.

Carcinoma, which is nearly always squamous cell carcinoma, can occur on the penis and is more common in areas where circumcision is uncommon. Human papillomavirus types 16 and 18 have been associated with some cases. The tumors are most often observed in patients between the ages of 40 and 70 years and form papillary or ulceroinvasive lesions that histologically resemble squamous cell carcinomas from other sites. The prognosis is worse when the cancers have invaded the penile shaft or metastasized to regional (inguinal and iliac) lymph nodes.

TESTES AND EPIDIDYMIS

Inflammations

Epididymitis is more common than orchitis. Syphilis characteristically produces orchitis before epididymitis; gonorrhea and tuberculosis characteristically produce epididymitis before orchitis.

Nonspecific Epididymitis and Orchitis

Bacterial lower urinary tract infections can pass through the vas deferens or the lymphatics of the spermatic cord to produce epididymitis, which may then be followed by orchitis. In children, a congenital genitourinary abnormality may be complicated by infection, usually with gram-negative rods, which subsequently spreads to the epididymis. *Chlamydia trachomatis* and *Neisseria gonorrhoeae* are spread by venereal transmission and can cause a nonspecific epididymitis seen most frequently in men younger than 35 years. *Escherichia coli, Pseudomonas,* and other urinary tract pathogens are most commonly observed in men older than 35 years.

The acute inflammation in nonspecific epididymitis and orchitis usually begins in the epididymis and may subsequently spread to the testes via direct continuity, through tubular channels, or through lymphatics. The inflammation typically begins in the interstitial connective tissue with a nonspecific acute inflammation exhibiting edema, congestion, and leukocytic (neutrophils, macrophages, lymphocytes) infiltration. Spread of the infection soon involves the tubules, permitting spread to the testes. The infection may be complicated by abscess formation or even complete suppurative necrosis of the epididymis or testes (or both). The inflammatory involvement usually resolves with fibrous scarring that can cause permanent sterility. Sterility can also occur as a consequence of testicular edema in the confined space enclosed by the tunica albuginea. Leydig cells are often relatively preserved, permitting continued sexual activity even if the patient is sterile.

Chlamydia, Neisseria, **and many urinary tract pathogens can cause nonspecific epididymitis.**

Granulomatous Orchitis

Rarely, a nontuberculous, granulomatous orchitis of unknown (possibly autoimmune) etiology causes unilateral testicular enlargement in a middle-aged man. The disease presents as a moderately tender to painless testicular mass of sudden onset that is clinically important because it mimics a testicular tumor. Histologically, granulomas resembling tubercules are seen in both the interstitium and the spermatic tubules.

Granulomatous orchitis of unknown etiology may affect middle-aged men.

Specific Inflammations

The epididymis and testes are also vulnerable to specific inflammations. **Gonorrhea** can cause nonspecific inflammation with abscess development that can destroy the epididymis and, less commonly, the testes. **Mumps** causes orchitis in about one-fifth of males over age 10 who seek medical attention for the condition. The orchitis may be unilateral or, somewhat less commonly, bilateral. It usually appears 1 week after parotid gland involvement. Acutely, the testis shows interstitial edema and a patchy leukocytic infiltration composed of lymphocytes, plasma cells, macrophages, and, in severe cases, neutrophils. Pus may fill tubular lumina. Most cases heal successfully; in a few bilateral lesions, the patient is subsequently infertile. **Tuberculosis,** usually of pulmonary, but sometimes of renal origin, can infect the epididymis and subsequently spread to the testis. The tubercules resemble those seen in other sites. **Syphilis,** in both acquired and congenital forms, is distinctive in that the testis is involved first, and the infection often does not spread to the epididymis. The orchitis can be characterized either by gumma forma-

Specific inflammations of the epididymis and testes can be caused by gonorrhea, mumps, tuberculosis, and syphilis.

tion or by a diffuse interstitial inflammation accompanied by obliterative endarteritis with perivascular lymphocytic and plasmacytic cuffing. With time, the testes become scarred and show considerable tubular atrophy, which may cause sterility.

A variety of **miscellaneous** infectious diseases can involve the testis and epididymis as a small component of a systemic disease. Examples include meningococcal infections, rickettsial infections, leprosy, brucellosis, typhoid fever, blastomycosis, and actinomycosis.

Diseases

Cryptorchidism

Testes that fail to descend may be found in the abdomen, pelvis, or inguinal canal.

The only common congenital anomaly of the testes is a failure of one or both testes to descend **(cryptorchidism),** which is observed in about 1 in 200 adult men. Rare congenital anomalies include testicular absence, testicular fusion (synorchism), and congenital testicular cysts.

The testes arise in the coelomic cavity and subsequently normally appear to move, as a result of differential growth rates of the body, first into the lower abdomen or pelvic brim (internal descent), and then through the inguinal canal into the scrotal sac (external descent). A failure in this process can produce malpositioned testes that may be found at any point along the apparent lines of internal and external descent.

Most cases of cryptorchidism are idiopathic, possibly the result of subtle hormonal deficiencies. Some cases are associated with mechanical factors, such as narrow inguinal canals or short spermatic cords; with genetic factors, notably trisomy 13; or with hormonal factors, including a rare deficiency of luteinizing hormone-releasing hormone. Cryptorchidism may be unilateral or, less commonly, bilateral and is usually identified on physical examination of the scrotal sac by the patient or a physician. The malpositioned testes are initially histologically normal, but by age 2 begin to develop pathology that eventually includes arrested development of germ cells. The spermatic tubular changes begin as hyalinization of the tubule and thickening of the tubular basement membrane and then progress until the tubules become hyaline cords of connective tissue surrounded by prominent basement membranes. The interstitial stroma is increased, often with Leydig cell hyperplasia. In cases of unilateral cryptorchidism, the contralateral descended testes may also, surprisingly, have decreased numbers of germ cells. Testicular trauma may be due to crushing against ligaments and bones if the testes lies in the inguinal canal. Sterility (bilateral cases) or infertility (many unilateral cases) are common in uncorrected cases. A significantly increased risk of later development of testicular carcinoma is substantially reduced, but not completely eliminated, if surgical repositioning is performed before age 2 years.

Testicular Atrophy

Testicular atrophy can occur in a variety of settings.

Testicular atrophy, with a histologic pattern similar to that described in cryptorchidism, occurs in a variety of other clinical settings including chronic testicular ischemia (atherosclerosis), severe inflammatory orchitis, hormonal disturbances (hypopituitarism, prolonged administration of estrogens, prolonged high levels of follicle-stimulating hormone), obstruction of semen outflow, severe malnutrition, and irradiation. In addition to testicular atrophy as a consequence of regression of a previously functional testes, testicular atrophy or improper development is observed in the sex chromosomal disorder Klinefelter syndrome. Severe bilateral testicular atrophy causes sterility. Unilateral testicular atrophy may be asymptomatic or cause infertility.

Testicular Torsion

A testes can occasionally twist on its spermatic cord tightly enough to cut off the arterial supply, causing the acute ischemic emergency known as testicular torsion. Precipitating causes usually consist of violent movement or physical trauma to the testes. A variety of anatomic abnormalities predispose for testicular torsion, including incomplete testicular descent, testicular atrophy, and abnormal or absent scrotal ligaments or gubernaculum testes. The morphologic changes produced vary with the duration and severity of the ischemia; they range from congestion to interstitial hemorrhage to infarction. Therapy is by prompt manual or, if necessary, surgical decompression of the torsion.

Testicular torsion is an acute ischemic emergency.

Miscellaneous Lesions of Tunica Vaginalis

The tunica vaginalis is a serosa-lined sac that lies proximal to the testis and epididymis. It is vulnerable to accumulation of serous fluid (**hydrocele**) secondary to neighboring infections or tumors; systemic edema; or peritoneal fluid entry consequent to failure of the processus vaginalis to close. The tunica vaginalis is also vulnerable to accumulation of blood (**hematocele**) secondary to trauma, testicular torsion, bleeding diatheses, or tumorous invasion. Lymphatic fluid can also accumulate (**chylocele**) if the lymphatic channels are obstructed, as in elephantiasis. Hydrocele, hematocele, and chylocele are clinically significant primarily because they may be mistaken for testicular enlargement. In most cases, the fluid accumulation can be relieved by removal with a syringe.

Serous fluid, blood, and lymph can accumulate within the tunica vaginalis.

Testicular Tumors

A surprising variety of tumors can occur in the testes. Testicular tumors are classified as either arising from germ cells (95 percent) or from sex cord stroma. The germinal tumors include seminoma, spermatocytic seminoma, embryonal carcinoma, yolk sac tumor (embryonal carcinoma infantile type), polyembryoma, choriocarcinoma, tetratoma, and germinal tumors with more than one histologic pattern. Sex cord-stromal tumors include Leydig cell tumor, Sertoli cell tumor, granulosa cell tumor, mixed forms, and incompletely differentiated forms. The clinical behavior of testicular tumors will be discussed after the histologic types are presented.

Testicular tumors are classified as arising from germ cells or sex cord stroma.

Seminoma

Slightly less than one-third of germinal tumors are seminomas, which almost never occur in infants and have a peak incidence in the fourth decade. Seminomas are composed of distinctive cells ("seminoma cells") with abundant, watery-appearing cytoplasm and a large hyperchromatic nucleus that often contains one or two prominent nucleoli. The cells grow in poorly defined lobules separated by delicate fibrous tissue stroma. Histologic variants include typical seminoma (over three-fourths), anaplastic seminoma, and an uncommon variant discussed later known

Seminomas are composed of cells with abundant, watery-appearing cytoplasm.

as spermatocytic seminoma. The **typical seminoma** is characterized by infrequent mitoses; relatively little cellular atypia; giant cells that may either be typical tumor giant cells or may resemble syncytiotrophoblast; and lymphocytic (common) or granulomatous (uncommon) (or both) reactions of the septa. Typical seminomas that contain large numbers of syncytial giant cells are often associated with elevated levels of serum human chorionic gonadotropins. **Anaplastic seminoma** is characterized by frequent tumor giant cells; many mitoses, (3 or more/high power field); and prominent cellular and nuclear atypia. Well-developed lymphocytic or granulomatous reactions are observed less commonly than in the typical variant.

Spermatocytic Seminoma

Spermatocytic seminoma has a more favorable clinical behavior than other forms of seminoma.

Spermatocytic seminoma is an uncommon (about 1 in 20 of seminomas) tumor that has been separated from other seminomas because its clinical and pathologic behaviors are very different. Unlike typical seminoma, spermatocytic seminoma has an excellent prognosis because it grows slowly and only rarely (if ever) produces metastases. The tumor usually grows as a large, pale gray mass with a friable cut surface. Spermatocytic seminomas have intermixed populations of cells including cells resembling secondary spermatocytes, cells with round nuclei and eosinophilic cytoplasm, and a few giant cells that may be multinucleated. Compared with typical seminomas, spermatocytic seminomas have more mitoses and do not show lymphocytic infiltration.

Embryonal Carcinoma

Embryonal carcinomas are a form of mixed tumors.

The peak incidence of the aggressive and often lethal **embryonal carcinoma** is between 20 and 30 years of age. At the time of diagnosis, the tumor is often a small, gray-white, testicular lesion with poorly demarcated margins and foci of hemorrhage and necrosis. Embryonal carcinoma is composed of large, anaplastic, immature cells with indistinct cell borders (unlike seminoma) and prominent nucleoli in hyperchromatic nuclei. The cells can grow in a variety of patterns, including glandular, alveolar, tubular, papillary, and sheetlike. Embryonal carcinomas contain frequent mitotic figures and tumor giant cells. These tumors are a form of mixed tumor, since in most embryonal carcinomas, both cells containing α-fetoprotein (yolk sac origin) and syncytial cells containing human chorionic gonadotropin (trophoblastic origin) can be demonstrated with immunoperoxidase techniques.

Yolk Sac Tumor

Yolk sac tumors may occur in pure form or as a component of mixed tumors.

Yolk sac tumor (infantile embryonal carcinoma or endodermal sinus tumor) is a common testicular tumor that occurs in pure form in infants and children and as a component of mixed tumors in adults. The pure form of the tumor forms a nonencapsulated, homogeneous, yellow-white mass with a mucinous appearance. Histologically, the tumor usually forms epithelial-lined spaces of varying sizes. Papillary structures, solid cords of cells, and structures resembling primitive glomeruli (endodermal sinuses) can also be found in some tumors. Typical tumor cells are flattened-to-cuboidal epithelial cells with vacuolated cytoplasm that contains eosinophilic, hyalinelike globules. These globules stain by immunohistochemical techniques for α-fetoprotein, indicating yolk cell differentiation, and α_1-antitrypsin.

Polyembryoma

Polyembryoma is rare in a pure form but is a common component of embryonal carcinoma and teratomas. The tumor forms distinctive structures that resemble embryonic discs ("embryoid bodies") with undifferentiated, large epithelial cells. The discs are often partially surrounded by cavities lined by flattened epithelial cells that resemble amniotic spaces. The embryoid bodies are found in a loose mesenchyma that may contain trophoblastic elements.

Polyembryoma forms structures resembling embryonic discs.

Choriocarcinoma

Choriocarcinoma is a highly malignant testicular tumor that is indistinguishable from choriocarcinomas in other sites such as the placenta, ovary, mediastinum, or abdomen. Choriocarcinomas characteristically form both cytotrophoblasts and syncytiotrophoblasts. At the time of detection, when metastases may have already occurred, the primary tumor is often only a small, palpable, testicular nodule, which may even have been replaced by a small fibrous scar. Alternatively, the primary tumor may be a large hemorrhagic and necrotic mass in which only tiny fragments of viable tumor can be found. Two cell types are present. Syncytiotrophoblastic cells are multinucleated giant cells that contain human chorionic gonadotropin and have abundant eosinophilic vacuolated cytoplasm and multiple irregular hyperchromatic nuclei. Cytotrophoblastic cells are uninucleate cells that have a regular, polygonal shape, clear cytoplasm with distinct cell borders, and fairly uniform nuclei. The cytotrophoblastic cells tend to grow in cords or masses that may be "capped" by syncytiotrophoblastic cells; well-formed placental villi are not seen. Choriocarcinoma tends to outgrow its blood supply rapidly, and consequently only small areas of viable tumor cells are found within large areas of hemorrhage and necrotic tumor.

Choriocarcinomas form both cytotrophoblast and syncytiotrophoblast.

Teratoma

Teratomas are complex tumors characterized by the growth of tissues from more than one germ layer. The tumors can occur from infancy to adulthood but are most often identified in childhood. Teratomas can be either benign or malignant and have been subdivided into mature teratomas, immature teratomas, and teratomas with malignant transformation. Mature teratomas are composed of a disorganized collection of mature tissues that may include nerve, muscle, cartilage, thyroid tissue, squamous epithelium, bronchial or bronchiolar epithelium, intestinal wall, or brain. Most mature teratomas occur in children. In adults, apparently mature teratomas should be carefully studied to detect any small foci of immature or malignant tissues. In immature teratomas, tissues are observed that are similar to those seen in the mature teratomas, but are characteristically incompletely differentiated and have a more disorganized arrangement. Immature teratomas behave malignantly, but do not appear cytologically malignant. Teratomas with malignant transformations are distinguished by the presence of obvious cytologic malignancies in cells from one or more germ cell layers. Examples include foci of squamous cell carcinoma, adenocarcinoma, or sarcoma. Both immature teratomas and teratomas with malignant transformation occur more commonly in adults.

Teratomas contain tissues from more than one germ layer.

Mixed Tumors

> **Mixed tumors are common among germ cell tumors.**

Over one-half of germ cell tumors are composed of mixtures of the tumors described above. The most prevalent pattern includes teratoma, embryonal carcinoma, yolk sac tumor, and human chorionic gonadotropin-containing syncytiotrophoblast. Other common patterns include seminoma with embryonal carcinoma and embryonal carcinoma with teratoma, sometimes called teratocarcinoma. Metastases from mixed tumors may contain multiple neoplastic components and may even show a new line of differentiation.

Clinical Features of Germ Cell Tumors

> **The histology of metastases may show a different line of differentiation from the primary tumor.**

Testicular tumors usually present with painless enlargement of the testis. Metastasis through the lymphatic system is first to the retroperitoneal para-aortic nodes; metastasis through the vascular system is mainly to the lungs, with other commonly affected sites including the liver, brain, and bones. In a few cases, the histology of the metastases may show a line of differentiation different from the primary tumor. Seminomas tend to have a better prognosis because they remain localized longer, are highly radiosensitive, and, when they do metastasize, spread to regional lymph nodes. Nonseminomatous germ cell tumors tend to behave more aggressively and to respond more poorly to therapy; choriocarcinoma is the most aggressive of these tumors.

Staging of testicular tumors is based on the presence of metastasis and tumor spread beyond the retroperitoneal nodes below the diaphragm. Germ cell tumors may secrete a variety of hormones and enzymes, of which the most useful markers are human chorionic gonadotropin and α-fetoprotein. Human chorionic gonadotropin is normally secreted by placental syncytiotrophoblasts. Its elaboration by a germ cell tumor suggests some syncytiotrophoblastic differentiation, as seen in almost all choriocarcinomas, as well as in many teratomas, embryonal carcinomas, and teratocarcinomas. α-Fetoprotein is produced by many yolk sac tumors, teratomas, embryonal carcinomas, and teratocarcinomas. The serum levels of these tumor markers are used primarily to monitor body tumor burden during staging and therapy.

Non-Germ Cell Tumors of the Testes

> **Other testicular tumors include Leydig cell tumors, Sertoli cell tumors, lymphomas, and adenomatoid tumors.**

Other important tumors of the testes include Leydig cell and Sertoli cell tumors (both derived from sex cord-gonadal stroma), testicular lymphoma, and the benign adenomatoid tumors. **Leydig (interstitial) cell tumors** are usually benign but sometimes malignant tumors composed of cells resembling Leydig cells. They can produce androgens, estrogens, or corticosteroids and have a distinctive yellow-brown hue on gross examination. **Sertoli cell tumors** (androblastoma) are usually benign but sometimes malignant tumors composed of cells resembling Sertoli cells and, in some cases, also granulosa cells. The tumors are gray-white to yellow, and some will secrete relatively small amounts of estrogens or androgens. Histologically, the growth pattern is often in cords reminiscent of spermatic tubules. **Testicular lymphoma** presents with a testicular mass and is the most common testicular cancer to affect men over age 60. The lymphoma is usually of the diffuse, large cell type and has a poor prognosis because disseminated disease occurs early. **Adenomatoid tumors** are benign nodules found in the epididymis; they contain stroma admixed with epithelial cuboidal cells that grow in glands, cords, or nests and may line cystic spaces.

PROSTATE

Prostatitis

Inflammations of the prostate can be classified as acute bacterial prostatitis, chronic bacterial prostatitis, and chronic abacterial prostatitis.

Acute bacterial prostatitis is an exquisitely tender prostatic inflammation caused by organisms similar to those that cause urinary tract infections. *Escherichia coli* is the most common pathogen; other commonly encountered bacteria include *Klebsiella, Proteus, Pseudomonas, Enterobacter, Serratia, Enterococcus,* and *Staphylococcus aureus.* The usual route of infection is by direct extension from a bladder or urethral source (often following surgical manipulation of the bladder, urethra, or prostate), but hematogenous or lymphatic spread from more distant sites can also occur. Histologically, acute prostatitis is characterized by abscess (either minute or large) formation with minimal to severe stromal leukocytic infiltration. Depending upon the severity of the infection, the prostatitis may heal with only minimal fibrous scarring or may progress to chronic prostatitis with continued infection in tiny, walled-off abscesses.

> **Acute bacterial prostatitis is typically due to urinary tract pathogens.**

Chronic bacterial prostatitis may be asymptomatic or may cause low back pain, perineal tenderness, or dysuria. Often, the patient experiences recurrent urinary tract infections by the same organism, which presumably seeds the urinary tract from a prostatic source. While some cases of chronic bacterial prostatitis follow acute bacterial prostatitis or surgical manipulations, chronic prostatitis most often develops insidiously without obvious predisposing factors. The infecting organisms are usually similar to those seen in acute bacterial prostatitis. Histologically, the prostate contains an inflammatory infiltrate composed of lymphocytes, plasma cells, macrophages, and neutrophils, which should be distinguished from the relatively pure lymphocytic infiltration seen in normal aging.

> **Chronic bacterial prostatitis may cause recurrent urinary tract infections.**

Chronic abacterial prostatitis clinically and pathologically resembles chronic bacterial prostatitis, but no pathogen is cultured. Chronic abacterial prostatitis is the most common form of prostatitis encountered today, and is most often seen in sexually active men. It is suspected that chronic abacterial prostatitis is, in most cases, actually a form of bacterial prostatitis in which the pathogen is difficult to culture. Suspected pathogens include *Chlamydia trachomatis* and *Ureaplasma urealyticum.*

> **Chronic abacterial prostatitis is suspected of being due to organisms that are difficult to culture such as *Chlamydia* or *Ureaplasma*.**

Nodular Hyperplasia

Nodular hyperplasia (benign prostatic hypertrophy or hyperplasia) is a common disorder after age 50 in men, and becomes nearly universal by the eighth decade. However, only about one-tenth of men with nodular hyperplasia have disease with sufficiently severe symptoms (difficulty in urination with or without urinary retention) to require cor-

> **Nodular hyperplasia is nearly universal in men in their eighth decade.**

rective surgery. In contrast to prostatic carcinoma, which usually involves the posterior lobe, the nodular hyperplasia usually originates in the preprostatic region adjacent to the urethra of the classically defined middle and lateral lobes. With continued growth, the nodular enlargements may compress the urethra, causing difficulty in urination. Alternatively, middle lobe enlargement can act as a ball valve at the bladder mouth of the urethra.

Histologically, the prostatic nodules show proliferation of both glands and stroma. In some cases, fibromuscular hypertrophy may be more prominent than glandular hyperplasia, producing almost pure aggregates of spindle-shaped cells without enclosed glands. The hyperplastic glands may be either large or small. When small, they may resemble prostatic adenocarcinoma. When prostatic hypertrophy is sufficiently severe to cause urinary retention, the residual urine is vulnerable to infection. The bladder may also develop secondary changes including hypertrophy, trabeculation, and formation of diverticula. Nodular hyperplasia does not appear to predispose for prostatic adenocarcinoma, although a carcinomatous nodule may be difficult to palpate in a prostate enlarged by nodular hyperplasia. Therapy of symptomatic nodular hyperplasia is usually by transurethral resection of the hypertrophied tissue.

Nodular hyperplasia may histologically resemble prostatic adenocarcinoma.

Prostate Cancer

Prostatic cancer is the most common cancer and the third leading cause of cancer death in men. In addition to carcinoma large enough to cause symptomatic diseases, microscopic foci of cancer are often found incidentally at postmortem examination or in prostatic resections for nodular hyperplasia. The significance of these occult carcinomas is still not clear, since in many cases the typically elderly patients die of unrelated causes before the occult carcinomas become large enough to produce symptoms. Symptomatic prostatic carcinoma is usually observed in men over age 50, with peak incidence in the eighth decade of life. For unknown reasons, possibly related to both genetics and environment, prostatic carcinoma is very uncommon in Orientals living in Asia and is particularly high in American blacks. White American men have an intermediate incidence of prostatic carcinoma.

Occult prostatic carcinoma is very common, and frank prostatic cancer is an important cause of death in men.

Prostatic cancer usually arises in the periphery of the gland, typically in a posterior location where it can be palpated on rectal examination. The carcinoma may be unifocal, multifocal, or a coalesced mass of previously multifocal lesions. The vast majority of prostate cancers are adenocarcinomas; rare forms include epidermoid carcinoma, adenoid cystic carcinoma, and transitional cell carcinoma. The most common pattern of growth for well-differentiated adenocarcinomas is in clusters of small to medium-sized glands lined by cuboidal or low columnar epithelium. This growth pattern can closely resemble that seen in some cases of nodular hyperplasia of the prostate. However, the neoplastic glands are usually lined by only a single layer of cells, the basement membrane may not be intact, and back-to-back glands may be found. Invasion beyond the capsule or perineural invasion are also helpful. The neoplastic cells often have pale, granular cytoplasm and round or oval nuclei. Mitotic figures are rare. Less commonly, well-differentiated adenocarcinomas grow in papillary or cribiform patterns; more than one growth pattern may be present in a single area of tumor. The neoplastic cells in poorly differentiated adenocarcinomas may grow in cords, nests, or sheets. In these poorly differentiated tumors, mitoses may be common, and the cells may be pleomorphic and have prominent acidophilic nucleoli.

Well-differentiated prostatic adenocarcinomas tend to have a better prognosis than poorly differentiated ones. The Gleason system of grading prostatic adenocarcinomas uses the tumor growth pattern and degree of glandular differentiation; the Gaeta system uses nuclear cytology and degree of glandular differentiation. Staging of prostatic cancer is based upon the presence or absence of features including palpable tumor, tumor extension beyond the prostatic capsule, and distant metastases. Therapy of prostatic cancer is by surgery, radiotherapy, or hormonal manipulations, including orchiectomy or administration of estrogens or synthetic agonists of luteinizing hormone-releasing hormone. Radiotherapy can be particularly useful in palliation of the pain of bone metastases. The 10-year survival rate for treated disseminated disease is now between 10 and 40 percent.

Therapy of prostatic cancer is often effective.

15

Breast and Female Genital System

BREAST

CONGENITAL ANOMALIES

Congenital anomalies of the breast are common but usually of little clinical significance. **Supernumerary nipples or breasts** can sometimes be found both above the breast in the anterior axillary fold and below it in the sagittal plane of the nipple. Diseases of the normally situated breast and nipple occasionally affect supernumerary nipples or breasts. **Accessory axillary breast tissue** may become clinically important if it gives rise to carcinoma, which may appear to be metastatic. **Congenital inversion of the nipples** is common, particularly in large breasts and is clinically important because it may make nursing difficult and may be confused with the nipple retractions sometimes encountered in breast cancer.

INFLAMMATIONS

A relatively few forms of inflammation affect the breasts, including acute mastitis, mammary duct ectasia, fat necrosis, and galactocele.

Acute Mastitis

Acute mastitis refers to bacterial infection of the breast, usually by staphylococci or less commonly streptococci. It is usually unilateral and is most often seen in conditions in which the skin is cracked or fissured, as in the first few weeks of nursing or in patients with eczema or other dermatologic conditions of the nipples. Staphylococci tend to produce single or multiple breast abscesses; streptococci usually produce a diffuse spreading infection. Therapy is with antibiotics and surgical drainage if an abscess is present. Mastitis may heal with a dense scar and skin retraction that may later be confused with breast cancer.

Congenital anomalies of the breast usually have little clinical significance.

Staphylococci and streptococci can cause acute mastitis.

323

Mammary Duct Ectasia

Mammary duct ectasia is a usually localized, chronic inflammation of the breast that is thought to be due to duct obstruction by inspissated secretions; it is most often observed in multiparous women in the fifth or sixth decade of life. Dilated ducts contain inspissated secretions. A marked chronic inflammatory reaction is most prominent around ducts and may contain granulomas, neutrophils, lymphocytes, and sometimes prominent plasma cells (plasma cell mastitis). Mammary duct ectasia is sometimes associated with pituitary adenomas, suggesting that prolactin secretion may contribute to its development. Mammary duct ectasia can resemble carcinoma by physical examination and by mammography.

Fat Necrosis

Fat necrosis is a usually sharply localized breast inflammation that can occur following (sometimes relatively minor) breast trauma. The breast adipose tissue is initially hemorrhagic, then undergoes central liquefactive necrosis, and finally develops granuloma formation and scarring with small foci of calcification. The necrotic focus eventually heals by either scar tissue replacement or encystment.

Galactocele

Galactocele is observed during lactation when one or more ducts become cystically dilated with milk. A galactocele may be secondarily infected, causing acute mastitis with or without abscess formation.

BREAST TUMORS

The breast is vulnerable to both benign and malignant tumors, of which the most clinically significant are fibroadenoma, phyllodes tumor, intraductal papilloma, and carcinoma.

Fibroadenoma

Fibroadenoma is a benign tumor that usually grows as a sharply circumscribed, freely movable, gray-white, spherical nodule within the breast tissue of women of reproductive age, usually below age 30 years. Glandular and cystic spaces, which may be compressed to slits, are lined by single or multiple layers of epithelial cells. The spaces are separated by a delicate stoma containing prominent fibroblastic cells. Several variants occur. **"Giant fibroadenoma"** (see phyllodes tumor below), may be up to 10 to 15 cm in diameter. **Tubular adenoma** is composed of densely packed glandular or acinar spaces within scant stroma. **Lactating adenoma** resembles tubular adenoma but shows epithelium with prominent secretory activity and is observed most often in lactating breasts. **Fibroadenomatosis** is a component of fibrocystic disease characterized by multiple small areas resembling fibroadenomas. Fibroadenomas are clinically significant because they form palpable breast nodules that must be biopsied to prove their benign character. Fibroadenomas change in size through the menstrual cycle and in pregnancy; regression or calcification may occur postmenopausally. Uncommonly, carcinoma in situ or ductal carcinoma may arise in a fibroadenoma.

Phyllodes Tumor

Some giant fibroadenomas undergo histologic malignant transformation characterized by increased stromal cellularity, increased mitoses, and cellular anaplasia. These tumors are then called **phyllodes tumors** (cystosarcoma phyllodes). The phyllodes tumors present a clinical problem, since, even in the presence of significant anaplasia, the tumors may behave in a completely benign fashion; may locally recur after excision; or may develop late metastases. Clinically malignant transformation is accompanied by rapid increase in tumor size, often with invasion of adjacent breast tissue.

Malignant transformation of a giant fibroadenoma produces a phyllodes tumor.

Intraductal Papilloma

Small (usually less than 1 cm), benign neoplastic papillary growths can develop within a principal lactiferous duct (**intraductal papilloma**) and cause serous or bloody nipple discharge; a small, palpable, subareolar tumor; or nipple retraction. Intraductal papillomas form delicate branching structures composed of fibrovascular cores covered by cuboidal or cylindrical epithelial cells that often fill a dilated duct. Intraductal papillomas must be distinguished from papillary carcinoma. Histologic features favoring a diagnosis of intraductal papilloma include the presence of both epithelial and myoepithelial cells in the papillary fronds; the absence of severe cytologic atypia or abnormal mitotic figures; and the absence of abnormal growth patterns such as cribiform formation, apocrine metasplasia, or absence of a vascular connective tissue core. Solitary intraductal papillomas are not considered precursors of papillary carcinomas; multiple intraductal papillomas appear to be associated with increased risk of carcinoma. Treatment of intraductal papillomas is by complete excision of the duct system to avoid local recurrence.

Intraductal papillomas develop within lactiferous ducts.

FIBROCYSTIC DISEASE OF THE BREAST

Female breasts may undergo a variety of morphologic changes that are loosely classified as **fibrocystic change or disease.** These changes may vary from location to location within a breast, and different women may have breasts with differing morphologic patterns. With the understanding that fibrocystic change can be strikingly pleomorphic, it is convenient to discuss this disorder in terms of the following dominant patterns of morphologic change.

Fibrocystic disease of the breast is a pleomorphic group of morphologic patterns.

   Simple fibrocystic change is the most common pattern, is usually multifocal, and affects both breasts. Cystic dilation of ducts produces epithelial-lined cysts that may be either microscopic or grossly observable. The cysts are usually surrounded by an increased fibrous stroma. The term **"blue-dome cyst"** is sometimes used for large cysts (up to 5 cm in diameter) that contain semitranslucent fluid and grossly appear brown or blue when unopened. The cyst lining is usually cuboidal or columnar in smaller cysts but may be flattened or atrophic in larger cysts. The usual lining epithelium has cells whose cytoplasm stains blue with hematoxylin and eosin, similar to normal duct epithelium. A variant, **apocrine metaplasia** of the epithelial lining, is characterized by

Simple fibrocystic change and apocrine metaplasia are not associated with increased risk of carcinoma.

large cells with strikingly eosinophilic cytoplasm and small deeply chromatic nuclei. The epithelium in apocrine metaplasia may also show epithelial overgrowth with papillary projection formation. The stroma around the cysts is characteristically compressed and may be infiltrated by lymphocytes. Despite sometimes florid changes, the apocrine metaplasia is almost always benign. Simple fibrocystic change is not associated with increased risk of carcinoma of the breast.

Epithelial hyperplasia within the ducts and ductules can accompany simple fibrocystic change and is associated with an increased risk of subsequently developing carcinoma of the breast. Not all foci of hyperplasia appear to be premalignant; the risk of subsequently developing cancer is greater with more severe or atypical hyperplasia. Microscopically, the duct epithelium is thicker than the normal two layers. The thickened epithelium may partially obliterate the duct lumen and grow in the form of solid masses, fenestrated masses with irregular openings, or papillary epithelial projections (ductal papillomatosis). The epithelial cells may show varying degrees of atypia. When the epithelium grows in a fenestrated pattern, it may be difficult to distinguish from the cribiform pattern of some intraductal carcinomas. In general, the hole in the benign fenestrated pattern are more irregularly shaped than those in the malignant cribiform pattern. Hyperplasias involving the terminal duct and ductules (acini) that resemble lobular carcinoma in situ (but do not have all the features of carcinoma in situ) are called **atypical lobular hyperplasia** and are associated with an increased risk of invasive carcinoma.

Sclerosing adenosis is a less common form of fibrocystic change characterized by collections of small glands, nests, or cords of epithelial cells within a dense fibrous stroma. This can be attributed to a combination of ductule proliferation and compression by the dense fibrous stroma. Sclerosing adenosis is clinically important because it may mimic carcinoma both grossly and microscopically. While these benign glands may look bizarre at high-power magnification, low-power magnification usually demonstrates a lobular organization. Sclerosing adenosis is not associated with an increased risk for carcinoma.

Infrequent variants of fibrocystic disease include pure **fibrosis,** characterized by dense stromal fibrous tissue without enclosed cysts or endothelial hyperplasia; and **radial scar** (benign sclerosing ductal proliferation), which is a proliferation of ducts around a central area of fibrosis and elastosis that may resemble the tubular form of breast carcinoma.

BREAST CANCER

Carcinoma of the breast causes approximately one-fifth of cancer deaths in women. Factors associated with a higher risk of breast cancer include increasing age, increasing lifetime exposure to estrogens (early menarche, late menopause, nulliparity, older age at birth of first child), obesity, exogenous estrogens, fibrocystic breast disease (when associated with atypical epithelial hyperplasia), breast cancer in other breast, and breast cancer in first-degree relatives.

In Situ Breast Cancer

Breast cancer can be either in situ or invasive. In situ carcinoma can be either intraductal or lobular.

Intraductal carcinoma is carcinoma that arises in ductal epithelium but remains confined within the ductal basement membrane. The gross appearance of intraductal carcinoma is of necrotic, cheeselike material filling cordlike ducts within the breast. The term **comedocarcinoma** is sometimes used since the necrotic material can be easily extruded by gentle squeezing (analogous to squeezing a pimple). Histologically, the dilated ducts are filled with neoplastic epithelial cells that may grow in a cribiform or, less commonly, a predominantly papillary pattern (intraductal papillary carcinoma). Approximately one-fourth of patients with intraductal carcinoma that are treated with biopsy alone subsequently (up to 15 years) develop invasive carcinoma, often in the same breast quadrant as the original intraductal carcinoma.

Intraductal carcinoma is confined to a duct.

Lobular carcinoma in situ is much less common than intraductal carcinoma and is characterized by proliferation of neoplastic cells with oval or round nuclei and small nucleoli in one or more terminal ductules. Lobular carcinoma in situ is associated with increased risk of subsequently developing, in either breast, both ductal and lobular infiltrative carcinomas. Lobular carcinoma in situ is sometimes observed in fibrocystic breasts and near areas of invasive or intraductal carcinoma.

Lobular carcinoma in situ is associated with increased risk of developing both ductal and lobular carcinoma.

Invasive Breast Cancer

Invasive breast carcinoma can be subdivided into a variety of histologic types.

Invasive ductal carcinoma, not otherwise specified, is the most common type of breast cancer, and consists of those ductal breast cancers that do not meet the specific criteria for any of the other histologic types described below. Grossly, the tumor usually forms fairly sharply circumscribed nodules with a hard consistency (scirrhous carcinoma) because of a marked increase in dense fibrous tissue stroma. The nodules may be fixed to the underlying chest wall and may also contain small foci of calcification, which facilitate their visualization by mammography. The fibrous stroma contains small to large anaplastic duct epithelial cells with hyperchromatic nuclei that can form a variety of structures including nests, cords, glands, and tubes. Invasion of ducts, lymphatics, blood vessels, perineural spaces, and perivascular spaces may be seen.

Invasive ductal carcinoma, not otherwise specified, is the most common type of breast cancer.

Medullary carcinoma is an uncommon form of ductal carcinoma characterized by a scant fibrous tissue stroma that contains sheets of large cells; these cells do not form glands but do appear to form syncytia. A moderate to marked lymphocytic infiltration is usually present. Medullary carcinoma has a better prognosis than do most infiltrating duct carcinomas, possibly because of the prominent immune response to the tumor.

Medullary carcinoma is composed of sheets of large cells.

Colloid or mucinous carcinoma is an unusual variant that grows slowly and produces gelatinous tumor masses composed of amorphous mucin "lakes" in which float small numbers of often vacuolated neoplastic cells. Colloid carcinoma can occur either in pure form or in combination with other forms of infiltrative carcinoma. In pure form, it has a better prognosis, with much less risk of metastasis than most infiltrative ductal carcinomas.

Tumor masses in colloid carcinoma appear to float in mucin "lakes."

Paget's disease of the nipple refers to the presence of isolated, anaplastic, malignant cells (Paget's cells) within the epidermis above areas of ductal carcinoma, with or without obvious invasion of the surrounding parenchyma. The Paget's cells are characteristically surrounded by a clear halo that can be stained for mucopolysaccharides by alcian blue. The involved skin, usually around the nipple and areola, causes

Paget's disease refers to the presence of isolated tumor cells in epidermis.

eczematoid changes and may be fissured, ulcerated, or oozing. About one-third of patients with Paget's disease of the nipple have metastases at the time of diagnosis.

Lobular carcinoma apparently arises in the terminal ductules of the breast lobule and is of particular clinical interest because the tumors tend to be multicentric and, in about one-fifth of cases, occur in both breasts. The tumors are poorly circumscribed and characteristically contain narrow strands of small, infiltrating tumor cells ("Indian files"). The tumor cells can also form concentric rings around ducts and irregularly shaped solid nests. Some tumors show coexisting features of both lobular and ductal carcinomas.

Uncommon forms of breast carcinoma include tubular carcinoma, adenoid cystic carcinoma, invasive comedocarcinoma, apocrine carcinoma, and invasive papillary carcinoma.

Invasive breast carcinomas of all histologic types tend to have certain features in common. Roughly one-half of the carcinomas arise in the **upper outer quadrants of the breasts,** with the remainder being distributed in other quadrants and beneath the nipples. Breast carcinomas are often initially mobile masses, but often later become fixed by infiltration into the fascia of the chest wall. Retraction and dimpling may be a consequence of tumor involvement of the dermis. Blocking of lymphatics by tumor can cause lymphedema with associated thickening and erythema of the skin, so that it resembles an orange peel **(peau d'orange).** Nipple retraction can occur if the tumor involves the main excretory ducts. Widespread tumor dissemination within a breast (often seen in pregnancy) can cause acute swelling, erythema, and tenderness, known clinically as inflammatory carcinoma.

Staging of breast cancer is based on tumor size, involvement of axillary nodes, tumor extension to skin or chest wall, and the presence of distant metastases. Breast carcinomas are usually initially identified by breast self-examination, by physician examination, or by mammography. They are most common around or shortly after menopause, but are observed at any age after 20 to 25 years. Early treatment of localized disease is much more successful than is treatment of disease that has spread to multiple axillary nodes. The prognosis is also more favorable if the tumor contains high numbers of estrogen or progesterone receptors, since hormonal manipulation by oophorectomy or the antiestrogen agent **tamoxifen** may then cause tumor regression. The specific therapy of breast carcinomas at different stages of disease progress is still an active area of research. Therapeutic approaches currently in use include many combinations of chemotherapy, radiotherapy, and resections of either the mass ("lumpectomy") or breast (simple mastectomy) with or without axillary disection. A few cancers recur as many as 10 or 20 years after initial therapy.

Miscellaneous Malignant Tumors

Rarely, other malignant tumors can occur in the breast. Carcinomas can arise in the breast skin or its adnexal structures. A variety of sarcomas (fibrosarcomas, myxosarcomas, liposarcomas, angiosarcomas, chondrosarcomas, osteogenic sarcomas) can arise in the breast stroma; of these, angiosarcomas are the most rapidly fatal. Malignant lymphomas also occasionally arise in the breast.

Lobular carcinoma is often multicentric.

Invasive breast carcinoma can involve structures adjacent to the breast.

Other malignant tumors rarely occur in the breast.

DISEASES OF THE MALE BREAST

The male breast can be affected by gynecomastia and by carcinoma. **Gynecomastia** is a unilateral or bilateral enlargement of the breast that often takes the form of a buttonlike subareolar mass. Gynecomastia is characterized histologically by proliferation of dense collagenous connective tissue with marked hyperplasia of the ductal epithelium. Gynecomastia can be observed at puberty, in the elderly, in hepatic cirrhosis (probably due to a failure of liver to metabolize estrogens), in Klinefelter syndrome, in testicular neoplasms, in chronic illegal drug users (marijuana, heroin), and, occasionally, idiopathically. Most cases of gynecomastia are related to either excess estrogen or a relative increase of estrogen compared with androgen hormonal levels. **Carcinoma** of the male breast has approximately 1 percent of the incidence of carcinoma of the female breast and is usually observed in the very elderly. These cancers resemble those of the female breast, but tend to disseminate more rapidly since the male breast is much smaller than the female, and the tumors rapidly involve the axillary nodes, skin, or chest wall. Distant metastases are also common.

Gynecomastia and carcinoma are the most important diseases of the male breast.

VULVA, VAGINA, AND CERVIX

DISEASES OF THE VULVA

The skin of the vulva is vulnerable to many diseases.

The vulva is vulnerable to diseases similar to those seen in other areas of hair-bearing skin including infections, inflammatory dermatologic diseases (psoriasis, eczema, allergic dermatitis), skin cysts (epidermal inclusion cysts), and tumors (moles, squamous cell carcinoma, melanomas). **Nonspecific vulvitis** is most often encountered in patients with predisposing conditions, including malnutrition, diabetes mellitus, uremia, and blood dyscrasias. **Bartholin's cyst** is a locally painful, cystic dilation (up to 5 cm) of Bartholin's vulvovaginal glands that occurs after blockage of the main duct of the gland. **Vulvar dystrophy** refers to abnormal vulvar epithelium accompanied by dermal changes and is subdivided into two forms, lichen sclerosis and squamous hyperplasia. **Lichen sclerosis** (chronic atrophic vulvitis) is most common after menopause and is characterized by thin, hairless skin overlying atrophic labia. Histologically, the epidermis is thinned but hyperkeratotic and shows disappearance of rete pegs and dermal adnexal structures. The underlying dermis becomes replaced by dense, collagenous fibrous tissue. Lichen sclerosis does not appear to predispose for cancer. **Squamous hyperplasia** (hyperplastic dystrophy) presents as a white plaque (leukoplakia) characterized histologically by marked epithelial hyperplasia and hyperkeratosis with increased mitotic activity in both basal and prickle cell layers. A prominent leukocytic infiltration of the dermis is sometimes present. If the epithelium does not show cellular atypia, the lesion is considered to have no predisposition for cancer; if cellular atypia is present, the lesion is considered dysplastic, with the potential to progress to squamous cell carcinoma.

Vulvar Tumors

A wide variety of benign and malignant tumors have been described in the vulva; most of them closely resemble their counterparts in other locations. Tumors most apt to be clinically important or that are distinctive of the vulva include the following.

Condyloma acuminata are associated with papillomavirus infection.

Condyloma acuminata (venereal wart) is a benign tumor induced by sexually transmitted human papillomavirus (mostly types 6 and 11); it becomes incorporated into the human genome and can be identified by molecular hybridization techniques as being localized to epithelial cells. The gross appearance is of a distinctly verrucous, frequently multiple, lesion on external surfaces of the genitalia, perianal region, vagina, or, rarely, cervix. (The lesions can also be found on the external genitalia or perianal region of infected men; see p. 111) Histologically, condyloma acuminatum shows a branching proliferation of stratified squamous epithelium that covers a fibrous stroma. The epithelial hyperplasia has perinuclear cytoplasmic vacuolization (koilocytosis) through most layers of the epithelium and oval nuclei in the superficial layers. Condyloma acuminatum is not considered precancerous but may coexist with human papillomavirus infection of other genital sites, which may consequently develop dysplasia or carcinoma.

Other benign verrucous protuberances of the vulva that may resemble condyloma acuminatum but that are not associated with human papillomavirus infection include **squamous papilloma,** which is not sexually transmitted and usually occurs as a single lesion in an older patient, and **condyloma latum,** due to syphilis.

Papillary hidradenoma is a rare, benign tumor of the modified apocrine sweat glands of the vulva composed of tubular ducts, resembling those of sweat glands, that are lined with one or two layers of nonciliated columnar epithelium with an underlying layer of flattened myoepithelial cells. Hidradenoma can be mistaken for carcinoma because it tends to ulcerate and has a complex histologic picture.

Papillary hidradenoma is composed of ducts that resemble sweat glands.

Vulvar dysplasia (vulvar intraepithelial neoplasia [VIN]) is a premalignant, white or dark, epithelial lesion characterized by cellular atypia, increased mitotic activity, and a failure of the surface cells of the epithelium to show normal differentiation. The dysplasia can range from mild dysplasia (VIN I), to moderate dysplasia (VIN II), to severe dysplasia including carcinoma in situ (VIN III), which is also known as Bowen's disease. It is thought that about 1 in 20 cases of carcinoma in situ, mostly in older patients, later progress to invasive carcinoma. In most lesions, human papillomavirus, most often types 16 and 18, can be demonstrated by molecular hybridization techniques. Vulvar dysplasia is occurring with increasing frequency in sexually active women below age 40 years. Patients with vulvar dysplasia should be carefully evaluated for other human papillomavirus-related tumors, since nearly one-third of cases have coexisting in situ or invasive cervical or vaginal carcinoma.

Patients with vulvar dysplasia may have coexisting cervical or vaginal carcinoma.

Vulvar squamous cell carcinoma can arise from any area of the vulva. The lesions begin as small areas of thickened epithelium that progress to form larger tumors that may be either exophytic or endophytic. The histology is almost always well-differentiated squamous cell carcinoma. While the tumor forms obvious lesions on the external genitalia, it is often neglected because it is misinterpreted as being due to dermatitis, eczema, or leukoplakia. Large lesions with regional lymph node metastasis have a less than 10 percent 5-year survival. Roughly three-fourths of patients who are treated for smaller lesions that have not metastasized survive more than 5 years. **Verrucous carcinoma** is a variant of well-differentiated squamous cell carcinoma that forms a large fungating tumor resembling condyloma acuminatum grossly and histologically. Verrucous carcinoma is usually locally invasive, resistant to radiotherapy, and only rarely metastasizes.

Squamous cell carcinoma can arise from any area of the vulva.

Extramammary Paget's disease resembles Paget's disease of the breast, although, unlike the breast form, it does not usually have an underlying adenocarcinoma. Extramammary Paget's disease presents as a maplike area of erythematous, crusted epithelium usually located on the labia majora. Histologically, isolated or small groups of large, anaplastic tumor cells, with clear halos due to cytoplasmic mucopolysaccharide, are found within the epidermis or its appendages. In some cases

Extramammary Paget's disease, unlike Paget's disease of the breast, is not always associated with an underlying adenocarcinoma.

of extramammary Paget's disease, carcinoma of the breast, bladder, or vulva may coexist for unknown reasons. Extramammary Paget's disease associated with carcinoma has a poor prognosis. Cases without associated carcinoma may persist without invasion for years, but a few untreated cases do eventually develop invasive disease.

Basal cell carcinomas, adenocarcinomas, and **malignant melanoma** also uncommonly arise in the vulva.

LESIONS OF THE VAGINA

Rarely, the vagina may be absent, atretic, or doubled; severe vaginal malformations are often accompanied by severe malformations elsewhere in the genital tract. **Gartner's duct cysts** arise from wolffian duct rests in the lateral walls of the vagina. They form benign, 1 to 2 cm (or uncommonly larger) cysts lined by a variety of epithelia that are clinically important because they must be distinguished from more ominous tumor masses. Other benign vaginal lesions that may simulate tumors are uncommon and include endometriosis, fibromas, leiomyomas, hemangiomas, and papillomas. Important cancers of the vagina include squamous cell carcinoma, adenocarcinoma, and embryonal rhabdomyosarcoma.

Squamous cell carcinoma of the vagina is seen in older women (peak incidence between 60 and 70 years), and most commonly arises in the upper posterior vagina near the exocervix. Cancers in the upper third of the vagina metastasize first to the iliac nodes; cancers in the lower two-thirds metastasize first to inguinal nodes. **Adenocarcinomas** uncommonly arise in the vagina. One subgroup, **clear cell adenocarcinoma,** is observed in about 0.1 percent of young women whose mothers had received diethylstilbestrol during pregnancy. Clear cell adenocarcinoma is composed of vacuolated, glycogen-containing cells. **Vaginal adenosis,** in which glandular columnar epithelium, either ciliated or mucous secreting, replaces or appears below the normal squamous epithelium, is commonly observed in daughters of women treated with diethylstilbestrol and may represent a precursor to clear cell adenocarcinoma.

Embryonal rhabdomyosarcoma (sarcoma botryoides) is an aggressive tumor that rarely forms polypoid masses resembling a bunch of grapes, most commonly in the vaginas of infants and children less than 5 years of age. Histologically, the tumor is a form of rhabdomyosarcoma composed of embryonal rhabdomyoblasts. These small tumor cells have cytoplasmic protrusions that cause them to resemble tennis rackets, and they may rarely contain cytoplasmic striations. Therapy is by radical surgery coupled with chemotherapy.

DISEASES OF THE CERVIX

Cervicitis

The cervix is vulnerable to inflammations caused both by the normal flora of the vagina (nonspecific cervicitis) and organisms that cause specific cervical inflammations (gonorrhea, syphilis, chancroid, tuberculosis). Specific syndromes are discussed elsewhere (see p. 40, 52). Nonspecific cervicitis can be either acute or chronic. **Acute cervicitis** is

---

Gartner's duct cysts arise from wolffian duct nests.

Squamous cell carcinoma and adenocarcinoma can both arise in the vagina.

Embryonal rhabdomyosarcoma is an aggressive childhood tumor.

The cervix is vulnerable to inflammation.

usually encountered (with the exception of gonorrhea) in the postpartum period and is characterized by neutrophil infiltration, stroma edema, and focal disruption of the cervical mucosa. Staphylococci and streptococci are the most common organisms isolated. **Chronic cervicitis** is very common, and minimal degrees of cervical inflammation are probably not clinically significant. Chronic cervicitis is characterized histologically by a mononuclear cell infiltrate and grossly by a reddened, granular swelling that is found around the margins of the external cervical os. The cervical and endocervical mucosa may show epithelial disorganization and nuclear alterations **(reactive atypia)** that are not premalignant and should therefore not be considered dysplastic. Schiller's solution can identify chronically inflamed areas of the cervix, based on the observation that the normal glycogen content of cervical cells is absent in chronic cervical inflammation, and consequently chronically inflamed areas fail to stain brown with the iodine-based solution. **Nabothian cysts** are cystic dilations of the cervical glands caused by inflammatory stenosis. **Follicular cervicitis** is a form of chronic cervicitis characterized by accumulation of chronic inflammatory cells into lymphoid follicles. **Squamous metaplasia** of endocervical glands refers to the extension of tongues of stratified squamous epithelium from the surface into the endocervical glands; this epithelial alteration is benign but can be mistaken for carcinoma.

Benign Cervical Tumors

The most important benign cervical tumorlike conditions are endocervical polyps and microglandular endocervical hyperplasia. **Endocervical polyps** are common inflammatory masses composed of dilated, mucus-secreting glands in loose fibromyxomatous stroma. The polyps usually arise in the endocervical canal, may form masses up to 5 cm that protrude through the canal, and are clinically significant primarily because they may cause irregular vaginal bleeding. **Microglandular endocervical hyperplasia** is a benign cervical lesion that grossly resembles an endocervical polyp but is composed of tightly packed glands and tubules that may contain focal areas of epithelial atypia and squamous metaplasia. Most of these lesions are seen in women taking progestogen-containing oral contraceptives. The lesions are important primarily because they resemble endocervical adenocarcinoma.

Endocervical polyps and microglandular endocervical hyperplasia are the most important benign tumorlike conditions of the cervix.

Cervical Dysplasia and Cancer

The cervical endothelium is vulnerable to dysplasia and carcinoma. Many cases of both cervical dysplasia and cervical carcinoma appear to be related to human papillomavirus infection, which is also associated with cervical condylomas. Cervical squamous cell carcinoma is associated with integration into the human DNA genome of types 16, 18, or 31, which are considered "high-risk" types of human papillomavirus. Cervical condylomas, which resemble those of the vulva and can be either verrucous or flat, are associated with the low-risk types 6 and 11, which occur in host cells as episomal viral DNA that is not integrated into the human genome. Cervical dysplasia may be associated with either low-risk or high-risk types of human papillomavirus.

   Cervical dysplasia, also known as cervical intraepithelial neoplasia, is classified as grades I (very mild to mild dysplasia), II (moderate dysplasia), and III (severe dysplasia and carcinoma in situ) based on the

Many cases of cervical dysplasia and carcinoma are related to papillomaviruses.

Cervical dysplasia is graded based on the proportion of squamous epithelium above the atypical cells.

Invasive cervical cancer may be squamous cell carcinoma, adenocarcinoma, adenosquamous carcinoma, or undifferentiated carcinoma.

proportion of the thickness of the squamous epithelium above the basal layer that contains atypical cells. Sample areas of the cervix for evaluation of dysplasia or carcinoma in situ can be identified with the Schiller test, in which the cervix is painted with an iodine-containing solution; areas in which most of the epithelial cells have been depleted of glycogen (due to inflammation, severe dysplasia, or carcinoma in situ) fail to stain brown. Cervical dysplasia can also be suspected if a Papanicolaou (Pap) smear contains cytology suggestive of dysplasia or carcinoma; definitive evaluation requires colposcopic biopsy of suspicious lesions.

Three-fourths or more of cases of **invasive cervical cancer** are due to squamous cell carcinoma, which may occur in fungating (exophytic), ulcerating, and infiltrative forms. Histologically, the squamous tumor cells can be nonkeratinizing large cells, keratinizing large cells, or small undifferentiated squamous cells. Staging is based on the depth of invasion into the cervix, extension to or beyond other pelvic structures, and the presence of metastases. Somewhat less than one-fourth of cervical cancers are other tumors including **adenocarcinomas, adenosquamous carcinomas,** or **undifferentiated carcinomas. Clear cell adenocarcinomas** of the cervix, like those of the vagina, are observed in some daughters of women treated with diethylstilbesterol during pregnancy.

The overall prognosis for cervical carcinoma has been improved through the use of the Papanicolaou (Pap) smear, which facilitates early identification of dysplastic lesions and carcinoma, and which consequently should be periodically performed on all sexually active women. Many preinvasive lesions can be treated with outpatient techniques such as laser ablation, cryotherapy, or electrocoagulation. The peak incidence of invasive cervical carcinoma occurs in women in their forties, and more advanced lesions are treated with surgery, radiotherapy, or both. Almost all patients with early lesions who are treated survive for 5 or more years; patients with widely disseminated disease have a dismal survival rate.

UTERUS

NON-NEOPLASTIC DISEASES OF THE UTERUS AND ENDOMETRIUM

Congenital Anomalies

The uterus is vulnerable to congenital anomalies or acquired defects. Hypoplasia is usually secondary to ovarian or pituitary hypofunction. A variety of anomalies related to imperfect fusion of the primitive müllerian ducts also occur, including simple fundal notching; partial division of the fundus by a septum; complete division of the uterus but not the cervix (septate uterus); and completely double uterus with double cervix. Uterine congenital anomalies may be compatible with normal menstruation and fertility but may cause difficulties during pregnancy and delivery.

Imperfect fusion of the primitive müllerian ducts can produce a variety of congenital anomalies.

Inflammations

The endometrium, and secondarily the myometrium, while relatively resistant to infections, do sometimes develop acute and chronic inflammations. **Acute endometritis** and myometritis are almost always seen following delivery or miscarriage, usually as a consequence of bacterial (group A hemolytic streptococci, staphylococci, others) colonization of a retained gestational fragment. Removal of the fragment by curettage is usually curative. **Chronic endometritis** is most often a secondary disease in which obvious predisposing factors are present, such as chronic pelvic inflammatory disease, tuberculosis, retained gestational fragments, or intrauterine contraceptive devices. In about one-seventh of cases, no obvious predisposing factor is identified, although chlamydial infection is suspected since many of these cases respond to antibiotic therapy. Patients with such "nonspecific" chronic endometritis can experience abnormal bleeding, pain, and infertility and have sometimes (unfortunately) been treated with hysterectomy for relief of chronic pain.

While endometrium is relatively resistant to infections, both acute and chronic endometritis can occur.

Adenomyosis

Nests of endometrium (**adenomyosis**) are sometimes found within the myometrium of the uterine wall, possibly as a consequence of an abnormal, downwardly directed growth of the basal zone of the endometrium. Subclinical adenomyosis is common (up to one-fifth of uteri at postmortem examination). Clinically significant adenomyosis is less common, and may produce pelvic pain, dysmenorrhea, dyspareunia, and

Nests of endometrium within the uterine wall are termed adenomyosis.

menorrhagia. Histologically, nests of typical endometrial glands surrounded by spindle cell stroma are found between the muscle bundles of the myometrium at least one power field below the endomyometrial junction. Relatively uncommonly, the glands included menstruate and may cause cysts filled with red-brown pigmentation caused by decomposed blood.

Endometriosis

Functional endometrium is sometimes found outside the uterus.

Relatively normal, functional endometrial glands and stroma are sometimes found outside the uterus **(endometriosis),** possibly as a consequence of menstrual regurgitation through fallopian tubes; abnormal differentiation of coelomic epithelium; or vascular/lymphatic dissemination. Sites for endometriosis include almost anywhere in the pelvis (ovaries, uterine ligaments, rectovaginal septum, vagina, vulva) and, less commonly, in the abdominal cavity (pelvic peritoneum, appendix, laparotomy scars, small and large intestine, umbilicus). The foci of endometrium undergo normal cyclical menstrual changes and appear as discrete red-blue to yellow-brown nodules often found on or just below the serosal surfaces of the sites noted above. Clinical signs and symptoms of endometriosis vary with the sites involved and include severe dysmenorrhea, pelvic pain, dyspareuria, pain on defecation, dysuria, intestinal disturbances, menstrual irregularities, and (commonly) infertility. Surgical or laser ablation of foci of endometriosis may be helpful in controlling the symptoms.

Dysfunctional Uterine Bleeding

Dysfunctional uterine bleeding has many causes.

Abnormal uterine bleeding, usually in the form of excessive bleeding during or between menstrual periods, has many causes. Precocious puberty, due to hypothalmic, pituitary, or ovarian disease, is the most common cause of abnormal uterine bleeding in children. Anovulatory cycles can cause dysfunctional bleeding in menstruating women of any age. Inadequate luteal phase is important in the reproductive age group. Organic lesions, including leiomyoma, adenomyosis, carcinoma, endometrial hyperplasia, and polyps, are important in both reproductive age and peri- and postmenopausal women. Complications of pregnancy that can cause dysfunctional bleeding include abortion, trophoblastic disease, and ectopic pregnancy. Irregular shedding and endometrial atrophy can cause abnormal uterine bleeding in, respectively, perimenopausal and postmenopausal women. Of the above, the most common causes of abnormal bleeding are anovulatory cycles and inadequate luteal phase.

Anovulatory cycles are an important cause of irregular bleeding.

Anovulatory cycles cause dysfunctional bleeding by prolonged estrogenic stimulation that is not interrupted by the normal progestational phase of the menstrual cycle. At irregular intervals, the proliferative endometrium will then break down, causing irregular bleeding. Most anovulatory cycles are idiopathic, possibly as the result of subtle hormonal imbalances. Causes of anovulatory cycles that have been implicated in some patients include endocrine disorders (thyroid, adrenal, pituitary diseases); primary ovarian disease (tumors, polycystic ovaries); and almost any severe chronic systemic disease. Anovulatory cycles are common around menarche and menopause. The repeated prolonged estrogen stimulation can adversely affect the endometrium since a history of repeated anovulatory cycles is often reported in patients with endometrial carcinoma.

Inadequate luteal phase is the term used when the corpus luteum fails to secrete adequate amounts of progesterone, and usually occurs in the setting of an irregular ovulatory cycle. Inadequate luteal phase produces postovulatory endometrium that lags behind its expected secretory characteristics. Clinically, infertility is accompanied by either amenorrhea or increased bleeding.

Reactive Endometrial Changes

Senile cystic endometrial atrophy refers to the benign occurrence in postmenopausal women of cystically dilated endometrial glands lined by flattened, atrophic epithelium. Endometrial changes induced by **oral contraceptives** vary with the specific hormones and dosing schedules, but commonly include a discordance between the physiologic state of the glands and the stroma. For example, inactive, nonsecretory glands might be surrounded by a stroma resembling that of the decidua of pregnancy, with large, mitotically active stromal cells. These endometrial changes are reduced when low-dose contraceptives are used.

ENDOMETRIAL HYPERPLASIA

Endometrial hyperplasia is clinically important both as a cause of abnormal uterine bleeding and because the hyperplasia is associated with increased risk of later developing endometrial carcinoma. This increased risk appears most closely associated with the degree of cellular atypia present. **Simple hyperplasia without atypia** (cystic or mild hyperplasia) rarely progresses to adenocarcinoma and is characterized by cystically dilated glands of varying sizes lined by sometimes multilayered cuboidal or tall columnar epithelium. **Complex hyperplasia without atypia** (moderate or adenomatous hyperplasia without atypia) is associated with an incidence of about 1 in 20 of progression to carcinoma. Complex hyperplasia is characterized by the presence of increased numbers of large, irregular endometrial glands lined by hyperplastic epithelium that often contains papillary buddings and small outpouchings. **Atypical hyperplasia** (complex or adenomatous hyperplasia with atypia) is associated with a close to 1 in 4 progression to carcinoma. Atypical hyperplasia resembles complex hyperplasia without atypia, but is additionally characterized by the presence of epithelial cells showing features of cellular atypia, including cytomegaly, increased nuclear cytoplasmic ratio, prominent nucleoli, and increased mitotic activity.

Endometrial hyperplasia is usually a perimenopausal disease that results from prolonged estrogen stimulation not interrupted by progestational activity. Endometrial hyperplasia can also be encountered in patients with functioning granulosa or thecal cell tumors of the ovary; Stein-Leventhal syndrome; adrenocortical hyperfunction; and exposure to prolonged, high levels of pharmaceutical estrogens. Abnormal bleeding (either excessive menstrual flow or spotting between periods) is produced by all types of hyperplasia.

UTERINE TUMORS

Benign Uterine Tumors

Commonly encountered benign uterine tumors include benign endometrial polyps and leiomyoma. **Benign endometrial polyps** are masses

---

Failure of the corpus luteum to secrete adequate amounts of progesterone can produce an abnormal endometrium.

The endometrium can be altered by aging and oral contraceptives.

Endometrial hyperplasia is subclassified as simple hyperplasia without atypia, complex hyperplasia without atypia, and atypical hyperplasia.

Endometrial polyps and leiomyomas are the most common benign uterine tumors.

of endometrial tissue that project from the endometrium into the uterine cavity. The endometrium of the polyps may be either hyperplastic or similar to that of the surrounding endometrium. Endometrial polyps are more common around menopause and may coexist with generalized endometrial hyperplasia. Rarely, an initially benign endometrial polyp may undergo malignant change.

Leiomyomas (myomas, "fibroids") are benign, usually roughly spherical, and often pedunculated, tumor masses composed of whorling bundles of smooth muscle cells with ovoid nuclei and long, bipolar cytoplasmic processes. Leiomyomas are very common tumors that occur in about one-fourth of women in active reproductive life and are often multiple. Their development appears to be related to hormonal (estrogen?) stimulation, since most leiomyomas regress, and may even calcify, following menopause. Leiomyomas may range in size from tiny to massive and can arise from almost any location in the myometrium. Symptoms, if present, tend to be related to the size and location of leiomyomas. Subserosal and intramural leiomyomas are often asymptomatic; submucosal leiomyomas may cause profuse menstrual bleeding and a variety of complications associated with pregnancy (when the leiomyomas often enlarge), including spontaneous abortion, fetal malpresentation, poorly formed uterine contractions, and postpartum hemorrhage. Other complications sometimes encountered include urinary frequency and infertility. Malignant transformation has been reported, but is rare.

Endometrial Carcinoma

Endometrial carcinoma is the most common invasive cancer of the female reproductive tract.

Carcinoma arising in the uterine endometrium is the most common invasive cancer of the female reproductive tract, principally as a consequence of the marked decrease in invasive cervical carcinoma following the widespread use of Papanicolau smears. The carcinomas are often identified at an early stage, when the prognosis with surgery or radiotherapy is good, because they cause abnormal bleeding, usually in a postmenopausal woman. The peak incidence for endometrial carcinoma is between ages 55 and 65. Other risk factors include obesity, diabetes, and hypertension. Additionally, any condition associated with prolonged estrogen stimulation, particularly when not interrupted by progesterone stimulation, tends to have an increased risk for development of carcinoma of the endometrium. Conditions associated with prolonged estrogen stimulation include a history of multiple anovulatory cycles; estrogen-secreting tumors; and use of exogenous estrogen (without progesterone) to control menopausal symptoms. A subset of patients, who often have aggressive endometrial carcinomas, do not have a history of hyperestrinism.

OVARIES AND FALLOPIAN TUBES

OVARIAN TUMORS

Ovarian tumors are relatively common and can exhibit a wide variety of histologic patterns. It is convenient to classify ovarian tumors as tumors of surface epithelium, germ cell tumors, sex cord-stroma tumors, unclassified tumors, and metastatic tumors.

Ovarian tumors may have many histologic patterns.

Tumors of Ovarian Surface Epithelium

A variety of tumors can arise in the coelomic surface epithelium, which embryologically has the potential to differentiate into a variety of epithelia, including fallopian tube epithelium, endometrial lining, and endocervical glands. These tumors include serous tumors (serous cystadenoma, borderline serous tumor, serous cystadenocarcinoma, adenofibroma, and cystadenofibroma), mucinous tumors (mucinous cystadenoma, borderline mucinous tumor, mucinous cystadenocarcinoma), endometrial carcinoma, clear cell adenocarcinoma, Brenner tumor, and undifferentiated carcinoma.

Tumors can arise from the coelomic surface epithelium of the ovaries.

Serous tumors are neoplasms containing one or multiple cysts and lined by a single layer of tall, columnar, ciliated epithelial cells reminiscent of those that line the fallopian tubes. Somewhat over one-half of these tumors are benign **(serous cystadenoma);** the remainder are split between borderline **(borderline serous tumor)** and clearly malignant **(serous cystadenocarcinoma)** histologic patterns. Features suggesting malignancy include cytologic atypia; epithelium lining more than one cell thick; papillary projections or solid projections into the cyst lumen; completely solid locales; and invasion of the cyst wall. **Cystadenofibroma** is a variant of serous cystadenoma characterized by pronounced proliferation of the fibrous stroma surrounding the cysts.

Serous tumors can be benign or malignant.

Mucinous tumors resemble their serous counterparts but are filled with sticky, gelatinous fluid that contains glycoproteins. Mucinous ovarian tumors are usually benign and sometimes produce enormous cystic masses (over 25 kg). Ovarian mucinous tumors are uncommonly complicated by a condition known as **pseudomyxoma peritonei,** in which rupture of a malignant mucinous cyst leads to seeding of peritoneal surfaces with small tumor implants, which then fill the peritoneal cavity with mucinous material. Histologically, the cyst lining is composed of nonciliated, mucin-secreting, tall columnar cells reminiscent of the lining of endocervical glands.

Mucinous tumors can also be benign or malignant.

Endometrial tumors usually contain both solid and cystic areas that form tubular glands reminiscent of benign or malignant endometri-

Tumors derived from ovarian surface epithelium can also resemble endometrium.

Clear cell adenocarcinoma may be a variant of endometrial adenocarcinoma.

Brenner tumors contain tissue resembling transitional epithelium.

Germ cell tumors are most often benign cystic teratomas.

The presence of immature tissues suggests that a teratoma is malignant.

Dysgerminomas can be considered the ovarian form of testicular seminoma.

um. Most endometrioid tumors are malignant, although benign and borderline forms also exist. Some tumors have foci of squamous differentiation or foci resembling serous or mucinous carcinomas. Up to one-third of endometrioid carcinomas are accompanied by carcinoma of the endometrium; in these cases, it is usually unclear whether the tumors represent double primary tumors or whether metastasis from one site to the other has occurred.

Clear cell adenocarcinoma is an uncommon pattern composed of large epithelial cells with abundant clear cytoplasm that can grow in sheets, tubules, or lining cystic spaces. The tumor may be a variant of endometrioid adenocarcinoma, since it resembles clear cell carcinoma of the endometrium and sometimes occurs in association with endometriosis or endometrioid carcinoma of the ovary.

Brenner tumor is a usually solid, but occasionally cystic, ovarian neoplasm composed of nests of transitional epithelium (rarely columnar, mucin-secreting epithelium) embedded in a dense fibrous stroma that usually resembles the stroma of the normal ovary, but infrequently contains plump fibroblasts resembling theca cells. Brenner tumors are almost always benign, but borderline and malignant Brenner tumors have been reported. Brenner tumors occasionally produce very large (up to 30 cm diameter) ovarian masses.

Germ Cell Tumors

Roughly one-fifth of ovarian tumors are germ cell tumors. Over nine-tenths are benign cystic teratomas (dermoids). The remainder are more frequently malignant or borderline and occur mainly in children and young adults. Germ cell tumors of the ovary strongly resemble those of the testes and are described in detail here only when they differ from their testicular counterparts.

Teratomas are tumors that can contain a variety of tissues including stratified squamous epithelium with skin adnexal structures (teeth, cartilage, bone, thyroid tissue, or tissues resembling other organs). Most teratomas of the ovary are benign cystic teratomas known as dermoids or dermoid cysts. Dermoids have a characteristic gross appearance in which a cystic cavity is filled with hair and cheesy sebaceous secretions and lined by what appears histologically to be skin. While dermoids are almost always benign, about 1 percent undergo malignant transformation of one element, most commonly producing squamous cell carcinoma and less often other tumors such as thyroid carcinoma or melanoma. In contrast to dermoids, teratomas composed of immature tissues are almost always malignant. In addition to dermoids and immature teratomas, a few teratomas are composed mainly of only one mature tissue. The most notable of these are **stroma ovarii,** which is composed of mature thyroid tissue and may cause hyperthyroidism; **ovarian carcinoid,** which arises in intestinal epithelium in a teratoma and may produce enough 5-hydroxytryptamine to cause the carcinoid syndrome; and **stromal carcinoid,** which is a combination of stroma ovarii and carcinoid.

Dysgerminomas are malignant tumors that can be considered the ovarian form of testicular seminoma (see p. 315). Dysgerminoma is composed of cells with abundant clear cytoplasm, central nuclei, and sharply defined cell boundaries. The cells are arranged in sheets or cords in a scant fibrous stroma that may be infiltrated with lymphocytes and occasional granulomas. Small dysgerminomas are occasionally found in the walls of dermoid cysts. About one-third of dysgerminomas are highly aggressive; the remainder are less so and can nearly always be successfully treated with simple salpingo-oophorectomy. Dysgerminomas, including those with aggressive behavior, are usually radiosensitive.

Endodermal sinus (yolk sac) tumor is the second most common malignant germ cell tumor and is analogous to its testicular counterpart (see p. 316). The characteristic histologic feature is a central blood vessel covered by immature epithelium to form papillary projection; this structure resembles the yolk sac endodermal sinus of Duval described in the rat placenta. Endodermal sinus tumors often contain α-fetoprotein and $α_1$-antitrypsin. The tumors most often occur in children and young women. Their formerly dismal prognosis has been somewhat improved by combination chemotherapy.

Choriocarcinoma, similar to that which can arise in placenta and testes, can arise in the ovary either as the result of an ovarian ectopic pregnancy or from the teratogenous development of germ cells. Choriocarcinomas commonly occur as one component in a mixed neoplasm containing another germ cell tumor. Ovarian choriocarcinomas elaborate high levels of chorionic gonadotropins. They are much more aggressive tumors than those that arise in placenta and have commonly widely metastasized at the time of diagnosis.

Embryonal carcinoma is a highly malignant tumor that resembles its testicular counterpart. **Polyembryoma** is a malignant tumor with a testicular counterpart; it produces structures called "embryoid bodies" that resemble embryonic discs. **Mixed germ cell tumors** contain two or more germ cell tumors, usually dysgerminoma, teratoma, endodermal sinus tumor, or choriocarcinoma.

Sex Cord-Stromal Tumors

Ovarian neoplasms that differentiate along lines of tissues derived from embryonic sex cord or from ovarian stroma are classified as sex cord-stromal tumors.

Granulosa-theca cell tumors form a spectrum of tumors ranging from pure granulosa cell tumors through mixed variants to pure thecomas. The tumors that are composed predominantly of theca cells are almost always benign; the others have biologic behavior that can be difficult to predict but should be considered potentially malignant. The tumors can occur at any age, but most are discovered in postmenopausal women. Prepubertal girls with granulosa-theca cell tumors may have precocious sexual development. Histologically, the theca cell component of these tumors consists of large sheets of cells whose shape ranges from cuboidal to spindle-shaped cells resembling those in fibromas, but they are distinguished by the fact that even pure thecomas produce estrogens. The granulosa cell component is composed of small, cuboidal-to-polygonal cells that grow as cords, sheets, strands, or small, glandlike structures filled with acidophilic material **(Call-Exner bodies).**

Fibromas are benign tumors (except for rare fibrosarcomas) composed of well-differentiated fibroblasts separated by scant collagenous connective tissue. In pure form, fibromas do not produce hormones. Some may contain cells resembling theca cells and are called **fibrothecomas.** For unknown reasons, ovarian fibromas may commonly be accompanied by ascites and hydrothorax in a triad known as **Meigs syndrome.** Also, ovarian fibromas may be a component in the **basal cell nevus syndrome.**

Endodermal sinus tumor resembles its testicular counterpart.

Choriocarcinoma resembles that of placenta and testes.

Granulosa-theca cell tumors produce estrogens.

Fibromas do not produce hormones.

Sertoli-Leydig cell tumors may produce hormones with either androgenic or estrogenic effects.

Sertoli-Leydig cell tumors (androblastomas) contain tissue resembling testicular tissue and are usually benign but have some malignant potential. The tumors resemble granulosa-theca cell tumor but contain varying amounts of large, eosinophilic **Leydig cells** and tubules reminiscent of seminiferous tubules composed of **Sertoli cells.** Some of the tumors contain heterologous elements (mucinous glands, bone, cartilage). Most of these tumors secrete hormones that usually produce masculinization but occasionally have estrogenic effects.

Other sex cord-stromal tumors include hilus cell tumor, luteoma, lipid cell tumor, and gonadoblastoma.

Other sex-cord stromal tumors are also observed. **Hilus cell tumor** is nearly always benign and is composed of cells resembling Leydig cells that can secrete 17-ketosteroids. Benign **stromal luteoma** is composed of cells resembling lutein cells that may secrete products causing androgen, estrogen, or progesterone effects. **Pregnancy luteoma** is a lesion (probably not a true neoplasm) composed of cells resembling the corpus luteum of pregnancy that is associated with virilization of pregnant patients or their infants. **Lipid cell tumor** contains large, vacuolated cells, may be virilizing, and may be either benign or malignant. **Gonadoblastoma** is observed in individuals with abnormal sexual development and is composed of a mixture of germ cells and sex cord derivatives (immature Sertoli and granulosa cells). Gonadoblastoma may be associated with dysgerminoma.

Metastatic Tumor

Metastases to ovary may be from pelvic organs, gastrointestinal tract, or breast.

Metastases to ovary are most commonly from carcinomas of other pelvic organs; carcinomas of the upper gastrointestinal tract; and carcinoma of the breast. **Krukenberg's tumor** refers to enlargement of the ovaries by bilateral metastatic disease composed of mucin-producing signet-ring cells, often from a gastric adenocarcinoma.

NON-NEOPLASTIC OVARIAN CYSTS

Cysts can arise from graafian follicles and corpus luteum.

The ovary is vulnerable to non-neoplastic cystic disease. **Follicular cysts** are usually multiple; can be up to 8 cm in diameter; arise in unruptured (or ruptured and immediately resealed) graafian follicles; and are composed of cysts filled with serous fluid and lined by granulosa cells that may have atrophied. Follicular cysts uncommonly cause pelvic pain or produce sufficient estrogen to stimulate endometrial hyperplasia. **Luteal cysts** are analogous to follicular cysts but are formed from sealing of a corpus hemorrhagicum and are lined by bright yellow luteal tissue. **Polycystic ovaries** (Stein-Leventhal syndrome) are large ovaries with multiple subcortical cysts roughly 1 cm in diameter and lined by granulosa cells with hypertrophic luteinized theca interna. The ovarian outer tunica is thickened and fibrosed ("cortical stromal fibrosis"), and corpora lutea are absent. Polycystic ovaries are clinically associated with persistent anovulation secondary to high levels of androgens and luteinizing hormone, possibly as a result of primary pituitary or hypothalmic dysfunction.

Polycystic ovaries may cause persistent anovulation.

DISEASES OF THE FALLOPIAN TUBES

The fallopian tubes are most commonly affected by inflammations, ectopic pregnancy, and endometriosis. **Suppurative salpingitis** (pelvic inflammatory disease) is most commonly caused by gonorrhea, but can also be caused by streptococci, staphylococci, coliforms, or other organisms. Salpingitis usually occurs concurrently with other manifestations of pelvic inflammatory disease. **Tuberculous salpingitis** is due to spread from other sites to the fallopian tubes, where the tuberculosis produces characteristic granulomas. Tuberculous salpingitis is relatively uncommon in the United States, but is an important cause of infertility in many parts of the world. **Tumors** do not usually arise in the fallopian tubes. Of the few that do arise, the most common are tiny, serous-filled, paraovarian cysts (hydatids of Morgagni) that are thought to arise from wolffian duct remnants and that are found in the broad ligaments and near the fimbriated end of the fallopian tube. Other tumors of the fallopian tubes that are rarely encountered include benign mesothelioma (adenomatoid tumor) and adenocarcinoma.

The fallopian tubes are most commonly affected by inflammations, ectopic pregnancy, and endometriosis.

16

Endocrine System

PITUITARY GLAND

The clinical presentation of most diseases of the pituitary gland is dominated by changes in the gland's endocrine functioning. The anterior lobe of the pituitary gland is composed of epithelial cells that secrete (under the influence of the hypothalamus) thyrotropin, luteinizing hormone, follicle-stimulating hormone, corticotropin, growth hormone, and prolactin. The posterior lobe of the pituitary is composed of nerve fibers from the hypothalamus with occasional pituicytes; vasopressin (antidiuretic hormone) and oxytocin are released from these fibers.

> **Changes in endocrine function dominate the clinical presentation of pituitary diseases.**

PITUITARY ADENOMAS

Hormone-secreting adenomas are virtually the only cause of hyperfunctioning of the anterior pituitary since pituitary carcinomas are very rare. The adenomas typically secrete a single tropic hormone, which is commonly prolactin, growth hormone, or corticotropin (ACTH). Clinical symptoms are produced by the excessive hormones. Excess prolactin in women produces amenorrhea, galactorrhea, and infertility; in men it produces impotence. Excess growth hormone produces acromegaly or gigantism. Excess corticotropin produces Cushing or Nelson syndromes. Excess thyrotropin produces hyperthyroidism. Excess gonadotropin is usually clinically silent. A few adenomas do not secrete hormone (**nonsecretory pituitary adenomas**) and present as space-occupying lesions or in syndromes associated with hypofunctioning of the pituitary. While the different types of pituitary adenomas cannot be clearly distinguished by routine tissue stains, immunohistochemical techniques can clearly identify the product produced by an adenoma. Pituitary adenomas (of all cell types) may form masses ranging in size from microscopic up to 10 cm in diameter. **Microadenomas** are very common and can be identified in approximately one-fourth of autopsied patients. **Large pituitary adenomas,** while benign, may enlarge the sella turcica; compress the optic nerve or vessels; and penetrate into surrounding structures including the base of the brain, nasal sinuses, and cavernous sinuses. Large pituitary adenomas may also undergo focal or total ischemic necrosis as they compress their blood supply.

> **Hormone-secreting pituitary adenomas usually produce prolactin, growth hormone, or corticotropin.**

345

Pituitary adenomas can be composed of cells containing eosinophilic granules (which often secrete growth hormone or prolactin), cells containing basophilic granules (which often secrete corticotropin), or sparsely granulated cells (which often do not secrete significant amounts of any hormone). Therapy of symptomatic pituitary adenomas is by surgical removal.

ANTERIOR PITUITARY INSUFFICIENCY

The most common causes of **anterior pituitary insufficiency** are non-secretory pituitary adenomas (discussed in the preceding section), Sheehan syndrome, and the empty sella syndrome. Hypothalmic supracellar tumors are an uncommon cause of anterior pituitary insufficiency.

Sheehan syndrome is a shock- or hemorrhage-induced ischemic necrosis of the pituitary.

Sheehan syndrome referred originally to the sudden ischemic necrosis of the pituitary occasionally precipitated by hemorrhage or shock associated with obstetric delivery (postpartum pituitary necrosis). The pituitary enlarges during pregnancy and may partially compress its vascular system, leaving it more vulnerable to shock. However, ischemic necrosis of the pituitary has also been observed in men and nonpregnant women, so Sheehan syndrome has been extended to include these cases. Risk factors in these patients include shock, disseminated intravascular coagulation, sickle cell anemia, cavernous sinus thrombosus, and temporal arteritis.

Empty sella syndrome has a variety of causes.

Empty sella syndrome is an uncommon condition with a number of etiologies characterized by the absence or near absence of the pituitary gland. Causes of empty sella syndrome include pressure atrophy of the pituitary; Sheehan syndrome; infarction of an adenoma; and surgery or radiotherapy. Usually sufficient pituitary tissue remains to prevent pituitary insufficiency, although both panhypopituitarism and inadequate secretion of one or more hormones can also occur.

Tumors involving the hypothalamus may affect pituitary hormone secretion.

Hypothalamic suprasellar tumors are very uncommon but, when present, can cause either hypofunction or hyperfunction of the pituitary. Tumors that can be found in this area include gliomas, craniopharyngiomas, germ cell tumors (see p. 315), and lipomas (see p. 123). **Craniopharyngiomas** (adamantinomas, ameloblastomas) are usually benign tumors that are most commonly seen in children and young adults and are found either in a suprasellar or infrasellar location. The craniopharyngiomas can be either solid or cystic, and, when cystic, contain dark oily fluid with granular debris and cholesterol crystals. Calcification is common. Craniopharyngiomas arise in remnants of Rathke's pouch and have a variable histologic pattern that resembles tooth enamel organ. A loose, fibrous stroma contains nests or cords of stratified squamous or columnar epithelium (or both), which are sometimes arranged in a characteristic pattern in which central squamous cells are surrounded by columnar cells. When cysts are present, they can be lined with either stratified squamous or columnar epithelium. While panpituitary insufficiency leads to a deficiency of a variety of tropic hormones, the most clinical significant deficits are usually of thyroid-stimulating hormone, leading to hypothyroidism, and ACTH, leading to adrenocortical insufficiency.

POSTERIOR PITUITARY SYNDROMES

Clinically significant disease of the **posterior pituitary** is rare and is usually the consequence of a primary suprasellar **hypothalamic lesion.** Changes in **oxytocin** secretion do not produce clinically significant disease, since the only known functions of oxytocin are to potentiate uterine contraction and contraction of breast lactating glands. Antidiuretic hormone (ADH) deficiency causes polyuria and excessive thirst **(diabetes insipidus).** ADH deficiency can be caused by involvement of the hypothalamus or by tumor, inflammation, surgery, radiotherapy, trauma, or idiopathic causes. **Persistent, inappropriate release of ADH** causes inappropriate water retention, with edema, hyponatremia, and hemodilation. Inappropriate ADH secretion is usually a paraneoplastic syndrome involving either a nonendocrine tumor (often oat cell bronchogenic tumor, but also thymoma, carcinoma of the pancreas, or lymphoma) or a non-neoplastic pulmonary disorder (pneumonia, tuberculosis) that does not involve the hypothalamus or pituitary gland. Central nervous system diseases that may infrequently cause inappropriate ADH secretion include hemorrhages and thromboses (intracerebral, subarachnoid, or subdural) and infections in and around the brain.

Clinically significant disease of the posterior pituitary may produce ADH deficiency or excess.

THYROID GLAND

TUMORS OF THE THYROID GLAND

Evaluation of Thyroid Nodules

Thyroid nodules are very common, but most nodules contain benign rather than malignant tissue. The clinical evaluation of a thyroid nodule usually begins with scintiscan of the thyroid following radioiodine administration, since nodules that accumulate radioiodine (**"hot" nodules**) are much less apt to contain carcinoma than are those that do not accumulate significant amounts of radioiodine (**"cold" nodules).** Once a cold nodule is demonstrated, the next step is usually fine-needle aspiration of the nodule for cytology, since only about one-fifth of cold nodules are malignant, or, more commonly, suspicious for malignancy or indeterminant for some other reason. In those cases in which the aspirate was considered unsuitable for definitive interpretation, surgical biopsy then establishes the diagnosis. Clinical factors associated with increased risk that the nodule is carcinoma include a solitary nodule, age less than 40 years, and male sex.

Thyroid Adenomas and Other Benign Tumors

Thyroid adenomas are usually small (less than 4 cm), solitary nodules that contain follicles of varying size and in variable proportions. Papillary neoplasms of the thyroid are now considered to be carcinomas. Since many thyroid carcinomas are composed of deceptively mature cells forming well-organized follicles, the distinction between adenomas and carcinomas can be difficult. Thyroid adenomas are distinguished from thyroid carcinoma by complete fibrous encapsulation of the nodules with compression of the adjacent thyroid parenchyma. Thyroid adenomas are distinguished from multinodular goiter by a clear distinction between the histologic architecture within and outside the nodule and by the lack of multinodularity of the surrounding thyroid parenchyma.

    Embryonal or trabecular adenoma is reminiscent of embryonic thyroid parenchyma and is characterized by cords or trabeculae of cells with only occasional abortive follicles. **Fetal adenoma** is reminiscent of the fetal thyroid and is characterized by small follicles with little or no colloid in a loose connective tissue stroma. **Simple adenoma** is composed of normal-sized, closely packed follicles. **Colloid adenoma** is composed of large, colloid-filled follicles lined by flattened epithelium. Since the clinical significance is similar for all of the above patterns, some pathologists prefer to use a simpler histologic classification, in which adenomas are divided into **microfollicular** and **macrofollicular** patterns. One additional variant, the **Hürthle cell adenoma,** is worth mentioning because it is the only variant in which the cells do not resemble normal follicular cells. The Hürthle cell adenoma is composed of large cells with brightly eosinophilic granular cytoplasm packed with mitochondria and lysosomes similar to the Hürthle cells sometimes seen in Hashimoto's thyroiditis and some other non-neoplastic thyroid diseases.

Thyroid adenomas are principally important because they must be distinguished from thyroid carcinomas. They may additionally become clinically significant if they (uncommonly) cause hyperthyroidism; cause pressure symptoms in the neck; or bleed, causing rapid, painful enlargement of the thyroid. It is now thought that true thyroid adenomas are not a precursor for carcinoma, and that previous studies suggesting that they might be were erroneous due to biopsy sampling errors of well-differentiated follicular carcinomas. Other nodules that can affect the thyroid gland include solitary cysts arising in multinodular goiters or from cystic degeneration of a follicular adenoma, as well as a variety of rare tumors including dermoid cysts, teratomas, lipomas, and hemangiomas.

True thyroid adenomas are now thought not to be a precursor of carcinoma.

GOITER

Derangements that hamper thyroid hormone production or release tend to produce compensatory hypertrophy of the follicular epithelium that manifests as a **goiter.** The goitrous enlargement tends initially to be diffuse, but often later becomes nodular.

Diffuse Nontoxic Goiter

Diffuse nontoxic (simple) **goiter** refers to diffuse enlargement of the thyroid gland in a patient who is clinically euthyroid. Diffuse nontoxic goiter has many etiologies, which are conveniently subdivided into those that cause endemic and sporadic cases. **Endemic goiter** can be caused by either iodine deficiency or by goitrogenic substances, including calcium, fluorides, cabbage, cassava, cauliflower, brussel sprouts, and turnips. In general, large quantities of goitrogenic substances must be consumed before goiter is produced. **Sporadic simple goiter** is less common than endemic goiter, has a marked female predominance, and is most often observed in the second or third decade of life. The mechanism causing most sporadic cases is still undetermined but may be due to either transitory elevations of thyroid-stimulating hormone (TSH) or an intrathyroidal mechanism. Rarely, autosomal recessive biosynthetic defects can be identified, which may involve almost any stage in thyroid hormone formation from iodide absorption to final synthesis of thyroid hormone.

Diffuse nontoxic goiter usually evolves in two stages. The **hyperplastic stage** is characterized by modest enlargement of the thyroid gland (up to about 150 g) and many small, newly formed follicles lined by columnar epithelium. The stage of **colloid involution** (colloid goiter) occurs as large amounts of colloid accumulates within some follicles, and the epithelium of the larger follicles becomes progressively flattened. The goiter at this stage may be up to 500 g. Most patients with diffuse nontoxic goiter remain euthyroid, although a few patients do become

Diffuse nontoxic goiter can be subdivided into endemic and sporadic cases.

Follicles in diffuse nontoxic goiter are initially hyperplastic but develop flattened epithelium as colloid accumulates.

hypothyroid. Early iodine administration will cause regression of the goiter. Long-standing goiters do not regress with iodine therapy and tend to progress to multinodular goiter.

Multinodular Goiter

Multinodular goiter (adenomatous or multiple colloid adenomatous goiter) usually arise as an end stage of long-standing diffuse goiters. Patients with multinodular goiters may be either euthyroid or hyperthyroid. Hyperthyroid patients with multinodular goiters tend to have less severe hypermetabolism than do those with Graves disease and do not develop dermopathy or ophthalomopathy. Multinodular goiters can produce extreme (up to 2,000 g) enlargements of the thyroid and can be mistaken for tumor masses. Histologically, the goiter is composed of masses of colloid-filled or hyperplastic follicles separated by random irregular scarring. Focal hemorrhages, hemosiderin deposition, focal calcification, and microcyst formation may be present. If the goiter grows behind the sternum, it is called an **intrathoracic** (plunging) **goiter.** A very large multinodular goiter, particularly if intrathoracic, can cause cosmetic disfigurement, dysphagia, inspiratory stridor, or superior vena caval symptoms with distention of neck veins. Hemorrhage within the goiter can cause a sudden, painful enlargement.

THYROIDITIS

Hashimoto's Thyroiditis

Hashimoto's thyroiditis (autoimmune thyroiditis, stroma lymphomatosa) is a chronic form of autoimmune thyroiditis that has a strong female predominance, with most cases occurring between the ages of 30 and 40. It is characterized by an intense lymphocytic and plasmacytic infiltrate, with formation of lymphoid germinal centers, that destroys most of the thyroid parenchyma. The few remaining follicles tend to be atrophic and to be lined by large cells with abundant eosinophilic granular cytoplasm (Hürthle cells or oncocytes). The resulting thyroid is usually rubbery, firm, and symmetrically enlarged.

A histologic variant, **fibrosing Hashimoto's thyroiditis,** is characterized by more intense fibrosis and a less prominent lymphocytic infiltrate. Hashimoto's thyroiditis usually produces hypothyroidism, but may, for short intervals, produce hyperthyroidism **(hashitoxicosis).** The basic defect appears to be a genetic predisposition for a deficiency in some suppressor T cells, so that the thyroid can be attacked by both cytoxic T cells and autoantibodies. There is an association with HLA-DR5, and patients with Hashimoto's thyroiditis sometimes have other autoimmune diseases, such as systemic lupus erythematosus, Sjögren syndrome, rheumatoid arthritis, or adult onset diabetes. Hashimoto's thyroiditis can also coexist with Graves disease. Hashimoto's thyroiditis may predispose for lymphoma arising in the thyroid gland but does not have an increased incidence of thyroid carcinoma.

Subacute Granulomatous Thyroiditis

Subacute granulomatous (de Quervain's) **thyroiditis** is observed in young to middle-aged adulthood and has a female predominance. The thyroiditis is characterized by an early active inflammatory phase followed by characteristc aggregations of macrophages and multinucleate giant cells around damaged thyroid follicles and pools of colloid. Later, the sites of injury become replaced by fibrosis with a chronic inflammatory infiltrate. Many cases of subacute thyroiditis are preceded by viral infection (mumps, influenza, others). The clinical presentation is variable; common presentations include fever with elevated sedimentation rate, painful thyroid enlargement, and transient hyperthyroidism. Recovery usually occurs within 5 or 6 months, with nearly complete healing of the thyroid except for focal areas of fibrosis.

Subacute granulomatous thyroiditis may be preceded by viral infection.

Subacute Lymphocytic Thyroiditis

Subacute lymphocytic (painless) **thyroiditis** is similar to subacute granulomatous thyroiditis but differs in that the thyroid gland enlargement is painless, and the only histologic changes observed are small foci of lymphocytic infiltration. Subacute lymphocytic thyroiditis causes transient hyperthyroidism and tends to resolve without sequelae. Subacute lymphocytic thyroiditis is most common in the postpartum period, but may occur at any age.

Subacute lymphocytic thyroiditis causes transient hyperthyroidism.

Riedel's Thyroiditis

Riedel's thyroiditis (stroma ligneous thyroiditis) is a rare form of chronic thyroiditis of unknown etiology that is characterized by destruction of most or all of the thyroid gland by a marked fibrous reaction usually extending beyond the thyroid gland to involve adjacent structures. The thyroid in Riedel's thyroiditis has a distinctive "woody" hardness. Riedel's thyroiditis affects middle-aged and older adults, with a female predominance. Riedel's thyroiditis clinically resembles a neck malignancy, sometimes presenting with symptoms such as stridor, dysphagia, laryngeal nerve paralysis, and dyspnea. Patients may be either euthyroid or hypothyroid. Needle biopsy may be difficult. In severe cases, surgical decompression of the trachea may be required.

Riedel's thyroiditis is a fibrous replacement of the thyroid gland.

HYPERTHYROIDISM

Increased serum levels of the thyroid hormones T3 and T4 cause a hypermetabolic state called **hyperthyroidism.** Cardiac manifestations include tachycardia, palpitations, cardiomegaly, and arrhythmias. **Ophthalmic manifestations** are most marked in the autoimmune syndrome Graves disease; they include a periorbital edema that causes protrusion of the eyeball accompanied by retraction of the upper eyelid. The skin is usually moist and flushed as a consequence of both the generally **increased metabolic rate** and **peripheral vasodilation.** Skeletal muscle may undergo atrophy, fatty infiltration, and sometimes lymphocytic infiltration, and the patient may experience fatigue, muscular weakness, and hand **tremor.** Other symptoms the patient may experience include **emotional lability,** nervousness, excessive perspiration, heat intolerance, menstrual changes, and weight loss with good appetite. Other pathologic changes sometimes observed include minimal hepatic fatty change, osteoporosis, and lymphadenopathy.

Hyperthyroidism has many clinical manifestations.

Hyperthyroidism is a clinical syndrome that can be caused by many thyroid diseases. Common causes include diffuse toxic hyperplasia (Graves disease), toxic multinodular goiter, and toxic adenoma. Other thyroid causes of hyperthyroidism include thyroiditis and thyroid carcinoma. Nonthyroid causes include pituitary adenoma that secretes TSH, choriocarcinoma, stroma ovarii, and iatrogenic hyperthyroidism.

HYPOTHYROIDISM

Severe hypothyroidism that begins in infancy produces cretinism; severe hypothyroidism in adults produces myxedema.

Markedly insufficient thyroid hormone in infancy causes cretinism, and at older ages causes myxedema. **Cretinism** usually begins to develop shortly after birth; early manifestations include feeding problems, somnolence, failure to thrive, and constipation. Later, the child develops impaired skeletal growth, with a protruding abdomen, dry skin, and, most seriously, retarded development of the brain (deaf-mutism, spasticity, and mental retardation). Less severe deficiency of thyroid hormone produces milder manifestations. **Myxedema** refers to the clinical pattern produced by hypothyroidism in older children and adults. In adults, clinical manifestations develop insiduously and consist of slowed speech and mental activity, fatigue, lethargy, cold intolerance, thickened dry skin, coarsened facial features, periorbital edema, constipation, and decreased cardiac output with a large, flabby heart. Older children have clinical manifestations intermediate between those of adults and infants.

Both cretinism and myxedema can be confirmed with laboratory studies showing subnormal serum levels of T3 and T4. If the hypothyroidism is the result of primary thyroid disease, TSH levels may be elevated; TSH levels are depressed if the hypothyroidism is due to pituitary or hypothalmic disease. Inadequate thyroid parenchyma can be due to agenesis, dysplasia, surgery, radiotherapy, or primary idiopathic myxedema. Hypothyroidism associated with goiter can be due to Hashimoto's thyroiditis, iodine deficiency, or goitrogenic agents (including iodide). Other causes include hypopituitarism, hypothalamic lesions, and decreased peripheral responsiveness to thyroid hormones. The most common of these causes are ablation of the thyroid by surgery or radiation and primary idiopathic myxedema, which is now thought to be due in many cases to autoantibodies that block TSH receptors in the thyroid gland.

GRAVES DISEASE

Graves disease is a form of autoimmune hyperthyroidism.

Graves disease is a form of autoimmune hyperthyroidism. The thyroid is diffusely hyperplastic (up to 80 or 90 g) with excessive cellularity of the follicular epithelium so that the epithelium contains tall columnar cells piled up into simple, nonbranching papillary projections. Other histologic changes include markedly diminished colloid and increased number of lymphocytes (and even lymphoid follicles) in the thyroid stroma. An **ophthalmopathy** is usually present (but may not be readily evident) that is thought to arise because of chronic immune-mediated edema of extraorbital tissues. The ophthalmopathy is characterized clinically by periorbital edema, weakness of eye muscles, and a marked proptosis of the eyeball that may prevent lid closure. A **dermopathy,** characterized by localized edema of the skin of legs or feet, is present in about one-tenth of cases. Graves disease usually presents with persistent thyrotoxicosis. The diagnosis is confirmed by demonstrating increased radioactive iodine uptake or elevated levels of serum T3 or T4.

While the thyrotoxicosis can be treated with a variety of techniques, these do not usually modify the ophthalmopathy, which may either spontaneously remit or may worsen, leading to corneal ulceration with risk of loss of one or both eyes. Graves disease sometimes coexists with Hashimoto's thyroiditis or with a variety of other autoimmune diseases. The pathogenesis appears to involve autoantibodies to TSH receptors that cause the receptors to trigger T3 and T4 release inappropriately.

THYROID CARCINOMA

Thyroid adenocarcinoma has a modest male predominance. People who have been exposed to therapeutic neck irradiation have a significantly increased risk of developing thyroid cancer, with more than 1 in 20 individuals who had neck irradiation in childhood (often for trivial conditions such as tonsillar enlargement or acne) subsequently developing thyroid carcinoma after a mean latent period of 20 years. Fortunately, most of these "iatrogenic" carcinomas are more easily treated than the aggressive undifferentiated thyroid carcinomas. Thyroid adenocarcinomas can be subclassified into papillary carcinoma, follicular carcinoma, and medullary carcinoma.

Previous neck irradiation is an important risk factor for thyroid cancer.

Papillary Carcinoma

Papillary carcinoma, including mixed papillary and follicular types, is observed in approximately two-thirds of cases. Any thyroid neoplasm that contains branching, papillary fronds with a fibrovascular core, usually covered by a cuboidal epithelium (even if the bulk of the tumor forms follicles), is classified as a papillary carcinoma. All degrees of cellular atypia may be encountered. Papillary carcinomas can contain areas of squamous metaplasia; laminated calcific spherules known as psammoma bodies; and nuclei with a distinctive "ground-glass" appearance. Papillary carcinomas usually grow slowly and tend to metastasize, while still small, to lymph nodes in the neck; distant metastases are less common.

Papillary carcinomas tend to metastasize early to regional lymph nodes.

Follicular Carcinoma

Follicular carcinomas are observed in approximately one-fourth of cases and are characterized by the presence of follicular structures and the absence of the features associated with papillary carcinomas described above. Pure follicular carcinomas tend to behave more aggressively than papillary carcinomas, and only about one-third of patients survive for 5 years. Follicular carcinomas tend to form either a single, small, apparently encapsulated nodule or an obvious invasive mass that irregularly enlarges the thyroid gland. Histologic patterns resembling those described above for thyroid adenomas may be observed, or the tumors may form very well-defined colloid follicles that are quite difficult to distinguish from normal thyroid tissue. In these difficult cases, the diagnosis of carcinoma is established by a careful search for penetration of the apparent capsule or vascular invasion (or both). Rare histo-

Pure follicular carcinomas behave more aggressively than papillary carcinomas.

logic variants with biologic behavior similar to that of other follicular carcinomas include those composed of **clear cells,** which resemble clear cell renal carcinoma, and those composed of large cells with abundant eosinophilic cytoplasm (**Hürthle cells** or oxyphil cells).

Medullary Carcinoma

Medullary carcinoma is a neuroendocrine neoplasm.

Medullary carcinoma is a neuroendocrine neoplasm derived from the thyroid parafollicular (C) cells and is the histologic pattern observed in about one-tenth of cases. Medullary carcinomas are distinctive because they contain amyloid; they can also secrete calcitonin and other biologically active products (somatostatin, gastrin-releasing peptide, histaminase, prostaglandins, ACTH, vasoactive intestinal peptide, and serotonin). Medullary carcinoma of the thyroid appears to be linked to a specific genetic defect on chromosome 10 and can be associated with other tumors. Sipple syndrome is the association of pheochromocytoma with medullary carcinoma of the thyroid, also known as **multiple endocrine neoplasia type IIa.** An adenoma or hyperplasia of the parathyroid glands may also be present. In **multiple endocrine neoplasia type IIb,** pheochromocytoma and medullary carcinoma of the thyroid are associated with a Marfanoid habitus and mucosal neuromas. Familial clusterings of medullary carcinoma without accompanying pheochromocytoma have also been described.

Medullary carcinoma may be a component in multiple endocrine neoplasia syndromes.

Medullary carcinoma of the thyroid can occur either as a discrete nodule or, particularly in familial cases, as numerous nodules, usually involving both thyroid lobes. Hemorrhage, necrosis, and spread outside the thyroid capsule may be present, as may metastases. The cells may be either round to polygonal, resembling those of other neuroendocrine tumors, or spindle-shaped, resembling sarcomas. The cells tend to be arranged in nests or sheets, and the intervening fibrovascular stroma characteristically contains amyloid deposits. Sporadic lesions tend to present late in life (fifth or sixth decade) and be solitary lesions; familial lesions are usually observed in the second or third decade and are typically multiple. Both types can produce persistent diarrhea as a consequence of calcitonin (or possibly some other substance) secretion. The sporadic lesions tend to be diagnosed later, and patients have a mean survival of about 5 years, compared with the over four-fifths of patients with familial disease who are disease-free 10 years after diagnosis.

Undifferentiated Carcinoma

Undifferentiated carcinomas are very aggressive.

More than one-tenth of thyroid carcinomas are highly aggressive, **undifferentiated carcinomas** that have usually produced bulky masses possibly extending beyond the thyroid gland by the time of diagnosis. **Small cell carcinomas** are composed of closely packed cuboidal cells growing in cords or clusters within a fibrous stroma. Mitotic figures are common. A variant of small cell carcinoma, which may actually be a malignant lymphoma in at least some cases, is composed of sheets of extremely small cells with dark, round nuclei. **Giant cell carcinoma** is a very aggressive neoplasm composed of highly anaplastic, pleomorphic tumor giant cells; spindle cells; and cells resembling cytoplasmic ribbons. These tumors apparently often arise in previously existing low-grade thyroid carcinomas and may consequently contain foci of papillary or follicular formation.

Other Malignant Tumors

Other malignant tumors that can affect the thyroid include Hodgkin's disease and non-Hodgkin's lymphomas; sarcomas, including fibrosarcoma, hemangiosarcoma, and osteogenic sarcoma; and squamous cell carcinoma.

MISCELLANEOUS THYROID LESIONS

Most congenital anomalies of the thyroid occur as a result of abnormalities in the downward growth of the thyroid from its original position in the foramen cecum at the back of the tongue to its final position in the anterior neck. **Thyroglossal cysts** and segments of thyroglossal duct are the most common clinically significant congenital anomalies; they arise in vestigial remnants of the tubular tract left as the thyroid grows downward. The cysts are located in the anterior midline, usually contain mucous secretion (unless superinfected), and tend to be lined by stratified squamous epithelium if located high in the neck or by epithelium resembling thyroidal acinar epithelium if located low in the neck. Thyroglossal cysts and ducts are clinically important because they form nodules that must be distinguished from tumor masses; they may form sinuses that drain to the skin or base of the tongue, and they may rarely develop malignancy.

Ectopic thyroid tissue rests are uncommonly found at the base of the tongue or along the course of the thyroglossal duct; they become clinically important because they must be distinguished from metastatic well-differentiated thyroid cancer. **Agenesis and dysgenesis** of the thyroid occur uncommonly. The thyroid gland is also vulnerable to **atrophy,** in which, possibly as a result of many different etiologies, the thyroid parenchyma becomes completely replaced by fibrous tissue. **Systemic diseases** that can affect the thyroid include amyloidosis, hemochromatosis, metastatic cancers, and blood-borne infections.

Congenital anomalies of the thyroid include thyroglossal cysts, ectopic thyroid tissue, and agenesis.

PARATHYROID GLANDS

Parathormone regulates serum calcium and phosphate levels.

Parathyroid glands secrete **parathyroid hormone,** which tends to increase serum calcium levels by reducing renal excretion of calcium, increasing dissolution of bone, and increasing renal synthesis of an active form of vitamin D, calcitriol, which in turn increases gut absorption of calcium. Parathyroid diseases are clinically important primarily because they produce either **hyperparathyroidism** or **hypoparathyroidism.** Hyperparathyroidism is conveniently subdivided into primary and secondary forms. Persistent hyperparathyroidism can produce elevated serum levels of parathyroid hormone and calcium, decreased serum levels of phosphate, and excessive urinary excretion of calcium. Other clinical manifestations include weakness, neuropsychiatric symptoms, renal calculi, and osteitis fibrosa cystica. Elevation of serum calcium levels is not sufficient to diagnosis primary hyperparathyroidism, since nonparathyroid diseases, notably malignancies (multiple myeloma and carcinomas of breast, lung, or kidney), cause osteolytic metastases or release calcium-mobilizing factors (prostaglandins, vitamin D-like substances, parathyroid hormone-like substances) that elevate serum calcium.

PRIMARY HYPERPARATHYROIDISM

Primary hyperparathyroidism can be caused by parathyroid adenomas, carcinomas, or hyperplasia.

Primary hyperparathyroidism can be caused by parathyroid adenomas, carcinomas, or hyperplasia.

Parathyroid adenomas are benign, usually single, tumors with a peak incidence in middle-aged adults of either sex. The adenomas are often tiny and may be difficult to identify at surgical exploration since they may be located either in normally situated (often inferior) parathyroids or in a variety of ectopic locations including thyroid, thymus, or pericardium. Parathyroid adenomas may contain either a single cell population (often chief cells) or mixed cell populations. The cells are usually arranged in sheets or bands but occasionally develop follicular structures that resemble thyroid tissue. A rim of normal or atrophic parathyroid tissue may surround the adenoma, facilitating the distinction from diffuse parathyroid hyperplasia.

Parathyroid carcinoma is rare and may either be nonfunctioning or may cause primary hyperparathyroidism. Distinguishing parathyroid carcinoma from a parathyroid adenoma may be difficult; features strongly suggesting malignancy include the presence of metastases, capsular invasion, or local recurrence after surgery.

Primary hyperplasia of the parathyroid is a diffuse process of unknown etiology that, unlike parathyroid adenoma, characteristically affects all of the patient's parathyroid glands, although one or two glands may be more severely involved. Chief cell hyperplasia is the most common form, although clear cell hyperplasia is also encountered. The numbers of stromal fat cells are usually markedly decreased. The chief cells usually grow in cords or sheets and may contain foci of oxyphil cells or a mixture of cells. When hyperplasia of clear cells occurs, the parathyroid glands become nearly completely replaced by enlarged cells with vacuolated cytoplasm.

SECONDARY HYPERPARATHYROIDISM

Secondary hyperparathyroidism is characterized by (sometimes mild) decreased serum calcium levels. Often, the serum calcium levels are decreased because of end-organ resistance to parathyroid hormone, and the parathyroids secondarily increase secretion of parathyroid hormone. Secondary hyperparathyroidism is encountered most commonly in chronic renal insufficiency. Other causes include vitamin D deficiency and intestinal malabsorption. Chief cell hyperplasia is usually present in all of the glands but is sometimes asymmetric. With appropriate therapy of the primary disease (renal transplantation, vitamin D supplementation), the secondary hyperplasia usually resolves. When it does not and the hyperparathyroidism persists, the resulting condition is sometimes called **"tertiary" hyperparathyroidism.**

> **Secondary hyperparathyroidism is most commonly encountered in renal insufficiency.**

HYPOPARATHYROIDISM

Inadequate secretion of biologically effective parathyroid hormone is observed when the delicate blood supply to the parathyroids is interrupted (thyroid surgery); in familial (posibly autoimmune) syndromes; in thymic dysplasia (DiGeorge syndrome, in which the parathyroids may also be hypoplastic); and due to diverse causes including radiotherapy and metastatic disease. Mild **hypoparathyroidism** produces hypocalcemia unaccompanied by overt clinical manifestations. More severe and persistent hypoparathyroidism can cause neuromuscular and central nervous system manifestation, including tetany, muscle cramps, cardiac arrhythmias, and increased cerebrospinal fluid pressure. Also seen are manifestations of abnormal calcification, and abnormal teeth.

> **Hypoparathyroidism has diverse causes.**

PSEUDO- AND PSEUDOPSEUDOHYPOPARATHYROIDISM

Pseudohypoparathyroidism is a genetic disease (possibly X-linked dominant) that clinically resembles hypoparathyroidism, but in which parathyroid hormone levels are normal or elevated. The defect may be a failure of end-organ tissues to respond to parathyroid hormone. Some patients have skeletal abnormalities (short stature, short neck, short metacarpals) that may or may not be accompanied by mental retardation. **Pseudopseudohypoparathyroidism** clinically resembles pseudohypoparathyroidism, but the patients have normal serum calcium and phosphate levels.

> **Pseudo- and pseudopseudohypoparathyroidism clinically resemble hypothyroidism.**

ENDOCRINE PANCREAS

ISLET CELL TUMORS

Islet cell tumors may produce insulin, gastrin, glucagon, or somatostatin.

Tumors of the islet cells of the pancreas are much less common than tumors of the exocrine pancreas. Islet cell tumors are described in terms of the hormone products they produce. Islet cell tumors may produce clinically significant disease while being so small as to be difficult to find. β-**Cell tumors** (insulinomas) produce insulin and are the most common islet cell tumors. The erratic insulin release causes attacks of hypoglycemia that are relieved by oral or parenteral glucose administration but they may be severe enough to cause confusion, stupor, or even coma. Most insulinomas are benign, but some are malignant. Similar clinical symptoms can sometimes be produced by islet cell hyperplasia. **Gastrinomas** produce gastrin, and both benign and malignant gastrinomas are common. Gastrinomas characteristically produce Zollinger-Ellison syndrome, with the triad of pancreatic islet cell tumor, gastric hypersecretion with hyperplasia of acid-secreting parietal cells, and severe peptic ulcer disease. The ulcers are commonly multiple gastric or duodenal ulcers and may be highly resistant to therapy. Similar clinical symptoms can sometimes be produced by islet cell hyperplasia. α-**Cell tumors** (glucagonomas) are rare tumors that produce glucagon and cause mild diabetes mellitus, anemia, and a necrotizing skin erythema. δ-**Cell tumors** (somatostatinomas) are rare tumors that produce somatostatin and cause diabetes mellitus, gallstones with steatorrhea, and hypochlorhydria. δ-Cell tumors can be a component of multiple endocrine neoplasia type I, in which patients have a predisposition for tumor or hyperplasia of parathyroids, pancreatic islet cells, pituitary, adrenal cortex, and thyroid. In contrast, pancreatic islet cell disease is not a component of multiple endocrine neoplasia (MEN) type IIa (pheochromocytoma, medullary carcinoma of thyroid, parathyroid disease) or MEN type IIb (medullary carcinoma of thyroid, pheochromocytoma, mucocutaneous neuromas).

DIABETES MELLITUS

Diabetes mellitus is actually a cluster of related diseases.

Diabetes mellitus is characterized by abnormal control of carbohydrate metabolism by insulin. Diabetes mellitus is actually a cluster of related diseases, of which the **type I** (juvenile onset or insulin-dependent) and **type II** (adult onset or insulin-independent) forms are most important. Type II diabetes is the more common of the two forms and is observed most often in older adults who may be obese. It is apparently related to a failure of often near normal serum levels of insulin to have adequate hypoglycemic effect, possibly because of end-organ resistance, which is exacerbated in obese individuals. Type I diabetes is less common, typically begins in childhood or adolescence (possibly following an unspecified viral illness), and is usually associated with decreased serum insulin levels. Type I diabetics classically require insulin by injection. Type II diabetics usually respond for many years to weight loss, dietary therapy, and oral hypoglycemic agents; eventually, some type II diabetics do require insulin to control their diabetes.

While the underlying defect in diabetes is disordered carbohydrate metabolism, diabetes is best understood as a systemic disorder that affects virtually the entire body. This relationship is most obvious when late complications are considered (see next section). Diabetes classically presents with **polyuria** and **polydipsia** as a consequence of the osmotic diuretic effect produced by glucose in urine. However, many patients are now identified by serum or urine glucose screening tests before the clinical symptoms become prominent. Diabetics also experience increased urinary tract and other **infections,** poor wound healing, and fatigue. Type I (juvenile) diabetics often have weight loss; type II diabetics are often obese. **Ketoacidosis** is usually observed in poorly controlled type I diabetics who have inadequate insulin therapy and is characterized by increased fat catabolism with production of ketone bodies. Other features include increased serum osmolality, hypovolemia, acidosis, and loss of electrolytes that may induce coma. Type II diabetics whose diabetes is inadequately controlled but who have some insulin activity are more apt to develop **hyperosmolar coma,** in which very high serum glucose levels produce sufficient dehydration to induce coma. Lactic acidosis leading to coma is also occasionally observed in diabetics. Coma can also be produced when insulin intake is greater than needed and the patient develops profound hypoglycemia (hypoglycemic coma).

Type I diabetics often have weight loss, while type II diabetics are often obese.

Diabetes mellitus types I and II are the classic forms of diabetes mellitus. Diabetes mellitus may also complicate pregnancy; primary pancreatic disease (chronic pancreatitis, mumps, cystic fibrosis); other endocrine diseases (acromegaly, Cushing syndrome, Conn syndrome); other systemic diseases (hemochromatosis); and pharmacotherapy (steroids, thiazide diuretics).

Diabetes may complicate many other diseases.

Late Complications of Diabetes Mellitus

By 10 to 15 years after onset of either type I or type II diabetes mellitus, most patients have begun to develop pathologic changes in many organs. The **pancreatic islets** may show very little change or may show fewer and smaller islets than normal, β-cell degranulation, islet fibrosis, amyloid deposition in islets, or lymphocytic or eosinophilic infiltration of islets. Both diabetic and nondiabetic children of diabetic mothers may show more and larger islets.

Late complications of diabetes are dominated by vascular changes in many organs.

Diabetic microangiopathy refers to the small vessel changes that are seen throughout the body of diabetics and are most obvious in skin, kidney, skeletal muscle, and retina. The capillary basement membranes become diffusely thickened, and, despite the thickening, the capillaries tend to leak plasma proteins into adjacent interstitial spaces. Similar thickening of other, nonvascular, basement membranes is also seen, notably in renal tubules, Bowman's capsule, peripheral nerves, and placenta. Arterioles show hyaline arteriosclerosis in which the arteriolar wall becomes thickened with amorphous hyaline material, usually causing lumenal narrowing. Hyaline arteriosclerosis is also seen in hypertensive patients without diabetes, but tends to be more severe in diabetics.

Atherosclerosis tends to be more florid and to cause significant disease at a younger age in diabetics compared with nondiabetics. The lesions are also more apt to be ulcerated or calcified, or to have superimposed thromboses. Diabetics with other risk factors for atherosclerosis (hyperlipidemia, obesity, hypertension, smoking) are at particular risk for severe atherosclerosis. Atherosclerotic narrowing or occlusion of arteries can cause many diabetic complications, including myocardial infarction, stroke, and gangrene of the legs.

Diabetic nephropathy, which may cause renal failure and contribute to the patient's poor health, is due to glomerular disease, arteriosclerosis, and frequent upper urinary tract infections.

Diabetic ocular complications can cause visual impairment and sometimes blindness secondary to retinopathy, cataract formation, or glaucoma.

Diabetic neuropathy can damage peripheral nerves, brain, or spinal cord. The mechanism of damage is unclear, but may be related to either microangiopathy or direct damage by disordered glucose metabolism (possibly via sorbitol accumulation). The peripheral neuropathy can be either symmetric, affecting both motor and sensory nerves of the legs, or one or more mononeuropathies affecting specific peripheral nerves. Nerve dysfunction can also cause bowel, bladder, and sexual dysfunction. Loss of neurons in brain and spinal cord also sometimes occur, and diabetics have an increased incidence of stroke, brain hemorrhage, and damage to neurons by ketoacidosis or hypoglycemia during insulin reactions.

ADRENAL GLANDS

DEVELOPMENTAL ANOMALIES OF THE ADRENAL CORTEX

The adrenal cortex is vulnerable to congenital hyperplasia (discussed on p. 362), congenital hypoplasia, and ectopic accessory adrenal tissue. Two forms of congenital hypoplasia are observed in newborns and young children. **Anencephalic congenital adrenal hypoplasia** occurs in anencephalic fetuses and is characterized by bilateral small adrenals (or sometimes completely absent adrenals) usually composed of adult cortex. **Cytomegalic congenital adrenal hypoplasia** is a possibly familial hypoplasia in which the small adrenal glands have a distinctive histologic pattern with abnormally large, eosinophilic cells. The condition is not related to viral cytomegalic inclusion disease and, if recognized promptly, can be treated with replacement steroid therapy.

Ectopic adrenal tissue can be found throughout the retroperitoneum; in subcapsular sites of the kidneys, testes, and ovaries; or in inguinal hernias. Most ectopic adrenal tissue consists of adrenal cortex, but adrenal medullary tissue can also occasionally be found. Ectopic adrenal tissue may become hyperplastic, and tumors will rarely arise in the ectopic tissue.

Congenital hyperplasia, congenital hypoplasia, and ectopic adrenal tissue can all affect the adrenal cortex.

HYPERFUNCTION OF THE ADRENAL CORTEX

The adrenal cortex produces glucocorticoids, mineralocorticoids, and sex steroids. Excessive production of these products is seen in Cushing's syndrome, aldosteronism, and adrenogenital syndromes with production of excess sex steroids, respectively.

Cushing Syndrome

Overproduction of cortisol produces **Cushing syndrome,** which is characterized clinically by deranged glucose metabolism that may manifest either as impaired glucose tolerance or overt diabetes. Altered fat metabolism produces obesity, "buffalo hump," and "moon facies." Other manifestations include mental disorders, easy bruisability, and osteoporosis. In women, abnormalities related to excess production of testosterone and cortisol inhibition of pituitary gonadotropin release include hirsutism, acne, and menstrual irregularities; in men, impotence and oligospermia are seen.

When the overproduction of cortisol is caused by pituitary disease, the term **Cushing's disease** is used, and the adrenal cortex usually shows

Overproduction of cortisol produces Cushing syndrome.

diffuse cortical hyperplasia that may contain small areas of nodularity. Cushing syndrome can also be caused by adrenal adenomas or carcinomas; diffuse cortical hyperplasia secondary to ectopic production of ACTH or corticotropin-releasing hormone by tumors; or multinodular adrenal disease. The multinodular adrenal disease may have the morphologic form of either multinodular hyperplasia, characterized by diffuse hyperplasia with nodules up to 3 cm, or microadenomatous dysplasia, characterized by atrophy of most of the adrenal cortex except for small pigmented nodules.

Hyperaldosteronism

Hyperaldosteronism may be primary or secondary.

Conn syndrome (**primary hyperaldosteronism**) can be caused by adrenal adenomas (or rarely carcinoma), or by hyperplasia of the zona glomerulosa of the adrenal cortex. Clinically, the elevated aldosterone levels produce renal potassium wasting, neuromuscular symptoms, and hypertension as a consequence of sodium and fluid retention. **Secondary hyperaldosteronism** occurs as a result of overproduction of renin by renal ischemia, renal juxtaglomerular cell hyperplasia (Bartter syndrome), edema, or renin-producing neoplasma. Secondary hyperaldosteronism clinically resembles primary hyperaldosteronism, with the combination of sodium retention and potassium wasting, but renin levels are high rather than low.

Congenital Adrenal Hyperplasia

The congenital adrenal hyperplasias are genetic enzymatic defects in hormone synthesis.

The adrenal cortex can produce sex steroids, and androgen-secreting adenomas or carcinomas may cause **adrenal virilism,** most easily recognizable in women. Rare cortical neoplasms may also produce feminization. Abnormal quantities of sex steroids can also be produced by enzymatic defects in steroid synthesis by the adrenals, which cause normally minor biochemical pathways to be stimulated when the normal synthetic pathways are blocked. People with these congenital enzymatic defects characteristically have hyperplastic adrenal glands, since the decreased synthesis of cortisol leads to adrenal stimulation by pituitary ACTH. These genetic diseases, of which at least eight have been described, are collectively called **congenital adrenal hyperplasia.** Different enzymatic defects produce somewhat different clinical presentations.

The congenital adrenal hyperplasias are genetic enzymatic defects in hormone synthesis.

Deficiency of 21-hydroxylase is the most common defect and has a higher incidence in some Alaskan-Eskimo tribes than in most other populations. The enzyme converts 17-α-hydroxyprogesterone to 11-deoxycortisol, and blocking of this conversion causes the biochemical pathway leading from 17-α-hydroxyprogesterone to androgen synthesis (starting with androstenedione) to be stimulated. Girls are born with normal internal reproductive organs but with external organs that have been stimulated by excess testosterone, typically showing at birth clitoral enlargement, fused labioscrotal folds, and a phallic urethra. Newborn boys may have bilateral cryptorchidism and hypospadias. Three variants of 21-hydroxylase deficiency have been described.

21-Hydroxylase deficiency is the most common genetic defect.

Classic 21-hydroxylase deficiency produces simple virilization in infancy; is not life-threatening; and is associated with HLA-Bw51. 21-Hydroxylase deficiency, with additional **deficient aldosterone synthesis,** produces severe salt wasting with hyponatremia and hyperkalemia; can cause death if untreated in early infancy; and is associated with HLA-Bw60. The decreased aldosterone synthesis occurs because 21-hydroxylase also converts progesterone to 11-deoxycorticosterone, which is an intermediary in aldosterone production. **Nonclassical 21-hydroxylase deficiency** produces virilization in late childhood; is not life-threatening; is more common in European Jews; and is associated with HLA-B14.

Deficiency of 11-hydroxylase is the second most common defect, and has a higher incidence among Moroccan Jews. 11-Hydroxylase normally converts 11-deoxycorticosterone to corticosterone in aldosterone synthesis and 11-deoxycortisol to cortisol. 11-Hydroxylase deficiency is not HLA linked and appears to have heterogenous clinical presentations. Accumulated cortisol precursors cause stimulation of androgen synthesis, resulting in virilization. Additionally, the accumulated deoxycorticosterone has a mineralocorticoid effect, causing hypokalemia and hypertension.

Other enzymatic deficiencies are uncommon. **17-Hydroxylase deficiency** causes decreased secretion of glucocorticoids and sex steroids, as well as increased mineralocorticoids. **Desmolase deficiency** causes decreased synthesis of testosterone. Biochemical analysis of urinary steroids, and, if necessary, adrenal tissue can be helpful in determining the enzymatic defect present in a particular case of congenital adrenal hyperplasia.

HYPOFUNCTION OF THE ADRENAL CORTEX

The adrenal cortex normally synthesizes both corticosteroids and mineralocorticoids. **Adrenocortical hypofunction** is deficient secretion of corticosteroids with or without deficient secretion of mineralocorticoids. **Hypoaldosteronism** is isolated aldosterone (mineralocorticoid) deficiency with normal cortisol production. Adrenocortical hypofunction has many causes, but can be conveniently discussed in terms of three clinical patterns: chronic primary adrenocortical insufficiency, acute primary adrenocortical insufficiency, and secondary adrenocortical insufficiency. Secondary adrenocortical insufficiency is due to a lack of ACTH, usually as a consequence of pituitary disease (see p. 346), and will not be discussed here.

Chronic Primary Adrenocortical Insufficiency

Chronic primary adrenocortical insufficiency (**Addison's disease**) occurs when disease damages the adrenal cortex sufficiently that appropriate amounts of steroid hormones cannot be secreted. **Idiopathic adrenal atrophy,** which may be an autoimmune disease, is the most important cause and is characterized by small adrenal glands with normal medulla and collapsed cortex. The cortex contains relatively small numbers of enlarged cells with eosinophilic cytoplasm and large irregular nuclei. The cells are embedded in a loose fibrous stroma with an often heavy lymphocytic infiltration.

Tuberculosis causes Addison's disease by replacing the adrenal tissue with granulomas. Tuberculosis was formerly the most important cause of

11-Hydroxylase deficiency is the second most common defect.

Other enzymes that may be deficient include 17-hydroxylase and desmolase.

Adrenocortical hypofunction may affect corticosteroids or mineralocorticoids, or both.

Destruction of the adrenal cortex by a variety of agents can produce chronic Addison's disease.

Addison's disease, and remains, despite modern antituberculosis therapy, the second most important cause. **Autoimmune Addison's disease** refers to the combination of adrenocortical insufficiency and any of many autoimmune diseases including insulin-dependent diabetes mellitus, pernicious anemia, hypoparathyroidism, or autoimmune thyroid disorders. Autoimmune Addison's disease can be a component in **polyglandular deficiency syndrome** (Schmidt syndrome), in which at least two of several endocrine organs (adrenal, thyroid, parathyroid, gonads, pancreas) have an apparently autoimmune-mediated hormonal deficiency.

Uncommon causes of Addison's disease include fungi, amyloidosis, sarcoidosis, hemochromatosis, metastatic tumor, hemorrhagic necrosis, and surgery. **Metabolic causes** of Addison's disease include congenital adrenal hyperplasia and drug-induced inhibition of cortical cell function, notably by the enzyme inhibitor metyrapone and the cytotoxic agent mitotase.

> **The symptoms of Addison's disease tend to be nonspecific.**

The symptoms experienced by patients with Addison's disease vary with the degree of adrenocortical insufficiency. Fatigue, progressive weakness, and weight loss are prominent symptoms in almost all patients. The weakness may be profound, affecting the patient's ability to perform even minimal tasks, including speech. Gastrointestinal symptoms can include nausea, vomiting, diarrhea, and constipation. Abdominal pain may be present that is occasionally sufficiently severe to mimic an acute abdominal emergency. Hyperpigmentation of the skin and sometimes mucous membranes occurs as a side effect of high levels of ACTH secreted by the pituitary to stimulate the failing adrenal cortex.

Clinical problems related to insufficient mineralocorticoids are observed only when the adrenal insufficiency is profound. These include severe salt wasting with lowered circulating volume, hypotension (sometimes less than 80/50 mmHg) with syncope, and elevated serum potassium, which may cause cardiac arrhythmias. Stress, including illness, may precipitate life-threatening superimposed acute adrenal insufficiency, cardiac arrhythmias, or hypoglycemic cerebral crises.

Acute Primary Adrenocortical Insufficiency

> **Acutely developing adrenocortical insufficiency most often follows steroid withdrawal, stress, or hemorrhagic destruction of the adrenals.**

Acutely developing insufficiency of adrenal steroids is seen most often in three settings. Too rapid **withdrawal from steroid therapy** for other diseases is the most common cause. This occurs because chronic therapy with exogenous steroids can cause suppression of the synthetic functions of the adrenal cortex, which may take some time to reverse when the exogenous steroids are discontinued. **Stress,** including illness, which normally triggers an immediate increased steroid output, can precipitate acute exacerbation in patients with Addison's disease, whose adrenal glands are not able to respond.

Massive hemorrhagic destruction of the adrenal glands can occur in several clinical settings. **Neonates** who have experienced trauma and hypoxia during a difficult delivery can have extensive adrenal hemorrhages. In adults, the **Waterhouse-Friderichsen syndrome** refers to the hemorrhagic destruction of the adrenals observed in some overwhelming bacterial infections, notably meningococcemia. Meningococcemia can develop very rapidly, causing skin and systemic hemorrhagic manifestations that are related to the development of disseminated intravascular coagulation. These hemorrhages often involve the adrenal gland, and the resulting adrenal necrosis causes rapidly developing acute adrenal insufficiency that contributes, together with the sepsis, to circulatory collapse that may cause death within 24 hours of the beginning of infectious symptoms.

Hypoaldosteronism

Isolated **aldosterone deficiency** is characterized clinically by an inability of the adrenal cortex to increase aldosterone secretion appropriately during salt restriction. Causes include deficient renin production ("hyporeninemic hypoaldosteronism") in conditions such as mild renal failure and diabetes mellitus; an inherited biosynthetic defect, usually a deficiency of 18-hydroxysteroid dehydrogenase, which catalyzes the transformation of the C-18 aldehyde of aldosterone; postoperatively following ablation of an aldosterone-secreting adenoma; and several miscellaneous causes including protracted heparin therapy, severe postural hypotension, and diseases of the nervous system that affect the pretectum. Isolated hypoaldosteronism produces hyperkalemia with normal cortisol levels. The renin levels are low if the cause is deficient renin production and high in other settings. Treatment can be either with oral mineralocorticoid (fludrocortisone) or with the potassium-wasting diuretic furosemide.

Isolated aldosterone deficiency produces hyperkalemia.

NONFUNCTIONAL MASS LESIONS OF THE ADRENAL GLAND

In addition to hyperplasia and tumors that produce steroid hormones, the adrenal cortex is vulnerable to **nonfunctional lesions** including the relatively common benign adrenal adenoma or nodule, which forms poorly encapsulated masses up to several centimeters in diameter; the highly malignant cortical carcinomas, not all of which produce hormones; metastatic, particularly bronchogenic, carcinomas; adrenal cysts, which may arise from necrosis of neoplastic masses or be of parasitic origin; and adrenal myelolipoma, which is an unusual benign tumor composed of hematopoietic cells embedded in mature adipose tissue.

Nonfunctional lesions can also affect the adrenal gland.

DISEASES OF THE ADRENAL MEDULLA

The paraganglionic system consists of the adrenal medulla and similar neuroendocrine tissue, which is widely distributed in paraganglia adjacent to organs throughout the body. The most important diseases of the adrenal medulla are **neoplasms,** and similar neoplasms can uncommonly arise in paraganglia in other sites. The most important tumors of the adrenal medulla are pheochromocytoma, neuroblastoma (see p. 195), and ganglioneuroma (see p. 195).

Pheochromocytoma

Pheochromocytomas secrete catecholamines.

Pheochromocytoma is an uncommon neuroendocrine tumor of the adrenal medulla that often secretes **catecholamines** (usually both norepinephrine and epinephrine) and is consequently significant as a cause of either sustained or paroxysmal hypertension. **Other hormones** that can be produced by pheochromocytomas include dopamine and ACTH. Pheochromocytomas are usually benign and uncommonly malignant tumors; however, even the benign tumors are potentially fatal as a consequence of uncontrollable hypertension. Technically, only those tumors that arise in the adrenal medulla are called pheochromocytomas. Similar tumors less commonly arise in other sites and are called **extra-adrenal paragangliomas.**

Pheochromocytomas and extra-adrenal paragangliomas are encountered most frequently in middle-aged adults, but can occur at any age. Paragangliomas are often found in the abdomen, particularly along the aorta. Retroperitoneal extra-adrenal paragangliomas are more apt to be malignant. Most pheochromocytomas and paragangliomas occur as sporadic, solitary neoplasms. Bilateral neoplasms and neoplasms associated with familial syndromes (multiple endocrine neoplasia types IIa and IIb, neurofibromatosis, von Hippel-Lindau syndrome) also occur. Pheochromocytomas can range in size from one to thousands of grams, with typical weights around 100 g.

Pheochromocytomas may be associated with familial syndromes.

Pheochromocytomas (and related extra-adrenal paragangliomas) are composed of chromaffin cells with abundant basophilic cytoplasm that contains secretory granules. The chromaffin cells can be arranged in either trabecular or alveolar patterns, and groups of cells are characteristically surrounded by a fibrovascular stroma. Both benign and malignant pheochromocytomas can contain pleomorphic cells and mitotic figures. Clinically malignant pheochromocytomas are consequently diagnosed only if distant metastases (lymph nodes, liver, lungs, or bones) are identified. A diagnosis of pheochromocytoma is usually confirmed by demonstrating elevated urinary levels of the catecholamine metabolites, metanephrine, and vanillylmandelic acid. Most patients with clinically malignant pheochromocytoma die within 3 years.

PINEAL GLAND AND THYMUS

PINEAL GLAND

The pineal gland produces melatonin, whose biologic actions are still not understood. While calcification of the pineal gland with increasing age is common, clinically significant pineal disease is rare and is most often due to germinoma, pineoblastoma, or pineocytoma. **Germinomas** and other tumors arising from embryonic germ cells (embryonal carcinomas, choriocarcinomas, teratomas) account for over one-half of pineal tumors and resemble their counterparts in testes and ovaries. **Pineoblastomas** are aggressive malignant tumors encountered in younger persons that tend to invade surrounding structures and cause death within 1 to 2 years. Pineoblastomas are usually composed of masses of pleomorphic cells with hyperchromatic nuclei that resemble neuroblastoma and may grow in poorly formed rosettes. **Pineocytomas** are observed in adults and tend to grow more slowly (average 7-year survival) than pineoblastomas. Both glial and neuronal differentiation may be present, and the cells may grow in large rosettes.

> **Tumors of the pineal gland include germinomas, pineoblastomas, and pineocytomas.**

THYMUS

While the thymus is also clearly a lymphoid organ, it is included in this section because it secretes hormones that facilitates the growth and differentiation of T-cell lymphocytes, including thymosin and thymopoietin. The thymus is vulnerable to agenesis and hypoplasia, hyperplasia, and tumors.

Agenesis and hypoplasia of the thymus can occur in several congenital forms (reticular dysgenesis, combined immunodeficiency disease, DiGeorge syndrome) that are characterized by profound T-cell deficiency and variable B-cell deficiency. Acquired hypoplasia occurs normally after puberty, but may be seen earlier in patients who have had malnutrition, radiotherapy, cytotoxic therapy, or glucocorticoid therapy. Acquired hypoplasia is usually asymptomatic.

> **Thymic agenesis occurs in several congenital forms.**

Hyperplasia of the thymus (thymic follicular hyperplasia) is characterized by the presence of germinal lymphoid centers that are usually located in the thymic medulla and may compress the cortex. Thymic hyperplasia is most commonly encountered in myasthenia gravis, but may also be seen in other chronic inflammatory and immunologic diseases, including Graves disease, Addison's disease, systemic lupus erythematosus, and others. The relationship between the inflammatory diseases and the thymic hyperplasia is still unclear.

> **Thymic hyperplasia is observed in myasthenia gravis.**

Both lymphomas and thymomas can arise in the thymus.

Malignant thymomas often extend beyond the thymic capsule.

Tumors can arise in the thymus in conditions including Hodgkin's disease, non-Hodgkin's lymphoma, and tumors of thymic epithelial cells known as thymomas. Rarely, other tumors can arise in germ cells, neuroendocrine cells, fibroblasts, vessels, or other minor components of the thymus.

Thymomas are usually benign but are sometimes malignant. The cells of both benign and malignant thymomas most often have large, pale nuclei and cytoplasm with poorly defined cell outlines. Variants may have spindle-shaped epithelial cells (that may sometimes appear similar to sarcoma cells), or cells with squamoid or reticular differentiation. Ultrasound studies demonstrate the epithelial nature of the cells by the presence of desmosomes and tonofilaments. A rich or scant lymphocytic infiltrate composed of T cells is present in all thymomas; this infiltrate, when extensive, can cause the thymoma to be mistaken for non-Hodgkin's lymphoma. **Malignant thymomas** are distinguished from benign thymomas by the presence of metastases or extension beyond the thymic capsule. If the cells appear cytologically malignant, as occurs only rarely, the term **"thymic carcinoma"** rather than malignant thymoma is used. The thymus can also contain thymic neuroendocrine tumors that histologically resemble carcinoid tumors or oat cell carcinoma of the lung and that may secrete ectopic hormones, including ACTH.

Thymomas are observed most often in middle-aged patients of both sexes. Some thymomas are found incidentally at surgery or chest radiography. Others cause symptoms due to pressure on the airways, esophagus, or vena cava. Somewhat less than one-half of patients have associated systemic disease, often the muscular weakness known as **myasthenia gravis.**

Other diseases sometimes associated with thymoma include bone marrow cytopenias, carcinoma, and many systemic diseases with autoimmune components. Most thymomas are benign and are cured by resection. The uncommon malignant thymomas and thymic carcinomas often cause death within 5 to 10 years. The presence of a concomitant systemic disorder is associated with a worse prognosis.

Suggested Readings

GENERAL PATHOLOGY TEXTS

The following books are standard pathology texts and contain additional factual information and some photographs.

Anderson JR: Muir's Textbook of Pathology. 12th Ed. Williams & Wilkins, Baltimore, 1988

Cotran RS et al: Robbins Pathological Basis of Disease. 3rd Ed. WB Saunders, Philadelphia, 1989

Rubin E et al: Pathology. JB Lippincott, Philadelphia, 1988

GENERAL SURGICAL PATHOLOGY TEXTS

Surgical pathology texts are written for pathology residents and contain detailed information about the histologic appearance of different diseases.

Rosai J: Ackerman's Surgical Pathology. 7th Ed. CV Mosby, St Louis, 1989

Silverberg SG: Principles and Practice of Surgical Pathology. Churchill Livingstone, New York, 1990

Sternberg SS: Diagnostic Surgical Pathology. Raven Press, New York, 1989

GENERAL ATLASES

General pathology atlases are usually affordable and are a source of pathology pictures. The Netter series of books, while somewhat older and too expensive for most medical students to buy, is commonly available in medical libraries and contains classic drawings of gross and microscopic pathology.

Curran RC: Color Atlas of Histopathology. 3rd Ed. Oxford University Press, New York, 1985

Gresham GA: A Color Atlas of General Pathology. 2nd Ed. Mosby Year Book, St Louis, 1992

Netter FH: The Ciba Collection of Medical Illustrations. 12 books. Ciba Medical, West Caldwell, NJ, 1970s and 1980s

Sandritter T: Macropathology: Text and Color Atlas. 5th Ed. Mosby Year Book, St Louis, 1990

SPECIALTY ATLASES

Specialty atlases are usually beautiful (but very expensive) books that contain large numbers of color photographs. If you have time, they are worth seeing in your medical school or pathology departmental libraries.

Atkinson BF: Atlas of Diagnostic Cytopathology. WB Saunders, Philadelphia, 1992

Begemann H, Rasketter J: Atlas of Clinical Hematology. Springer-Verlag, New York, 1989

Churg J et al: Renal Disease: Classification and Atlas of Glomerular Diseases (1982). Renal Disease: Classification and Atlas of Tubulointerstitial Diseases (1985). Igaku-Shoin, New York

Colby TV et al: Atlas of Pulmonary Surgical Pathology. WB Saunders, Philadelphia, 1991

Marcove RC, Arlen M: Atlas of Bone Pathology. JB Lippincott, Philadelphia, 1992

Mitros FA: Atlas of Gastrointestinal Pathology. JB Lippincott, Philadelphia, 1988

Olsen EG: Atlas of Cardiovascular Pathology. Kluwer Academic, Norwell, MA, 1987

Royal College of Surgeons of Edinburgh: Color Atlas of Demonstrations in Surgical Pathology. Williams & Wilkins, Baltimore, 1983

Skarin AT: Atlas of Diagnostic Oncology. JB Lippincott, Philadelphia, 1991

True LD: Atlas of Diagnostic Immunohistopathology. JB Lippincott, Philadelphia, 1990

Weller RO: Color Atlas of Neuropathology. Oxford University Press, New York, 1984

Wenig BM: Atlas of Head and Neck Pathology. WB Saunders, Philadelphia, 1993

Wold LE et al: Atlas of Orthopedic Pathology. WB Saunders, Philadelphia, 1991

Woodruff JD, Parmley TH: Atlas of Gynecologic Pathology. Grower, 1988

Woods GL, Gutierrez Y: Diagnostic Pathology of Infectious Diseases. Lea & Febiger, Philadelphia, 1993

Index

A

Abdomen, actinomycosis lesions involving, 56
Aberrant locations, of gallbladder, 277
Abetalipoproteinemia, 246
Abortion, in congenital syphilis, 53
Abscesses
   of brain, 180
   Brodie's, in pyogenic osteomyelitis, 140
   hepatic, 261
   injection, atypical mycobacteria causing, 55
   perinephric, 304
   pulmonary, 169–170
     "primary cryptogenic," 169
   of spleen, in nonspecific acute splenitis, 104
   subperiosteal, in pyogenic osteomyelitis, 140
Absidia infections, 60
Acanthamoeba infections, 63–64
Acanthosis nigricans, 114
Accessory axillary breast tissue, 323
Acetaminophen toxicity, 10–11
Achalasia, 232
Achondroplasia, 3, 146
Acinar cell carcinomas, pancreatic, 281
Acne
   conglobata, 111
   vulgaris, 110–111
Acoustic neuromas, 152
Acquired immunodeficiency syndrome (AIDS), 23–24
   central nervous system in, 181, 182
   Pneumocystis carinii infections in, 65
Acrochordon (fibroepithelial polyps; skin tags; squamous papilloma), 114
Actinic keratoses, 115–116
Actinomyces infections, 56
Actinomycetes, 56
Actinomycosis, 56
   cervicofacial, 56
Acute tubular necrosis. *See* Tubular necrosis, acute.
Adamantinomas (craniopharyngiomas; ameloblastomas), 346
Addison's disease (chronic primary adrenocortical insufficiency), 363–364
   autoimmune, 364
   in tuberculosis, 55
Adenocarcinomas

   of bile ducts, 277
   of bladder, 309
   bronchogenic, 170
   cervical, 334
     clear cell, 334
   colonic, 254
   esophageal, 234
   gastric, 239
   ovarian, clear cell, 340
   pancreatic, 281
   prostatic, 320–321
   small intestinal, 248
   thyroid, 353
   vaginal, 332
     clear cell, 332
   vulvar, 332
Adenomas. *See also* Fibroadenomas.
   of bile ducts, 269
   of breasts, tubular, 324
   colonic
     tubular, 253
     tubulovillous, 253
     villous, 253–254
   of gallbladder, 276
   gastric
     tubular, 239
     villous, 239
   lactating, 324
   parathyroid, 356
   pituitary. *See* Pituitary gland, adenomas of.
   renal, 269
     cortical, 300
   thyroid, 348–349
     colloid, 348
     embryonal (trabecular), 348
     fetal, 348
     Hürthle cell, 349
     microfollicular and macrofollicular patterns of, 349
     simple, 348
Adenomatoid tumors, testicular, 319
Adenomatous (multinodular; multiple colloid adenomatous) goiter, 350
   intrathoracic (plunging), 350
Adenomatous hyperplasia
   with atypia (complex endometrial hyperplasia with atypia), 337
   without atypia (complex endometrial hyperplasia without atypia), 337
Adenomatous polyps, small intestinal, 248
Adenomyomas, of gallbladder, 276
Adenomyosis, 335–336

Adenosis, vaginal, 332
Adenosquamous carcinomas
   of bile ducts, 277
   bronchogenic, 170
   cervical, 334
   colonic, 255
   pancreatic, 281
Adenoviruses
   digestive tract infections caused by, 28
   respiratory infections caused by, 28
Adenylate cyclase, in *Vibrio cholerae* infections, 45
ADH (antidiuretic hormone), persistent, inappropriate secretion of, 347
Adhesions, intestinal, 246–247
Adhesive mediastinopericarditis, 229
Adnexal tumors, of skin, 115
Adrenal glands, 361–366
   adrenal cortex
     developmental anomalies of, 361
     hyperfunction of, 361–363
     hypofunction of, 363–365
     idiopathic atrophy of, 363
   adrenal medulla, tumors of, 365–366
   nonfunctional mass lesions of, 365
Adrenal hyperplasia, congenital, 362–363
Adrenal hypoplasia
   congenital, anencephalic, 361
   cytomegalic, 361
Adrenal tissue, ectopic, 361
Adrenal virilism, 362
Adrenocortical hypofunction, 363
Adrenocortical insufficiency, primary
   acute, 364–365
   chronic (Addison's disease), 363–364
     autoimmune, 364
     in tuberculosis, 55
Adrenoleukodystrophy/adrenomyeloneuropathy, 179
Adult hemolytic uremic syndrome, 288
Adult onset (insulin-independent; type II) diabetes mellitus, 358, 359
Adult polycystic kidney disease, 284
Adult respiratory distress syndrome, 161
Adult T-cell leukemia/lymphoma, 92–93, 121
Adverse drug reactions, 10–11
Aeromonas hydrophila infections, gastroenterocolitis and, 243
African trypanosomiasis, 66–67
Agenesis
   esophageal, 231

Agenesis *(Continued)*
  of gallbladder, 277
  renal, 283
  thymic, 367
  of thyroid gland, 355
Agyria (lissencephaly), 177
AIDS (acquired immunodeficiency syndrome), 23–24
  central nervous system in, 181
  Pneumocystis carinii infections in, 65
AIDS-related complex (ARDS), 24
AIDS-related dementia, 182
Air conditioner lung, 167
Albers-Schönberg disease ("marble bones"; osteopetrosis), 146
  adult pattern of, 146
Albinism, 6, 117
Albright (McCune-Albright) syndrome, 145
Alcohol
  ethyl
    central nervous system and, 178
    toxicity of, 9
  methyl
    central nervous system and, 178
    toxicity of, 9
Alcoholic steatosis (fatty liver), 262
  macrovesicular, 262
  microvesicular, 262
Alcoholism
  chronic pancreatitis and, 280
  dilated cardiomyopathy and, 220
  liver disease and. *See* Liver diseases, alcoholic.
  neuropathy in, 19
Aldosterone
  deficiency of, 365
  deficient synthesis of, 362–363
  sodium homeostasis and, 286
"Aleukemic" anemia, 80
Alkaline phosphatase
  in chronic myeloid leukemia, 96
  leukocyte, in myeloid metaplasia, 99
Alkaptonuria, 7
Allergic aspergillosis, 60
Allergic (atopic; reagin-mediated) asthma, 165
Allergic granulomatosis/angiitis (Churg-Strauss syndrome), 204
Allergic rhinitis (hay fever), 152–153
Allergies, atopic, 20
Alport syndrome, 295
Alveolar rhabdomyosarcomas, 125
Alzheimer's disease, 190–191
Amebiasis, 63
Amebic hepatitis (amebic liver abscess), 262
Amebic meningoencephalitis, 63–64
Ameloblastomas (adamantinomas; craniopharyngiomas), 346
American trypanosomiasis. *See* Chagas disease.
Ampulla of Vater, carcinoma of, 277
Amputation (traumatic) neuromas, 197
Amyloid angiopathy, 190
Amyloidosis, 26
  cardiac, restrictive cardiomyopathy and, 221

  familial, 26
  glomerular lesions associated with, 295
  liver and, 273
  localized, 26
  primary systemic, 26
  secondary systemic, 26
  in tuberculosis, 55
  tumor amyloid, 26
Amylopectinosis (type IV glycogen storage disease), 4–5, 273
Amyotrophic lateral sclerosis, 192–193
Anaerobes
  gram-negative, 42
  gram-positive, 46
Analgesic abuse nephropathy, 298
Anaphylaxis (type I hypersensitivity), 19–20
  local reactions, 20
  systemic, 20
Ancylostoma infections
  Ancylostoma duodenale, 69
  hepatic abscesses and, 262
Andersen's disease (type IV glycogen storage disease), 4–5, 273
Androblastomas (Sertoli cell tumors)
  ovarian, 342
  testicular, 318
Anemias
  "aleukemic," 80
  aplastic, 80
  of blood loss, 77
  in chronic myeloid leukemia, 96
  of diminished erythropoiesis, 78–79
    megaloblastic, 79
  Fanconi's, 80
  hemolytic. *See* Hemolytic anemias.
  immunohemolytic. *See* Hemolytic anemias, autoimmune (immunohemolytic).
  iron deficiency, 17, 79–80
  megaloblastic, 16, 79
  microcytic, iron deficiency and, 17
  pernicious, 79
    juvenile, 79
  pure red cell aplasia, 80
  sickle cell, 4
Anemic anoxia, 186
Anemic infarcts, 187–188
Anencephaly, 176
Aneurysm(s), 201–203
  aortic dissection (dissecting aneurysm; dissecting hematoma), 188, 202–203
    type A, 202–203
    type B, 203
  atherosclerotic, 201–202
  Charcot-Bouchard, 185
  cystic medial necrosis and, 202
  syphilitic, 202
Aneurysmal vessel, 185
"Angel dust" (phencyclidine hydrochloride), adverse effects of, 11
Angiitis
  allergic (Churg-Strauss syndrome), 204
  hypersensitivity (leukocytoclastic angiitis; microscopic polyarteritis), 204
Angina pectoris, 215
  Prinzmetal's variant, 215
  stable (typical), 215

  unstable (crescendo), 215
Angiodysplasias, 250
Angioedema, 107
Angiofibromas, nasopharyngeal, 153
Angiolipomas, 123
Angiomas
  of eye, 155
  small intestinal, 248
Angiomyolipomas, renal, 300
Angioneurotic edema, hereditary, 107
Angiopathy, amyloid, 190
Angiosarcomas
  cardiac, 223
  hepatic, 271
Anitschkow cells, 224
Ankylosing spondylitis (Marie-Strümpell disease; rheumatoid spondylitis), 131
Ankylosis
  bony, 130
  fibrous, 130
Anogenital warts, 111
Anopheles mosquitoes, 65
Anovulatory cycles, 336
Anoxia, 186–187
  anemic, 186
  histotoxic, 186
  stagnant (ischemic), 186
Anterior pituitary insufficiency, 346
Anterior spinal artery, 188
Anthrax, 48
Antibiotics, toxicity of, 11
Antibody-dependent cell-mediated cytotoxicity reactions, 20
Anticancer agents. *See* Antineoplastic agents.
Antidiuretic hormone (ADH), persistent, inappropriate secretion of, 347
Antigen-antibody complexes, circulating, deposition of, 20–21
Antineoplastic agents
  central nervous system and, 178
  cystitis and, 308
  toxicity of, 11
  vitamin A as, 14
Antioxidants, vitamin E as, 14
Antireceptor antibodies, 20
Antitoxin
  for botulism, 47
  for tetanus, 46
α^1-Antitrypsin deficiency, 265
Antoni A areas, 198
Antoni B areas, 198
Aorta
  coarctation of, 214
    postductal ("adult form"), 214
    preductal ("infantile form"), 214
  double-barreled, 203
  in tertiary syphilis, 53
  transpositions of the great arteries and, 212
Aortic arch, syphilitic aneurysms of, 202
Aortic dissection (dissecting aneurysm; dissecting hematoma), 188, 202–203
  type A, 202–203
  type B, 203

Aortic valvular atresia, 214
Aortic valvular stenosis, 214
    calcific, 223–224
Aphthous ulcers (canker sores), 154
Aplastic anemia, 80
Aplastic crises, in sickle cell disease, 83
Appendicitis, 249
    acute, simple, 249
    chronic, 249
    gangrenous, 249
    suppurative, 249
Arachnodactyly, 3
Arbovirus (arthropod-borne virus) infections, 31
    encephalitis and, 180–181
ARDS (AIDS-related complex), 24
Ariboflavinosis, 15
Arnold-Chiari malformations, 176
    type I, 176
    type II, 176
    type III, 176
Arteries
    arteriosclerosis and, 199–200
    congenital diseases of, 199
Arteriolitis, hyperplastic, 287
Arteriolosclerosis, 200
    hyaline, 200
    hyperplastic, 200
Arteriopathy, pulmonary, plexogenic, 163
Arteriosclerosis. See also Arteriolosclerosis;
    Atherosclerosis.
    hyaline, 286
    hyperlipidemia and, 201
    Mönckeberg's (medial calcific sclerosis),
      199–200
Arteriovenous malformations, 186
    fistulas, 199
Arteritis
    pulmonary, in schistosomiasis, 76
    rheumatoid, in rheumatic heart disease,
      225
    Takayasu's (pulseless disease), 205–206
    temporal (giant cell), 205
Arthritis
    acute, in gout, 133
    in acute rheumatic fever, 134
    chronic, in gout, 133
    gonococcal, 40
    in inflammatory bowel disease, 134
    in Lyme disease, 132
    migratory polyarthritis, acute, 224–225
    osteoarthritis, 129
    in psoriasis, 134
    in Reiter syndrome, 134
    rheumatoid, 129–131
      cardiac involvement in, 223
      variants of, 131
    suppurative, 131–132
      in pyogenic osteomyelitis, 140
    in systemic lupus erythematosus, 24
    tuberculous, 134
Arthropathy, hydroxyapatite, 134
Arthropod-borne viruses (arboviruses), 31
    encephalitis and, 180–181
Arthus reaction, 21
Arylsulfatase A (cerebroside sulfatase) defi-

ciency, 178
Ascaris lumbricoides infections, 68–69
Aschoff bodies, 224
Aschoff cells, 224
Ascorbic acid (vitamin C) deficiency, 16
Aspergillomas (fungus balls), 60
Aspergillosis, 60
    allergic, 60
    localized involvement in, 60
    pulmonary, invasive, 60
    rhinocerebral form of, 60
Aspergillus infections
    Aspergillus flavus, hepatocellular carcinoma and, 269
    Aspergillus fumigatus, 60
    Aspergillus niger, 60
    encephalitis and, 183
    endocarditis and, 226
    myocarditis and, 219
    orbital, 156
    pulmonary, 168
Aspirin
    Reye syndrome caused by, 28, 183, 272
    toxicity of, 11
Asteroid bodies, in sarcoidosis, 58
Asthma. See Bronchial asthma.
Astrocytomas, 193
    anaplastic, 193
Asymmetric septal hypertrophy (hypertrophic cardiomyopathy; hypertrophic obstructive cardiomyopathy; idiopathic hypertrophic subaortic stenosis), 221
Ataxia
    Friedrich's, 190
    telangiectasia, 23
Atelectasis, 159–160
Atheroembolic renal disease, 288
Atheromatous plaques, 200–201
    "complicated," 201
    renal, 288
Atherosclerosis, 200–201
    acute myocardial infarction and, 216
    aneurysms and, 201–202
    in diabetes mellitus, 360
    hypertension and, 217
Athlete's foot (tinea pedis), 112
Atopic (allergic; reagin-mediated) asthma,
    165
Atresia
    esophageal, 231
    small intestinal, 242
Atrial septal defect, 213
Atrophic vulvitis, chronic (lichen sclerosis),
    330
Atrophy
    adrenal, idiopathic, 363
    endometrial, cystic, senile, 337
    testicular, 314–315
Atypical lobular hyperplasia, of breast, 326
Atypical mycobacteria, 55
Autoantibodies, in systemic lupus erythematosus, 24
Autoimmune Addison's disease, 364
Autoimmune diseases, 19. See also specific
    diseases.
Autoimmune hemolytic anemias. See

Hemolytic anemias, autoimmune
    (immunohemolytic).
Autoimmune thyroiditis (Hashimoto's thyroiditis; stroma lymphomatosa), 350
    fibrosing, 350
Autosomal chromosomal abnormalities. See
    Chromosomal diseases, autosomal.
"Autosplenectomy," in sickle cell disease, 83
Axon(s)
    degeneration of, 197
    regeneration of, 197
Axonal injury, diffuse, 184

B

Babesia bovis infections, 66
Babesia microti infections, 66
Bacillary dysentery, 44
Bacillus anthracis infections, 48
Bacteremia, atypical mycobacteria causing,
    55
Bacterial endocarditis. See Endocarditis,
    infective (bacterial).
Bacterial infections, 32–58. See also specific
    bacteria and infections.
    actinomycetes, 56
    acute calculous cholecystitis and, 274
    acute endometritis and, 335
    in AIDS, 23–24
    in children, 42–43
    chlamydial. See Chlamydia infections.
    cholangitis and, 261
    clostridial. See Clostridium infections.
    cystitis and, 308
    encephalitis and, 180
    endocarditis and, 225–226
    enteric, 43–46
      bacillary dysentery, 44
      Helicobacter, 45
      cholera, 45
      Escherichia coli, 43
      Salmonella, 43–44
      Yersinia, 45–46
    epididymal, 313
    gastroenterocolitis and, 243
    gonococcal, 40
    gram-negative bacilli, 40–42
    hepatic abscesses and, 261
    meningitis and, 179
    meningococcal, 39–40
    mycobacterial. See Mycobacterium infections.
    mycoplasmal. See Mycoplasma infections.
    myocarditis and, 219
    in needle users, 11
    pneumococcal, 39
    prostatitis and, 319
    pseudomembranous colitis and, 252–253
    pulmonary, 168, 169
    pyogenic osteomyelitis and, 140
    rapidly progressive glomerulonephritis
      and, 292
    rickettsial. See Rickettsia infections.
    sarcoidosis, 58
    staphylococcal. See Staphylococcus infections.

Bacterial infections *(Continued)*
  streptococcal. *See Streptococcus* infections.
  testicular, 313
  treponemes. *See* Treponemal infections.
  uncommon, 56–58
    bartonellosis, 58
    chancroid, 57
    granuloma inguinale, 57
    ozena, 57
    rhinoscleroma, 56–57
  ureteral, 307
  urinary, 303
  urolithiasis and, 303
Bacterial invasive enterocolitis, 243
Bacterial overgrowth syndrome, 244–245
Bacteroides fragilis infections, 42
  of brain, 180
Bacteroides melaninogenicus infections, 42
Baker's cysts, 136
Balanoposthitis, 311
Balantidium coli infections, 63
Barrett's mucosa, 234
Bartholin's cyst, 330
Bartonella bacilliformis infections, 58
Basal cell carcinomas
  of skin, 116
  vulvar, 332
Basal cell nevus syndrome
  basal cell carcinoma of skin and, 116
  ovarian fibromas and, 341
Basal ganglia, degenerative diseases of, 191–192
Basement membrane, of glomerular capillaries, thickening of, 294
Becker muscular dystrophy, 138
Bejel, 53
Bence Jones proteins, in multiple myeloma, 100
Benign fibrous histiocytoma, 119
Benign prostatic hypertrophy/hyperplasia (nodular hyperplasia), 319–320
Benign sclerosing ductal proliferation (radial scar), 326
Berger's disease (IgA nephropathy), 296
Beriberi
  "dry," 15
  "wet," 15
Bernard-Soulier syndrome, 87
Bile canaliculi, hepatocellular carcinoma and, 269
Bile ducts
  adenomas of, 269
  carcinomas of, 277
Bile pigment, hepatocellular carcinoma and, 269
Bilharziasis, hepatic abscesses and, 262
Biliary atresia, extrahepatic, 272
Biliary cirrhosis
  primary, 265–266
    florid inflammation in, 265
    proliferation of ducts in, 265–266
  secondary, 266
Biliary system
  chronic pancreatitis and, 280
  extrahepatic, 274–278. *See also* Gallbladder.

cholelithiasis and, 275–276
  tumors of, 276–277
Binswanger's disease (subcortical leukoencephalopathy), 188
Binucleate plasma cells, in multiple myeloma, 100
Bird fancier's disease (pigeon breeder's lung), 167
Blackwater fever, 66
Bladder, 307–309
  congenital anomalies of, 307–308
  cystitis and, 308
  in schistosomiasis, 76
  tumors of, 308–309
    benign, 309
    malignant, 308–309
"Blast crisis", in chronic myeloid leukemia, 97
Blastomyces infections
  Blastomyces dermatitidis, 61
  encephalitis and, 183
  myocarditis and, 219
Blastomycosis, 61
  cutaneous, 61
  pulmonary, 61
Bleeding. *See also* Hemorrhage; *headings beginning with term* Hemorrhagic.
  uterine, dysfunctional, 336–337
Blepharoblasts, 194
Blisters, 112. *See also* Skin, blistering diseases of.
  in erythema multiforme, 108
  fever (cold sore; herpes labialis), 154
  microscopic, in dermatitis herpetiformis, 113
Blood. *See* Anemias; Hematopoietic system, erythrocyte disorders.
Blood dyscrasias. *See also* Plasma cell dyscrasias.
  drug-induced, 10
Blood loss
  acute, 77
  chronic, 77
Blood vessels. *See* Arteries; Vasculature; Veins.
"Blue-dome cysts," 325
Blue nevus, 118
Blue sclera, in osteogenesis imperfecta, 145
Bone(s), 140–149
  defects in maturation of, 144–145
    fibrous cortical defects, 145
    fibrous dysplasia, 144–145
  fractures of. *See* Fractures.
  hereditary disorders of, 145–147
    achondroplasia, 146
    exostoses, 146–147
    osteogenesis imperfecta, 145–146
    osteoporosis, 146
  infections of, 140–141
    pyogenic osteomyelitis, 140–141
    syphilis, 141
    tuberculosis, 141
  one, secondary diseases of, 143–144
    hyperparathyroid-induced skeletal changes, 143–144
    osteomalacia, 143

osteoporosis and, 142
    Paget's disease of (osteitis deformans), 142–143
  secondary diseases of
    hypertrophic osteoarthropathy, 144
    renal osteodystrophy, 144
    rickets, 143
  tumors of, 147–149
    chondromatous, 148–149
    osteoblastic, 147–148
    of unknown origin, 149
Bone marrow
  in aplastic anemia, 80
  failure of, 81
  in hemolytic anemias, 77–78
  in leukemias, 95, 97–98
    depression of normal function of, 95
  in megaloblastic anemias, 79
  in neutropenia, 89
  transplantation of, transplant rejection and, 22
Bony ankylosis, 130
Border zone (watershed) infarcts, 187
Bordetella pertussis infections, 42
Borrelia infections
  Borrelia burgdorferi. See Lyme disease.
  Borrelia recurrentis, 50–51
  myocarditis and, 219
Botryoid rhabdomyosarcomas, 125
Botulism, 46–47
Bowel. *See* Colon; Small intestine.
Bowenoid papulosis, 312
Bowen's disease, 312
Brain. *See also* Central nervous system.
  abscesses of, 180
  healing of, 12
  left-sided congestive heart failure and, 218
  Wilson's disease and, 265
Brainstem
  degenerative diseases of, 191–192
  gliomas of, 194
Branhamella catarrhalis infections, conjunctival, 155
Breakbone fever, 31
Breasts, 323–343
  congenital anomalies of, 323
  fibrocystic disease of, 325–326
    simple fibrocystic change, 325–326
  inflammations of, 323–324
    acute mastitis, 323
    fat necrosis, 324
    galactocele, 324
    mammary duct ectasia, 324
  male, diseases of, 329
  supernumerary, 323
  tumors of, 324–325
    carcinomas, 326–328
    fibroadenoma, 324
    intraductal papilloma, 325
    phyllodes tumor (cystosarcoma phyllodes), 325
Brenner tumors, 340
Brill-Zinsser disease, 35
"Brittle bones," 145
Brodie's abscess, in pyogenic osteomyelitis, 140

Bronchial asthma, 165–166
  atopic (allergic; reagin-mediated), 165
  nonreaginic, 165
  occupational, 165
  pharmacologic, 165
Bronchial carcinoids, 171
Bronchiectasis, 166
Bronchiolitis fibrosa obliterans, 165
Bronchioloalveolar carcinomas, 170
Bronchitis, chronic, 164–165
  obstructive, 165
  simple, 165
Bronchogenic carcinomas, 170–171
  adenosquamous, 170
  small cell, 170
  squamous cell (epidermoid), 170
Bronchogenic cysts, 159
Bronchopneumonia, 167–168
Bronchopulmonary sequestration, 159
"Brown tumors" (reparative giant cell granulomas), 144
Brucella abortus infections, 49
Brucella melitensis infections, 49
Brucellosis
  acute self-limited, 49
  carrier state in, 49
  chronic, 49
Brugia malayi infections, 71
Bruton's hypogammaglobulinemia, 23
Bubonic plague, 48–49
Buboes
  in bubonic plague, 49
  in chancroid, 57
Budd-Chiari syndrome, 267
Buerger's disease (thromboangiitis obliterans), 206
Bulbar palsy, progressive, 192–193
Bullae, 112
Bullous emphysema, 164
Bullous pemphigoid, 113
Burkitt's lymphoma, 92
  in Epstein-Barr virus infections, 31
Bursitis, 135–136
Buschke-Lowenstein tumor (giant condyloma; verrucous carcinoma), 312
Byssinosis, 167

C

Calcific aortic valve stenosis, 223–224
Calcification, of mitral annulus, 227
Calcific sclerosis, medial (Mönckeberg's arteriosclerosis), 199–200
Calcium crystal deposition arthritis, 134
Calcium metabolism, vitamin D and, 14
Calcium oxalate urolithiasis, 302–303
Calculi, urinary, 302–303
Call-Exner bodies, 341
Callus
  fibrocartilaginous, 142
  osseous, 142
  procallus, 142
Calymmatobacterium donovani infections, 57

Helicobacter infections
  Helicobacter jejuni, 45
  Helicobacter pylori, 45
  enteric, 45
Cancer. *See* Tumor(s).
Candida infections
  Candida albicans, 59
    cystitis and, 308
    of oral cavity, 154–155
  Candida glabrata (Torulopsis glabrata), 59
  encephalitis and, 183
  endocarditis and, 226
  gastroenterocolitis and, 243
  myocarditis and, 219
  oral (moniliasis; thrush), 59, 154–155
  orbital, 156
  pseudomembranous colitis and, 252
  pulmonary, 168
  urinary, 304
Canker sores (aphthous ulcers), 154
Capillaria hepatica infections, hepatic abscesses and, 262
Capillaria philippinensis infections, 70
Capillary basement membrane, glomerular, thickening of, 294
Capillary hemangiomas, 186, 207
Carbon monoxide, toxicity of, 10
Carbuncle, 37
Carcinogens, 10
Carcinoids (endocrine cell tumors; neuroendocrine tumors)
  bronchial, 171
  cardiac, 227
  gastric, 241
  ovarian, 340
  small intestinal, 248
    foregut, 248
    hindgut, 248
    midgut, 248
  stromal, 340
Carcinomas. *See also* Adenocarcinomas; Cholangiocarcinomas; Choriocarcinomas; Comedocarcinomas; Cystadenocarcinomas.
  acinar cell, pancreatic, 281
  adenosquamous. *See* Adenosquamous carcinomas.
  basal cell
    of skin, 116
    vulvar, 332
  of bile ducts
    adenosquamous, 277
    squamous cell, 277
  of bile ducts and ampulla of Vater, 277
  of bladder, 309
    squamous cell, 309
    transitional cell, 309
  of breast, 326–328, 329
    colloid (mucinous), 327
    ductal, invasive, not otherwise specified, 327
    lobular, 327, 328
    in males, 329
    medullary, 327

  in situ, 326–328
  uncommon forms of, 328
  bronchioloalveolar, 170
  bronchogenic. *See* Bronchogenic carcinomas.
  cervical, 334
    invasive, 334
    undifferentiated, 334
  clear cell. *See* Clear cell carcinomas.
  colloid (mucinous), of breast, 327
  colonic
    adenosquamous, 255
    poorly differentiated, 255
    small cell undifferentiated, 255
  embryonal. *See* Embryonal carcinomas.
  endometrial, 338
  esophageal, squamous cell, 233
  of gallbladder, 276–277
  gastric, 239–240
    expanding, 240
    "gastric-infiltrative," 239
    infiltrative, 240
    "intestinal-type," 239
    undifferentiated, 240
  hepatocellular, 269–270
    drug-induced, 273
    fibrolamellar variant of, 270
  intraductal, 326–327
    of breast, 326–328
  large cell, bronchogenic, 170
  laryngeal, 154
  lobular, of breast, 327
    in situ, 327
  medullary. *See* Medullary carcinomas.
  Merkel cell, 117
  ovarian, embryonal, 341
  pancreatic, 281
    acinar cell, 281
    adenosquamous, 281
  parathyroid, 356
  penile
    in situ, 312
    squamous cell, 312
    verrucous (Buschke-Lowenstein tumor; giant condyloma), 312
  prostatic, 320–321
  renal cell, 301
  of renal pelvis, urothelial, 302
  in situ. *See* In situ carcinomas.
  of skin
    basal cell, 116
    in situ, 116
    squamous cell, 116
  small intestinal, 248
  squamous cell (epidermoid). *See* Squamous cell (epidermoid) carcinomas.
  testicular, embryonal, infantile (endodermal sinus tumors; yolk sac tumors), 316
  "thymic," 368
  thyroid, 353–354
    follicular, 353–354
    medullary, 354. *See also* Multiple endocrine neoplasia.

Carcinomas *(Continued)*
    papillary, 353
    undifferentiated, 354
   undifferentiated. *See* Undifferentiated
    carcinomas.
   ureteral, 307
   verrucous
    penile (Buschke-Lowenstein tumor;
      giant condyloma), 312
    vulvar, 331
   vulvar, verrucous, 331
Carcinomatous cirrhosis, 266
Cardiac amyloidosis
   restrictive cardiomyopathy and, 221
   senile isolated, 221
Cardiac failure. *See also* Congestive heart
    failure.
   in Chagas disease, 67
Cardiac rhabdomyomas, 124
Cardiac sclerosis, 267
   cirrhosis and, 266
Cardiomyopathy, 220–222
   dilated (congestive cardiomyopathy;
    Keshan disease), 18, 220
   hypertrophic (asymmetric septal hyper-
    trophy; hypertrophic obstructive car-
    diomyopathy; idiopathic hypertrophic
    subaortic stenosis), 221
   restrictive (infiltrative; obliterative),
    221–222
   secondary, 222
Cardiovascular diseases, 186–187, 199–229.
    See also Aneurysm(s); Arteries;
    Heart; Vasculature; Veins; *specific
    diseases.*
Carditis, acute, rheumatic fever and, 224
Caroli's disease, 268
Carrier state
   in brucellosis, 49
   in viral hepatitis, 259
Carrión's disease (Oroya fever), 58
Caruncles, ureteral, 307
Caseous pericarditis, 228–229
Cataracts, 156–157
Catecholamines, pheochromocytoma secre-
    tion of, 366
Cat-scratch disease, 52
Cauliflower ear, 151
Cavernous hemangiomas, 186, 207–208
   hepatic, 269
Cecum, malignant tumors of, 254
Celiac sprue (celiac disease; gluten-sensitive
    enteropathy; nontropical sprue), 113,
    245
Cellulitis, necrotizing, 47
Central core disease, 139
Central nervous system, 175–196. *See also*
    Brain; Spinal cord.
   cerebral edema and, 175–176
   degenerative diseases of, 190–193
    of basal ganglia and brainstem,
     191–192
    of cerebral cortex, 190–191
    of motor neurons, 192–193
    spinocerebellar degeneration, 190
   demyelinating diseases of, 189–190

multiple sclerosis, 189
   perivenous encephalomyelitis, 189–190
   encephalitis and. *See* Encephalitis.
   environmental disorders and, 178
   hydrocephalus and, 176
   inborn errors of metabolism and, 178–179
   increased intracranial pressure and, 175
   intracranial hemorrhage and. *See*
    Intracranial hemorrhage.
   left-sided congestive heart failure and,
    219
   malformations and developmental dis-
    eases of, 176–177
   meningitis and. *See* Meningitis.
   meningovascular syphilis and, 53
   nutritional disorders and, 177–178
   in tertiary syphilis, 53
   trauma to, 183–184
   tumors of, 193–196
    astrocytoma, 193
    choroid plexus papilloma, 194–195
    ependymoma, 194
    glioblastoma multiforme, 193–194
    lymphomas and leukemias, 196
    of meninges, 195–196
    of neuronal origin, 195
    oligodendroglioma, 194
    of primitive or undifferentiated cells,
     195
   vascular diseases of, 186–188
    cerebral infarction, 187–188
    hypertensive, 188
    ischemic encephalopathy, 187
    of spinal cord, 188
Central pontine myelinolysis, 178
Centriacinar (centrilobular) emphysema,
    164
Centronuclear (myotubular) myopathy, 139
Cercariae, free-swimming, 75
Cerebral cortex, degenerative diseases of,
    190–191
Cerebral edema, 175–176
   cytotoxic, 175–176
   interstitial, 176
   vasogenic, 175
Cerebral infarction, 187–188
   anemic, 187–188
   hemorrhagic, 188
Cerebroside sulfatase (arylsulfatase A) defi-
    ciency, 178
Cervical dysplasia (cervical intraepithelial
    neoplasia), 333–334
Cervical tumors
   benign, 333
   malignant, 333–334
Cervicitis, 332–333
   acute, 332–333
   chlamydial, 32
   chronic, 333
   follicular, 333
Cervicofacial actinomycosis, 56
Cestodes, 72–73
   cysticercosis, 72–73
   echinococcosis, 73
   hepatic abscesses and, 262
   intestinal tapeworms, 72–73

Chagas disease (American trypanosomia-
    sis), 67–68
   achalasia and, 232
   hepatic abscesses and, 262
   megacolon and, 249
   myocarditis and, 219
Chalazion, 155
Chancre, in African trypanosomiasis, 66
Chancroid (soft chancre), 57
Charcot-Bouchard aneurysms, 185
Charcot-Marie-Tooth disease, hypertrophic
    type (peroneal muscular atrophy; sen-
    sory motor neuropathy, type I heredi-
    tary), 198
Charcot type multiple sclerosis, 189
Chemicals, hepatitis induced by, 260
Chemotherapy. *See* Antineoplastic agents.
Chickenpox (varicella), 30
Childhood hemolytic uremic syndrome,
    287–288
Childhood polycystic kidney disease, 284
Children. *See also* Infant(s); Neonates;
    headings beginning with term
    Juvenile.
   bacterial infections in, 42–43
   suppurative arthritis in, 131–132
Chlamydia infections
   cervicitis and, 32
   Chlamydia psittaci, 32
   Chlamydia trachomatis, 33–34
    conjunctival, 155, 156
    epididymal, 313
    prostatitis and, 319
   cystitis and, 308
   inclusion conjunctivitis and, 33
   lymphogranuloma venereum and, 33–34
   pulmonary, 169
   trachoma and, 33
   ureteral, 307
   urethritis and, 32
Cholangiocarcinomas, 270
Cholangitis, 261
   ascending, 261
   sclerosing, primary, 261
Cholecystitis, 274–275
   acute
    acalculous, 274–275
    calculous, 274
   chronic, 275
Cholelithiasis (gallstones), 275–276
   cholesterol and mixed stones, 275–276
   pigment stones, 276
Cholera, 45
Cholestasis, neonatal, 272
Cholesteatomas, 152
Cholesterolosis, 278
Cholesterol stones, 275
Chondroblastomas, 148
Chondrocalcinosis (pseudogout), 134
Chondrodermatitis nodularis helicis, 151
Chondromas, 148
Chondromatous tumors, 148–149
Chondromyxoid fibromas, 148
Chondrosarcomas, 148–149
   clear cell variant of, 149
   primary, 148

secondary, 148–149
Chorea
    Huntington's, 3
    Sydenham's, in rheumatic heart disease, 225
Choriocarcinomas, 317
    ovarian, 341
Choroid plexus papilloma, 194–195
Christmas disease (factor IX deficiency; hemophilia B), 7, 88
Chromomycosis, 62
Chromosomal diseases, 2–7
    autosomal abnormalities, 3–7
        dominant, 3, 191
        intermediate, 4
        recessive, 4–7, 146
    sex chromosome abnormalities, 2
    X-linked, 7, 179
Chromosomes, double, minute, in neuroblastomas, 127
Chronic interstitial pneumonitis (cryptogenic fibrosing alveolitis; Hamman-Rich syndrome; idiopathic pulmonary fibrosis; usual interstitial pneumonitis), 166
Chronic obstructive pulmonary disease, 163–166
    bronchial asthma, 165–166
    bronchiectasis, 166
    chronic bronchitis, 164–165
    emphysema, 164
Churg-Strauss syndrome (allergic granulomatosis/angiitis), 204
Chylocele, 315
Chylothorax, 174
Cigarette smoking, 9
Cirrhosis, 257, 263–266
    alcoholic, 263
        early, 263
        late, 263
    α^1-antitrypsin deficiency and, 265
    biliary
        primary, 265–266
        secondary, 266
    carcinomatous, 266
    cryptogenic, 266
    drug-induced, 273
    hemochromatosis and, 264
    hepatic, congestive splenomegaly caused by, 104
    macronodular, 257
    micronodular, 257
    postnecrotic, 263–264
    Wilson's disease and, 265
Civatte (colloid) bodies, in lichen planus, 110
Clear cell adenocarcinomas
    cervical, 334
    ovarian, 340
    vaginal, 332
Clear cell carcinomas, thyroid, 354
Clear cell chondrosarcomas, 149
Clonorchis sinensis infections, 74
    hepatic abscesses and, 262
Closed (simple) fractures, 141
Clostridium infections, 46–47

botulism and, 46–47
Clostridium botulinum, 46–47
    gastroenterocolitis and, 243
Clostridium difficile, 47
    pseudomembranous colitis and, 251–252
Clostridium perfringens (welchii), 47
Clostridium tetani, 46
    pseudomembranous colitis and, 47
    septic, 47
    tetanus and, 46
Clotting factor abnormalities, 87–88
    acquired, 87
    factor IX deficiency (Christmas disease; hemophilia B), 7, 88
    factor VIII deficiency (classic hemophilia; hemophilia A), 7, 87–88
    hereditary, 87
    vitamin K and, 15
Coagulopathy, consumption, disseminated intravascular coagulation and, 85
Coarctation of the aorta, 214
    postductal ("adult form"), 214
    preductal ("infantile form"), 214
Cobalamin (vitamin B^{12}) deficiency
    central nervous system and, 177–178
    megaloblastic anemia caused by, 16
Cocaine, adverse effects of, 11
Coccidioides infections
    Coccidioides immitis, 61–62
        myocarditis and, 219
    encephalitis and, 183
Coccidioidomycosis, 61–62
Colchicine, in gout, 133
Cold agglutinin autoimmune hemolytic anemia, 82
Cold hemolysin autoimmune hemolytic anemia, 82
    idiopathic form of, 82
Cold sore (fever blister; herpes labialis), 154
Colitis
    collagenous, 253
    necrotizing enterocolitis, 253
    pseudomembranous, 47, 251–252
    ulcerative, idiopathic, 251
Collagenous colitis, 253
Collateral sprouts, in denervation atrophy, 137
Colloid adenomas, thyroid, 348
Colloid (Civatte) bodies, in lichen planus, 110
Colloid (mucinous) carcinoma, of breast, 327
Colloid cysts, 196
Colloid involution (colloid goiter), 349–350
Colon, 249–255
    angiodysplasias and, 250
    appendiceal diseases of, 249
    ascending, malignant tumors of, 254–255
    congenital anomalies of, 249–250
    diverticular disease of, 250–251
    hemorrhoids and, 250
    inflammations of, 251–252
        collagenous colitis, 252
        necrotizing enterocolitis, 252
        pseudomembranous colitis, 251–252
        ulcerative colitis, 251

left side, tumors arising in, 254–255
    malignant tumors of, 254–255
    melanosis coli and, 250
    polyps of, 252–254
        benign, 252–253
        hamartomatous, 253
        hyperplastic, 253
        inflammatory (pseudopolyps), 253
        juvenile, 253
        lymphoid, 253
        neoplastic, 253–254
        Peutz-Jeghers, 253
Colorado tick fever, 31
Color blindness, 7
Coma
    hyperosmolar, 359
    hypoglycemic, 359
Comedocarcinomas, of breast, 327
Comedones
    closed, 111
    open, 110–111
Comminuted fractures, 141
Common acquired nevus, 117
Common wart (verruca vulgaris), 111
Compensatory emphysema, 164
Complement-mediated reactions, 20
Complete fractures, 141
Compound (open) fractures, 141–142
Compound nevus, 118
    of Spitz, 118
Concretocordis, 229
Concussion, 184
Condyloma
    acuminata (venereal warts), 111
        penile, 312
        vulvar, 330–331
    giant (Buschke-Lowenstein tumor; verrucous carcinoma), 312
    lata, 52
    vulvar, 331
Congenital adrenal hyperplasia, 362–363
Congenital diseases, 1. *See also specific disorders*.
    of adrenal cortex, 361
    of arteries, 199
    of breasts, 323
    cardiac. *See* Heart disease, congenital.
    of central nervous system, 176–177
    colonic, 249–250
    esophageal, 231
    of gallbladder, 277
    gastric, 235
    glaucoma, 156–157
    of oral cavity, 154
    pancreatic, 278
    penile, 311
    renal, 283
    of respiratory system, 159
    simple congenital lymphedema, 211
    of small intestine, 242
    of spleen, 103
    syphilis, 53
    thyroid, 355
    ureteral, 306
    uterine, 335
Congenital fiber-type disproportion, 139

Congenital lobar overinflation, 164
Congenital myopathies, 139
Congenital nevocellular nevus, 118
Congestion, acute, of spleen, 103
Congestive cardiomyopathy (dilated cardiomyopathy; Keshan disease), 18, 220
Congestive heart failure, 218–219
    insidiously developing, 215
    left-sided, 218
    right-sided, 218–219
Congestive splenomegaly, 104
Coning, 175
Conjunctivitis
    acute, 155
    chronic, 155–156
    gonococcal, neonatal, 40
    inclusion, 33
Connective tissue. See also Arthritis; Bone; Dermatoses; Lyme disease; Muscle; Skin.
    Baker's cyst and, 136
    bursitis and, 135–136
    degenerative joint disease and, 129
    ganglion and, 136
    gout and, 132–134
    tenosynovitis and, 135
    tumorlike conditions of, 127–128
        desmoids, 127
        fibromatosis, 127
        nodular fasciitis, 127–128
        traumatic myositis ossificans, 128
    tumors of. See Bone(s), tumors of; Skin; Soft tissue, tumors of.
Conn syndrome (primary hypoaldosteronism), 362
Constrictive pericarditis, 229
Consumption coagulopathy, disseminated intravascular coagulation and, 85
Contrecoup lesions, 184
Contusions, of brain, 184
Coombs antiglobulin test, in autoimmune hemolytic anemias, 81
Copper
    deficiency of, 17–18
    Wilson's disease and, 4, 17, 265
"Cor bovinum," 202
Cori's disease (type III glycogen storage disease), 4, 273
Cor pulmonale (pulmonary heart disease), 217
    acute, 217
    chronic, 217
Cortical adenomas, renal, 300
Cortical necrosis, diffuse, 288–289
Corynebacterium infections
    Corynebacterium diphtheriae, 42–43
    myocarditis and, 219
Coup lesions, 184
Cowdry type A (intranuclear) inclusions, in herpesvirus infections, 29
Coxiella infections, 34
    Coxiella burnetii, 36, 169
Coxsackie viruses, respiratory infections caused by, 27
Crack, adverse effects of, 11

Cranial encephalocele, 176
Cranial meningocele, 176
Craniopharyngiomas (adamantinomas; ameloblastomas), 346
Crescentic (rapidly progressive) glomerulonephritis, 292
    idiopathic, 292
CREST syndrome, 26
Cretinism, 7, 352
Creutzfeldt-Jakob disease (subacute spongiform encephalopathy), 183
"Crew haircut" appearance, in syphilis osteomyelitis, 141
Cri du chat syndrome (5p- syndrome), 3
Crigler-Najjar syndrome
    type I, 271
    type II, 271
Crohn's disease, 247
Crushing injury, splenic rupture and, 105
Cryoglobulinemia, essential mixed, glomerular lesions associated with, 295
Cryptococcosis, 60–61
Cryptococcus infections
    Cryptococcus neoformans, 60–61
    cystitis and, 308
    encephalitis and, 183
    myocarditis and, 219
    orbital, 156
    pulmonary, 168
Cryptogenic cirrhosis, 266
Cryptogenic fibrosing alveolitis (chronic interstitial pneumonitis; Hamman-Rich syndrome; idiopathic pulmonary fibrosis; usual interstitial pneumonitis), 166
Cryptorchidism, 314
Cryptosporidium infections, 64
    gastroenterocolitis and, 243
Cunninghamella infections, 60
Cushing's disease, 361–362
Cushing's ulcers, 238
Cushing syndrome, 361
Cutaneous blastomycosis, 61
Cutaneous leishmaniasis (tropical sore), 67–68
    diffuse, 67–68
Cutaneous lupus erythematosus, subacute, 25
Cutaneous lymphomas, 120–121
Cyclops, 70
Cylindromas, 115
Cystadenocarcinomas
    pancreatic, 281
    serous, ovarian, 339
Cystadenofibromas, ovarian, 339
Cystadenomas, serous
    ovarian, 339
    pancreatic, 281
Cysticercosis, 72–73
    hepatic abscesses and, 262
Cystic fibrosis, 4
    cirrhosis and, 266
    liver and, 279
    lungs and, 278–279
    pancreas and, 278

salivary glands and, 279
    testes and, 279
Cystic medial necrosis, 202
Cystine stones, 303
Cystitis, 303, 308
    chronic, 308
    cystica, 308
    emphysematous, 308
    eosinophilic, 308
    hemorrhagic, 308
    polypoid, 308
    suppurative, 308
    ulcerative, 308
        interstitial (Hunner's ulcer), 308
Cystosarcoma phyllodes (phyllodes tumors), 325
Cysts
    Baker's, 136
    "blue-dome," 325
    bronchogenic, 159
    colloid, 196
    dermoid
        ovarian (benign cystic teratomas), 340
        of skin, 115
    epithelial (wens), 114–115
    Gartner's duct, 332
    hepatic, 268
        choledochal, 268
        simple, 268
    horn, 114
    hydatid, 262
    inclusion, epidermal, 115
    Nabothian, 333
    ovarian, 342
        follicular, 342
        luteal, 342
    pancreatic, congenital, 278
    paraovarian (hydatids of Morgagni), 343
    in Pneumocystis carinii infections, 65
    renal. See Renal cysts.
    thyroglossal, 355
    in toxoplasmosis, 68
    trichilemmal (pilar), 115
Cytomegalic inclusion disease, 30
Cytomegalovirus infections, 30
    encephalitis and, 181–182
    orbital, 156
Cytoplasmic granules, in granular cell tumors, 122
Cytoplasmic vacuolization (koilocytosis), 111
Cytotoxicity, T cell-mediated, 21
Cytotrophoblastic cells, 317

D

Dandy-Walker malformation, 177
Darier's sign, 121
Dawson's encephalitis (subacute sclerosing panencephalitis), 182
Decay accelerating factor, in paroxysmal nocturnal hemoglobinuria, 81
Deeply ulcerating lesions, esophageal, 233
Degeneration, axonal, 197
Degenerative diseases
    of central nervous system. See Central

nervous system, degenerative diseases of.
of joints (osteoarthritis), 129
primary, 129
secondary, 129
of muscle, 136
of peripheral nervous system, 196–197
Delayed-type (type IV) hypersensitivity, 21
Dementia, AIDS-related, 182
Demineralization, hyperparathyroidism-induced, 143
Demyelinating diseases, 189–190
multiple sclerosis, 189
neuropathy, acute, 197
perivenous encephalomyelitis, 189–190
Denervation atrophy, of muscle, 137
group, 137
Dengue fever, 31
de Quervain's (subacute granulomatous) thyroiditis, 350–351
Dermal nevus, 118
Dermatitis
eczematous, acute (eczema; spongiotic dermatitis), 107–108
herpetiformis, 113
Dermatofibroma, 119
Dermatofibrosarcoma protuberans, 119
Dermatographism, 121
Dermatoses
acute inflammatory, 107–109
acute eczematous dermatitis, 107–108
erythema induratum, 108, 109
erythema multiforme, 108
erythema nodosum, 108–109
urticaria (hives), 107
chronic inflammatory, 109–111
acne vulgaris, 110–111
lichen planus, 109–110
lupus erythematosus, 110
psoriasis, 109
papulosa nigra (seborrheic keratoses; senile keratoses), 114
Dermoids
ovarian (benign cystic teratomas), 340
of skin, 115
Dermopathy, in Graves disease, 352
des-γ-carboxy prothrombin, hepatocellular carcinoma and, 270
Desmoids, 127
Desmolase deficiency, 363
Desquamative interstitial pneumonitis, 166–167
Developmental diseases, of central nervous system, 177
Devic's disease (neuromyelitis optica), 189
Dextrinosis, limited (type III glycogen storage disease), 4, 273
Dextrocardia, 214
Diabetes insipidus, 347
Diabetes mellitus, 358–360
glomerulosclerosis and, 294–295
diffuse, 294
nodular (intercapillary glomerulosclerosis; Kimmelstiel-Wilson syndrome), 294–295
late complications of, 359–360

neuropathy in, 197
retinopathies caused by, 156–157
type I (insulin-dependent; juvenile onset), 358–359
type II (adult onset; insulin-independent), 358, 359
Dialysis, renal cysts associated with, 285
Diaphragmatic hernias, 235
Diarrhea, acute, viral causes of, 28
Dicrocoelium dendriticum infections, hepatic abscesses and, 262
Diethylstilbestrol toxicity, 11
Diffuse axonal injury, 184
Diffuse cortical necrosis, 288–289
Diffuse infiltrative lesions, esophageal, 233
Diffuse nontoxic (simple) goiter. See Goiter, diffuse nontoxic (simple).
Diffuse sclerosis (Schilder's disease), 189
DiGeorge syndrome (thymic dysplasia), 23, 357
Digestive system. See also specific organs and disorders.
viral infections of, 28
Dilated cardiomyopathy (congestive cardiomyopathy; Keshan disease), 18, 220
Dipetalonema streptocerca infections, 72
Diphtheria, 42–43
Diphtheria pseudomembrane, 43
Diphyllobothrium latum infections, 72
Dirofilaria immitis infections, 72
Dirofilaria tenuis infections, 72
Disaccharidase deficiency, 246
Discoid lesions, in discoid lupus erythematosus, 110
Discoid lupus erythematosus, chronic, 25
Dissecting aneurysms (aortic dissection; dissecting hematomas), 188, 202–203
type A, 202–203
type B, 203
Disseminated encephalomyelitis, acute (postinfectious encephalitis; postvaccinal encephalitis), 189
Disseminated intravascular coagulation, 85
in African trypanosomiasis, 66
in leukemias, 95
Distal acinar (paraseptal) emphysema, 164
Diverticula
of bladder
acquired, 307
congenital, 307
colonic, 250–251
esophageal. See Esophagus, diverticula of.
small intestinal, 242
Meckel's, 242
ureteral, congenital, 306
Diverticular disease, colonic, 250–251
Diverticulitis, 250
Diverticulosis, 250
Donath-Landsteiner antibodies, in cold hemolysin autoimmune hemolytic anemia, 82
Double-barreled aorta, 203
Down syndrome (mongolism; trisomy 21), 3
Alzheimer's disease in, 191
Dracunculus medinensis (guinea worm)

infections, 70
Drugs. See also specific drugs and drug types.
gastric ulcers and, 238
hepatic injury induced by, 273
hepatitis induced by, 260
illicit
adverse effects of, 11–12
infections associated with needle use and, 11
suppurative arthritis and, 131
lupus erythematosus syndromes induced by, 25
resistance of gram-negative bacilli to, 41
tubulointerstitial nephritis caused by, 297–298
"Dry beriberi," 15
D trisomy (Patau syndrome; 13-15 trisomy), 3
Dubin-Johnson syndrome, 271–272
Duchenne muscular dystrophy, 7, 138
Ductal proliferation, benign sclerosing (radial scar), 326
Ductus arteriosus, patent, 213
Duodenum, peptic ulcers of, 238
Duplications, of small intestine, 242
Dysgenesis, of thyroid gland, 355
Dysgerminomas, 340–341
Dysplastic nevus, 118
Dystrophin, 138

E

Ear(s), 151–152
cauliflower, 151
external, 151
inner, 152
middle, 152
Eaton agents, 36–37
Eaton-Lambert syndrome, 137
Ebola virus, 31
Eburnation, in osteoarthritis, 129
Eccrine poromas, 115
Echinococcosis, 262
Echinococcus infections
Echinococcus granulosus
European strain of, 73
northern strain of, 73
Echinococcus multilocularis, 73
Echinococcus vogeli, 73
hepatic abscesses and, 262
myocarditis and, 219
Echoviruses, respiratory infections caused by, 28
Ectopia cordis, 214
Eczematous dermatitis, acute (eczema; spongiotic dermatitis), 107–108
Edema. See also Lymphedema; Papilledema.
angioneurotic, hereditary, 107
cerebral. See Cerebral edema.
pulmonary, 160
hemodynamic, 160
microvascular injury and, 160
Edwards syndrome (E trisomy; 16-18 trisomy), 3

Eggs, of schistosomes, 75
Ehrlichia infections, 34
Elastosis, solar, 115–116
Electron-dense deposits, in lupus renal disease, 293
Elephantiasis (lymphatic filariasis), 33, 71
Embolism, pulmonary, 161–162
Embolus(i)
    atheroembolic, renal, 288
    septic, 162
Embryonal (trabecular) adenomas, thyroid, 348
Embryonal carcinomas, 316
    infantile (endodermal sinus tumors; yolk sac tumors), testicular, 316
    ovarian, 341
    testicular, 316
        infantile (endodermal sinus tumors; yolk sac tumors), 316
Embryonal rhabdomyosarcoma (sarcoma botryoides), 332
Emotional lability, in hyperthyroidism, 351
Emphysema, 164
    bullous, 164
    centriacinar (centrilobular), 164
    compensatory, 164
    interstitial, 164
    panacinar (panlobular), 164
    paraseptal (distal acinar), 164
    senile (senile hyperinflation), 164
Emphysematous cystitis, 308
Empty sella syndrome, 346
Empyema
    subdural, 179
    thoracic (suppurative pleuritis), 173
Encephalitis, 180–183
    bacterial, 180
    Dawson's (subacute sclerosing panencephalitis), 182
    fungal, 183
    parasitic infections and, 183
    postinfectious (acute disseminated encephalomyelitis; postvaccinal encephalitis), 189
    subacute, in AIDS, 182
    viral, 180–183
        slow virus infections and, 182–183
Encephalocele, cranial, 176
Encephaloclastic porencephaly, 177
Encephalomyelitis, disseminated, acute (postinfectious encephalitis; postvaccinal encephalitis), 189
Encephalopathy
    hepatic, 257
    hypertensive, 188
    hypoxic (ischemic), 187
    subacute spongiform (Creutzfeldt-Jakob disease), 183
    transmissible, 183
Enchondromas, 148
Enchondromatosis (Ollier's disease), 148
Endemic goiter, 349
Endocardial fibroelastosis, restrictive cardiomyopathy and, 222
Endocarditis, 225–227
    Candida, 59

infective (bacterial), 225–226
    acute, 225
    glomerular lesions associated with, 294
    gonococcal, 40
    staphylococcal, 38
    subacute, 225–226
    Löffler's, restrictive cardiomyopathy and, 221
    of systemic lupus erythematosus, 226–227
    thrombotic, nonbacterial (marantic), 226
Endocervical hyperplasia, microglandular, 333
Endocervical polyps, 333
Endocrine cell tumors. *See* Carcinoids (endocrine cell tumors; neuroendocrine tumors).
α-Cell tumors (glucagonomas), 358
β-Cell tumors (insulinomas), 358
δ-Cell tumors (somatostatinomas), 358
Endocrine disorders. *See specific endocrine glands and disorders.*
    muscle and, 139
Endocrine pancreas, 358–360. *See also* Diabetes mellitus.
    islet cell tumors of, 358
Endocrinopathies, polyostotic fibrous dysplasia in association with, 145
Endodermal sinus tumors (infantile embryonal carcinomas; yolk sac tumors)
    ovarian, 341
    testicular, 316
Endometrial atrophy, cystic, senile, 337
Endometrial hyperplasia, 337
    atypical (complex or adenomatous hyperplasia with atypia), 337
    complex, without atypia (moderate or adenomatous hyperplasia without atypia), 337
    simple, without atypia (cystic or mild hyperplasia), 337
Endometrial polyps, benign, 337–338
Endometrial tumors, 339–340
Endometriosis, 336
Endometritis, 335
    acute, 335
    chronic, 335
Endomyocardial fibrosis, restrictive cardiomyopathy and, 221
Endophthalmitis, 156
Entamoeba histolytica infections, 63
    gastroenterocolitis and, 243
Enteritis
    Helicobacter, 45
    clostridial, 47
    cryptosporidial, 64
    enteroadhesive, 43
    isosporal, 64
    Listeria monocytogenes, 48
    Yersinia enterocolitica, 45–46
Enteroadhesive enteritis, 43
Enterobacter infections
    cholangitis and, 261
    cystitis and, 308
    Enterobacter aerogenes, 41
    hepatic abscesses and, 261
    prostatitis and, 319

urinary, 303
Enterobius vermicularis (pinworm) infections, 69
Enterococcus infections, prostatitis and, 319
Enterocolitis
    bacterial, invasive, 243
    necrotizing, 253
Enteropathogenic bacteria. *See* Bacterial infections, enteric.
Enteropathy, gluten-sensitive (celiac disease; celiac sprue; nontropical sprue), 113, 245
Enterotoxins
    Escherichia coli, 43
    Vibrio cholerae, 45
Environmental disorders, central nervous system and, 178
Enzyme deficiencies
    muscle and, 139
    red cell, 83
Eosinophilia, pulmonary infiltration with, 167
    secondary, chronic, 167
    simple, 167
Eosinophilic cystitis, 308
Eosinophilic gastritis, 237
Eosinophilic granuloma, 102
Eosinophilic leukocytosis, 90
Eosinophilic pneumonia, chronic, 167
Ependymomas, 194
    myxopapillary, 194
    posterior fossa, 194
    spinal cord, 194
Ephelis (freckles), 117
Epidemic typhus, 34–35
Epidermal hyperplasia, papillomatous, 111
Epidermal inclusion cysts, 115
Epidermidalization, 156
Epidermodysplasia verruciformis, 111
Epidermoid carcinomas. *See* Squamous cell (epidermoid) carcinomas.
Epidermolysis bullosa, 114
Epididymis, inflammation of, 312–314
    epididymitis, 312–313
Epidural hematomas, 184
Epiglottitis, *Haemophilus influenzae*, 42
Episcleritis, 156
Epispadias, 311
Epithelial cells
    viral epithelial growths and, 28
    vitamin A and, 14
Epithelial hyperplasia, of breast, 326
Epithelioid hemangioendotheliomas, 209
Epstein-Barr virus infections, 30–31
Eruptive xanthoma, 120
Erythema
    induratum, 108, 109
    infectiosum, 29
    multiforme, 108
    nodosum, 108–109
Erythrocytes. *See also* Anemias; Hematopoietic system, erythrocyte-disorders.
    decreased deformability of, 83
Erythroplasia of Queyrat, 312
Erythropoiesis

diminished, 78–79
 megaloblastic anemias and, 79
 ineffective, megaloblastic anemia caused
  by, 79
Eschar
 in rickettsial infections, 34
 in Rocky Mountain spotted fever, 35
Escherichia coli infections, 40–41
 cholangitis and, 261
 cystitis and, 308
 endocarditis and, 226
 enteric, 43
  gastroenterocolitis and, 243
  invasive, 43
 epididymal, 313
 hemolytic uremic syndrome and, 288
 meningitis and, 179
 prostatitis and, 319
 pulmonary, 169
 pyogenic osteomyelitis and, 140
 tropical sprue and, 245
 ureteral, 307
 urinary, 303
Esophageal (Schatzki's) rings, 231
Esophageal webs, 231
Esophagitis, 234
Esophagus, 231–234
 achalasia of, 232
 acquired anatomic defects of, 231–232
 benign, esophageal, 233
 congenital anomalies of, 231
 diverticula of, 232
  pulsion (Zenker's), 232
  traction, 232
  Zenker's (pulsion), 232
 esophagitis and, 233
 lacerations of, 232
 malignant, esophageal, 233–234
 tumors of, 233–234
 varices of, 232
Espundia (mucocutaneous leishmaniasis),
 67
Essential mixed cryoglobulinemia, glomerular lesions associated with, 295
Esthiomene, 33
Estrogens, toxicity of, 11
État marbre, 177
Ethyl alcohol
 central nervous system and, 178
 toxicity of, 9
E trisomy (Edwards syndrome; 16-18 trisomy), 3
Ewing's sarcomas, 149
Exocrine pancreas, 278–281. *See also*
 Pancreatitis.
 congenital anomalies of, 278
 cystic fibrosis and, 278–279
 pseudocysts of, 280–281
 tumors of, 281
  benign, 281
  malignant, 281
Exoerythrocytic cycle, in malaria, 65
Exostoses (osteochondromas), 146–147,
 148
 multiple, hereditary (osteochondromatosis), 146

Exotoxin, type A, of *Clostridium botulinum*, 46
Exstrophy, of bladder, 307
External otitis, malignant, 151
Extramedullary hematopoiesis, in myeloid
 metaplasia, 99
Extravascular hemolysis, 77–78
Extravascular hemolytic anemias, 83
Eye(s), 155–157
 cataracts and, 157
 in congenital syphilis, 53
 conjunctival diseases of, 40, 155–156
 corneal diseases of, 156
 in diabetes mellitus, 360
 eyelid diseases and, 155
 glaucoma and, 156–157
 in Graves disease, 352
 in hyperthyroidism, 351
 inflammatory orbital diseases of, 156
 neoplasms of, 155
 papilledema and, 157
 retinal detachment and, 157
 retinopathies and, 157
 retrolental fibroplasia and, 156
 vitamin A and, 14
Eyelid, diseases of, 155
"Eye worm" (loa loa), 72

F

Fabry's disease (glycosphingolipidosis), 5,
 273
Factor IX deficiency (Christmas disease;
 hemophilia B), 7, 88
Factor VIII deficiency (classic hemophilia;
 hemophilia A), 7, 87–88
Fallopian tube diseases, 343
Familial polyposis coli, 254
Fanconi's anemia, 80
Farmer's lung, 167
Fasciola gigantica infections, 74
Fasciola hepatica infections, 73–74
 hepatic abscesses and, 262
Fasciolopsis buski infections, 74
Fascioscapulohumeral dystrophy, 138
Fat necrosis, of breast, 324
Fatty liver (alcoholic steatosis), 262
 macrovesicular, 262
 microvesicular, 262
Fatty streaks, 200
Felons, 37
Felty syndrome, 131
Females. *See also* Ovarian tumors; Uterus;
 headings beginning with term
 Cervical.
 fallopian tube diseases in, 343
 sex chromosome abnormalities in, 2
 vaginal lesions of, 332
 vulvar diseases in, 330–332
  tumors, 330–332
Fetal adenomas, thyroid, 348
Fetuses, toxoplasmosis in, 68
Fever, in rheumatic heart disease, 224
Fever blister (cold sore; herpes labialis), 154
Fiber splitting, 136
Fibrinous pericarditis, 228

Fibroadenomas, of breasts, 324
 "giant," 324
Fibroadenomatosis, 324
Fibroblastic meningiomas, 195
Fibrocartilaginous callus, 142
Fibrocystic disease of breast, 325–326
 simple fibrocystic change, 325–326
Fibroelastic hyperplasia, renal, 286–287
Fibroelastosis
 endocardial, restrictive cardiomyopathy
  and, 222
 papillary, 223
Fibroepithelial polyps (acrochordon; skin
  tags; squamous papilloma), 114
"Fibroids" (leiomyomas; myomas), 338
Fibrolipomas, 123
Fibromas, 125
 chondromyxoid, 148
 ovarian, 341
 pleural (benign mesotheliomas), 172
Fibromatosis, 127
Fibrosarcomas, 125–126
Fibrothecomas, ovarian, 341
Fibrous ankylosis, 130
Fibrous cortical defects (nonossifying fibromas), 145
Fibrous dysplasia, 144–145
 monostotic, 145
 polyostotic, 145
  in association with endocrinopathies,
   145
Fibrous histiocytomas, 122–123
 benign, 122–123
 malignant, 122–123
  myxoid, 123
  storiform-pleomorphic, 123
Filariasis, 71–72
 lymphatic (elephantiasis), 33, 71
Fistulas
 arteriovenous, 199
 of bladder, 308
 esophageal, 231
5p- syndrome (cri du chat syndrome), 3
Flat warts (verruca plana), 111
Flatworms. *See* Cestodes; Trematodes.
"Fleur-de-lis" pattern, in gram-negative
  bacilli infections, 41
Flukes. *See* Trematodes.
Flying squirrel typhus, 35
Focal necrotizing vasculitis, 205
Focal nodular hyperplasia, 268
Focal proliferative glomerulonephritis, 297
 primary, 297
 secondary, 297
Focal segmental glomerulosclerosis,
  290–291
 idiopathic, 291
 secondary, 291
Focal vascular inflammation, in rickettsial
  infections, 34
Folded fundus, of gallbladder, 277
Folic acid (folate) deficiency, 16
 megaloblastic anemia caused by, 79
Follicular carcinomas, thyroid, 353–354
Follicular cervicitis, 333
Follicular cysts, 342

Follicular hyperplasia, 90
  thymic, 137, 367
Follicular lymphomas. *See* Lymphomas, follicular.
Food poisoning, staphylococcal, 38
Forbes disease (type III glycogen storage disease), 4, 273
Foregut carcinoids, 248
"Fort Bragg fever," 50
Fractures, 141–142
  closed (simple), 141
  comminuted, 141
  complete, 141
  compound (open), 141–142
  incomplete (greenstick), 141
  of skull, 183–184
  spiral, 141
Fragile vessels, 86
Fragile X syndrome, 2
Francisella tularensis infections, 49
Freckles (ephelis), 117
Free-swimming cercariae, 75
"Fried egg" cells, in oligodendrogliomas, 194
Friedrich's ataxia, 190
Fulminant hepatitis, 259
Fungal infections, 59–62. *See also specific infections and fungi.*
  in AIDS, 24
  coccidioidomycosis, 61–62
  cystitis and, 308
  deep, unusual, 62
  encephalitis and, 183
  endocarditis and, 225, 226
  gastroenterocolitis and, 243
  hepatic abscesses and, 261
  histoplasmosis, 62
  mucormycosis, 60
  myocarditis and, 219
  in needle users, 11
  of oral cavity, 154–155
  paracoccidioidomycosis, 61
  prostatitis and, 319
  pseudomembranous colitis and, 253
  pulmonary, 169
  pyogenic osteomyelitis and, 140
  superficial, 62, 112
  ureteral, 307
  urinary, 303, 304
Fungus balls (aspergillomas), 60
Furuncle, 37

G

Galactocele, 324
Galactosemia, 4, 272–273
Gallbladder
  anatomic variants of, 277
  carcinoma of, 276–277
  cholecystitis and. *See* Cholecystitis.
  cholesterolosis and, 278
  polyps of, 278
  "porcelain," 275
  strawberry, 278
  tumors of, benign, 276
"Gallstone ileus," 275

Gallstones (cholelithiasis), 275–276
  cholesterol and mixed stones, 275–276
  pigment stones, 276
Gandy-Gamma nodules, in congestive splenomegaly, 104
Ganglion(s), 136
Ganglioneuroblastomas, 126
Ganglioneuromas (gangliocytomas), 126, 195
Gangliosidoses
  GM^1 (generalized), 6
  GM^2 (Tay-Sachs disease), 5–6
  liver and, 273
Gangrenous appendicitis, 249
Gardner syndrome, 3, 127, 254
Garré's sclerosing osteomyelitis, 140
Gartner's duct cysts, 332
Gas gangrene (clostridial myonecrosis), 47
Gastric atrophy, chronic, 236
Gastric dilatation, massive, 235
Gastric mucosal defects, focal, 237
Gastric rupture, 235
Gastrinomas (Zollinger-Ellison syndrome), 237, 358
Gastritis, 235–237
  acute, 235–236
    erosive, hemorrhagic, 235–236
  chronic, 236
    atrophic, 236
    eosinophilic, 237
    granulomatous, 237
    Helicobacter, 237
    hypersecretory, 236
    hypertrophic, 237
    superficial, 236
    type A (fundal), 236
    type AB (environmental), 236
    type B (antral), 236
Gastroenterocolitis, infective, 243–245
Gastropathy, hypersecretory, 237
Gaucher's disease, 5, 273
Generalized (GM^1) gangliosidoses, 6
Genetic diseases. *See* Chromosomal diseases.
Genetic influences
  dilated cardiomyopathy and, 220
  neonatal cholestasis and, 272
German measles (rubella), 29
Germ cell tumors
  ovarian, 340–341
    mixed, 341
  testicular, 315–318
    clinical features of, 318
    mixed, 318
Germinomas, pineal, 367
Ghon complex, 54
Ghon focus, 54
Giant cell(s) (polykaryons), in herpesvirus infections, 29
Giant cell (temporal) arteritis, 205
Giant cell carcinomas, thyroid, 354
Giant cell granulomas, reparative ("brown tumors"), 144
Giant cell tumors
  of bone (osteoclastomas), 149
  of tendon sheath (nodular tenosynovitis),

135
Giant condyloma (Buschke-Lowenstein tumor; verrucous carcinoma), 312
"Giant fibroadenomas", of breasts, 324
Giant osteoid osteomas (osteoblastomas), 147
Giardia lamblia infections, 64
  gastroenterocolitis and, 243
Gilbert's syndrome, 271
Gingivostomatitis, herpetic, primary, 154
Glanders, 50
Glandular tularemia, 49
Glaucoma, 156–157
  congenital, 156–157
  primary angle closure, 156
  primary open-angle, 156–157
  secondary, 156–157
Glial cells, healing of brain and, 12
Glial nodules, 180
Glioblastoma multiforme, 193–194
Gliomas, brainstem, 194
Globoid cell leukodystrophy (Krabbe's disease), 5, 178
Glomangiomas (glomus tumors), 208
Glomerular diseases, 289–297. *See also* Glomerulonephritis.
  associated with systemic disease, 292–295
    amyloidosis, 295
    bacterial endocarditis, 294
    diabetic glomerulosclerosis, 294–295
    essential mixed cryoglobulinemia, 295
    Goodpasture syndrome, 295
    Henoch-Schönlein purpura, 294
    plasma cell dyscrasias, 295
    polyarteritis nodosa, 295
    systemic lupus erythematosus, 292–294
    Wegener's granulomatosis, 295
  focal segmental glomerulosclerosis, 290–291
  lipoid nephrosis (minimal change disease), 290
  nephrotic syndrome, 289
  in schistosomiasis, 76
Glomerulitis, necrotizing, 287
Glomerulonephritis
  acute poststreptococcal, 291–292
  Alport syndrome and, 295
  chronic, 297
  focal proliferative, 297
  IgA nephropathy (Berger's disease), 296
  lupus, mesangial, 293
  membranoproliferative. *See* Membranoproliferative glomerulonephritis.
  membranous (membranous nephropathy), 289–290, 293
  poststreptococcal, acute, 291–292
  proliferative
    diffuse, 293
    focal, 293
  rapidly progressive (crescentic), 292
Glomerulosclerosis
  diabetic, 294–295
    diffuse, 294
    nodular (intercapillary glomerulosclerosis; Kimmelstiel-Wilson syndrome),

294–295
focal segmental, 290–291
idiopathic, 291
secondary, 291
Glomus tumors (glomangiomas), 208
Glucagonomas (α-cell tumors), 358
Glucose-6-phosphate dehydrogenase deficiency, 7, 83
A-variants of, 83
Mediterranean variant of, 83
Glutathione synthetase deficiency, 83
Gluten-sensitive enteropathy (celiac disease; celiac sprue; nontropical sprue), 113, 245
Glycogen storage diseases (glycogenoses), 4–5
type I (von Gierke's disease, hepatorenal form), 4, 273
type Ib, 4
type II (Pompe's disease, generalized or cardiac form), 4
type III (Cori's disease; Forbes disease; limited dextrinosis), 4, 273
type IV (amylopectinosis; Andersen's disease), 4–5, 273
type V (McArdle's disease; muscle glycogenosis), 5
type VI (Hers disease; liver glycogenosis), 5, 273
type VII, 5
type VIII, 5
Glycosphingolipidosis (Fabry's disease), 5, 273
GM2 gangliosidosis (Tay-Sachs disease), 5–6
Goiter
diffuse nontoxic (simple), 349–350
colloid, 349–350
endemic, 349
hyperplastic stage of, 349
sporadic, 349
multinodular (adenomatous; multiple colloid adenomatous), 350
intrathoracic (plunging), 350
Gonadoblastomas, 342
Gonorrhea, 40
endocarditis and, 226
epididymis and, 313
Goodpasture syndrome, 162
glomerular lesions associated with, 295
Gout, 132–134
primary, idiopathic, 132
secondary, 133–134
Gram-negative organisms
bacilli, 40–42
anaerobic, 42
endocarditis and, 226
pulmonary infections and, 168
rods
epididymitis and, 313
pulmonary infections and, 168
Gram-positive anaerobes, 46
Gram-positive shock (staphylococcal septicemia), 38
Granular cell tumors, 122
Granulocytes. See Hematopoietic system, granulocyte and lymphocyte disorders.

Granulocytopoiesis, failure of, neutropenia caused by, 89
Granulomas
eosinophilic, 102
giant cell, reparative ("brown tumors"), 144
gravidarum (pregnancy tumor), 208
inguinale, 57
necrotizing, acute, 205
noncaseating
in Crohn's disease, 247
in sarcoidosis, 58
pyogenicum (granulation tissue-type hemangioma), 208
Granulomatosis
allergic (Churg-Strauss syndrome), 204
infantiseptica, 48
lymphomatoid, 205
Wegener's, 204–205
Granulomatous diseases
gastritis and, 237
liver and, 273
orchitis, 313
Granulosa-theca cell tumors, 341
Granulovacuolar degeneration, 190–191
Graves disease, 352–353
Great arteries, transpositions of. See Transpositions of the great arteries.
Greenstick (incomplete) fractures, 141
Group A streptococci, 38–39
acute endometritis and, 335
acute poststreptococcal glomerulonephritis and, 291–292
Group atrophy, of muscle, 137
Group B streptococci, 39
pyogenic osteomyelitis and, 140
Group D streptococci, 39
rheumatic fever and, 224
Growth retardation, zinc deficiency causing, 17
Guinea worm (Dracunculus medinensis) infections, 70
Gummas, syphilitic, 53
in congenital syphilis, 53
Gynecomastia, 329

H

Haemophilus infections
conjunctival, 155
Haemophilus ducreyi, 57
Haemophilus influenzae, 42
laryngeal, 153
meningitis and, 179
of middle ear, 152
pulmonary, 168
pyogenic osteomyelitis and, 140
suppurative arthritis and, 131
Hairy cell leukemia, 97
Halo nevus, 118
Halothane toxicity, 10
Hamartomas, pulmonary, 171
Hamartomatous polyps, colonic, 253
Hamman-Rich syndrome (chronic interstitial pneumonitis; cryptogenicfibrosing

alveolitis; idiopathic pulmonary fibrosis; usual interstitial pneumonitis), 166
Hand-Schüller-Christian triad, 102
Hansen's disease. See Leprosy (Hansen's disease).
Hartnup's disease, 16
Hashimoto's thyroiditis (autoimmune thyroiditis; stroma lymphomatosa), 350
fibrosing, 350
Hashitoxicosis (hyperthyroidism), 350, 351–352
Haverhill fever (rat-bite fever, streptobacillary form), 51, 52
Hay fever (allergic rhinitis), 152–153
HDL (high-density lipoprotein), 201
Head. See specific organs.
Healing, 12
of brain, 12
primary, 12
secondary union, 12
Heart, 212–229. See also Heart disease; headings beginning with term Cardiac; specific diseases.
enlargement of, 202
in Lyme disease, 132
malpositions of, 214
tumors of, 222–223
Heart disease. See also Cardiomyopathy; Endocarditis; Ischemic heart disease; Pericardial disease; Pericarditis; Valvular heart disease.
carcinoid, 227
congenital, 212–214
left-to-right shunts, 213
malpositions, 214
obstructive noncyanotic congenital anomalies, 214
right-to-left shunts, 212
congestive heart failure, 218–219
left-sided failure, 218
right-sided failure, 218–219
cor pulmonale (pulmonary heart disease), 217
hypertensive, 217
myocarditis, 219–220
rheumatic, 224–225
chronic, 225
rheumatoid, 223
tumors, 222–223
Heart valves, prosthetic. See also Valvular heart disease.
complications of, 227
infective endocarditis and, 226
Heavy chain disease, 101
Heavy egg burdens, of schistosomes, 75
Heberden's nodes, 129
Heinz bodies, 83
Helicobacter jejuni infections, gastroenterocolitis and, 243
Helicobacter pyloris infections, gastritis and, 237
Helminths. See Parasitic infections, helminthic.
Hemangioendotheliomas, 209
epithelioid, 209

Hemangiomas, 207–208
    capillary, 186, 207
    cavernous, 186, 207–208
        hepatic, 269
    glomus tumor (glomangioma), 210
    granulation tissue-type (granuloma pyogenicum), 210
    juvenile ("strawberry"), 207
    pregnancy tumor (granuloma gravidarum), 208
    renal, 300
    sclerosing, 119
Hematoceles, 315
Hematologic disorders, in systemic lupus erythematosus, 24
Hematomas, 128
    dissecting (aortic dissection; dissecting aneurysms), 202–203
        type A, 202–203
        type B, 203
    epidural, 184
    subdural, 184
        acute, 184
        chronic, 184
Hematopoiesis, extramedullary, in myeloid metaplasia, 99
Hematopoietic system, 77–105
    erythrocyte disorders, 77–88
        anemias. See Anemias; Hemolytic anemias.
        clotting factor abnormalities, 87–88
        defective platelet function, 87
        disseminated intravascular coagulation, 85
        paroxysmal nocturnal hemoglobinuria, 81
        polycythemia, 81
        red cell enzyme deficiency, 83
        structurally abnormal hemoglobin synthesis, 83–84
        thalassemias, 4, 84–85
    granulocyte and lymphocyte disorders, 89–102. See also Leukemias; Lymphomas.
        histiocytoses, 101–102
        leukopenia, 89
        myeloproliferative disorders, 98–99
        plasma cell dyscrasias, 99–101
        reactive proliferations of white cells and nodes, 89–91
    hemorrhagic diatheses, 85–87
Hemochromatosis, 3, 264
Hemoglobin
    C (HbC), sickle cell disease and, 84
    β-chain of, valine substitution for glutamic acid in, 83
    D (HbD), sickle cell disease and, 84
    H (HbH) disease, 85
Hemoglobinopathies, 83–84
Hemoglobin S (HbS), in sickle cell disease, 83–84
Hemoglobinuria, paroxysmal nocturnal, 81
Hemolysis
    extravascular, 77–78
    ineffective, megaloblastic anemia caused by, 79

intravascular, 77
Hemolytic anemias, 77–78
    autoimmune (immunohemolytic), 81–82
        in chronic lymphocytic leukemia, 97
        cold agglutinin, 82
        cold hemolysis, 82
        warm body, 82
    extravascular, 83
    hereditary, 78
        red cell membrane disorders, 78
    microangiopathic, 78, 287–288
    traumatic, 78
Hemolytic uremic syndrome
    adult, 288
    childhood, 287–288
Hemopericardium, 228
Hemophilia
    B (Christmas disease; factor IX deficiency), 7, 88
    classic (hemophilia A; factor VIII deficiency), 7, 87–88
Hemorrhage
    of adrenal glands, 364–365
    intracranial. See Intracranial hemorrhage.
    pulmonary, 162
    Virchow-Robin, 185
Hemorrhagic cystitis, 308
Hemorrhagic diatheses, 85–87
    fragile vessels, 86
    thrombocytopenia, 86–87
Hemorrhagic erosive gastritis, acute, 235–236
Hemorrhagic infarcts, 188
Hemorrhagic necrosis, central, 267
Hemorrhagic pancreatitis, acute, 279
Hemorrhagic pericarditis, 228
Hemorrhagic pleuritis, 173
Hemorrhoids, 250
Hemothorax, 174
Henoch-Schönlein purpura, 86
    glomerular lesions associated with, 294
Hepatic abscesses, 261
Hepatic artery, occlusion of, 267
Hepatic cirrhosis, congestive splenomegaly caused by, 104
Hepatic encephalopathy, 257
Hepatic infarction, 267
Hepatic vein thrombosis, 267
Hepatitis, 258–262
    acute viral, 258–259
        convalescent phase of, 258
        incubation period of, 258
        symptomatic icteric phase of, 258
        symptomatic preicteric phase of, 258
    alcoholic, 262–263
    amebic (amebic liver abscess), 262
    chronic viral, 259–260
        active, 259–260
        "carriers" and, 259
        persistent, 259
    drug-induced, 273
    fulminant, 259
    hepatitis A, 258
    hepatitis B, 258
    hepatitis C, 258

    hepatitis D, 258
    neonatal
        idiopathic, 272
        infectious, 272
    non-A, non-B, 258
    nonviral causes of, 260
Hepatoblastomas, 270–271
Hepatocellular carcinomas, 269–270
    drug-induced, 273
    fibrolamellar variant of, 270
Hepatocyte plasma membrane, 256
Hepatomegaly, in leukemia, 98
Hepatorenal syndrome, 257
Hepatosplenomegaly, in chronic lymphocytic leukemia, 97
Hereditary angioneurotic edema, 107
Hereditary hemolytic anemias, spherocytosis, 78
Heritable melanoma syndrome, 118
Hermaphrodites, true, 2
Hernias
    diaphragmatic, 235
    hiatal
        paraesophageal, 232
        sliding, 231–232
    of small intestine, 246
Heroin, adverse effects of, 11
Herpes labialis (cold sore; fever blister), 154
Herpes simplex virus
    type I, 29–30
        encephalitis and, 181
        of oral cavity, 154
    type II
        encephalitis and, 181
        herpes genitalis and, 29–30
Herpesviruses, 29–31. See also specific viruses.
    encephalitis and, 181
Herpes zoster (shingles), 30, 181
Herpes zoster-varicella virus, encephalitis and, 181
Herpetic gingivostomatitis, primary, 154
Herpetic stomatitis, 154
Hers disease (type VI glycogen storage disease), 5, 273
Herxheimer reaction, 50
"Heterogeneous system degeneration" (olivopontocerebellar atrophy), 190
Heterophil (Paul-Bunnell) antibodies, in infectious mononucleosis, 31
Hexokinase deficiency, 83
Hiatal hernias
    paraesophageal, 232
    sliding, 231–232
Hidradenitis suppurativa, 37
Hidradenomas, papillary, 331
High-density lipoprotein (HDL), 201
Hilus cell tumor, 342
Hindgut carcinoids, 248
Hirano bodies, 191
Hirschsprung's disease (congenital megacolon), 249–250
Histiocytoma, fibrous, benign, 119
Histiocytoses, 101–102
    Langerhans cell
        acute disseminated (Letterer-Siwe dis-

ease), 102
unifocal and multifocal, 102
sinus, 90
Histiocytosis X bodies, 102
Histoplasma infections
encephalitis and, 183
Histoplasma capsulatum, 62
Histoplasma duboisii, 62
Histoplasmosis, 62
Histotoxic anoxia, 186
Hives (urticaria). *See* Urticaria (hives).
Hodgkin's disease, 93–94
lymphocyte depletion, 93
lymphocyte-predominant, 93
mixed cellularity, 93
nodular sclerosing, 93–94
Holoprosencephaly, 177
"Honeycombed" lungs, in idiopathic pulmonary fibrosis, 166
Hookworm disease, 69
Hormonal reactions, drug-induced, 10
Horn cysts, 114
Horseshoe kidneys, 283
"Hourglass" deformity, 308
HSV. *See* Herpes simplex virus.
Hunner's ulcer (ulcerative interstitial cystitis), 308
Hunter syndrome (type II mucopolysaccharidosis), 6
Huntington's disease (chorea), 3, 191
Hurler syndrome (type I mucopolysaccharidosis), 6
Hürthle (oxyphil) cell(s), in follicular thyroid carcinomas, 354
Hürthle cell adenomas, thyroid, 349
Hutchinson's teeth, in congenital syphilis, 53
Hutchinson-type neuroblastomas, 126
Hyaline arteriolosclerosis, 200
Hyaline arteriosclerosis, 286
Hyaline membrane disease (respiratory distress syndrome of newborn), 160–161
Hydatid cysts, 262
Hydatids of Morgagni (paraovarian cysts), 343
Hydrocele, 315
Hydrocephalus, 176
communicating, 176
noncommunicating, 176
vacuo, 176
Hydroencephaly, 177
Hydrolysis, inadequate, 244
Hydrops
fetalis, 85
of gallbladder (mucocele), 275
Hydrothorax, 174
Hydroureter, 306
Hydroxyapatite arthropathy, 134
11-Hydroxylase deficiency, 363
17-Hydroxylase deficiency, 363
21-Hydroxylase deficiency, 362–363
classic, 362–363
nonclassic, 363
Hymenolepis nana infections, 72
Hyperaldosteronism, 362
primary (Conn syndrome), 362

secondary, 362
Hyperbilirubinemias, hereditary, 271–272
Hypercontraction, of myofibers, 136
"Hyperinfection", *Strongyloides stercoralis*, 70
Hyperlipidemia, 201
Hyperlipoproteinemias
type 1, 201
type 3, 201
type 4, 201
type 5, 201
type 2a, 201
type 2b, 201
Hyperosmolar coma, 359
Hyperparathyroidism
primary, 356–357
secondary, 357
skeletal changes induced by, 143–144
Hyperplastic arteriolitis, 287
Hyperplastic arteriolosclerosis, 200
Hyperplastic dystrophy, vulvar (squamous hyperplasia), 330
Hyperplastic polyps
colonic (pseudopolyps), 253
gastric (inflammatory polyps), 239
Hypersecretory gastritis, 236
Hypersecretory gastropathy, 237
Hypersensitivity
type I (anaphylaxis), 19–20
type II, 20
in systemic lupus erythematosus, 24
type III, 20–21
type IV (delayed-type), 21
Hypersensitivity angiitis (leukocytoclastic angiitis; microscopic polyarteritis), 204
Hypersensitivity pneumonitis, 167
Hypersomnolence (pickwickian syndrome), 13
Hypersplenism, 103, 104
thrombocytopenia and, 86
Hypertension, 188
heart disease and, 217
early compensated, 217
late compensated, 217
intraparenchymal hemorrhage related to, 185
malignant, 285
portal. *See* Portal hypertension.
renal failure and, 285–287
benign nephrosclerosis and, 286–287
malignant nephrosclerosis and, 287
renin-angiotensin system and, 285
secondary forms of hypertension and, 286
sodium homeostasis and, 286
vasopressor substances and, 286
retinopathies caused by, 156–157
Hypertensive encephalopathy, 188
Hyperthyroidism (hashitoxicosis), 350, 351–352
Hypertrophic cardiomyopathy (asymmetric septal hypertrophy; hypertrophic obstructive cardiomyopathy; idiopathic hypertrophic subaortic stenosis), 221

Hypertrophic gastritis, 237
Hypertrophic osteoarthropathy, 144
Hypertrophic subaortic stenosis, idiopathic (asymmetric septal hypertrophy; hypertrophic cardiomyopathy; hypertrophic obstructive cardiomyopathy; idiopathic hypertrophic subaortic stenosis), 221
Hyperuricemia, 132–134
Hypoaldosteronism, 363, 365
Hypogammaglobulinemia
acquired, 23
Bruton's, 23
in chronic lymphocytic leukemia, 97
transient, of infancy, 23
Hypoglycemic coma, 359
Hypoparathyroidism, 356, 357
Hypoplasia
renal, 283
thymic, 367
Hypospadias, 311
Hypothalamus
posterior pituitary syndromes and, 347
suprasellar tumors of, 346
Hypothyroidism, 352
Hypoxanthine-guanine phosphoribosyltransferase deficiency, partial, in gout, 132
Hypoxia, mucosal, Cushing's ulcers causing, 238
Hypoxic (ischemic) encephalopathy, 187

I

I cell disease (type II mucolipidosis), 7
Icterus (jaundice), 256
Idiopathic pulmonary fibrosis (chronic interstitial pneumonitis; cryptogenic fibrosing alveolitis; Hamman-Rich syndrome; usual interstitial pneumonitis), 166
Idiopathic pulmonary hemosiderosis, 162
Idiopathic thrombocytopenic purpura, 87
IDL (intermediate-density lipoprotein), 201
IgA nephropathy (Berger's disease), 296
Ileus, gallstone, 275
Illicit drugs. *See* Drugs, illicit.
Immature infants, 1–2
Immune diseases, 19–25
autoimmune, 19. *See also specific diseases.*
mechanisms of tissue injury in, 19–22. *See* Hypersensitivity.
transplant rejection and, 22
primary immunodeficiency disorders, 22–24
AIDS, 23–24
systemic lupus erythematosus, 24–25
Immune-mediated reactions, myocarditis and, 220
Immunocompromised adults, suppurative arthritis in, 131
Immunodeficiency syndromes, 22–24
AIDS, 23–24

Immunoglobulins
  IgA
    celiac sprue and, 245
    α-chain disease and, 101
    in monoclonal gammopathy of undetermined significance, 101
    in multiple myeloma, 100
    selective deficiency of, 23
    type III hypersensitivity and, 21
    in Wiskott-Aldrich syndrome, 23
  IgA nephropathy (Berger's disease) and, 296
  IgD, in multiple myeloma, 100
  IgE
    hypersensitivity reaction mediated by, tubulointerstitial nephritis caused by, 297–298
    in multiple myeloma, 100
    urticaria and, 107
    in Wiskott-Aldrich syndrome, 23
  IgE antibodies, type I hypersensitivity and, 19–20
  IgG
    γ-chain disease and, 101
    hypogammaglobulinemia and, 23
    in monoclonal gammopathy of undetermined significance, 101
    in multiple myeloma, 100
    selective deficiency of, 23
    type III hypersensitivity and, 21
    in Wiskott-Aldrich syndrome, 23
  IgG antibodies
    in pemphigus, 113
    type II hypersensitivity and, 20
    warm antibody autoimmune anemia caused by, 82
  IgG autoantibodies, cold hemolysin autoimmune hemolytic anemia caused by, 82
  IgM
    μ-chain disease and, 101
    in monoclonal gammopathy of undetermined significance, 101
    in multiple myeloma, 100
    selective deficiency of, 23
    type III hypersensitivity and, 21
    in Wiskott-Aldrich syndrome, 23
  IgM antibodies, cold agglutinin autoimmune hemolytic anemia caused by, 82
Immunohemolytic anemias. See Hemolytic anemias, autoimmune (immunohemolytic).
Immunosuppressants, toxicity of, 11
Immunosuppressed patients
  basal cell carcinoma of skin in, 116
  pneumonia in, 168
  toxoplasmosis in, 68
Impetigo, 112
Inborn errors of metabolism
  central nervous system and, 178–179
  cirrhosis and, 266
Inclusion conjunctivitis, 33
Incomplete (greenstick) fractures, 141
Infants. See also Neonates.
  embryonal carcinomas endodermal sinus tumors; yolk sac tumors) in, 316
  immature, 1–2
  infant respiratory distress syndrome and, 1
  progressive spinal muscular atrophy in (Werdnig-Hoffman disease), 193
  sickle cell disease in, 84
  small for gestational age, 1–2
  sudden infant death syndrome and, 2
  toxoplasmosis in, 68
  transient hypogammaglobulinemia in, 23
Infarctions
  cerebral, 187–188
    anemic, 187–188
    hemorrhagic, 188
  hepatic, 267
  mucosal, of small intestine, 244
  mural, of small intestine, 244
  myocardial, 216
    subendocardial, 216
    transmural, 216
  pulmonary, 162
  renal, 289
  of renal tissue, 287
  splenic, 104–105
  transmural, of small intestine, 243–244
Infarct of Zahn, 267
Infections. See also Bacterial infections; Fungal infections; Parasitic infections; Viral infections; specific infections and infectious agents.
  in AIDS, 182
  of bone. See Bone, infections of.
  of central nervous system, 179–183
  in diabetes mellitus, 359
  paroxysmal cold hemoglobinuria following, 82
  pulmonary. See Pneumonia; Pulmonary infections.
  of skin. See Skin, infections of.
  of thrombi, 210
  urinary. See also Pyelonephritis.
    cystitis and, 303
  venereal, suppurative arthritis and, 131
Infectious mononucleosis, 30–31
Infective endocarditis. See Endocarditis, infective (bacterial).
Infective gastroenterocolitis, 243–245
Infiltrative (obliterative; restrictive) cardiomyopathy, 221–222
Inflammation
  of air sinuses, 153
  of bladder. See Cystitis.
  of breasts. See Breasts, inflammations of.
  of bursa, 135–136
  colonic. See Colon, inflammations of.
  dermatoses and. See Dermatoses.
  epididymal, 312–314
    epididymitis, 312–313
  florid, in primary biliary cirrhosis, 265
  hepatic, 258–262. See also Hepatitis.
  of lymph nodes, nonspecific, chronic, 90
  of nasal cavities, 152–153
  of oral cavity, 154–155
  of orbit, 156
  orbital, 156
  pelvic inflammatory disease and, 40, 343
  penile, 311
  of sinuses, 153
  testicular, 312–314
    orchitis, 312, 313
  ureteral, 307
  urethras, 307
  uterine, 335
  vascular, focal, in rickettsial infections, 34
Inflammatory bowel disease, 247
  arthritis in, 134
Inflammatory polyps
  colonic (pseudopolyps), 253
  gastric (hyperplastic polyps), 239
Influenza viruses, respiratory infections caused by, 27–28
Inhalant illicit drugs, adverse effects of, 12
Inhalation, Legionella infection acquired by, 41
Injection abscesses, atypical mycobacteria causing, 55
In situ carcinomas
  of breast, 326–328
    lobular, 327
  penile, 312
  of skin, 116
Insulinomas (β-cell tumors), 358
Intercapillary glomerulosclerosis (Kimmelstiel-Wilson syndrome; nodular glomerulosclerosis), 294
Intermediate-density lipoprotein (IDL), 201
Interstitial (Leydig) cell tumors, 318
Interstitial emphysema, 164
Interstitial fibrosis, 215
Interstitial pneumonitis, 169
  chronic (cryptogenic fibrosing alveolitis; Hamman-Rich syndrome; idiopathic pulmonary fibrosis; usual interstitial pneumonitis), 166
  desquamative, 166–167
Intestinal flukes, 74
Intestine. See Colon; Small intestine.
Intracerebral hemorrhage, traumatic, 184
Intracranial hemorrhage, 184–186
  intraparenchymal, 185
    larger, 185
    mild, 185
    subarachnoid hemorrhage and, 186
  subarachnoid, 185–186
    intraparenchymal hemorrhage and, 186
Intracranial lesions, gastric erosions and ulcers and, 237–238
Intracranial pressure, increased, 175
Intraductal carcinomas, 326–327
Intraductal papillomas, 325
Intraepithelial neoplasia, cervical (cervical dysplasia), 333–334
Intraerythrocytic asexual cycle, in malaria, 65
Intranuclear (Cowdry type A) inclusions, in herpesvirus infections, 29
Intraparenchymal hemorrhage. See Intracranial hemorrhage, intraparenchymal.
Intrathoracic (plunging) goiter, 350
Intravascular hemolysis, 77
Intravenous drug abusers, infective endocarditis in, 226

Iridocyclitis, 156
Iron deficiency, 17
Iron deficiency anemia, 17, 79–80
Irradiation, central nervous system and, 178
Ischemic (stagnant) anoxia, 186
Ischemic atrophy, patchy, renal, 286
Ischemic bowel disease, small intestinal, 242–243
  mucosal and mural infarctions, 243
  transmural infarction, 242–243
Ischemic (hypoxic) encephalopathy, 187
Ischemic heart disease, 215–216
  angina pectoris, 215
  chronic, 215
  myocardial infarction, 216
  sudden cardiac death and, 215
Ischemic renal injury, 288–289
Islet cell tumors, 358
Isoniazid toxicity, 10
Isospora belli infections, 64

J

Jansky-Bielschowsky disease, 6
Jaundice (icterus), 256
Joint(s)
  arthritis and. *See* Arthritis.
  bursitis of, 135–136
  tenosynovitis of, 135
"Joint mice," 129
Junctional nevus, 117–118
Juvenile amaurotic idiocy of Spielmeyer-Vogt, 6
Juvenile ("strawberry") hemangiomas, 207
Juvenile onset (insulin-dependent; type I) diabetes mellitus, 358–359
Juvenile pernicious anemia, 79
Juvenile polyp(s), colonic, 253
Juvenile polyposis syndrome, 253
Juvenile rheumatoid arthritis (Still's disease), 131
Juxtaglomerular tumors, renin-producing, 300–301

K

Kala-azar (visceral leishmaniasis), 67
Kaposi's sarcoma, 23, 120
Kartagener syndrome, 153, 214
Kawasaki syndrome (disease), 31, 206
Keratin pearls, 116
Keratoacanthomas, 115
Keratoses
  actinic, 115–116
  follicular, inverted, 114
  seborrheic (dermatosis papulosa nigra; senile keratoses), 114
Keshan disease (congestive cardiomyopathy; dilated cardiomyopathy), 18, 220
Ketoacidosis, in diabetes mellitus, 359
Kidneys, 283–305. *See also headings beginning with term* Renal.
  congenital anomalies of, 283
  cystic diseases of. *See* Renal cysts.

ectopic, 283
glomerular diseases of. *See* Glomerular diseases; Glomerulonephritis.
horseshoe, 283
left-sided congestive heart failure and, 218, 219
medullary sponge, 284
pyelonephritis and, 303–305
  acute, 304
  chronic, 304–305
transplantation of, transplant rejection and, 22
tubulointerstitial nephritis and, 297–298
  analgesic abuse nephropathy, 298
tumors of, 300–302
  benign, 300–301
  malignant, 301–302
urinary tract obstruction and, 302
urolithiasis and, 302–303
vascular diseases of. *See* Hypertension, renal failure and; Renal vascular diseases.
Kimmelstiel-Wilson syndrome (intercapillary glomerulosclerosis; nodular glomerulosclerosis), 294
Klatskin tumor, 277
Klebsiella infections
  cholangitis and, 261
  cystitis and, 308
  Klebsiella ozaenae, 57
  Klebsiella pneumoniae, 41
    pulmonary, 168, 169
  Klebsiella rhinoscleromatis, 56–57
  prostatitis and, 319
  pyogenic osteomyelitis and, 140
  urinary, 303
Klinefelter syndrome (47,XXX), 2
Koilocytosis (cytoplasmic vacuolization), 111
Koplik's spots, 29
Krabbe's disease (globoid cell leukodystrophy), 5, 178
Krukenberg tumors, 240, 342
Kuru, 183
Kwashiorkor, 13

L

Labyrinthitis, 152
Lacerations
  of brain, 184
  esophageal, 232
Lactase deficiency, acquired, 246
Lactating adenomas, 324
Lacunae, 188
Lacunar cells, 93–94
Landry-Guillain-Barré syndrome (acute idiopathic polyneuritis), 198
Langerhans cell histiocytoses
  acute disseminated (Letterer-Siwe disease), 102
  multifocal, 102
  unifocal, 102
Large cell carcinomas, bronchogenic, 170
Larvae, in visceral larva migrans, 70
Larva migrans, visceral, 70

hepatic abscesses and, 262
Laryngitis, 153
Larynx, 153–154
Lassa virus, 31
Lateral sclerosis
  amyotrophic, 192–193
  primary, 192–193
Lead poisoning, 9–10
LE bodies, in systemic lupus erythematosus, 24
Left-to-right shunts, 213
Left ventricular hypertrophy, 217
Legionella pneumophila infections, 41, 168
Legionnaire's disease, 41
Leigh's disease, 178
Leiomyomas, 125
  ovarian ("fibroids"; myomas), 338
Leiomyosarcomas, 125
Leishmania brasiliensis infections, 67
  hepatic abscesses and, 262
Leishmania donovani infections, 67
  hepatic abscesses and, 262
Leishmania manor infections, 67–68
Leishmania mexicana infections, 67–68
Leishmaniasis, 67–68
  cutaneous (tropical sore), 67–68
    diffuse, 67–68
  mucocutaneous (espundia), 67
  visceral (kala-azar), 67
Lentiginous hyperplasia, 118
Leprosy (Hansen's disease), 55–56
  lepromatous, 56
  tuberculoid, 56
Leptomeningitis, in listeriosis, 48
Leptospira infections
  Leptospira interrogans, 50
  myocarditis and, 219
Leptospirosis
  immune phase of, 50
  mild, 50
  septicemic phase of, 50
Lethal midline granuloma (polymorphic reticulosis), 153
Letterer-Siwe disease (acute disseminated Langerhans cell histiocytosis), 102
Leukemias, 94–98. *See also* Leukemias, acute; Leukemias, chronic.
  adult T-cell leukemia/lymphoma, 92–93, 121
  "aleukemic," 94
  of central nervous system, 196
  morphology of, 97–98
  T-cell, 31
Leukemias, acute, 94–96
  clinical presentation and treatment of, 95–96
  lymphoblastic, 94
  myeloblastic, 95
    acute erythroleukemia, 95
    acute megakaryocytic leukemia, 95
    acute monocytic leukemia, 95
    acute myelocytic leukemia with differentiation, 95
    acute myelocytic leukemia without differentiation, 95
    acute myelomonocytic leukemia, 95

Leukemias, acute *(Continued)*
  acute promyelocytic leukemia, 95
  in polycythemia vera, 99
  myelocytic, 94
Leukemias, chronic, 96–97
  hairy cell, 97
  lymphocytic, 94, 97
  myelogenous, 94
  myeloid, 96–97
    "accelerated phase" of, 97
    "blast crisis" in, 97
Leukemic infiltration, in leukemias, 95
Leukemoid reaction, 90
Leukocyte alkaline phosphatase, in myeloid
    metaplasia, 99
Leukocytoclasis, 204
Leukocytoclastic angiitis (hypersensitivity
    angiitis; microscopic polyarteritis),
    204
Leukocytosis, 89–90
  eosinophilic, 90
  monocytic, 90
  neutrophilic, 89–90
Leukodystrophies, 178–179
  adrenoleukodystrophy/adrenomyeloneu-
    ropathy, 179
  globoid cell (Krabbe's disease), 178
  metachromatic (sulfatide lipidosis), 5, 178
Leukoencephalitis, hemorrhagic, necrotiz-
    ing, acute, 190
Leukoencephalopathy
  multifocal, progressive, 182
  subcortical (Binswanger's disease), 188
Leukomalacia, periventricular, 177
Leukopenia, 89
Lewy bodies, 192
Leydig cell(s), 342
Leydig (interstitial) cell tumors
  ovarian, 342
  testicular, 318
Libman-Sacks disease, 226–227
Lichen planus, 109–110
Lichen sclerosis (chronic atrophic vulvitis),
    330
Limb-girdle muscular dystrophy, 138
Lipid cell tumors, 342
Lipidosis, sulfatide (metachromatic leukody-
    strophy), 5, 178
Lipid storage diseases, 5–6
  liver and, 273
  sphingomyelin (Niemann-Pick disease), 5,
    273
  sulfatide (metachromatic leukodystro-
    phy), 5
Lipomas, 123–124
  cardiac, 223
Lipomatous masses, non-neoplastic,
    123–124
Lipoproteins
  abetalipoproteinemia and, 246
  hyperlipidemia and, 201
Liposarcomas, 124
  myxoid, 124
  pleomorphic, 124
  round cell, 124
  well-differentiated, 124

Lissencephaly (agyria), 177
Listeria monocytogenes infections, 48
Liver. *See also* Liver diseases; *headings
    beginning with term* Hepatic.
  cystic fibrosis and, 279
  Wilson's disease and, 265
Liver cell adenomas, 269
Liver diseases, 256–273. *See also specific
    diseases.*
  alcoholic, 262–263
    cirrhosis, 263
    fatty liver, 262
    hepatitis, 262–263
  cholestasis, neonatal, 272
  cirrhosis, 257. *See* Cirrhosis.
  cystic, 268
  drug-induced, 10
  drug-related, 273
  fatty liver (alcoholic steatosis), 262
    macrovesicular, 262
    microvesicular, 262
  hyperbilirubinemias, hereditary, 271–272
  inflammatory, 258–262. *See also*
    Hepatitis.
  jaundice (icterus), 256
  liver failure, 256–257
  polycystic, 268
  portal hypertension, 257
  Reye syndrome, 272
  tumors, 268–271
    benign, 268–269
    malignant, 269–271, 273
  vascular, 266–268
    hepatic infarction, 267
    hepatic vein thrombosis, 267
    hepatic veno-occlusive disease, 268
    passive congestion, 266–267
    portal vein obstruction, 268
Liver failure, 256–257
Liver flukes, 74
  cholangiocarcinomas and, 270
  cirrhosis and, 266
Liver glycogenosis (type VI glycogen storage
    disease), 5, 273
Loa loa ("eye worm"), 72
Lobar overinflation, congenital, 164
Lobar pneumonia, 167–168
Lobular carcinoma, of breast, 328
  ductal, not otherwise specified, 327
  in situ, 327
Lobular hyperplasia, atypical, of breast, 326
"Lockjaw," 46
Löffler's endocarditis, restrictive cardiomy-
    opathy and, 221
Löffler syndrome, 167
Lower respiratory viral infections, 27
Lues. *See* Syphilis (lues).
Lung(s). *See also headings beginning with
    terms* Pulmonary *and* Respiratory.
  air conditioner, 167
  cystic fibrosis and, 278–279
  drug-induced disease of, 10
  farmer's, 167
  paragonimiasis in, 74
  pigeon breeder's (bird fancier's disease),
    167

  tumors of, 170–172
    bronchial carcinoids, 171
    bronchogenic carcinomas, 170–171
    metastatic, 172
"Lupus-band test," 110
Lupus erythematosus, 110
  discoid, 110
  systemic. *See* Systemic lupus erythemato-
    sus.
Lupus profundus, 110
Luteal cysts, 342
Luteal phase, inadequate, 336–337
Luteomas
  pregnancy, 342
  stromal, 342
Lyme disease, 51, 132
  primary stage of, 51
  second stage of, 51
  tertiary neural and vascular lesions in, 51
Lymphadenitis
  acute nonspecific, 90–91
  atypical mycobacteria causing, 55
Lymphadenopathy, in chronic lymphocytic
    leukemia, 97
Lymphangitis, 210–211
Lymphatic filariasis (elephantiasis), 33, 71
Lymphatic obstruction, malabsorption syn-
    dromes and, 244
Lymphedema, 210–211
  praecox, 211
  simple congenital, 211
Lymph nodes. *See also specific lymph node
    disorders.*
  enlargement of, in leukemia, 98
  nonspecific inflammation of, chronic, 90
  swelling of, in African trypanosomiasis,
    66
Lymphocytes. *See* Hematopoietic system,
    granulocyte and lymphocyte disorders.
Lymphocytic infiltrate, in erythema multi-
    forme, 108
Lymphocytic lymphomas, 91–93
  high-grade, 92
  intermediate-grade, 92
  low-grade, 91–92
  small, 91–92
Lymphocytic thyroiditis, subacute (pain-
    less), 351
Lymphocytosis, 90
  in chronic lymphocytic leukemia, 97
  reactive, 90
Lymphoepitheliomas, inverted, 153
Lymphogranuloma venereum, 33–34
Lymphoid aggregates, in Crohn's disease,
    247
Lymphoid polyps, colonic, 253
Lymphomas, 91–94
  adult T-cell leukemia/lymphoma, 92–93,
    121
  Burkitt's, 92
    in Epstein-Barr virus infections, 31
  of central nervous system
    primary, 196
    secondary, 196
  diffuse
    large cell, 92

mixed small and large cell, 92
small cleaved cell, 92
follicular
mixed small and large cell, 91–92
predominantly large cell, 92
small cleaved cell, 91
gastrointestinal
Mediterranean, 240
primary, 240
sporadic (Western), 240
sprue-associated, 240
Hodgkin's disease, 93–94
immunoblastic, large cell, 92
lymphoblastic, 92
lymphocytic, 91–93
mycosis fungoides, 92
small noncleaved cell, 92
T cell, cutaneous, 120–121
testicular, 318–319
Lymphomatoid granulomatosis, 205
Lymphopenias, 89
Lymphoproliferative disorders
α-chain disease, 101
γ-chain disease, 101
μ-chain disease, 101

M

McArdle's disease (type V glycogen storage disease), 5
MacCallum's plaques, 224
McCune-Albright (Albright) syndrome, 145
Macroglobulinemia, Waldenström's, 91, 100–101
Macronodular cirrhosis, 257
Maffucci syndrome, 148
Malabsorption syndromes, 244–246
abetalipoproteinemia, 246
bacterial overgrowth syndrome, 244–245
celiac sprue (celiac disease; gluten-sensitive enteropathy; nontropical sprue), 245
disaccharidase deficiency, 246
tropical sprue, 245
Whipple's disease, 245–246
Malakoplakia, 308
Malaria, 65–66
benign
quartan, 65
tertian, 65
exoerythrocytic cycle in, 65
hepatic abscesses and, 262
intraerythrocytic asexual cycle in, 65
malignant, quartan, 65
Malassezia furfur infections, 112
Males
genital system of. *See specific organs.*
sex chromosome abnormalities in, 2
Malignant external otitis, 151
Malignant hypertension, 285
Malignant melanomas, 118–119
of eye, 155
radial growth pattern of, 119
variegated color of, 118
vertical growth pattern of, 119

vulvar, 332
Mallory bodies, in alcoholic hepatitis, 262
Mallory-Weiss syndrome, 232
Malnutrition, protein-energy, 13
Malrotations, of small intestine, 242
Mammary duct ectasia, 324
Marantic (nonbacterial thrombotic) endocarditis, 226
Marasmus, 13
"Marble bones" (Albers-Schönberg disease; osteopetrosis), 146
adult pattern of, 146
Marburg type multiple sclerosis, 189
Marburg virus, 31
Marfan syndrome, 3
Marie-Strümpell disease (ankylosing spondylitis; rheumatoid spondylitis), 131
Marijuana, adverse effects of, 11–12
Mask of pregnancy (melasma), 117
Mastitis, acute, 323
Mastocytomas, solitary, 121
Mastocytosis, 121
with systemic manifestations, 121
M component, in multiple myeloma, 100
Measles (rubeola), 29
Meckel's diverticulum, 242
Medial calcific sclerosis (Mönckeberg's arteriosclerosis), 199–200
Mediastinal tumors, 172
Mediastinopericarditis, 228
adhesive, 229
Mediterranean lymphomas, 240
Medullary carcinomas
of breast, 327
thyroid, 354. *See also* Multiple endocrine neoplasia.
Medullary sponge kidney, 284
Medulloblastomas, 195
Megacolon, 249–250
acquired, 249
in Chagas disease, 67
congenital (Hirschsprung's disease), 249–250
Megaesophagus, in Chagas disease, 67
Megalencephaly, 177
Megaloblastic anemias, 16, 79
Meigs syndrome, 341
Meissner's plexus, 250
Melanomas, malignant. *See* Malignant melanomas.
Melanosis coli, 250
Melasma (mask of pregnancy), 117
Melioidosis, 50
Membranoproliferative glomerulonephritis, 296
type I, 296
type II, 296
type III, 296
Membranous glomerulonephritis (membranous nephropathy), 289–290, 293
MEN (multiple endocrine neoplasia)
type IIa, 354, 358
type IIb, 354, 358
Menetrier's disease, 237
Ménière's disease, 152

Meningiomas, 195–196
benign, 195–196
fibroblastic, 195
malignant, 196
syncytial, 195
transitional, 195–196
Meningitis, 179
acute
lymphocytic, 179
pyogenic, 179
aseptic, in AIDS, 182
blood-borne route of transmission of, 179
chronic, 179
direct implantation and, 179
gonococcal, 40
Haemophilus influenzae, 42
local extension and, 179
meningococcal, 39
in tuberculosis, 55
Meningocele, 176
cranial, 176
Meningococcal infections, 39–40
Meningoencephalitis, amebic, 63–64
Menkes kinky hair disease, 17–18
Merkel cell carcinoma, 117
Mesotheliomas
benign (pleural fibromas), 172
malignant, 172–173
Metabolic diseases, secondary cardiomyopathy and, 222
Metabolic disorders, inborn errors of metabolism
central nervous system and, 178–179
cirrhosis and, 266
Metabolic factors
in Addison's disease, 364
neonatal cholestasis and, 272
Metabolic rate, in hyperthyroidism, 351
Metachromatic leukodystrophy (sulfatide lipidosis), 5, 178
Metastatic tumors. *See* Tumor(s), metastatic.
Methyl alcohol
central nervous system and, 178
toxicity of, 9
Microadenomas, pituitary, 345
Microangiopathic hemolytic anemias, 78, 287–288
Microangiopathy, diabetic, 359
Microcephaly, 177
Microcytic anemia, iron deficiency and, 17
Microglandular endocervical hyperplasia, 333
Micronodular cirrhosis, 257
Microscopic polyarteritis (hypersensitivity angiitis; leukocytoclastic angiitis), 204
Microvesicular steatosis, hepatitis induced by, 260
Midgut carcinoids, 248
Midsystolic click, 224
Migratory phlebitis, 210
Mikulicz cells, 57
Mikulicz syndrome, 58
Miliary tuberculosis, 55
Milroy's disease, 211
"Milwaukee shoulder syndrome," 134

Minimal change disease (lipoid nephrosis), 290
Mitral valve
  anulus of, calcification of, 227
  prolapse of, 224
Mixed connective tissue disease, 26
Mixed stones, 275–276
Moles. See Nevus(i), nevocellular (mole; pigmented nevus).
Molluscum bodies, 112
Molluscum contagiosum, 111–112
Mönckeberg's arteriosclerosis (medial calcific sclerosis), 199–200
Mongolism (Down syndrome; trisomy 21), 3
  Alzheimer's disease in, 191
Moniliasis (oral candidiasis; thrush), 59, 154–155
Monoclonal gammopathy of undetermined significance, 101
Monocytic leukocytosis, 90
Mononeuropathy, 197
Mononucleosis, infectious, 30–31
Monostotic fibrous dysplasia, 145
Motor neurons, degenerative diseases of, 192–193
Mucinous (colloid) carcinoma, of breast, 327
Mucinous tumors, ovarian, 339
Mucoceles, 153
  of gallbladder (hydrops), 275
Mucocutaneous leishmaniasis (espundia), 67
Mucocutaneous neuromas, 358
Mucolipidoses, 7
  type I (I Cell disease), 7
  type II (pseudo-Hurler syndrome), 7
Mucopolysaccharidoses, 6
  liver and, 273
  type I (Hurler syndrome), 6
  type II (Hunter syndrome; Sanfilippo syndrome), 6
Mucor infections, 60
  encephalitis and, 183
  pulmonary, 168
Mucormycetes infections, gastroenterocolitis and, 243
Mucormycosis (phycomycosis; zygomycosis), 60
Mucosal cells, small intestinal, abnormalities of, 244
Mucosal hypoxia, Cushing's ulcers causing, 238
Mucosal infarction, of small intestine, 244
Mucus production, copious, in bronchial asthma, 165
Multifocal growth pattern, in basal cell carcinoma of skin, 116
"Multiform" lesions, in erythema multiforme, 108
Multinodular (adenomatous; multiple colloid adenomatous) goiter, intrathoracic (plunging), 350
Multiple endocrine neoplasia (MEN)
  type IIa, 354, 358
  type IIb, 354, 358
Multiple myeloma, 100
Multiple sclerosis, 189

Charcot type, 189
  Marburg type, 189
Multisystem diseases, rapidly progressive glomerulonephritis and, 292
Mumps, 28
  orchitis and, 313
Munro's microabscesses, 109
Mural infarction, of small intestine, 244
Murine typhus, 35
Muscle(s)
  atrophy of, 136
    denervation, 137
    group, 137
    infantile progressive spinal muscular atrophy (Werdnig-Hoffman disease), 193
    peroneal (Charcot-Marie-Tooth disease, hypertrophic type; sensory motor neuropathy, type I hereditary), 198
    progressive, 192–193
  endocrine disorders of, 139
  enzyme deficiencies and, 139
  myopathic diseases of, 137–138
    centronuclear (myotubular), 139
    congenital, 139
    muscular dystrophies, 138
    nemaline (rod body), 139
    ocular, 138
  neurogenic diseases of, 136–137
    denervation atrophy, 137
    Eaton-Lambert syndrome, 137
    myasthenia gravis, 137
  pathologic reactions of, 136
  toxins and, 139
  type grouping of fibers, 137
Muscle glycogenosis (type V glycogen storage disease), 5
Muscular dystrophies, 138
  Becker, 138
  Duchenne, 7, 138
  fascioscapulohumeral, 138
  limb-girdle, 138
  myotonic, 138
Musculoskeletal system. See also Bone(s); Muscle(s); specific musculoskeletal disorders.
  rheumatoid arthritis and, 130
Myasthenia gravis, 137, 368
Mycetomas, 62
Mycobacterium infections, 54–56
  in AIDS, 24
  atypical, 55
  Mycobacterium avium-intracellulare, 55
  Mycobacterium chelonei, 55
  Mycobacterium fortuitum, 55
  Mycobacterium kansasii, 55
  Mycobacterium leprae, 55–56
  Mycobacterium marinum, 55
  Mycobacterium scrofulaceum, 55
  Mycobacterium tuberculosis, 55
  Mycobacterium tuberculosis bovis, 54
  Mycobacterium tuberculosis hominis, 54
  Mycobacterium ulcerans, 55
  myocarditis and, 219
Mycoplasma infections, 36–37
  cystitis and, 308

Mycoplasma hominis, 36
Mycoplasma pneumoniae, 36–37
  pulmonary, 169
  ureteral, 307
Mycosis fungoides, 92, 120–121
  d'emblée, 121
Myelinolysis, central pontine, 178
Myelocele, 176
Myelodysplastic syndromes, 96
Myelofibrosis, in myeloid metaplasia, 99
Myelolipomas, 123
Myeloma(s)
  multiple, 100
  solitary (plasmacytoma), 100, 153
Myeloma nephrosis, 100
Myeloproliferative disorders, 98–99. See also Leukemias, chronic, myeloid.
  myeloid metaplasia with myelofibrosis, 99
  polycythemia vera, 81, 98–99
Myocardial atrophy, 215
Myocardial infarction, acute, 216
  subendocardial, 216
  transmural, 216
Myocarditis, 219–220
  in Chagas disease, 67
  postviral, dilated cardiomyopathy and, 220
Myofibers, variation in diameter of, 136
Myomas ("fibroids"; leiomyomas), 338
Myonecrosis, clostridial (gas gangrene), 47
Myopathic changes, 136
Myopathies. See Muscle, myopathic diseases of.
Myositis ossificans, traumatic, 128
Myotonia, 138
Myotonic dystrophy, 138
Myotubular (centronuclear) myopathy, 139
Myxedema, 352
Myxoid liposarcomas, 124
Myxoid malignant fibrous histiocytomas, 123
Myxomas, 222–223
Myxopapillary ependymomas, 194

N

Nabothian cysts, 333
Naegleria fowleri infections, 63–64
Nasal cavities, inflammation of, 152–153
"Nasal polyps," 153
Nasal tumors, 153
Nasopharynx, tumors of, 153
Necator americanus infections, 69
Neck. See specific organs.
Necrosis
  papillary (necrotizing papillitis), 304
  submassive, 259
Necrotizing cellulitis, 47
Necrotizing enterocolitis, 253
Necrotizing glomerulitis, 287
Necrotizing granulomas, acute, 205
Necrotizing granulomatous sinusitis, 153
Necrotizing hemorrhagic leukoencephalitis, acute, 190
Necrotizing papillitis (papillary necrosis), 304

Necrotizing vasculitis, focal, 205
Needle users, infections in, 11
Neisseria infections
    myocarditis and, 219
    Neisseria gonorrhoeae, 40
        endocarditis and, 226
        epididymal, 313
    Neisseria meningitidis, 39–40
        meningitis and, 179
Nemaline (rod body) myopathy, 139
Nematodes, hepatic abscesses and, 262
Neonatal conjunctivitis, gonococcal, 40
Neonatal thrombocytopenia, 86
Neonates
    cholestasis in, 272
    hemorrhagic destruction of adrenal glands
        in, 364
    respiratory distress syndrome of (hyaline
        membrane disease), 160–161
Neoplastic disease. *See* Tumor(s).
Neoplastic polyps, colonic, 253–254
Nephritis
    interstitial, hypersensitivity, 297–298
    tubulointerstitial, 297–298
        analgesic abuse nephropathy, 298
        hypersensitivity interstitial nephritis,
            297–298
Nephroblastomas (Wilms tumors), 301–302
Nephrolithiasis, uric acid, in gout, 133
Nephronophthisis uremic medullary cystic
        disease complex, 284–285
Nephropathy
    analgesic abuse, 298
    diabetic, 360
    IgA (Berger's disease), 296
    membranous (membranous glomeru-
        lonephritis), 289–290
    reflux (chronic-reflux associated
        pyelonephritis), 304–305
    in sickle cell disease, 288
    urate, chronic, in gout, 133–134
    uric acid, acute, in gout, 133
Nephrosclerosis, 286–287
    benign, 286–287
    malignant, 287
Nephrosis
    lipoid (minimal change disease), 290
    myeloma, 100
Nephrotic syndrome, 289, 290
Nervous system, in Lyme disease, 132
Neurilemmomas (schwannomas), 127, 198
Neuroblastomas, 126–127, 195
    Hutchinson-type, 126
    olfactory, 153
Neuroendocrine cells, 248
Neuroendocrine tumors. *See* Carcinoids
        (endocrine cell tumors; neuroen-
        docrine tumors).
Neurofibrillary tangles, 190, 191
Neurofibromas, 127, 198
Neurofibromatosis, 177
    von Recklinghausen's, 195
Neurogenic muscle disease. *See* Muscle,
        neurogenic diseases of.
Neurologic disorders, in systemic lupus ery-
        thematosus, 24

Neuromas
    acoustic, 152
    mucocutaneous, 358
    traumatic (amputation), 197
Neuromuscular diseases, secondary car-
        diomyopathy and, 222
Neuromyelitis optica (Devic's disease), 189
Neuronophagia, 180
Neuropathies
    diabetic, 360
    peripheral, 197–198
        multiple, 197
Neurosyphilis, paretic, 180
Neutropenia, 89
Neutrophil(s), destruction of, neutropenia
        caused by, 89
Neutrophilic leukocytosis, 89–90
Nevocellular nevus. *See* Nevus(i), nevocellu-
        lar (mole; pigmented nevus).
Nevus(i), 117–119. *See also* Basal cell nevus
        syndrome.
    basal cell carcinoma of skin and, 116
    dysplastic, 118
    of eye, 155
    flammeus, 208
    malignant melanoma, 118–119
    nevocellular (mole; pigmented nevus),
        117–118
        blue, 118
        common acquired, 117
        compound, 118
        compound nevi of Spitz, 118
        congenital, 118
        dermal, 118
        halo, 118
        junctional, 117–118
Newborns. *See* Neonates.
Nezelof syndrome, 23
Niacin deficiency, 16
Niemann-Pick disease (sphingomyelin lipi-
        doses), 5, 273
Nigrostriatal dopaminergic system, 191
Nipples
    congenital inversion of, 323
    supernumerary, 323
Nocardia infections, 56
    Nocardia asteroides, 56
    Nocardia brasiliensis, 56, 62
Nodular (pseudosarcomatous) fasciitis,
        127–128
    cellular stage of, 128
    fascial form of, 127
    fibrosing stage of, 128
    intramuscular form of, 127
    myxoid stage of, 128
    subcutaneous form of, 127
Nodular hyperplasia
    hepatic, focal, 268
    prostatic (benign prostatic
        hypertrophy/hyperplasia), 319–320
Nodular lesions, in basal cell carcinoma of
        skin, 116
Nodular tenosynovitis (giant cell tumor of
        tendon sheath), 135
Nodules, thyroid, 348
    "cold," 348

"hot," 348
Noncaseating granulomas
    in Crohn's disease, 247
    in sarcoidosis, 58
Non-Hodgkin's lymphomas. *See*
        Lymphocytic lymphomas.
Nonossifying fibromas (fibrous cortical
        defects), 145
Nonreaginic asthma, 165
Nonspecific lymphadenitis, acute, 90–91
Nonthrombocytopenic purpura, 86
Nontropical sprue (celiac disease; celiac
        sprue; gluten-sensitive enteropathy),
        113, 245
North American Brugia, 72
Norwalk agents, digestive tract infections
        caused by, 28
Nuclei, centrally located, in muscle, 136
"Nurse cell," in trichinosis, 71
Nutritional diseases, 13–18
    of central nervous system, 177–178
    mineral deficiencies, 17–18
    protein-energy malnutrition, 13
    vitamin deficiencies
        of fat-soluble vitamins, 13–15
        of water-soluble vitamins, 15–16

O

Obesity, 13
Obliterative (infiltrative; restrictive) car-
        diomyopathy, 221–222
Obstructive lung disease. *See* Chronic
        obstructive pulmonary disease.
Obstructive overinflation, 164
Occupational asthma, 165
Ocular glandular syndrome (Parinaud syn-
        drome), 52
Ocular myopathy, 138
Ocular trauma, 156
Oculoglandular tularemia, 49
Oligodendrogliomas, 194
Olivopontocerebellar atrophy ("heteroge-
        neous system degeneration"), 190
Ollier's disease (enchondromatosis), 148
Onchocerca volvulus infections, 71
Onchocerciasis, 71
Oncocytomas, renal, 301
Onychomycosis, 112
Open (compound) fractures, 141–142
Ophthalmia, sympathetic, 156
Ophthalmopathy, in Graves disease, 352
Opisthorchis felineus infections, 74
    hepatic abscesses and, 262
Opisthorchis sinensis infections
    cholangiocarcinomas and, 270
    pigment stones and, 276
Opisthorchis viverrini infections, 74
Oral candidiasis (moniliasis; thrush), 59,
        154–155
Oral cavity, 154–155
    congenital anomalies of, 154
    inflammation of, 154–155
Oral contraceptives, endometrial changes
        induced by, 337

Orbit, inflammation of, 156
Orchitis, 312, 313
  granulomatous, 313
Ornithosis (psittacosis), 32, 169
Oroya fever (Carrión's disease), 58
Osseous callus, 142
Osteitis
  deformans. *See* Paget's disease, of bone (osteitis deformans).
  fibrosa
    cystica (von Recklinghausen's disease of bone), 144
    hyperparathyroidism-induced, 143–144
Osteoarthritis. *See* Degenerative diseases, of joints (osteoarthritis).
Osteoarthropathy, hypertrophic, 144
Osteoblastic tumors, 147–148
Osteoblastomas (giant osteoid osteomas), 147
Osteochondromas (exostoses), 146–147, 148
  multiple, hereditary (osteochondromatosis), 146
Osteochondromatosis (hereditary multiple exostoses), 146
Osteoclastomas (giant cell tumors), 149
Osteodystrophy, renal, 144
Osteogenesis imperfecta, 145–146
  type I, 145
  type II, 145–146
  type III, 146
  type IV, 146
"Osteogenic" sarcomas (osteosarcomas), 147–148
Osteoma(s), 147–148
  osteoid, 147
    giant (osteoblastomas), 147
Osteomalacia, 143, 144
  vitamin D and, 14
Osteomyelitis
  Garré's sclerosing, 140
  pyogenic, 140–141
  syphilis, 141
  tuberculous (Pott's disease), 55, 141
Osteopetrosis (Albers-Schönberg disease; "marble bones"), 146
  adult pattern of, 146
Osteophytes, 129
Osteoporosis, 142
  idiopathic, 142
  primary, 142
  secondary, 142
Osteosarcomas ("osteogenic" sarcomas), 147–148
Ostium primum defects, 213
Ostium secundum defects, 213
Otitis
  external, malignant, 151
  media
    acute suppurative, 152
    chronic, 152
    serous, 152
Otosclerosis, 152
Ovarian cysts, 342
  follicular, 342
  luteal, 342
Ovarian tumors, 339–342

germ cell, 340–341
  metastatic, 342
  sex cord-stromal, 341–342
  of surface epithelium, 339–340
Oxyphil (Hürthle) cells, in follicular thyroid carcinomas, 354
Oxytocin secretion, 347
Ozena, 57

P

Pachygyria, 177
Paget's disease
  of bone (osteitis deformans), 142–143
    initial osteolytic stage of, 143
    secondary osteoblastic activity in, 143
  of breast, 327–328
  extramammary, 331–332
Painless (subacute lymphocytic) thyroiditis, 351
Panacinar (panlobular) emphysema, 164
Pancreas. *See* Endocrine pancreas; Exocrine pancreas; Pancreatitis.
Pancreatic islets, in diabetes mellitus, 359
Pancreatic tissue, ectopic, 278
  in small intestine, 242
Pancreatitis, 279–280
  acute, 279–280
    hemorrhagic, 279
  chronic, 280
    calcifying, 280
    obstructive, 280
Pancytopenia, in leukemia, 98
Panencephalitis, sclerosing, subacute (Dawson's encephalitis), 182
Panniculitis, 108, 110
Pannus, in rheumatoid arthritis, 130
Papanicolaou (Pap) smear, 334
Papilla, sloughing of, in analgesic abuse nephropathy, 298
Papillary carcinomas, thyroid, 353
Papillary-cystic (solid-cystic) tumors, pancreatic, 281
Papillary fibroelastosis, 223
Papillary hidradenomas, 331
Papillary necrosis (necrotizing papillitis), 304
Papilledema, 156–157
Papillitis, necrotizing (papillary necrosis), 304
Papillomas
  of choroid plexus, 194–195
  of gallbladder, 276
  intraductal, 325
  inverted, nasal and paranasal, 153
  laryngeal, 154
  squamous, vulvar, 331
  transitional cell, of bladder, 309
Papillomatous epidermal hyperplasia, 111
Paracoccidioides brasiliensis infections, 61
Paracoccidioidomycosis, 61
Parafollicular hyperplasia, 90
Paragonimiasis, 74–75
Paragonimus westermani infections, 74–75
Parainfluenza viruses, respiratory infec-

tions caused by, 28
Paralysis agitans (idiopathic Parkinson's disease), 192
Paramyxovirus, digestive tract infections caused by, 28
Paraovarian cysts (hydatids of Morgagni), 343
Paraphimosis, 311
Paraseptal (distal acinar) emphysema, 164
Parasitic infections, 63–76
  in AIDS, 23
  encephalitis and, 183
  gastroenterocolitis and, 243–244
  helminthic, 68–76
    cestodes, 72–73
    hepatic abscesses and, 261
    intestinal roundworms, 68–70
    nematodes, hepatic abscesses and, 262
    tissue roundworms, 70–72
    trematodes, 73–76
  metazoal, myocarditis and, 219
  protozoal, 63–68
    of blood and tissues, 65–67
    encephalitis and, 183
    hepatic abscesses and, 261, 262
    intracellular, 67–68
    luminal, 63–65
    myocarditis and, 219
Parathyroid glands, 356–357. *See also* Multiple endocrine neoplasia.
  adenomas of, 356
  carcinomas of, 356
  hyperparathyroidism and
    primary, 356–357
    secondary, 357
  hypoparathyroidism and, 356, 357
  primary hyperplasia of, 356–357
  pseudo- and pseudopseudohypoparathyroidism and, 357
Parathyroid hormone, 356
Paretic neurosyphilis, 180
Parinaud syndrome (ocular glandular syndrome), 52
Parkinsonism, 191–192
  idiopathic Parkinson's disease (paralysis agitans), 192
  postencephalic, 183
  postencephalitic Parkinson's disease, 192
Paronychia, 37
Parotitis, mumps, 28
Paroxysmal nocturnal hemoglobinuria, 81
Passive congestion, 266–267
  active, 266
  passive, chronic, 267
Pasteurella multocida infections, 49
Patau syndrome (D trisomy; 13-15 trisomy), 3
Patchy ischemic atrophy, renal, 286
Patent ductus arteriosus, 213
Paul-Bunnell (heterophil) antibodies, in infectious mononucleosis, 31
Pautrier's microabscesses, 120
P blood group antigen, IgG autoantibodies against, in cold hemolysin autoimmune hemolytic anemia, 82
Peau d'orange, 328
Pellagra, 16

Pelvic inflammatory disease (suppurative salpingitis), 40, 343
Pemphigoid, bullous, 113
Pemphigus, 113
   erythematosus, 113
   foliaceus, 113
   vulgaris, 113
Penis, 311–312
   congenital anomalies of, 311
   inflammation of, 311
   tumors of, 311–312
Pepper-type syndrome, 126
Peptic ulcers, gastric and duodenal, 238
Perfusion, impaired, hepatitis induced by, 260
Pericardial disease, 227–229. See also Pericarditis.
   hemopericardium, 228
   pericardial effusions, 227–228
Pericardial effusions, 227–228
   serous, 226
Pericarditis, 228–229
   adhesive mediastinopericarditis, 229
   caseous, 228–229
   constrictive, 228, 229
   fibrinous, 228
   hemorrhagic, 228
   mediastinopericarditis, 228
   purulent (suppurative), 228
   serofibrinous, 228
   serous, 228
Pericholangitis, 261
Perinephric abscesses, 304
Peripartum period, dilated cardiomyopathy during, 220
Peripheral nervous system, 196–198
   degenerative diseases of, 196–197
   meningitis caused by infections of, 179
   peripheral neuropathies and, 197–198
   tumors of, 198
Peripheral neuropathies, 197–198
   in AIDS, 182
Perivenous demyelination, 189–190
Periventricular leukomalacia, 177
Perivenular demyelination, 189–190
Pernicious anemia, 79
   juvenile, 79
Peroneal muscular atrophy (Charcot-Marie-Tooth disease, hypertrophic type; sensory motor neuropathy, type I hereditary), 198
Peutz-Jeghers polyps, 253
Peyronie's disease, 127
Phacomatoses, 177
Pharmacologic asthma, 165
Phencyclidine hydrochloride ("angel dust"), adverse effects of, 11
Phenylketonuria, 6
Pheochromocytomas, 366. See also Multiple endocrine neoplasia.
   extra-adrenal, 366
Philadelphia chromosome, 96
Phimosis, 311
Phlebitis, migratory, 210
Phlebosclerosis, 209
Phlegmasia alba dolens, 210

5-Phosphoribosyl-1-pyrophosphate synthetase variants, in gout, 132
Phosphorus metabolism, vitamin D and, 14
Phycomycetes, 60
Phycomycosis (mucormycosis; zygomycosis), 60
Phyllodes tumors (cystosarcoma phyllodes), 325
Pick's bodies, 191
Pick's cells, 191
Pick's disease, 191
Pickwickian syndrome (hypersomnolence), 13
Pigeon breeder's lung (bird fancier's disease), 167
Pigmentary disorders, of skin, 117
Pigmented nevus. See Nevus(i), nevocellular (mole; pigmented nevus).
Pigmented villonodular synovitis, 135
Pigment stones, 276
Pilar (trichilemmal) cysts, 115
Pineal gland, 367
Pineoblastomas, 367
Pinguecula, 156
Pinta, 53
Pinworm (Enterobius vermicularis) infections, 69
Pipe stem fibrosis, in schistosomiasis, 76
Pituitary gland, 345–347
   adenomas of, 345–346
      hormone-secreting, 345
      large, 345
      microadenomas, 345
      non-secretory, 345
   anterior pituitary insufficiency and, 346
   posterior pituitary syndromes and, 347
Pituitary necrosis, postpartum, 346
Plague, 48–49
   bubonic, 48–49
   "plague minor," 48
   pneumonic, 48, 49
   septicemic, 48, 49
Plane xanthoma, 120
Plaques
   atheromatous, 200–201
      "complicated," 201
      renal, 288
   MacCallum's, 224
   in multiple sclerosis, 189
   senile, 191
Plasma cell dyscrasias, 99–101
   glomerular lesions associated with, 295
   heavy chain disease, 101
   monoclonal gammopathy of undetermined significance, 101
   multiple myeloma, 100
   solitary myeloma (plasmacytoma), 100
   Waldenström's macroglobulinemia, 91, 100–101
Plasmacytomas (solitary myelomas), 100, 153
Plasmodium falciparum infections, 66
Plasmodium malariae infections, 65
Plasmodium ovale infections, 65
Plasmodium vivax infections, 65
Platelets

decreased production of, thrombocytopenia due to, 86
   decreased survival of, thrombocytopenia due to, 86
   defective function of, 87
Platyhelminthes. See Cestodes.
Pleiotropy, 3
Pleomorphic liposarcomas, 124
Pleomorphic rhabdomyosarcomas, 125
Pleural diseases, 172–174
   noninflammatory pleural effusions, 174
   pleuritis, 173
   pneumothorax, 173–174
   tumors, 172–173
Pleural effusions, noninflammatory, 174
Pleuritis, 173
   hemorrhagic, 173
   serofibrinous, 173
   suppurative (empyema), 173
Pleuropneumonia-like organisms, 36–37
Plexogenic pulmonary arteriopathy, 163
Plummer-Vinson syndrome, 80, 231
Plunging (intrathoracic) goiter, 350
Pneumococcus infections, 39
   conjunctival, 155
   meningitis and, 179
Pneumocystis carinii infections, 65, 168
Pneumonia, 27
   eosinophilic, chronic, 167
   Haemophilus influenzae, 42
   hemorrhagic (woolsorter's disease), 48
   interstitial, 36–37
   lobar, 167–168
   in measles, 29
   Pneumocystis carinii, 65, 168
   staphylococcal, 37
Pneumonic plague, 48, 49
Pneumonitis
   hypersensitivity, 167
   interstitial, 169
      chronic (cryptogenic fibrosing alveolitis; Hamman-Rich syndrome; idiopathic pulmonary fibrosis; usual interstitial pneumonitis), 166
      desquamative, 166–167
   in rheumatic heart disease, 225
Pneumothorax, 173–174
   tension, 174
Poikilocytes, in myeloid metaplasia, 99
Poliomyelitis, encephalitis and, 181
Polyarteritis, microscopic (hypersensitivity angiitis; leukocytoclastic angiitis), 204
Polyarteritis nodosa, 203–204
   glomerular lesions associated with, 295
   healed, 204
Polyarthritis, in Lyme disease, 132
Polycystic kidney disease
   adult, 284
   childhood, 284
Polycystic liver disease, 268
Polycystic ovaries (Stein-Leventhal syndrome), 342
Polycythemia, 81
   absolute
      primary, 81
      secondary, 81

Polycythemia (Continued)
    relative, 81
    vera, 81, 98–99
Polydipsia, in diabetes mellitus, 359
Polyembryomas, 317
    ovarian, 341
Polyglandular deficiency syndrome
        (Schmidt syndrome), 364
Polykaryons (giant cells), in herpesvirus
        infections, 29
Polymicrogyria, 177
Polymorphic reticulosis (lethal midline
        granuloma), 153
Polymyositis-dermatomyositis, 26
    mixed connective tissue disease and, 26
Polyneuritis, acute idiopathic (Landry-
        Guillain-Barré syndrome), 198
Polyneuropathy, sensorimotor. See
        Sensorimotor polyneuropathy.
Polyostotic fibrous dysplasia, 145
    in association with endocrinopathies, 145
Polyp(s)
    adenomatous, small intestinal, 248
    colonic. See Colon, polyps of.
    endocervical, 333
    endometrial, benign, 337–338
    fibroepithelial (acrochordon; skin tags;
        squamous papilloma), 114
    inflammatory
        gastric (hyperplastic), 239
        mucosal, sessile, 278
    laryngeal, 153–154
    neoplastic, gastric, 239
Polypoid cystitis, 308
    interstitial (Hunner's ulcer), 308
Polypoid fungating lesions, esophageal, 233
Polyposis coli, familial, 254
Polyuria, in diabetes mellitus, 359
Pompe's disease, generalized or cardiac form
        (type II glycogen storage disease), 4
"Porcelain gallbladder," 275
Porencephaly, encephaloclastic, 177
Poromas, eccrine, 115
Porphyria, 113–114
Portal hypertension, 257
    intrahepatic, 257
    posthepatic, 257
    prehepatic, 257
Portal vein
    obstruction of, 268
        extrahepatic, 268
        intrahepatic, 268
    occlusion of, 267
Port-wine stain, 208
Posterior fossa ependymomas, 194
Posterior pituitary syndromes, 347
Postnecrotic cirrhosis, 263–264
Postpartum pituitary necrosis, 346
Poststreptococcal glomerulonephritis, acute,
        291–292
Post-transfusion thrombocytopenia, 86
Pott's disease (tuberculous osteomyelitis),
        55, 141
Preformed bacterial toxins, 243
Pregnancy, mask of (melasma), 117
Pregnancy luteomas, 342

Pregnancy tumor (granuloma gravidarum),
        208
Primary healing, 12
Primary lateral sclerosis, 192–193
Primitive cells, of central nervous system,
        tumors of, 195
Prinzmetal's variant angina, 215
Procallus, 142
Progressive bulbar palsy, 192–193
Progressive multifocal leukoencephalopa-
        thy, 182
Progressive muscular atrophy, 192–193
Progressive supranuclear palsy, 192
Progressive systemic sclerosis, 25
    scleroderma in, 25
Propionibacterium acnes infections, 110
Prostatic diseases, 319–321
    carcinoma, 320–321
    nodular hyperplasia (benign prostatic
        hypertrophy/hyperplasia), 319–320
    prostatitis, 319
        acute bacterial, 319
        chronic abacterial, 319
Prosthetic valves
    complications of, 227
    infective endocarditis and, 226
Protein
    malabsorption of, 244
    synthesis of, hepatic, diminished, 256
Protein-energy malnutrition, 13
Proteus infections
    cystitis and, 308
    prostatitis and, 319
    Proteus mirabilis, 41
    pulmonary, 168
    urinary, 303
    urolithiasis and, 303
Protozoal diseases. See Parasitic infections,
        protozoal.
Pseudocysts, pancreatic, 280–281
Pseudogout (chondrocalcinosis), 134
Pseudohermaphrodites
    female, 2
    male, 2
Pseudo-Hurler syndrome (type III mucolipi-
        dosis), 7
Pseudohypoparathyroidism, 357
Pseudomembranous colitis, 47, 251–252
Pseudomonas infections
    epididymal, 313
    hepatic abscesses and, 261
    prostatitis and, 319
    Pseudomonas aeruginosa, 41
        of external ear, 151
        pulmonary, 279
    Pseudomonas cepacia, pulmonary, 279
    Pseudomonas mallei, 50
    Pseudomonas pseudomallei, 50
        pulmonary, 168
        pyogenic osteomyelitis and, 140
Pseudomyxoma peritonei, 339
Pseudopolyps (inflammatory polyps),
        colonic, 253
Pseudopseudohypoparathyroidism, 357
Pseudosarcomatous fasciitis. See Nodular
        (pseudosarcomatous) fasciitis.

Psittacosis (ornithosis), 32, 169
Psoriasis, 109
    arthritis in, 134
Pterygium, 156
Pulmonary abscesses, 169–170
    "primary cryptogenic," 169
Pulmonary alveolar proteinosis, 162–163
Pulmonary arteriopathy, plexogenic, 163
Pulmonary arteritis, in schistosomiasis, 76
Pulmonary aspergillosis, invasive, 60
Pulmonary blastomycosis, 61
Pulmonary disease, atypical mycobacteria
        causing, 55
Pulmonary edema, 160
    hemodynamic, 160
    microvascular injury and, 160
Pulmonary embolism, 161–162
Pulmonary fibrosis, idiopathic (chronic
        interstitial pneumonitis; cryptogenic
        fibrosing alveolitis; Hamman-Rich
        syndrome; usual interstitial pneu-
        monitis), 166
Pulmonary hamartomas, 171
Pulmonary heart disease (cor pulmonale),
        217
    acute, 217
    chronic, 217
Pulmonary hemorrhage, 162
    diffuse, 162
    vasculitis-associated, 162
Pulmonary hypertension, 163
    primary, 163
    secondary, 163
Pulmonary infarction, 162
Pulmonary infections, 167–170
    interstitial pneumonitis, 169
    pneumonia, bronchopneumonia and lobar
        pneumonia, 167–168
    pulmonary abscess, 169–170
Pulmonary infiltration, with eosinophilia,
        167
    secondary, chronic, 167
    simple, 167
Pulmonary valvular stenosis/atresia, 214
Pulmonary vascular diseases, 160–163
    adult respiratory distress syndrome, 161
    diffuse pulmonary hemorrhage, 162
    newborn respiratory distress syndrome
        (hyaline membrane disease), 160–161
    pulmonary alveolar proteinosis, 162–163
    pulmonary congestion and edema, 160
    pulmonary embolism, hemorrhage, and
        infarction, 161–162
    pulmonary hypertension and vascular
        sclerosis, 163
Pulmonic circulation, left-sided congestive
        heart failure and, 218
Pulseless disease (Takayasu's arteritis),
        205–206
Pulsion (Zenker's) diverticula, 232
"Punched-out defects," in multiple myeloma,
        100
Pure red cell aplasia, 80
Purkinje cells, 187
Purpura
    Henoch-Schönlein, 86

glomerular lesions associated with, 294
nonthrombocytopenic, 86
thrombocytopenic
idiopathic, 87
thrombotic, 86–87, 287–288
Purulent (suppurative) pericarditis, 228
Pustules
malignant, in anthrax, 48
spongiform, in psoriasis, 109
Pyelonephritis, 303–305
acute, 304
acute renal failure and, 299
chronic, 304–305
obstructive, 304–305
reflux associated (reflux nephropathy), 304–305
xanthogranulomatous, 305
secondary, in analgesic abuse nephropathy, 298
Pyloric stenosis, hypertrophic, congenital, 235
Pylorotomy, 235
Pyogenic osteomyelitis, 140–141
Pyonephrosis, 304
Pyramidal cell(s), 187
Pyramidal cell layers, 187
Pyridoxine (vitamin B$_6$) deficiency, 16
Pyruvate kinase deficiency, 83

Q

Q fever, 36, 169

R

Rabies, encephalitis and, 181
RA cells, 130
Radial scar (benign sclerosing ductal proliferation), 326
Radiation, cystitis and, 308
Ramsay Hunt syndrome, 30
Rapidly progressive (crescentic) glomerulonephritis, 292
idiopathic, 292
Rash
in rickettsial infections, 34
in Rocky Mountain spotted fever, 35
in systemic lupus erythematosus, 24, 25
viral disorders with, 29
zinc deficiency causing, 17
Rat-bite fever, 51–52
spirillar form (sodoku), 51–52
streptobacillary form (Haverhill fever), 51, 52
Raynaud's disease/phenomenon, 206–207
Reactive atypia, cervical, 333
Reactive hyperplasia, of spleen, 104
Reactive lymphocytosis, 90
Reagin-mediated (allergic; atopic) asthma, 165
Red blood cells. See Anemias; Hematopoietic system, erythrocyte disorders.
Red cell enzyme deficiency, 83
Reed-Sternberg cells, 93–94

Reflux nephropathy (chronic-reflux associated pyelonephritis), 304–305
Regeneration
of axons, 197
of muscle, 136
Reiter syndrome, 134, 307
Relapsing fever, 50–51
Relapsing polychondritis, 151
Renal artery stenosis, unilateral, 285
Renal cell carcinomas, 301
Renal cysts, 283–285
adult polycystic kidney disease, 284
childhood polycystic kidney disease, 284
cystic renal dysplasia, 283–284
dialysis-associated, 285
of renal medulla, 284–285
simple, 285
Renal diseases. See also specific renal diseases.
acute necrotizing granulomas and, 205
atheroembolic, 288
chronic, osteodystrophy and, 144
drug-induced, 10
glomerular, in schistosomiasis, 76
in gout, 133–134
in systemic lupus erythematosus, 24
vascular. See Renal vascular diseases.
Renal dysplasia, cystic, 283–284
Renal failure
acute, 298–300
acute tubular necrosis, 299–300
glomerular, 299
intrarenal, 298–299
postrenal, 299
prerenal, 298
tubular, 299
chronic, in analgesic abuse nephropathy, 298
hypertension and. See Hypertension, renal failure and.
Renal infarctions, 289
Renal osteodystrophy, 144
Renal pelvis, urothelial carcinomas of, 302
Renal vascular diseases, 285–289
atheroembolic, 288
diffuse cortical necrosis, 288–289
microangiopathic hemolytic anemia, 287–288
renal infarction, 289
sickle cell nephropathy, 288
Renin-angiotensin system
hypertension and, 285–286
sodium homeostasis and, 286
Renin-producing juxtaglomerular tumors, 300–301
Renomedullary interstitial cell tumors, 300
Reparative giant cell granulomas ("brown tumors"), 144
Respiratory distress syndrome
adult, 161
infant, 1
of newborn (hyaline membrane disease), 160–161
Respiratory infections, viral, 27–28
Respiratory syncytial virus, respiratory infections caused by, 28

Respiratory system, 159–174. See also Lung(s); headings beginning with term Pulmonary; specific respiratory diseases.
atelectasis and, 159–160
chronic obstructive pulmonary disease and. See Chronic obstructive pulmonary disease.
congenital anomalies of, 159
infections of. See Pneumonia; Pulmonary infections.
lung tumors and. See Lung(s), tumors of.
mediastinal tumors and, 172
pleural diseases and. See Pleural diseases.
restrictive lung diseases and. See Restrictive lung diseases.
vascular diseases of. See Pulmonary vascular diseases.
Restrictive (infiltrative; obliterative) cardiomyopathy, 221–222
Restrictive lung diseases, 163, 166–167
desquamative interstitial pneumonitis, 166–167
hypersensitivity pneumonitis, 167
idiopathic pulmonary fibrosis, 166
pulmonary infiltration with eosinophilia, 167
Reticuloendothelial hyperplasia, 103
Reticulosis, polymorphic (lethal midline granuloma), 153
Retinal detachment, 156–157
Retinitis pigmentosa, 156–157
Retinoblastomas, 155
Retinopathies, 156–157
Retrolental fibroplasia, 156
Reye syndrome, 28, 272
encephalitis and, 183
Rhabdomyomas, 124
cardiac, 124, 223
extracardiac, 124
Rhabdomyosarcomas, 124–125
alveolar, 125
botryoid, 125
cardiac, 223
embryonal (sarcoma botryoides), 332
embryonal subtype of, 124–125
pleomorphic, 125
Rheumatic fever, 224
acute, arthritis in, 134
Rheumatic heart disease, 224–225
Rheumatoid arteritis, in rheumatic heart disease, 225
Rheumatoid arthritis, 129–131
cardiac involvement in, 223
variants of, 131
Rheumatoid spondylitis (ankylosing spondylitis; Marie-Strümpell disease), 131
Rhinitis
acute, 152
allergic (hay fever), 152–153
Rhinoscleroma, 56–57
Rhinoviruses, respiratory infections caused by, 27
Rhizopus infections, 60
Riboflavin deficiency, 15

"Rice-water" stools, in *Vibrio cholerae* infections, 45
Rickets, 143
Rickettsia infections, 34–36
  encephalitis and, 183
  myocarditis and, 219
  Rickettsia prowazekii, 34–35
  Rickettsia rickettsii, 35–36
  Rickettsia tsutsugamushi, 36
    myocarditis and, 219
  Rickettsia typhi (mooseri), 35
Riedel's (stroma ligneous) thyroiditis, 351
Right-to-left shunts, 212
Right ventricular hypertrophy, 217
Ring fibers, 136
Rocky Mountain spotted fever, 35–36
Rod body (nemaline) myopathy, 139
Roseola infantum, 29
"Rose spots," in typhoid fever, 44
Rotaviruses
  digestive tract infections caused by, 28
  gastroenterocolitis and, 243
Rotor syndrome, 272
Round cell liposarcomas, 124
Roundworms
  intestinal, 68–70
    ascariasis, 68–69
    enterobiasis, 69
    hookworm disease, 69
    strongyloidiasis, 69–70
    trichuriasis, 69
  tissue, 70–72
    filariasis, 71–72
    guinea worm infection, 70
    trichinosis, 70–71
    visceral larva migrans, 70
"Rubber hose" rigidity, in Crohn's disease, 247
Rubella (German measles), 29
Rubeola (measles), 29
Russell bodies, in multiple myeloma, 100

S

Saber shin
  in congenital syphilis, 53
  in syphilis osteomyelitis, 141
Saddle nose deformity, in congenital syphilis, 53
Salivary glands, cystic fibrosis and, 279
Salmonella infections
  enteric, 43–44
  gastroenterocolitis and, 243
  myocarditis and, 219
  pyogenic osteomyelitis and, 140
  Salmonella choleraesuis, 44
  Salmonella heidelberg, 43
  Salmonella newport, 43
  Salmonella paratyphi, 43, 44
  Salmonella typhi, 44
  Salmonella typhimurium, 43, 44
  suppurative arthritis and, 132
Salpingitis
  suppurative (pelvic inflammatory disease), 40, 343

tuberculous, 343
Sandhoff's disease, 6
Sanfilippo syndrome (type II mucopolysaccharidosis), 6
San Joachim Valley fever, 61–62
Sarcoidosis, 58
Sarcoma botryoides (embryonal rhabdomyosarcoma), 332
Sarcomas. *See also specific types of sarcoma.*
  Ewing's, 149
  Kaposi's, 23, 120
  "osteogenic" (osteosarcomas), 147–148
  synovial, 126
Scalded skin syndrome (toxic epidermal necrolysis), 37, 108
Scars, 12
Schatzki's (esophageal) rings, 231
Schaumann bodies, in sarcoidosis, 58
Scheie syndrome, 6
Schilder's disease (diffuse sclerosis), 189
Schistosoma infections
  enteric, 44
  hepatic abscesses and, 262
  Schistosoma haematobium, 74, 76
    carcinoma of bladder and, 309
  Schistosoma japonicum, 74–75
  Schistosoma mansoni, 74–75
    gastroenterocolitis and, 243
Schistosomiasis, 74–75
  cystitis and, 308
Schistosomula, 75
Schizencephaly, 177
Schmidt syndrome (polyglandular deficiency syndrome), 364
Schwannomas (neurilemmomas), 127, 198
Sclera, blue, in osteogenesis imperfecta, 145
Scleritis, 156
Scleroderma
  esophagus and, 232
  linear, 25–26
  morphea, 25–26
  in progressive systemic sclerosis, 25
Sclerosing hemangioma, 119
Scolex, of intestinal tapeworms, 72
Scrapie, 183
Scrub typhus (tsutsugamushi fever), 36
  myocarditis and, 219
Scurvy, 16
Seborrheic keratoses (dermatosis papulosa nigra; senile keratoses), 114
Secondary involvement, of spleen, in neoplastic disease, 104–105
Secondary union, 12
Segmental degeneration, 196–197
Selenium deficiency, 18
Seminomas, 315–316
  anaplastic, 316
  spermatocytic, 316
  typical, 316
Senile emphysema (senile hyperinflation), 164
Senile keratoses (dermatosis papulosa nigra; seborrheic keratoses), 114
Senile plaques, 191
Sensorimotor polyneuropathy
  chronic

acquired, 197
  inherited forms of, 197
  relapsing, 197
  subacute
    asymmetric, 197
    symmetric, 197
Sensory motor neuropathy, type I hereditary (Charcot-Marie-Tooth disease, hypertrophic type peroneal muscular atrophy), 198
Septic embolus, 162
Septicemia
  gonococcal, 40
  staphylococcal (gram-positive shock), 38
Septicemic plague, 48, 49
Sequestration crises, in sickle cell disease, 83
Sequestrum, in pyogenic osteomyelitis, 140
Serofibrinous pericarditis, 228
Serous cystadenocarcinomas, ovarian, 339
Serous cystadenomas
  ovarian, 339
  pancreatic, 281
Serous effusions, pericardial, 227
Serous pericarditis, 228
Serous tumors
  cervical, borderline, 339
  of ovarian surface epithelium, 339
Serratia infections
  prostatitis and, 319
  Serratia marcescens, 41
Sertoli cell(s), 342
Sertoli cell tumors (androblastomas)
  ovarian, 342
  testicular, 318
Serum sickness
  acute, 21
  chronic, 21
Sessile mucosal inflammatory polyps, 278
Severe combined immunodeficiency, 23
Sex chromosome abnormalities, 2
Sex cord-stromal tumors, 341–342
Sézary-Lutzner cells, 120
Sézary syndrome, 121
Sheehan syndrome, 346
Shigella infections, 44
  gastroenterocolitis and, 243
  pseudomembranous colitis and, 252
Shingles (herpes zoster), 30, 181
Shock, gram-positive (staphylococcal septicemia), 38
Shy-Drager syndrome, 192
Sialadenitis, suppurative, 37
Sickle cell anemia, 4
  suppurative arthritis in, 132
Sickle cell disease, 83
  nephropathy and, 288
Sickle cell trait, 84
Simon's foci, 54
Simple (closed) fractures, 141
Sinuses
  inflammation of, 153
  tumors of, 153
Sinus histiocytosis, 90
Sinusitis, 153
  granulomatous, necrotizing, 153

Situs inversus totalis, 214
16-18 trisomy (Edwards syndrome; E tri-
    somy), 3
Skin, 107–121. *See also* Dermatoses.
    benign epithelial tumors of, 114–115
        acanthosis nigricans, 114
        adnexal, 115
        epithelial cysts (wens), 114–115
        fibroepithelial polyps (acrochordon; skin
            tags; squamous papilloma), 114
        keratoacanthomas, 115
        seborrheic keratoses (dermatosis papu-
            losa nigra; senile keratoses), 114
    blistering diseases of, 112–114
        bullous pemphigoid, 113
        noninflammatory, 113–114
        pemphigus, 113
    drug-induced reactions and, 10
    in Graves disease, 352
    infections of, 111–112
        fungal, superficial, 112
        impetigo, 112
        molluscum contagiosum, 111–112
        verrucae, 111
    in Lyme disease, 132
    lymphomas of, 120–121
    mastocytosis and, 121
    nevi of. *See* Nevus(i).
    pigmentary disorders of, 117
    premalignant and malignant epidermal
        tumors of, 115–117
        actinic keratoses, 115–116
        basal cell carcinoma, 116
        Merkel cell carcinoma, 117
        squamous cell carcinoma, 116
    in rheumatic heart disease, 224–225
    in rheumatoid arthritis, 130
    tumors of dermis of, 119–120
        benign fibrous histiocytoma, 119
        dermatofibrosarcoma protuberans, 119
        Kaposi's sarcoma, 120
        xanthomas, 120
Skin tags (acrochordon; fibroepithelial
        polyps; squamous papilloma), 114
Skull fractures, 183–184
"Sleeping sickness," 66
"Slow viruses," 182–183
Small cell carcinomas
    bronchogenic, 170
    colonic, undifferentiated, 255
    thyroid, 354
Small for gestational age infants, 1–2
Small intestine, 242–248
    congenital anomalies of, 242
    Crohn's disease and, 247
    infective gastroenterocolitis and, 243–244
    ischemic bowel disease of, 242–243
        mucosal and mural infarctions, 243
        transmural infarction, 242–243
    malabsorption syndromes and. *See*
        Malabsorption syndromes.
    obstructive lesions of, 246–247
    tumors of, 248
        carcinoids, 248
        carcinomas, 248
Small lymphocytic lymphomas, 91

Smallpox (variola), 29
Smoking, 9
Sodium homeostasis, 286
Sodoku (rat-bite fever, spirillar form), 51–52
Soft chancre (chancroid), 57
Soft tissue
    tumorlike conditions of, 127–128
        desmoid, 127
        fibromatosis, 127
        nodular (pseudosarcomatous) fasciitis,
            127–128
        traumatic myositis ossificans, 128
    tumors of, 122–127
        benign fibrous histiocytoma, 122–123
        fibroma and fibrosarcoma, 125–126
        ganglioneuroma, 126
        granular cell, 122
        leiomyoma and leiomyosarcoma, 125
        lipoma and liposarcoma, 123–124
        malignant fibrous histiocytoma, 123
        neuroblastoma, 126–127
        rhabdomyoma and rhabdomyosarcoma,
            124–125
        synovial sarcoma, 126
Solar elastosis, 115–116
Solid-cystic (papillary-cystic) tumors, pan-
        creatic, 281
Solitary myeloma (plasmacytoma), 100, 153
Solubilization, inadequate, 244
Somatostatinomas (δ-cell tumors), 358
Spermatocytic seminomas, 316
Spherocytosis, hereditary, 78
Sphingomyelin lipidoses (Niemann-Pick dis-
        ease), 5, 273
Spider telangiectasias, 208
Spina bifida, 176
Spinal artery, anterior, 188
Spinal cord. *See* Central nervous system.
    ependymomas of, 194
    trauma to, 184
    vascular disease of, 188
Spindle (stromal) cell tumors
    benign, gastric, 239
    gastric, malignant, 240–241
Spinocerebellar degeneration, 190
Spiral fractures, 141
Spirillum minus infections, 51–52
Spleen, 103–105. *See also* Splenomegaly.
    abnormal lobulations of, 103
    accessory, 103
    complete absence of, 103
    hypersplenism and, 103, 104
    infarcts of, 104–105
    neoplasms of, 105
    nonspecific acute splenitis and, 103–104
    reactive hyperplasia of, 104
    rupture of, 105
        "spontaneous," 105
Splenitis, acute, nonspecific, 103–104
Splenomegaly, 103
    in chronic myeloid leukemia, 96
    congestive, 104
    in leukemia, 98
Spondylitis
    ankylosing (Marie-Strümpell disease;
        rheumatoid spondylitis), 131

    in inflammatory bowel disease, 134
Spongiosis, 108
Spongiotic dermatitis (eczematous dermati-
        tis), 107–108
Sporadic (Western) lymphomas, 240
Sporadic simple goiter, 349
Spotted fevers, 35–36
Sprue
    celiac (celiac disease; gluten-sensitive
        enteropathy; nontropical sprue), 113,
        245
    tropical, 245
Sprue-associated lymphomas, 240
Squamous cell (epidermoid) carcinomas
    of bile ducts, 277
    bronchogenic, 170
    cervical, 334
    esophageal, 233
    penile, 312
    of skin, 116
        invasive, 116
    vaginal, 332
    vulvar, 331
Squamous hyperplasia, vulvar (hyperplastic
        dystrophy), 330
Squamous metaplasia, cervical, 333
Squamous papillomas
    of skin (acrochordon; fibroepithelial
        polyps; skin tags), 114
    vulvar, 331
Staghorn calculi, 303
Stagnant (ischemic) anoxia, 186
Staphylococcus infections, 37–38
    acute endometritis and, 335
    of brain, 180
    conjunctival, 155
    endocarditis and, 225–226
    hepatic abscesses and, 261
    potentially life-threatening, 37
    pseudomembranous colitis and, 252
    pulmonary, 168
    Staphylococcus aureus, 37–38
        endocarditis and, 225, 226
        gastroenterocolitis and, 243
        prostatitis and, 319
        pulmonary, 168, 169, 278–279
        pyogenic osteomyelitis and, 140
    Staphylococcus epidermidis, 37, 38
    Staphylococcus saprophyticus, 38
    urolithiasis and, 303
"Starry sky" histologic pattern, in high-
        grade lymphomas, 92
Status asthmaticus, 166
Steatocystoma multiplex, 115
Steatosis
    alcoholic (fatty liver), 262
        macrovesicular, 262
        microvesicular, 262
    drug-induced, 273
    microvesicular, hepatitis induced by, 260
Stein-Leventhal syndrome (polycystic
        ovaries), 342
Stenotic valves, in rheumatic heart disease,
        225
Steroid therapy, withdrawal from, 364
Stevens-Johnson syndrome, 108

Still's disease (juvenile rheumatoid arthritis), 131
Stomach, 235–241. *See also* headings beginning with term Gastric.
 acute erosions of, 237–238
 congenital anomalies of, 235
 gastritis and. *See* Gastritis.
 rupture of, 235
 tumors of
  benign, 239
  malignant, 239–241
 ulcers of, 238
  Cushing's, 238
  peptic, 238
  stress, 238
Stomatitis, herpetic, 154
Storage diseases. *See also* Glycogen storage diseases (glycogenoses).
 lipid storage diseases, 5–6
  liver and, 273
  secondary cardiomyopathy and, 222
Storiform pattern, in dermatofibroma protuberans, 119
Storiform-pleomorphic malignant fibrous histiocytomas, 123
Strawberry gallbladder, 278
"Strawberry" (juvenile) hemangiomas, 207
"Strawberry mucosa," in *Trichomonas vaginalis* infections, 64
Streptobacillus moniliformis infections, 51, 52
Streptococcus infections, 38–39
 acute poststreptococcal glomerulonephritis and, 291–292
 of brain, 180
 conjunctival, 155
 β-hemolytic, pulmonary, 169
 hepatic abscesses and, 261
 myocarditis and, 219
 pulmonary, 168
 Streptococcus bovis, 39
 Streptococcus pneumoniae, 39
  endocarditis and, 226
  of middle ear, 152
  pulmonary, 168
 Streptococcus viridans, 39
Stress ulcers, 238
Striatonigral degeneration, 192
Strokes, 187
Stroma ligneous (Riedel's) thyroiditis, 351
Stromal tumors
 benign, gastric, 239
 benign, small intestinal, 248
 luteomas, 342
 malignant, gastric, 240–241
Stroma lymphomatosa (autoimmune thyroiditis; stroma lymphomatosa), 350
 fibrosing, 350
Stroma ovarii, 340
Strongyloides stercoralis infections, 69–70
 hepatic abscesses and, 262
Sturge-Weber disease (syndrome), 177, 208
Stye, 155
Subacute sclerosing panencephalitis (Dawson's encephalitis), 182
Subacute spongiform encephalopathy (Creutzfeldt-Jakob disease), 183
Subaortic stenosis, hypertrophic, idiopathic (asymmetric septal hypertrophy; hypertrophic cardiomyopathy; hypertrophic obstructive cardiomyopathy; idiopathic hypertrophic subaortic stenosis), 221
Subarachnoid hemorrhage, 185–186
 intraparenchymal hemorrhage and, 186
Subcortical leukoencephalopathy (Binswanger's disease), 188
Subcutaneous tissues, left-sided congestive heart failure and, 219
Subdural empyema, 179
Subdural hematomas, 184
 acute, 184
 chronic, 184
Subependymomas, 194
Subepithelial deposits, in nephrotic syndrome, 290
Subfalcine herniation, 175
Submassive necrosis, 259
Subperiosteal abscess, in pyogenic osteomyelitis, 140
Sudden death
 cardiac, 215
  hypertrophic cardiomyopathy and, 221
 pulmonary embolism and, 161–162
 sudden infant death syndrome and, 2
Sulfatide lipidosis (metachromatic leukodystrophy), 5, 178
Suppurative appendicitis, 249
Suppurative arthritis, 131–132
 in pyogenic osteomyelitis, 140
Suppurative cystitis, 308
Suppurative otitis media, acute, 152
Suppurative (purulent) pericarditis, 228
Suppurative pleuritis (empyema), 173
Suppurative salpingitis (pelvic inflammatory disease), 40, 343
Suppurative sialadenitis, 37
Suppurative tenosynovitis, 135
Supranuclear palsy, progressive, 192
Suprasellar tumors, hypothalamic, 346
Surfactant, reduced, in respiratory distress syndrome of newborn, 161
Surgical wounds, staphylococcal infection of, 37
Sydenham's chorea, in rheumatic heart disease, 225
Sympathetic ophthalmia, 156
Syncytial meningiomas, 195
Syncytiotrophoblastic cells, 317
Synovial sarcomas, 126
Synovitis
 pigmented villonodular, 135
 tenosynovitis, 135
Syphilis (lues), 52–53
 acquired primary, 52
 cirrhosis and, 266
 cold hemolysin autoimmune hemolytic anemia caused by, 82
 congenital, 53
  osteomyelitis and, 141
 encephalitis caused by, 180
 secondary, 52
 tertiary, 53
  aneurysms and, 202
  testes and, 313–314
Syphilis osteomyelitis, 141
Syringobulbia, 177
Syringomas, 115
Syringomyelia, 177
Systemic circulation, left-sided congestive heart failure and, 218
Systemic lupus erythematosus, 24–25, 110
 chronic discoid, 25
 drug-induced erythematosus syndromes and, 25
 endocarditis of, 226–227
 glomerular lesions associated with, 292–294
 subacute cutaneous, 25
Systemic reactions, drug-induced, 10

T

Tabes dorsalis, 180
Tachyzoites, in toxoplasmosis, 68
Taenia saginata infections, 72
Taenia solium infections, 72–73
 hepatic abscesses and, 262
Takayasu's arteritis (pulseless disease), 205–206
Tapeworms. *See* Cestodes.
"Target lesions", in erythema multiforme, 108
Taussig-Bing malformation, 212
Tay-Sachs disease (GM_2 gangliosidosis), 5–6
T-cell leukemia, 31, 92–93, 121
T cell-mediated cytotoxicity, 21
Telangiectasias (vascular ectasias), 208–209
 hereditary hemorrhagic telangiectasias (Osler-Weber-Rendu disease), 208–209
 spider, 208
Temporal (giant cell) arteritis, 205
Tendinous xanthoma, 120
Tenosynovitis
 nodular (giant cell tumor of tendon sheath), 135
 suppurative, 135
 traumatic, 135
 tuberculous, 135
Tension pneumothorax, 174
Teratomas
 ovarian, 340
  benign cystic (dermoids), 340
 testicular, 317
Testes
 atrophy of, 314–315
 cryptorchidism and, 314
 cystic fibrosis and, 279
 inflammation of, 312–314
  orchitis, 312, 313
 torsion of, 315
 tumors of, 315–319
  benign, 317, 318–319
  malignant, 315–319
Tetanus, 46
 clinical, 46

Tetanus toxoid, 46
Tetralogy of Fallot, 212
Thalassemias, 4
  α-, 84–85
    hemoglobin H disease, 85
    hydrops fetalis and, 85
    silent carrier state, 84
    α-thalassemia trait, 84
  β-, 84
    thalassemia intermedia, 84
    thalassemia major, 84
    thalassemia minor, 84
  sickle cell disease and, 84
Thiamine deficiency, 15
13-15 trisomy (D trisomy; Patau syndrome), 3
Thorax, actinomycosis lesions involving, 56
Thorotrast, cholangiocarcinomas and, 270
Thrombasthenia, 87
Thromboangiitis obliterans (Buerger's disease), 206
Thrombocytopenias, 86–87
  in chronic lymphocytic leukemia, 97
  neonatal, 86
  post-transfusion, 86
  thrombotic thrombocytopenic purpura and, 86–87
Thrombocytopenic purpura
  idiopathic, 87
  thrombotic, 86–87, 287–288
Thrombocytosis, in chronic myeloid leukemia, 96
Thrombophlebitis, 210
Thrombosis
  in disseminated intravascular coagulation, 85
  of hepatic vein, 267
Thrombotic endocarditis, nonbacterial (marantic), 226
Thrombotic thrombocytopenic purpura, 86–87, 287–288
Thrombus, infected, 210
Thrush (moniliasis; oral candidiasis), 59, 154–155
"Thymic carcinomas," 368
Thymomas, 137, 368
  malignant, 368
Thymus, 367–368
  agenesis of, 367
  dysplasia of (DiGeorge syndrome), 23, 357
  hyperplasia of (thymic follicular hyperplasia), 137, 367
  hypoplasia of, 367
  in leukemias, 95–96
  tumors of, 368
Thyroglossal cysts, 355
Thyroid gland, 348–355
  congenital anomalies of, 355
  evaluation of thyroid nodules and, 348
  goiter and. See Goiter.
  Graves disease and, 352–353
  hyperthyroidism (hashitoxicosis) and, 350, 351–352
  hypothyroidism and, 352
  systemic diseases affecting, 355
  thyroiditis and. See Thyroiditis.

  tumors of, 348–349
    benign, 348–349
    malignant, 353–355
Thyroiditis, 350–351
  Hashimoto's (autoimmune thyroiditis; stroma lymphomatosa), 350
  fibrosing, 350
  Riedel's (stroma ligneous), 351
  subacute
    granulomatous (de Quervain's), 350–351
    lymphocytic (painless), 351
Thyroid tissue rests, ectopic, 355
Tinea barbae, 112
Tinea capitis, 112
Tinea corporis, 112
Tinea cruris, 112
Tinea pedis (athlete's foot), 112
Tinea versicolor, 112
Tobacco smoking, 9
Tophi, in gout, 133
Torsion, testicular, 315
Torulopsis glabrata (Candida glabrata) infections, 59
Touton giant cells, 120
Toxic agents, secondary cardiomyopathy and, 222
Toxic epidermal necrolysis (scalded skin syndrome), 37, 108
Toxicity
  adverse drug reactions, 10–11
  of illicit drugs, 11–12
  of nontherapeutic agents, 9–10
Toxic shock syndrome, 37
Toxins
  bacterial, preformed, 243
  muscle and, 139
Toxocara infections
  hepatic abscesses and, 262
  Toxocara cani, 70
  Toxocara cati, 70
Toxoplasma infections, 183
  orbital, 156
  Toxoplasma gondii, 68
Toxoplasmosis, 68
  encephalitis and, 183
Trabecular (embryonal) adenomas, thyroid, 348
Trachoma, 33
Transfusions, thrombocytopenia following, 86
Transient hypogammaglobulinemia of infancy, 23
Transitional cell papillomas, of bladder, 309
Transitional meningiomas, 195–196
Transmissible encephalopathy, 183
Transplant rejection, 22
  acute, 22
    cellular, 22
    humoral, 22
  chronic, 22
  hyperacute, 22
Transpositions of the great arteries, 212
  common pattern of, 212
  "corrected," 212
  Taussig-Bing malformation, 212

Transtentorial herniation, 175
Transmural infarction, of small intestine, 243–244
Trauma
  to central nervous system, 183–184
  ocular, 156
Traumatic hemolytic anemia, 78
Traumatic myositis ossificans, 128
Traumatic (amputation) neuromas, 197
Traumatic tenosynovitis, 135
"Tree-barking," of aorta, 202
Trematodes, 73–76
  clonorchiasis, 74
  fascioliasis, 73–74
  fasciolopsiasis, 74
  hepatic abscesses and, 262
  opisthorchiasis, 74
  paragonimiasis, 74–75
  schistosomiasis, 75–76
Tremor, in hyperthyroidism, 351
Treponemal infections, 52–53
  bejel and, 53
  pinta and, 53
  syphilis. See Syphilis (lues).
  Treponema pallidum, 52–53
  yaws and, 53
Triatominae, 67
Trichilemmal (pilar) cysts, 115
Trichilemmomas, 115
Trichinella infections
  myocarditis and, 219
  Trichinella spiralis, 70–71
Trichoepitheliomas, 115
Trichomonas vaginalis infections, 64
Trichuris trichiura (whipworm) infections, 69
Tricuspid atresia, 213
"Triple stones," 303
"Triple X" females (47,XXX), 2
Trisomy 13-15 (D trisomy; Patau syndrome), 3
Trisomy 16-18 (Edwards syndrome; E trisomy), 3
Trisomy 21 (Down syndrome; mongolism), 3
  Alzheimer's disease in, 191
Trophozoites, of *Pneumocystis carinii*, 65
Tropical sore (cutaneous leishmaniasis), 67–68
  diffuse, 67–68
Tropical sprue, 245
Truncus arteriosus, 212
Trypanosoma infections
  myocarditis and, 219
  Trypanosoma cruzi. See Chagas disease.
  Trypanosoma gambiense, 66–67
  Trypanosoma rhodesiense, 66–67
Trypanosomiasis
  African, 66–67
  American. See Chagas disease.
Tsutsugamushi fever (scrub typhus), 36
  myocarditis and, 219
Tuberculin reaction, 21
Tuberculoid leprosy, 56
Tuberculomas, 180
Tuberculosis, 54–55
  Addison's disease caused by, 363–364

Tuberculosis *(Continued)*
  arthritis and, 134
  cystitis and, 308
  encephalitis caused by, 180
  epididymis and testes and, 313
  gastroenterocolitis and, 243
  miliary, 55
  osteomyelitis and (Pott's disease), 55, 141
  primary, 54
  salpingitis and, 343
  secondary, 54–55
  tenosynovitis and, 135
Tuberous sclerosis, 177
Tuberous xanthoma, 120
Tubular adenomas, 324
  colonic, 253
  gastric, 239
Tubular necrosis, acute, 299–300
  initiating phase of, 299
  ischemic tubulorrhectic, 299
  maintenance phase of, 299–300
  nephrotoxic, 299
  nonoliguric, 300
  pigment-induced, 299
  recovery phase of, 300
Tubulointerstitial nephritis, 297–298
  analgesic abuse nephropathy, 298
  hypersensitivity interstitial nephritis, 297–298
Tubulovillous adenomas, colonic, 253
Tularemia, 49
  glandular, 49
  oculoglandular, 49
  typhoidal, 49
  ulceroglandular, 49
Tumor(s). *See also* Antineoplastic agents; *specific tumors and anatomic sites.*
  in AIDS, 23
  benign
    adnexal, of skin, 115
    of bladder, 308
    of blood vessels, 207–209
    of bone, 147, 148, 149
    of breasts, 324, 325–326
    cardiac, 222–223
    of central nervous system, 195–196
    cervical, 333
    of endocrine pancreas, 358
    epithelial, 114–115
    of gallbladder, 276
    gastric, 239
    hepatic, 268–269
    pancreatic, 281
    penile, 311–312
    pleural, 172
    renal, 300–301
    small intestinal, 248
    of soft tissue, 122–124, 125
    splenic, 104–105
    testicular, 317, 318–319
    thymic, 368
    thyroid, 348–349
    ureteral, 306, 307
    uterine, 337–338
  malignant
    of adrenal medulla, 365–366

  benign, penile, 311–312
  of bile ducts and ampulla of Vater, 277
  of bladder, 308–309
  of blood vessels, 207, 209
  of bone, 147–149
  of breasts, 325, 326–328, 329
  cardiac, 223
  of central nervous system, 195, 196
  cervical, 333–334
  of endocrine pancreas, 358
  of gallbladder, 276–277
  gastric, 239–241
  hepatic, 269–271, 273
  of lung, 170–172
  neoplastic colonic polyps, 253–254
  pancreatic, 281
  parathyroid, 356
  of peripheral nerves, 198
  pineal, 367
  pleural, 172–173
  prostatic, 320–321
  renal, 301–302
  of skin, 118–119
  small intestinal, 248
  of soft tissue, 122–123, 124–127
  splenic, 104–105
  testicular, 315–319
  thymic, 368
  thyroid, 353–355
  ureteral, 306, 307
  metastatic
    of adrenal medulla, 366
    cardiac, 222
    of central nervous system, 196
    of eye, 155
    gastric, 241
    hepatic, 271
    of lungs, 172
    ovarian, 342
    testicular, 318
    ureteral, 306
  nonfunctional, of adrenal gland, 365
Tumorlike conditions
  of connective tissue. *See* Connective tissue, tumorlike conditions of.
  of external ear, 151
  soft tissue. *See* Soft tissue, tumorlike conditions of.
Tunica vaginalis lesions, 315
Turban tumor, 115
Turner syndrome (45,X0), 2
Type A exotoxin, of *Clostridium botulinum*, 46
Typhoidal tularemia, 49
Typhoid fever, 44
Typhoid nodules, 44
Typhus, 34–35
  Brill-Zinsser disease, 35
  epidemic, 34–35
  flying squirrel, 35
  murine, 35
  scrub (tsutsugamushi fever), 36
    myocarditis and, 219
Tyrosine metabolism abnormalities, 6–7
Tyrosinosis, 7
  liver and, 273

U

Ulcer(s)
  aphthous (canker sores), 154
  duodenal, peptic, 238
  elongated, in typhoid fever, 44
  esophageal, squamous cell carcinoma and, 233
  gastric. *See* Stomach, ulcers of.
  Hunner's (ulcerative interstitial cystitis), 308
  peptic, 238
  of skin, atypical mycobacteria causing, 55
Ulcerative colitis, idiopathic, 251
Ulcerative cystitis, 308
Ulceroglandular tularemia, 49
Ulegyria, 177
Umbilical cord stumps, in tetanus, 46
Uncinate herniation, 175
Undifferentiated carcinomas
  cervical, 334
  gastric, 240
  small cell, colonic, 255
  thyroid, 354
Undifferentiated cells, of central nervous system, tumors of, 195
Upper respiratory viral infections, 27
Upward herniation, 175
Urachus, 308
Urate nephropathy, chronic, in gout, 133–134
Ureaplasma urealyticum infections, 36
  prostatitis and, 319
Ureter(s), bifid, 306
Ureteral diseases, 306
  congenital, 306
  obstructive, 306
    extrinsic lesions and, 306
    intrinsic lesions and, 306
  tumors, 306
  ureteritis, 306
Ureteritis, 306
  chronic, 306
Ureteropelvic junction obstruction, 306
Urethra, 307
  inflammations of, 307
  tumors of, 307
Urethritis, 307
  chlamydial, 32
  gonococcal, 40
Uric acid nephrolithiasis, in gout, 133
Uric acid nephropathy, acute, in gout, 133
Uric acid stones, 303
Urinary bladder. *See* Bladder.
Urinary tract. *See also* specific organs and diseases.
  infections of. *See also* Pyelonephritis.
    cystitis and, 303
  obstruction of, 302
Urolithiasis, 302–303
Urothelial carcinomas, of renal pelvis, 302
Urticaria (hives), 107
  IgE-dependent, 107
  IgE-independent, 107
Urticaria pigmentosa, 121
Uterus, 335–338

adenomyosis and, 335–336
congenital anomalies of, 335
dysfunctional uterine bleeding and, 336–337
endometrial hyperplasia and, 337
endometriosis and, 336
inflammations of, 335
reactive endometrial changes and, 337
tumors of, 337–338
  benign, 337–338
  malignant, 338

V

Vaginal adenosis, 332
Vaginal lesions, 332
Valine, sickle cell disease and, 83
Valvular heart disease, 223–227
  calcific aortic valve stenosis, 223–224
  calcification of mitral annulus, 227
  complications of artificial valves, 227
  congenital
    aortic valvular stenosis/atresia, 214
    pulmonary valvular stenosis/atresia, 214
    tricuspid atresia, 213
  mitral valve prolapse, 224
  stenotic, in rheumatic heart disease, 225
Varicella (chickenpox), 30
Varicella-zoster virus infections, 30
Varices, esophageal, 232
Varicose veins, 209
Variola (smallpox), 29
Vascular diseases. See also specific vascular diseases.
  of brain, 186–187
  in diabetes mellitus, 359–360
  hepatic. See Liver diseases, vascular.
  pulmonary. See Pulmonary vascular diseases.
Vascular ectasias (telangiectasias), 208–209
  hereditary hemorrhagic telangiectasias (Osler-Weber-Rendu disease), 208–209
  spider telangiectasias, 208
Vasculature, 199–229. See also Aneurysm(s); Arteries; Veins.
  focal inflammation of, in rickettsial infections, 34
  tumors of, 207–209
    hemangioendotheliomas, 209
    hemangiomas, 207–208
    telangiectasias, 208–209
  vasculitides and, 203–207
    allergic granulomatosis and angiitis (Churg-Strauss syndrome), 204
    hypersensitivity angiitis (leukocytoclastic angiitis; microscopic polyarteritis), 204
    Kawasaki disease, 206
    polyarteritis nodosa, 203–204
    Raynaud's disease and Raynaud's phenomenon, 206–207
    secondary vasculitis, 206
    Takayasu's arteritis (pulseless disease), 205–206

temporal (giant cell) arteritis, 205
    thromboangiitis obliterans (Buerger's disease), 206
    Wegener's granulomatosis, 204–205
  veins, 209–210
    thrombophlebitis and, 210
    varicose, 209
Vasculitides. See Vasculature, vasculitides and.
Vasculitis
  acute, in rheumatoid arthritis, 130
  necrotizing, focal, 205
  pulmonary hemorrhage associated with, 162
  secondary, 206
Vasodilation, peripheral, in hyperthyroidism, 351
Vasoocclusive crises, in sickle cell disease, 83
Vasopressors, renal, 286
Veins, 209–210
  thrombophlebitis and, 210
  varicose, 209
Veneral infections
  suppurative arthritis and, 131
  Trichomonas vaginalis, 64
Venereal infections. See also Gonorrhea; Syphilis (lues).
Venereal warts (condyloma acuminata), 111
  penile, 312
  vulvar, 330–331
Veno-occlusive disease, hepatic, 268
Ventricular hypertrophy
  left, 217
  right, 217
Ventricular septal defect, 213
Verrucae (warts), 111
  palmaris, 111
  plana (flat wart), 111
  plantaris, 111
  in rheumatic heart disease, 224
  vulgaris (common wart), 111
Verrucous carcinomas
  penile (Buschke-Lowenstein tumor; giant condyloma), 312
  vulvar, 331
Very low-density lipoprotein (VLDL), 201
Vesicles, 112
Vesicoureteral reflux, 307–308
Vibrio cholerae infections, 45
  gastroenterocolitis and, 243
Villous adenomas
  colonic, 253–254
  gastric, 239
VIN (vulvar dysplasia; vulvar intraepithelial neoplasia), 331
Viral infections, 27–31. See also specific infections and viruses.
  acute, 258–259
    chronic, 259–260
  acute rhinitis caused by, 152
  in AIDS, 23
  arboviruses causing, 31
  cystitis and, 308
  of digestive tract, 28
  encephalitis and, 180–182

slow virus infections and, 182–183
  epithelial growths and, 28
  gastroenterocolitis and, 243
  hepatitis. See Hepatitis.
  herpesviruses causing, 29–31
  meningitis and, 179
  myocarditis and, 219
    dilated cardiomyopathy and, 220
  in needle users, 11
  pulmonary, 169
  respiratory, 27–28
  with skin rashes, 29
Virchow-Robin hemorrhages, 185
Virilism, adrenal, 362
Visceral larva migrans, 70
  hepatic abscesses and, 262
Visceral leishmaniasis (kala-azar), 67
Vision. See also Eye(s).
  vitamin A and, 14
Vitamin deficiencies
  central nervous system and, 177–178
  of fat-soluble vitamins, 13–15
    vitamin A, 14, 244
    vitamin D, 14, 244
    vitamin E, 14
    vitamin K, 15, 244
  subclinical, 16
  vitamin B₁₂
    central nervous system and, 177–178
    megaloblastic anemia caused by, 16, 79
  of water-soluble vitamins, 15–16
    vitamin B complex, 15–16
    vitamin C, 16
Vitiligo, 117
VLDL (very low-density lipoprotein), 201
von Gierke's disease, hepatorenal form (type I glycogen storage disease), 4, 273
von Hippel-Lindau disease (syndrome), 177, 208, 278
von Recklinghausen's disease of bone (osteitis fibrosa cystica), 144
von Recklinghausen's neurofibromatosis, 195
von Willebrand's disease, 87–88
Vulvar diseases, 330–332
  dysplasia (vulvar intraepithelial neoplasia [VIN]), 331
  dystrophy, 330
  tumors, 330–332
  vulvitis
    atrophic, chronic (lichen sclerosis), 330
    nonspecific, 330

W

Waldenström's macroglobulinemia, 91, 100–101
Wallerian degeneration, 196
"Walnut brain," 191
Warm antibody autoimmune anemia, 82
Wart(s) (verrucae), 111
  in rheumatic heart disease, 224
  venereal (condyloma acuminata), 312
    penile, 312
    vulvar, 330–331

Warthin-Finkeldey giant cells, 29
Waterhouse-Friderichsen syndrome, 39,
    364–365
Watershed (border zone) infarcts, 187
Wegener's granulomatosis, 204–205
    glomerular lesions associated with, 295
Weil's disease, 50
Wens (epithelial cysts), 114–115
Werdnig-Hoffman disease (infantile pro-
    gressive spinal muscular atrophy),
    193
Wernicke-Korsakoff syndrome, 15
Western (sporadic) lymphomas, 240
"Wet beriberi," 15
Whipple's disease, 245–246
Whipworm (*Trichuris trichiura*) infections,
    69
Whooping cough, 42
Wickham striae, 109
Wilms tumors (nephroblastomas), 301–302
Wilson's disease, 4, 17, 265
Wiskott-Aldrich syndrome, 23
Wolman's disease, 6
Woolsorter's disease (hemorrhagic pneumo-
    nia), 48
Working Formulation, for classification of
    non-Hodgkin's lymphomas, 91
Worms. *See* Parasitic infections, helminthic.

encephalitis and, 183
Wuchereria bancrofti infections, 71

X

Xanthelasmas, 120, 155
Xanthogranulomatous pyelonephritis, 305
Xanthomas, 120
    eruptive, 120
    plane, 120
    tendinous, 120
    tuberous, 120
Xeroderma pigmentosum, 116
    basal cell carcinoma of skin and, 116
45,X0 females (Turner syndrome), 2
X-linked genetic diseases, 7, 179
47,XXX females ("Triple X" females), 2
47,XXX males (Klinefelter syndrome), 2

Y

Yaws, 53
Yellow fever, 31
Yersinia enterocolitica infections, 45–46
    gastroenterocolitis and, 243
Yersinia pestis infections, 48–49

Yolk sac tumors (endodermal sinus tumors;
    infantile embryonal carcinomas)
    ovarian, 341
    testicular, 316

Z

Zinc deficiency, 17
Zollinger-Ellison syndrome (gastrinomas),
    237, 358
Zoonotic infections, 47–52
    anthrax, 48
    brucellosis, 49
    cat-scratch disease, 52
    glanders, 50
    leptospirosis, 50, 219
    listeriosis, 48
    Lyme disease, 51, 132
    melioidosis, 50
    plague, 48–49
    rat-bite fever, 51–52
    relapsing fever, 50–51
    tularemia, 49
    Weil's disease, 50
Zygomycosis (mucormycosis; phycomycosis),
    60